HODGKIN'S DISEASE:
THE CONSEQUENCES OF SURVIVAL

HODGKIN'S DISEASE:
THE CONSEQUENCES OF SURVIVAL

Mortimer J. Lacher, M.D., F.A.C.P.

Associate Clinical Member
Memorial Sloan-Kettering Cancer Center
New York, New York

John R. Redman, M.D., F.A.C.P.

Assistant Professor of Medicine
The University of Texas
M.D. Anderson Cancer Center
Houston, Texas

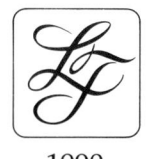

LEA & FEBIGER   PHILADELPHIA • LONDON
1990

Lea & Febiger
600 Washington Square
Philadelphia, PA   19106-4198
U.S.A.
(215) 922-1330

Lea & Febiger (UK) Ltd.
145a Croydon Road
Beckenham, Kent BR3 3RB
U.K.

Library of Congress Cataloging in Publication Data

Hodgkin's disease: the consequences of survival / [edited by]
   Mortimer J. Lacher, John Redman.
     p.   cm.
   Includes bibliographies and index.
   ISBN 0-8121-1204-0
   1. Hodgkin's disease—Treatment—Complications and sequelae.
I. Lacher, Mortimer J., 1930–   . II. Redman, John R.
   [DNLM: 1. Drug Therapy—adverse effects. 2. Hodgkin's Disease—
complications. 3. Hodgkin's Disease—therapy. 4. Radiotherapy—
adverse effects. WH 500 H68924]
RC644.H63   1989
616.99'44606—dc19
DNLM/DLC
for Library of Congress   89-2735
                                                                                   CIP

Copyright © 1990 by Lea & Febiger. Copyright under the International Copyright Union. All Rights Reserved. This book is protected by copyright. *No part of it may be reproduced in any manner or by any means without written permission from the publisher.*

PRINTED IN THE UNITED STATES OF AMERICA

Print number: 5   4   3   2   1

FOREWORD

"Would you tell me, please, which way I ought to go from here?"
"That depends a good deal on where you want to get to," said the Cat.
"I don't care much where . . . " said Alice.
"Then it doesn't matter which way you go," said the Cat.

Alice's Adventures in Wonderland—LEWIS CARROLL

Science does not tell us where to go, but once we have decided on a direction, it definitely can tell us the best way to get there. We scientists who are dedicated to the control and cure of all forms of cancer know exactly what we want to achieve. Through science we have the means to set the best pathway to reach our goal. We are dedicated at all levels of research to cure our patients without inflicting further harm. We are sensitive to the need to preserve and support the patient's psyche as well as the patient's physical system.

The role of the clinician is to see to it that the basic data of the research laboratory get translated in an appropriate and necessary process into the language of the clinic. The success achieved by the advances in treatment for Hodgkin's disease underscores this relationship. Laboratory physicists were responsible for the development of high-energy linear accelerators. Then this force was uniquely applied to deliver radiation therapy to the patient with Hodgkin's disease by the clinical radiation therapist. A dramatic increase in survival of the Hodgkin's patient was the net result.

The same developmental research sequence (from the laboratory to the bedside) is responsible for the extraordinary success of growing numbers of chemotherapeutic drugs discovered in only the past 30 years. Research laboratories around the world have developed individual new drugs for the treatment of Hodgkin's disease, but the ultimate success in significantly extending the useful lives of Hodgkin's patients was dependent on the clinical investigational application of the chemotherapeutic agents by the medical oncologists.

The movement from the use of single agents to the juggling application of multidrug chemotherapy for Hodgkin's disease was sparked by clinical observations and research initiated in the great clinical centers for cancer treatment at the Memorial Sloan-Kettering Cancer Center and the National Cancer Institute. It was extended to centers all around the United States and the world as the national commitment to the progressive improvement in our ability to control and cure cancers expanded the available resources to conduct clinical trials.

Some data can only be gathered at the bedside. Now that we have dramatically extended the lives of almost 90% of the patients with Hodgkin's disease, we recognize and are seeking ways to modify the side effects created by the therapy itself. *Hodgkin's Disease: The Consequences of Survival,* edited by Drs. Lacher and Redman, is a compendium of clinical observations that highlight this new set of challenges. With contributions by 37 outstanding clinicians and investigators, this book serves as a signal to all those who plan the future treatment of all cancer patients that once long-term survival is achieved, the job is not over. Constant careful follow-up attention to the patients' physical, emotional, and social problems is a life-long task of the clinical oncologist.

It is up to the clinician, directly interacting with the patient, to assure that the powerful new discoveries do not remain anchored to the laboratory bench. New methods of treatment, however, will bring new problems. In addition, the current methods must constantly be evaluated and reevaluated as a successfully treated Hodgkin's population lives on toward a record-setting life expectancy. As emphasized in *Hodgkin's Disease: The Consequences of Survival*, we can take credit for the long life of the majority of Hodgkin's patients and simultaneously be sure that we constantly adapt and change our methods to eliminate any of the problems we have induced on the road to success.

Paul A. Marks, M.D.
President
Memorial Sloan-Kettering Cancer Center

PREFACE

During the early years of successful Hodgkin's treatment, characterized by the introduction of high-energy, extended-field radiation therapy and later successful drug and multiple drug chemotherapy, little thought was given to the consequences of survival. The horror of the repeated deaths of patient after patient struck down in the prime of their life and frequently in the bloom of their youth, moved us to devise and accept any method that would stop that holocaust. High-dose radiation therapy with megavoltage machines proved to be an extraordinary addition to our armamentarium. After the introduction of high-energy, high-dose, large-field ("prophylactic") radiation, the survival rates of Hodgkin's patients improved dramatically.

Chemotherapy added to this survival boom when new drugs like vinblastine and chlorambucil proved to be so much more effective in combination than single agents. We then began using multidrugs in combinations, such as MOPP, C-MOPP, ABVD, TVPP, and then 8-drug and 10-drug combinations. Patients we thought would die in a few years or less, were now able to live past 10 years. Patients who relapsed after a remission induced by radiation therapy, were being "salvaged" with chemotherapy.

The joy of birth, even after radiation and chemotherapy, marked this new population of Hodgkin's patients. Many babies were born to mothers and fathers successfully treated with radiation and chemotherapy. A whole new generation has been spawned on the success of our treatment. Hodgkin's disease, a disease once almost uniformly fatal within a few years after diagnosis, can now be suppressed, allowing the majority of patients to lead a productive life.

In the flush of our success over the past 30 years, we lost sight of the double edge of our mighty treatment sword. Now is the time to pause, reconsider, count the effects and the side effects carefully, and start to think of new ways to modify our treatment to hold the line of long survival that we have painstakingly drawn. We must find ways to reduce the unwanted late side effects.

Hodgkin's Disease: The Consequences of Survival contains information that illustrates the late complications, induced by the therapy itself, which affect every organ system. By making clinicians aware that the number of complications observed are far greater than that expected by chance, we should be able to immediately save some lives through early diagnosis of treatment-induced second primary cancers and endocrine deficits. We must insist on the continuous diligent follow-up of the treated Hodgkin's patient.

Furthermore, the awareness that many of the induced complications cannot be reversed, except by changing our primary therapy, may be the start of a movement to refine or possibly even eliminate the use of large-field, high-dose radiation therapy. Thus, we may see the beginning of a trend toward using primary chemotherapy alone for all patients, providing we can be sufficiently secure that our choice of drugs will not lower our overall survival results or merely cause one set of complications to be exchanged for another more formidable set.

Chemotherapy does produce late side effects, just as radiation therapy does, but where the late effects of radiation may prove to be too difficult to control and the radiation treatment may be too difficult to modify effectively, chemotherapy and immunotherapy (and its variations) have boundless possibilities for development and variation.

Let us not leave the future to chance. By recognizing the problems associated with treatment-induced illness, and not denying their importance, we should feel free to modify our current methods to create more effective treatment devoid of unmanageable side effects. *Hodgkin's Disease: The Consequences of Survival* should excite, anger, give us pause for a few accolades, and stimulate us to modify what is harmful, promote what is useful, and push us to finding still better ways to treat the Hodgkin's patient.

New York, NY — Mortimer J. Lacher
Houston, TX — John R. Redman

ACKNOWLEDGMENTS

We are indebted to each of the individual authors who contributed their expert knowledge, time, and effort to produce *Hodgkin's Disease: The Consequences of Survival*. A special source of assistance and encouragement came from supporters of The Lymphoma Foundation; its executives, William D. Zabel and Martin Zausner; and its board members, William R. Gruver, Karen Hughes, Edward Moresco, and Edward Spiegel. Extraordinary contributions have been made by Robert and Joyce Menschel, who are committed to the support of numerous important causes that benefit the whole society. These individuals, their families, and friends have had the special vision to provide funds for scientists dedicated to cancer research. We also recognize that without the daily assistance of the staff, Myrna Rubin, Sr. Kathleen Toner, and Diana Berner, we would not have been able to fulfill our obligations and deadlines. We owe The Memorial Sloan-Kettering Cancer Center and the M.D. Anderson Hospital and Tumor Institute our gratitude for giving us the opportunity to study, to learn, to continue our clinical research, and to give back to patients and society the most advanced medical care that has allowed us to save so many lives in our lifetime.

Finally, we salute our patients, who with their powerful emotional support have given us the strength to continue our work and achieve success in the face of many failures.

M.J.L.
J.R.R.

CONTRIBUTORS

Teresa Alonso
  Director of Planning and Development
  FIDIA Pharmaceutical Corporation
  Washington, D.C.

Gretchen Anderson, M.D.
  Department of Dermatology
  Resident, Memorial Sloan-Kettering Cancer
    Center
  New York, New York

Donald Armstrong, M.D.
  Professor of Medicine
  Cornell University Medical College;
  Chief, Infectious Disease Service
  Director, Microbiology Laboratory
  Memorial Sloan-Kettering Cancer Center
  New York, New York

Daiva R. Bajorunas, M.D.
  Associate Professor of Clinical Medicine
  Cornell University Medical College;
  Associate Attending Physician, Memorial Hospital,
  Memorial Sloan-Kettering Cancer Center
  New York, New York

H. Richard Beresford, M.D., J.D.
  Professor of Neurology
  Cornell University Medical College;
  Director, Department of Neurology
  North Shore University
  Manhasset, New York;
  Attending Neurologist
  The New York Hospital
  New York, New York

Magnus Björkholm, M.D., Ph.D.
  Associate Professor of Medicine
  Head, Division of Hematology
  Department of Medicine
  Karolinska Hospital
  Stockholm, Sweden

Jeffrey S. Borer, M.D.
  Gladys and Roland Harriman Professor of
    Cardiovascular Medicine
  Cornell University Medical Center;
  The New York Hospital
  New York, New York

Kathy Clagett Carr
  Project Manager, AIDS Operations Office
  Social and Scientific Systems, Inc.
  Rockville, Maryland

Terrence L. Cascino, M.D.
  Assistant Professor
  Mayo Graduate School of Medicine;
  Consultant in Neurology
  Mayo Clinic and Foundation
  Rochester, Minnesota

Grace H. Christ, C.S.W.
  Director, Department of Social Work
  Memorial Sloan-Kettering Cancer Center
  New York, New York

Susan M. Diamond, M.D.
  Doctor's Hospital
  Dallas, Texas

Sarah S. Donaldson, M.D.
  Professor, Radiation Oncology
  Department of Radiation Oncology
  Stanford University School of Medicine
  Stanford, California

Barbara Gerling, M.D.
  Assistant Professor of Medicine
  Cornell University Medical College;
  Co-Director, Intermediate Cardiac Care Unit
  The New York Hospital
  New York, New York

CONTRIBUTORS

John S. Gottdiener, M.D.
Associate Professor of Medicine
University of Maryland School of Medicine;
Head, Echocardiography Research
Co-Director, Echocardiography Laboratory
University of Maryland Hospital
Baltimore, Maryland

Harry Griffiths, M.D.
Professor of Radiology
Director of Musculoskeletal Radiology
Director of MRI
Department of Radiology
University of Minnesota Hospital Center
Minneapolis, Minnesota

Samuel Hellman, M.D.
A.N. Pritzker Professor
Division of Biological Sciences
Dean, Pritzker School of Medicine
Vice President for the Medical Center
University of Chicago
Chicago, Illinois

Göran Holm, M.D., Ph.D.
Professor, Head of the Department of Medicine
Karolinska Hospital
Stockholm, Sweden

Sanford Kempin, M.D.
Associate Professor of Clinical Medicine
Cornell University Medical School;
Associate Attending Physician
Hematology/Lymphoma Service
Memorial Sloan-Kettering Cancer Center
New York, New York

Mortimer J. Lacher, M.D., F.A.C.P.
Clinical Associate Professor of Medicine
Cornell University College of Medicine;
Associate Attending Physician
Lymphoma/Hematology Service
Department of Medicine
Memorial Sloan-Kettering Cancer Center
New York, New York

Moshe Levi, M.D.
Assistant Professor of Internal Medicine
University of Texas Southwestern Medical
  Center at Dallas;
Chief, Home Dialysis
Dallas Veterans Administration Medical Center
Dallas, Texas

Brian Leyland-Jones, M.D.
Head, Developmental Chemotherapy Section
National Cancer Institute
Bethesda, Maryland

Jay S. Loeffler, M.D.
Assistant Professor
Joint Center for Radiation Therapy
Department of Radiation Therapy
Harvard Medical School
Boston, Massachusetts

Peter Mauch, M.D.
Associate Professor
Chief, Brigham and Women's Hospital Division
Joint Center for Radiation Therapy
Department of Radiation Therapy
Harvard Medical School
Boston, Massachusetts

Håkan Mellstedt, M.D., Ph.D.
Associate Professor
Deputy Director, Department of Oncology
Karolinska Hospital
Stockholm, Sweden

Grace Y. Minamoto
Instructor in Clinical Medicine
Columbia University College of Physicians and
  Surgeons;
St. Luke's-Roosevelt Hospital Center
New York, New York

Patricia L. Myskowski, M.D.
Assistant Professor of Medicine
Cornell University Medical College;
Associate Attending Physician, Dermatology
  Service
Department of Medicine
Memorial Sloan-Kettering Cancer Center
New York, New York

Peter O'Dwyer, M.D.
Associate Professor of Medicine
Temple University;
Director of Developmental Chemotherapy
Fox Chase Cancer Center
Philadelphia, Pennsylvania

Brian P. O'Neill, M.D.
Professor of Neurology
Mayo Medical School;
Consultant in Neurology
Mayo Clinic and Foundation
Rochester, Minnesota

John R. Redman, M.D., F.A.C.P.
Assistant Professor of Medicine
Hematology Department
The University of Texas
M.D. Anderson Cancer Center
Houston, Texas

Bijan Safai, M.D., D.S.
    Professor of Medicine
    Cornell University Medical College;
    Attending Physician, Division of Dermatology
    The New York Hospital;
    Chief, Dermatology Service, Memorial Hospital
    Memorial Sloan-Kettering Cancer Center
    New York, New York

David Schottenfeld, M.D.
    John G. Searle Professor and Chairman
    Department of Epidemiology
    School of Public Health;
    Professor of Internal Medicine
    Division of Hematology/Oncology
    Department of Internal Medicine
    Medical School
    The University of Michigan
    Ann Arbor, Michigan

Karolynn Siegel, Ph.D.
    Director of Research
    Department of Social Work
    Memorial Sloan-Kettering Cancer Center
    New York, New York

Moshe Shike, M.D.
    Associate Professor of Clinical Medicine
    Cornell University;
    Associate Attending Physician
    Memorial Hospital, Memorial Sloan-Kettering Cancer Center
    New York, New York

Julius Smith, M.D., M.R.C.P., F.R.C.R.
    Associate Professor of Radiology
    Cornell University Medical College;
    Attending Radiologist, Memorial Sloan-Kettering Cancer Center
    New York, New York

Nancy J. Tarbell, M.D.
    Assistant Professor
    Chief, The Children's Hospital Division
    Joint Center for Radiation Therapy
    Department of Radiation Therapy
    Harvard Medical School
    Boston, Massachusetts

Philip Terman, D.D.S.
    Director at Large
    American Cancer Society;
    Associate Attending, Dental Service
    Memorial Sloan-Kettering Cancer Center
    New York, New York

Eliot Zimbalist, M.D.
    Director, Gastrointestinal Education and Research
    Associate Attending Gastroenterology
    Maimonides Medical Center;
    Associate Attending Gastroenterology
    Health Science Center
    SUNY at Downstate
    Brooklyn, New York

CONTENTS

Introduction 1
Mortimer J. Lacher
John R. Redman

Chapter 1. Epidemiology of Second Primary Cancers in Patients with Hodgkin's Disease 11
David Schottenfeld

Chapter 2. Late Effects of Radiation Therapy in the Treatment of Hodgkin's Disease 27
Jay S. Loeffler
Peter Mauch
Samuel Hellman

Chapter 3. Late Effects of Chemotherapeutic Agents 47
Brian Leyland-Jones
Peter O'Dwyer
Teresa Alonso

Chapter 4. Late Hematologic Complications After Treatment of Hodgkin's Disease 63
Sanford Kempin

Chapter 5. Immunocompetence in Patients with Hodgkin's Disease 112
Magnus Björkholm
Göran Holm
Håkan Mellstedt

Chapter 6. Infectious Complications of Hodgkin's Disease 151
Donald Armstrong
Grace Y. Minamoto

Chapter 7. Late Infectious Complications: Viral Infections....................... 168
Brian Leyland-Jones
Kathy Clagett Carr
Peter O'Dwyer

Chapter 8. The Skeletal System 182
Julius Smith
Harry Griffiths

Chapter 9. Late Neurologic Complications of Hodgkin's Disease Treatment .. 203
Terrence L. Cascino
Brian P. O'Neill

Chapter 10. Therapy-Related Thyroid and Parathyroid Dysfunction in Patients with Hodgkin's Disease 222
John R. Redman
Daiva R. Bajorunas

Chapter 11. Hodgkin's Disease: Pregnancy and Progeny 244
John R. Redman
Daiva R. Bajorunas
Mortimer J. Lacher

Chapter 12. Cardiovascular Complications of the Treatment of Hodgkin's Disease 267
Barbara Gerling
John Gottdiener
Jeffrey S. Borer

Chapter 13. Pulmonary Complications of Hodgkin's Disease Treatment: Radiation Pneumonitis, Fibrosis, and the Effect of Cytotoxic Drugs 296
Nancy J. Tarbell
Peter Mauch
Samuel Hellman

Chapter 14. Renal and Genitourinary Complications from the Treatment of Hodgkin's Disease 306
Susan M. Diamond
Moshe Levi

Chapter 15. Gastrointestinal Complications of Staging and Treatment of Hodgkin's Disease 316
Eliot Zimbalist
Moshe Shike

Chapter 16. Cutaneous Sequelae of Hodgkin's Disease 331
Bijan Safai
Gretchen Anderson
Patricia L. Myskowski

Chapter 17. Dental Complications After Treatment for Hodgkin's Disease 346
Philip Terman
Mortimer J. Lacher

Chapter 18. Pediatric Hodgkin's Disease: The Uniqueness of the Pediatric Patient 363
Sarah S. Donaldson

Chapter 19. Hodgkin's Disease Survivorship: Psychosocial Consequences 383
Karolynn Siegel
Grace H. Christ

Chapter 20. Late Iatrogenesis: Legal Aspects 400
H. Richard Beresford

Summary and Analysis 410
Mortimer J. Lacher
John R. Redman

Index 435

HODGKIN'S DISEASE:
THE CONSEQUENCES OF SURVIVAL

Introduction

MORTIMER J. LACHER
JOHN R. REDMAN

Physicians now have the privilege of following a large cohort of long-surviving Hodgkin's patients after successful treatment with intensive radiation therapy and chemotherapy. In the process of achieving our current success, however, a price has been paid in unwanted, delayed side effects of treatment. These side effects impact in some way on every biologic system; the full impact of the effect of splenectomy, radiation therapy, and chemotherapy on the Hodgkin's population will not be fully determined until much more time goes by.

Hodgkin's Disease: The Consequences of Survival should serve as a benchmark on the road to a full analysis of what can happen to the surviving Hodgkin's patients. By analyzing the effects of therapy on Hodgkin's survivors, we should be able to better adjust or choose future treatment methods that will achieve long survival for the majority of Hodgkin's patients, while diminishing or ending the unwanted late side effects.

For the sake of simplicity, we have taken the view that it is reasonable to blame (almost) everything that happens to the survivors on the effects of the treatment itself (surgery, radiation therapy, and chemotherapy). It should be noted, however, that important constitutional (genetic) differences among individuals must, at least in part, account for the late changes. It is probable that these inherited differences play as important a role in the development of Hodgkin's disease, and the late side effects, as the environmental factors.

In this book we emphasize the late side effects, caused primarily by therapy, unrelated to relapse of the Hodgkin's tumor itself. It must be acknowledged, however, that one of the major consequences of survival that all Hodgkin's survivors must face is the possibility of a relapse. In that regard, Bjorkholm, Holm, and Mellstedt in their chapter titled "Immunocompetence in Patients with Hodgkin's Disease" (Chapter 5) have pointed out that not everything that occurs is necessarily only a result of the treatment. They observed: "Another, and in many aspects more important issue is whether treatment and its detrimental immunologic effects may enhance a conceivable constitutional risk to develop Hodgkin's disease. . . In other words," they queried with regard to the Hodgkin's patients' potential for relapse, "are Hodgkin's patients more prone to develop de novo Hodgkin's disease than the normal population? . . . This might be anticipated if there is a constitutional/genetic basis for the evolution of Hodgkin's disease. To fully resolve this issue, not only Hodgkin's disease specific markers in general, but also clonal markers will be needed. In the future, molecular genetic analyses will be demanded to differentiate between relapsing and de novo Hodgkin's disease."

LONG-SURVIVING HODGKIN'S PATIENTS FACE NEW PROBLEMS

Our limitations in analyzing the late effects of therapy or the nature of Hodgkin's disease itself is related, in part, to the fact that we are just beginning to deal with a substantial number of long survivors, and our total experience, so far, is minimal. While we enthusiastically congratulate ourselves on our current success, we must recognize that so far only "... limited numbers of patients have survived 15 years or more following the introduction of modern radiotherapy and chemotherapy. Consequently, it remains to be seen whether this patient category will retain its low probability of 'relapse'." (Chapter 5)

Although we have invited the authors to analyze the current problems associated with the long-surviving Hodgkin's patient, generally, as a system by system review, a certain amount of overlapping of data is inevitable. Certain themes, such as the inordinately strong (and hopefully now diminished) concern over the potential development of treatment-induced leukemia, dominate more than one chapter. (Chapters 1, 3, 4, and 20)

TREATMENT-INDUCED ACUTE LEUKEMIA

A somewhat hysterical fear has been generated among physicians that multidrug chemotherapy, as it is used in the treatment of Hodgkin's disease and especially when combined with radiation therapy, would lead to the development of an excessive number of cases of acute leukemia. By analysis of occurrence alone, acute leukemia, as a complication of the treatment of Hodgkin's disease, is definitely on the rise. Schottenfeld (Chapter 1) noted the following: "In comparison with the clinical reports of Hodgkin's disease patients treated and evaluated before 1970, the relative risk or cumulative actuarial risk of leukemia has been observed to increase significantly in cohorts studied during the past 15 years. Whereas less than 20 case reports were recorded before 1970, there are now reports of over 300 patients who have developed acute leukemia following chemotherapy alone, or more commonly, in conjunction with radiotherapy."

It should be emphasized that despite the attention given to the increase in cases of post-treatment leukemia, we are not currently dealing with large numbers of patients who have developed either acute leukemia or nonHodgkin's lymphoma. Furthermore, it is Kempin's view (Chapter 4), as well as almost all others reviewing this problem, that the development of acute leukemia or non-Hodgkin's lymphoma (usually large cell lymphomas) is related to the "... improvement in survival of patients whose lives have been prolonged sufficiently, so that the number of patients at risk has increased dramatically over the last two decades." Despite what has been noted to be a significant increase in numbers of cases of leukemia and nonHodgkin's lymphomas, the actual numbers are much less alarming. Kempin (Chapter 4) notes that the initial report of a nonHodgkin's lymphoma developing in a patient surviving after Hodgkin's disease appeared in 1977, and between 1977 and 1985 he reviewed 26 more reported cases.

It has also been observed that the cases of post-treatment leukemia have occurred particularly in Hodgkin's patients who are failing treatment and who require repeated courses of chemotherapy merely to slightly prolong survival. Therefore, the development of leukemia, although leading to certain death, has not impacted significantly on the overall survival figures.

Children successfully treated for Hodgkin's disease have the longest lifetime risk of exposure to developing any of the complications of survival. Despite this, Donaldson (Chapter 18) has pointed out, with regard to the risk of developing leukemia, that "Most studies have shown age to be a prognostic indicator, with an especially high risk of leukemia among older patients (over 40 years of age). Conversely, children less than 20 have faired most favorably."

LEUKEMIA AND THE INTENSIVELY TREATED HODGKIN'S PATIENT

The fear of an excessive number of deaths from treatment-induced leukemia in Hodgkin's patients is being dispelled in light of a recent report from the National Cancer Institute. The title of the paper published by Blayney et al. in the New England Journal of Medicine (1987) tells the story. "Decreasing Risk of Leukemia with prolonged follow-up after chemotherapy and radiotherapy for Hodgkin's disease."[1]

It had been anticipated that leukemia induced by treatment would develop progressively, so the investigators at the National Cancer Institute set up a prospective follow-up study of their patients treated with MOPP to record the morphologic changes in the bone marrow, which they anticipated would precede the development of the leukemia they predicted would occur. Instead of discovering that their initial ominous predictions were correct, they discovered that the rate of leukemia development faltered; now they are predicting that in the surviving patient, after eleven years of observation, the incidence of secondary acute nonlymphocytic leukemia (ANLL) and myelodysplastic syndromes approaches the background incidence rate anticipated in a normal cohort of individuals.

Succinctly put, Blayney et al. conclude the following: "The projection that an increasing fraction of long-term survivors would die from leukemia was premature. With longer follow-up it appears that the incidence of leukemia falls, following a second-order rather than a linear regression model. The decrease in treatment-related risk after 11 years should reinforce the aggressive approach to this once uniformly fatal disease [Hodgkin's disease]."[1] All of this indicates that, so far, long survival does not carry with it a unique seed of latent death by leukemia, even if long survival was achieved by using combined radiation therapy and multidrug chemotherapy.

Armed with this knowledge, combining multidrug chemotherapy plus a limited dose of radiation therapy as primary treatment of Hodgkin's disease in adults as well as children is now more readily accepted as a universal policy of treatment. By limiting the dose of radiation therapy to the still forming bone structure in children, the additional effect of reducing the chance for bone growth deformities is simultaneously achieved.

Beresford (Chapter 20), in his analysis of potential malpractice problems associated with the iatrogenic effects of treatment of Hodgkin's patients uses the late development of a secondary malignancy (acute leukemia) as his case point of reference.

SOLID TUMORS ARE A SERIOUS LATE-DEVELOPING COMPLICATION

It appears that the risk of developing a wide variety of solid tumors will be the true danger for the surviving Hodgkin's patient. Current evidence suggests that the delayed development of leukemia is limited, whereas the development of radiation-induced, late-onset solid tumors is on the rise; the incidence is far higher than would be expected in a normal population.

The lesson to be learned is that we must constantly accede to the application of reality testing as opposed to the guess work of projection analysis. We must always deal with actual results in preference to actuarial or projected analyses. Human biologic systems are not always mathematically ordered over the long term, so we cannot rely solely on projections or predictions. What actually exists must influence us the most, and all predictions must constantly be tested against reality. Therefore, even with regard to the late development of leukemia, we should not come to any firm conclusions until much more follow-up time goes by. We may yet live to see another period, late in the life of the long-surviving Hodgkin's patient, when another rise in secondary leukemia appears.

NEUROLOGIC SIDE EFFECTS OF TREATMENT

We are aware of how late neurologic complications may appear after successful treatment for Hodgkin's disease. Physical and emotional support is all that can be offered once the neurologic deficit has been established. Each patient must individually judge if the treatment for Hodgkin's disease was worth it. Typically, in radiation-induced neurologic syndromes the symptom-free interval from treatment to the onset of the neurologic symptoms varies enormously from patient to patient. Values of 1 to 31 years (median 5 years) have been found, and more immediate deficits have occurred at one month and three to six month intervals. In one of our patients, the time interval from the point of treatment to the point of the development of the symptoms of neurologic spinal cord damage occurred 23 years after the end of radiation treatment with the development of progressive lower-extremity paralysis. In this patient, no evidence of recurring Hodgkin's disease was present. She will become a paraplegic as a late consequence of radiation therapy to the spinal cord, which was delivered as part of her treatment for Hodgkin's disease. Overall, this patient's quality of survival was phenomenal. Until the onset and the insidious uncontrolled progression of her paralysis, starting 23 years after her primary radiation therapy, everything appeared fine. Unfortunately, this patient is not alone; others treated with "modern" radiation techniques have also developed progressive paraplegia, with a much earlier onset of neurologic deficit. We know of no effective therapy for this form of radiation damage to the spinal cord. Chapter 9, by Cascino and O'Neil, reviews the potential late neurologic complications that might be anticipated.

TREATABLE SIDE EFFECTS

HYPOTHYROIDISM

One of the side effects of radiation therapy now readily recognized and simply treated has been considered trivial by some. But until all of the long surviving Hodgkin's patients are found and continually monitored for thyroid function (after they have received radiation therapy to the neck area) what seems trivial may become disastrous. These patients, if allowed to go undetected and untreated, may develop myxedema or they may die from heart failure.

Hypothyroidism is usually diagnosed while the patient is in a state of compensated hypothyroidism, with primary thyroid failure having been induced by previous radiation therapy. The primary thyroid failure is corrected, temporarily at least, by natural forces that drive the thyroid-stimulating hormone (TSH) to varying heights above normal. Loeffler, Mauch, and Hellman (Chapter 2) have observed that the incidence of hypothyroidism following mantle-field radiation varied from 20 to 50%. With continuing follow-up and long survival this incidence figure may approach 100%.

The potential development of hypothyroidism requires constant observation and evaluation during the patient's lifetime. Replacement hormone therapy appears to be curative once the diagnosis is established. The fine points of this complication have still not been worked out. How often and when should testing for thyroid failure begin? Is it wise to start treatment immediately after discovering that the patient's TSH is elevated? Can we afford to wait for a spontaneous regression of this abnormality? Is waiting and watching a minimally elevated TSH over a period of months or years, in anticipation of its spontaneous regression, a wise approach or will this result in an excessively high risk for the development of thyroid cancer? These problem, still not solved, are a perfect example of the work that needs to be done, which will be generated by interest in one of the consequences of survival.

AVASCULAR NECROSIS AND RETARDATION OF BONE GROWTH

In patients receiving radiation or chemotherapy alone, or combinations of radiation and chemotherapy (especially when the therapy includes prednisone), the incidence of avascular necrosis of bone has been reported to be as high as 10% among long-term survivors, although in most series the actual incidence of avascular necrosis is much less than that.[2]

The problem with the development of avascular necrosis and radiation damage to the spine, with its associated retardation of growth, is addressed by Smith and Griffiths in Chapter 8. Effects of radiation therapy and chemotherapy on the development of the jaw (in children) and on tooth decay is addressed in Chapter 17 on dental complications. Since the problems associated with bone growth are especially important to the pediatric population, these issues are also addressed by Donaldson in Chapter 18. Recognition of the untoward effect of radiation therapy on the development of the spine in children has led to a change in the methods of treatment for the pediatric patient with Hodgkin's disease. Radiation doses have been decreased and chemotherapy has been increased.

The side effects of treatment in damaging bone growth are also not trivial, but at least they are not life threatening. Today, avascular necrosis of the femoral head can be corrected with surgical intervention. Patients who develop avascular necrosis of the femoral head (and in some instances this is bilateral), can be successfully and satisfactorily rehabilitated with the appropriate surgery and a prosthetic hip replacement.

Having followed some of these patients for over 10 years since their first hip replacement it must be noted that even these artificially operating joints wear out and require reoperative replacement. How often this may be required in one person's life remains to be seen. So far, the record is two times in the same person, but these persons have definitely not reached their old age and therefore the height of their disability has probably not yet been realized.

An even smaller percent of patients develop avascular necrosis of the humeral head; they must live with this disability because still no successful surgical solution to their disability exists. Some patients with avascular necrosis of the humeri have been able to adjust their lives to this unpleasant disability, even though no satisfactory surgical solution currently exists.

SOFT TISSUE AND OTHER BONE GROWTH ABNORMALITIES

Using "old" techniques of radiation therapy with children receiving over 3500 cGy to the axial skeleton, a disproportionate alteration in sitting height, as compared to standing height, among children receiving total nodal radiation has been observed. The growth defect is particularly significant among those children whose bone growth is still in the formative stage (usually below the age of 14). Once past that phase of growth, high dose radiation therapy does not appear to be an important factor in bone growth.

By reducing the doses and the volume of irradiation and combining the radiation therapy with multidrug chemotherapy, bone growth alterations are avoided in children effectively treated for Hodgkin's disease. The goal is keep the radiation dose less than 2500 cGy. This prevents the height alterations that had been observed when radiation therapy alone was relied on as the primary treatment of children.

CARDIOPULMONARY COMPLICATIONS

The emerging data on the delayed clinical and subclinical cardiovascular toxicity of Hodgkin's therapy are reviewed by Gerling, Gottdiener, and Borer in Chapter 12.

Emphasizing the need to keep a careful watch on long survivors, they note among other issues, that "Early reports of radiation-induced pericardial disease emphasized a relatively short interval of up to 48 months between radiotherapy and the onset of pericardial disease. The late appearance (later than 48 months), however, of chronic pericardial disease in patients treated with mediastinal irradiation is becoming increasingly recognized as a significant consequence of therapy for Hodgkin's disease."

Changes in left ventricular function after radiation therapy are also outlined. Although the follow-up time of current Hodgkin's survivors may still be too short to properly analyze the effects of radiation on coronary artery disease, they conclude that ". . . the occurrence of clinically important coronary artery obstruction in several large studies is relatively infrequent considering the number of individuals at risk. On the other hand, considerable evidence supports the association between radiation and accelerated coronary atherosclerosis as a clinical entity."

The effect of chemotherapy on the myocardium is also reviewed in Chapter 12. The immediate adverse chemical effect on the cardiac muscle of drugs such as doxorubicin (Adriamycin) is carefully outlined.

Tarbell, Mauch, and Hellman (Chapter 13) address, among other problems related to the effects of radiation therapy, the pulmonary complications of treatment that result in radiation pneumonitis and later fibrosis. It is their view that "There is no clear cut relationship between acute pneumonitis and the later development of fibrosis."

STERILITY, ALTERATIONS IN FERTILITY, AND POTENTIAL GONADAL INJURY

The physician should discuss the risks of sterility, alterations in fertility, and gonadal injury with the patient before therapy for Hodgkin's disease begins. Chapter 11, which reviews the effects of Hodgkin's disease on pregnancy and progeny, concludes that major suppressive effects on gonadal reproductive function occur in the male secondary to a wide variety of chemotherapy, and it is the male patient who has a higher incidence of sterility induced by chemotherapy than the female.

The pessimism that has been expressed concerning the "price" the female patient must pay for long survival by not being able to conceive and bear children is almost always associated with the relapsing Hodgkin's patient who requires repeated courses of "salvage" chemotherapy in the hope of achieving a remission and longer survival. Thoughts of pregnancy or concern over the presence or absence of the menstrual cycle are rarely an issue in the minds of these patients. Their goal is to survive at any cost.

In females, the likelihood of maintenance of ovarian function is directly related to gonadal exposure to radiation, the type of chemotherapy, and the age at treatment. The younger the woman at the time of therapy, the higher the probability of maintenance of regular menses following therapy. Damage imposed on ovarian function by aggressive therapy is less severe in girls and young women than in older women. Women in their child-bearing years with Hodgkin's—even after treatment with a wide variety of chemotherapy combinations and radiation therapy (as long as the radiation avoids a direct application to the ovaries)—can and do have children at a rate similar to that of their peers.

In contrast to females, male patients treated with radiation therapy or chemotherapy for Hodgkin's disease develop a much higher percentage of sterility. Germ cell depletion and dysfunction of Leydig's cells are expected and likely to be irreversible in adolescent and adult males following six cycles of MOPP chemotherapy. Because cytotoxic damage to the testicular germinal epithelium appears to be related to both the dose and the type of chemotherapy employed, different chemotherapies must be evaluated separately and no generalization can be made merely by extrapolating the data derived from a six cycle course of MOPP.* Radiation therapy delivered to the pelvis in males is not easily shielded from the testes and this alone may result in permanent sterility.

Although the total follow-up time that has been recorded is not long when one considers the span of a normal male's productive lifetime, it is likely that there is little hope for recovery once a man is rendered sterile at an early age. Merely having Hodgkin's disease may also have an adverse effect on a man's fertility before any form of staging or treatment. Males with HD are subfertile prior to initiation of therapy.

Chapter 11, on pregnancy and progeny, also addresses treating Hodgkin's disease and pregnancy when they occur simultaneously, including the potential side effects of radiation and chemotherapy on the fetus, the effects of pregnancy on the patient in remission of Hodgkin' disease, and what—if any—effects may be expected on children born to patients after treatment is complete.

GASTROINTESTINAL COMPLICATIONS

Gastrointestinal complications resulting from the treatment of Hodgkin's disease can be serious, but the incidence is low. Most of the problems are related to staging laparotomy and radiation therapy. According to Zim-

---
*Mechlorethamine hydrochloride, vincristine sulfate (Oncovin), procarbazine hydrochloride, prednisone.

balist and Shike, "The cyclic combination drug programs use in Hodgkin's disease rarely cause significant complications." This Chapter (15) reviews the effects of staging laparotomy from the gastroenterologist's viewpoint. Mortality from staging laparotomy for Hodgkin's disease amounted to 0.5%, similar to other groups undergoing elective abdominal exploration. "Mechanical small bowel obstruction secondary to adhesions, volvulus or intussusception, and prolonged paralytic ileus are well-known complications of any abdominal surgery, and have been reported in patients with Hodgkin's disease who have undergone a staging laparotomy." They also noted that "The staging laparotomy can result in adhesions and an immobility of the bowel, exposing some of its segments to high doses of irradiation. Thus, the staging laparotomy may contribute to the development of radiation enteropathy. In a report on patients with Hodgkin's disease undergoing subdiaphragmatic radiation, the incidence of radiation enteritis was 23% among patients who had exploratory laparotomy, significantly higher than the 7% in patients who had radiation alone."

RENAL DISEASE

Renal complications of radiation therapy have not become a major problem according to the review by Diamond and Levi (Chapter 14). "Despite the large number of drugs used in the treatment of Hodgkin's disease, nephrotoxicity is not a major complication of therapy."

SKIN

Anderson, Myskowski, and Safai (Chapter 16) review the cutaneous sequelae of therapy in Hodgkin's patients. "Since most of the treatments of Hodgkin's disease are aimed at rapidly dividing cells," they point out, "it is not surprising that the skin and mucous membranes are frequently affected by the complications of antitumor therapy. Indeed, it has been estimated that 15 to 30% of all patients with Hodgkin's disease will develop some sort of cutaneous disorder during the course of their illness." Their review covers chronic radiation injury to the skin and the most common cutaneous complications of chemotherapy, including alopecia, stomatitis, hyperpigmentation with local chemical injury, onychodystrophy, hypersensitivity reactions, and photosensitivity. Other complications, such as infection and second malignancies of the skin, are also reviewed.

IMMUNOCOMPETENCE IN HODGKIN'S DISEASE

Bjorkholm, Holm, and Mellstedt (Chapter 5) provide us with some insights into the immunologic puzzle of Hodgkin's disease. Long survivors, after treatment for Hodgkin's disease, have a T-cell lymphocytopenia and impairment of T-cell functions. Although it seems that this could be attributed primarily to the effects of therapy, these immunodeficiencies may actually be genetically determined.

Because of the high familial incidence of Hodgkin's disease, it has always been assumed that the cause of Hodgkin's disease is genetically determined, at least in part. One of the ways to approach this issue is through analyses of immunologic aberrations that characterize Hodgkin's disease. Bjorkholm, Holm, and Mellstedt pose the following questions:

1. Is the immunodefect in "cured" HD patients acquired? If so, is it secondary to the tumor- or disease-associated factors that may promote and perpetuate a state of immunologic imbalance in predisposed individuals?
2. Is the immunodeficiency an inherited (genetic?) characteristic of Hodgkin's disease patients? If so, it might be detected in relatives. Moreover, it may predispose one to developing the disease and may modulate its course. An inherited immunodeficiency may also be latent and precipitated by the disease or other factors. Early immunologic aging may contribute.

Bjorkholm, Holm, and Mellstedt have not completely answered their own questions but their conclusion, after studying healthy relatives of Hodgkin's patients, is that ". . . otherwise healthy persons with a first-degree relative with Hodgkin's disease display a significantly increased frequency of T-cell impairment. These findings have led us to hypothesize that a state of T-cell impairment existed in certain patients prior to the evolution of Hodgkin's disease."

The immunologic effects of pretreatment splenectomy are also reviewed by Bjorkholm, Holm and Mellstedt. They are concerned that "The asplenic state, reduced IgM levels, and possibly impaired B-cell responses contribute to the persistent, life-long threat of overwhelming postsplenectomy infections in splenectomized patients with Hodgkin's disease."

INFECTION

Armstrong and Minamoto concern themselves with the potential for serious bacterial infection in the Hodgkin's survivor. They review, among other problems, the delayed development of fatal infections in splenectomized patients unrelated to chemotherapy or relapsing Hodgkin's disease. They conclude: "Based on the available published data, postsplenectomy infection should be anticipated, even in patients in disease remission; however, recent chemotherapy and radiotherapy and the status of the disease are likely to be as important in determining the causative organisms, severity of infection, and empiric treatment."

Many of the serious infections encountered in adults treated for Hodgkin's disease, with or without their spleens intact, have been associated with periods of retreatment for relapsing or progressive tumor and associated with leukopenia and suppression of immune function. Many of these serious infections in adults occur in the already dying patient.

As Donaldson, in Chapter 18, has emphasized, ". . . in the Stanford series, 52% of the episodes of serious bacterial infection in [splenectomized] children occurred months or years following completion of treatment among a population presumed to be cured of Hodgkin's disease. Infection in this setting has been observed as an initial event at 13 years following therapy, with 4 of 12 of the treatment episodes being fatal."

Although it is recognized that splenic irradiation can produce splenic atrophy and dysfunction, which may also result in overwhelming infection, so far it is the splenectomized patient and not the merely irradiated patient that seems to be in danger of sudden, late fatal sepsis—most commonly inflicted by encapsulated bacteria, especially pneumococci. Because the predominant organisms for serious bacterial infections are penicillin sensitive, many investigators now recommend the routine use of prophylactic antibiotics for children who have had a previous splenectomy. The problems presented with long-term prophylactic antibiotic therapy center around the fact that neither the optimal dose nor the optimal duration of antibiotic administration is known. Armstrong and Minamoto (Chapter 6) comment: "Penicillin prophylaxis has many advocates, although no controlled studies support this recommendation."

Analyzing various reports concerning the pneumococcal vaccine, in addition to one that ". . . found that postimmunization antibody levels in patients with Hodgkin's disease were significantly lower than those of normal control subjects for 10 of 12 serotypes measured . . ." Armstrong and Minamoto concluded that "the efficacy of the vaccine is therefore questionable." Despite the limited scientific proof of usefulness, they still advocate that both prophylactic penicillin and the pneumococcal vaccine be used in all splenectomized patients with Hodgkin's disease. They do, however, qualify their recommendation with the following statement: "The duration of prophylaxis is not established."

The treatment of viral infections such as herpes zoster is still unsatisfactory, and although the use of zoster immune globulin (ZIG) or immune-compromised children exposed to chickenpox appears to be useful, the actual or observed experience in immune-compromised adults is extremely limited.

PSYCHOSOCIAL EFFECTS OF SURVIVING CANCER

Despite the persistence of certain lingering psychological effects associated with their disease and treatment, the adaptation of the surviving Hodgkin's patient to a "normal" life has been gratifying.

The existence of many long survivors among cancer victims is a new experience for society. Siegel and Christ (Chapter 19) explore the relatively new phenomenon of the recovered cancer patient. "Society," they point out, "continues to equate cancer with death. As a result there are no clear expectations or norms regarding how the cancer survivor should act, feel, or be treated by others. Finally, the fear of recurrence . . . prevents many individuals from accepting that they have recovered from the illness."

The enduring sense of enhanced vulnerability and of living a precarious existence, which has been noted in cancer survivors in general, is shared by the Hodgkin's survivor. But Siegel and Christ note that the worry about the possibility of recurrence diminishes when the Hodgkin's survivor lives two or more years after treatment. Unfortunately, most of the patients do not ever seem to dispel the lurking fear of recurrence or the development of a new cancer. Because of this enhanced sense of vulnerability, cancer survivors shift their life goals and general outlook. They tend to move away from purely materialistic goals, instead they emphasize humanistic values.

Attitudes of the Hodgkin's patient toward his own future are important to explore, but just as important are the attitudes of society toward the surviving Hodgkin's patient. "With the improved prognosis of Hodgkin's disease, health care staff have tended to focus on the optimistic prognosis, at times inadvertently denying the realities of the patient's experience subsequent to diagnosis and treatment. While it is appropriate for most patients with Hodgkin's disease to expect long-term survival, they cannot ignore the potentially fatal nature of this disease or its meaning to the patient, his family and friends, and society. The patient should become hopeful about the ultimate outcome; he is not likely to die. He must, however, also deal with the transition from being a healthy young adult to one who has the potential to be chronically or fatally ill. Cancer is not like a broken leg from which one can expect to recover fully with no possibility of later medical problems, side-effects, or psychological or social consequences."

Siegel and Christ review the problems that exist for Hodgkin's patients, health care professionals, and society. They emphasize that "Health care staff should avoid a tendency to focus exclusively on the good prognosis, which may inadvertently trivialize the patient's struggle." On the other hand, they report that "Society has been slow to integrate the improved prognosis of Hodgkin's disease patients into its perception of them and into its employment and insurance policies." Barriers to full participation in society definitely exist for the surviving Hodgkin's patient, but these barriers are surmountable; as we constantly improve absolute survival, they fall steadily.

FUTURE IMPLICATIONS

The good news is that for the majority of long survivors the complications of treatment have generally not been severe and the complications caused by treatment have not yet had a significant impact on decreasing the overall long survival of the Hodgkin's patient. That is the message of this book, coupled with a warning. There is a disturbing rising incidence of second primary tumors (of the lung, colon, breast) among the surviving Hodgkin's patients that cannot be adequately treated once they go beyond the point of simple surgical excision. These second primary tumors may be the ultimate killers of our Hodgkin's patients and every effort must be made to detect these second cancers in their earliest stages. If these tumors are caused primarily by the use of radiation therapy, every effort must be made to discover effective alternative therapies.

It should be clear that the final word is not in yet, and this cannot be overemphasized. The patients who contracted Hodgkin's disease in the early 1970s and who were the beneficiaries of the new wave of treatment using extended-field, high-dose radiation therapy and then multidrug chemotherapy are just now passing the 10- and 15-year survival mark. If the majority of these patients were between the ages of 20 and 40 when they were first treated, they are only now beginning to live their third through fifth decade. That is not exactly "old age"; therefore, it still remains to be seen what will happen to the heart, lungs, and the rest of the organ systems that were subjected to high doses of radiation and chemotherapy.

If the threat of acute leukemia, which haunts the Hodgkin's patient, has been dispelled, what will the final word be regarding other forms of secondary malignant tumors? Will a rising incidence of leukemia appear after much longer follow-up? What other side effects will occur later in their lives? Will the Hodgkin's relapse rate escalate 30 years after primary treatment? It remains to be seen.

No matter what problems have been created by our various treatment programs, the bottom line is that the Hodgkin's patient has enjoyed an increase in survival coupled with a generally good quality of life. Despite this rousing success for most Hodgkin's patients, which was accomplished over the past 25 years, we must still face the fact that a significant proportion of all Hodgkin's patients do not respond to our current treatment and do not enjoy a long survival. Furthermore, for a significant proportion of the patients, the effects of the treatment cause serious consequences, resulting in unwanted pain, deficiencies, and an early death.

Our job is clear. We must continue to analyze our results and constantly monitor the effects of our treatment over time. In this way we will learn to adjust our treatment to continually decrease the unwanted side effects and continue to improve the overall survival of the Hodgkin's patient.

REFERENCES

1. Blayney, D.W., et al. Decreasing risk of leukemia with prolonged follow-up after chemotherapy for Hodgkin's disease. N. Engl. J. Med. *316*(12):710, 1987.
2. Prosnitz, L.R., Lawson, J.P., Friedlander, G.E., et al. Avascular necrosis of bone in Hodgkin's disease patients treated with combined modality treatment. Cancer *47*:2793–2797, 1981.

CHAPTER 1

Epidemiology of Second Primary Cancers in Patients with Hodgkin's Disease

DAVID SCHOTTENFELD

The use of high-dose extended field or total nodal radiation therapy, and/or cyclical multidrug chemotherapy, have dramatically improved the survival rates of patients with Hodgkin's disease. Combination chemotherapy can cure more than half of the patients with stages III and IV disease; it has also contributed, in the past decade, to the 50 to 55% decline in United States mortality resulting from Hodgkin's disease. Intensive, combined modality therapy or intensive multidrug chemotherapy, however, are associated with significant long-term sequelae.[1]

An increasingly important manifestation of the toxic potential of antineoplastic agents is the induction of leukemias and related myelodysplastic disorders, nonHodgkin's lymphomas, carcinomas, and sarcomas. The improving survival of patients with Hodgkin's disease has made it possible to assess the incidence of second primary cancers. If the subsequent incidence or risk of second primary cancers is increased significantly one may infer that common pathogenic factors are operating in both neoplasms, or that one or more agents used in the treatment of the index cancer are oncogenic. Helpful epidemiologic features for judging the biologic plausibility of a common pathogenesis for cancers of different organ sites would be the demonstration of reciprocally excessive occurrences of second primary cancers in patient cohorts and a demonstration of risk factors common to both organ sites.[2] This chapter examines methodologic approaches to studies of incident malignant neoplastic events in Hodgkin's disease patients and the role of radiotherapy, chemotherapy, and host factors in their development.

METHODOLOGY

PERSON-YEARS AT RISK

While observations on prevalence and proportional frequencies of specific combinations of multiple primary cancers are of historical interest, they do not enable as precise a determination of risk as studies based on incidence within a cohort of patients after the diagnosis of a particular index cancer. In order to determine whether combinations of index and second primary cancers are occurring more frequently than might be expected by chance, the observed number of second primary cancers in a cohort of cancer patients is summarized in relation to the person-years of observation accumulated from a specified point in time after the diagnosis of the index cancer. The expected number is derived by multiplying the person-years at risk, which are stratified by age, sex, and calendar period, by age-, sex-, and calendar period-specific incidence rates for cancers of all sites and selected sites reported by a population-based cancer registry. The ratio of the observed to expected number of second primary cancers is used as a measure of relative risk. Since the probability of a subsequent or metachronous primary cancer is relatively small, the number of subsequent primary cancers can be expected to follow a Poisson distribution. The statistical significance of the standardized ratio of the observed to the expected number of cancers can be tested readily. A unique advantage of a cohort study that is developed from a population-based cancer registry, as distinguished from one in which the patient population is limited to one or more hospital cancer registries, is that the populations yielding observed and expected numbers of multiple primary cancers are derived from the same reference population.

The denominator—person-years—increases either with longer follow-up or with use of a larger sample, and treats equivalently the exposure time of five persons for one year, one person for five years, or ten persons for six months. As a measure of risk, which is expressed as the observed crude incidence of second primary cancers per cumulative person-years of observation, this index assumes that each patient has a constant risk during the entire post-treatment period, and that an adequate number of patients in various subgroups can be followed for sufficient and comparable periods of time. If this is not the case, then a method of survival analysis that uses a life-table approach would be more appropriate for the comparison of patients with different periods of follow-up or different risks over time.[3]

One bias that may operate in the selection of cases for study from major cancer treatment centers is the "healthy person-years" bias, which is defined as the cancer-free interval between primary diagnosis and treatment and referral to a specialized center, in which the preceding person-years at risk for a study subject inflate the calculation of the expected number of cancers. In effect, these patients must survive to enable subsequent referral. If one decides to include referral patients and to accumulate patient-years at risk toward the development of subsequent primary cancers from the date of diagnosis or date of first treatment, then "healthy person-years at risk" would be selected into the study. One can adjust for this by accumulating patient-years of observation from the date first seen at the referral institution. Such individuals should be considered late entries into follow-up after an appropriate interval of time, which is equivalent to the period from diagnosis or first treatment to the date first seen at the referral center. Although "healthy person-years" can be accounted for with such an approach, one cannot disregard the implications of ignoring the potential oncogenic effects of previous treatment factors.

As suggested previously, use of person-years at risk may not always be appropriate in studies of multiple primaries, since a major assumption of the approach requires that the risk following a putative causal exposure remains constant over time. The standard approach in which all person-years of observation are allocated to a single exposure category, such as a course of treatment, fails to take into account the transient or changing nature of the exposure. Misclassification errors result from such an approach because all person-years at risk are assigned to a single treatment classification. A method of analysis proposed by Mantel and Byar[4] may be employed; it allocates person-years of exposure to different treatment categories as a patient's course of treatment changes, and it takes into account the interval of follow-up since initial treatment exposure, the interval from diagnosis of the index disease, and the different degrees of censoring among treatment groups.

LIFE-TABLE SURVIVAL METHODS

Life-table methods and actuarial survival curves have been used to calculate the cumulative probabilities of site-specific second primary cancers in a cohort of Hodgkin's disease patient who were identified by calendar period, nature of initial course of therapy, and duration of follow-up. In general, the quantitative assessment of risk of treatment-induced cancers has been based on the incidence of metachronous primary cancers, which become clinically apparent following completion of the initial course of treatment. An implicit assumption of the life-table methods, with respect to the probability of developing second primary cancers, is that subjects who are censored as losses, withdrawals, or transfers are comparable to subjects who remain under observation. Therefore, the occurrence of a censored observation is viewed as a random event, unrelated to the risk of developing a second primary cancer.

The earlier methodology for estimating survival curves (i.e., Berkson-Gage) employed preset intervals of time into which vital events and censoring were grouped. Currently, the more common practice is to base the analysis on precise, observed individual end points, rather than preset grouped data, and to derive (by the method of Kaplan and Meier[5]) an estimate of the probability of an event over time. Other methods are then used to compare cumulative risks in different cohorts. For example, the log-rank or Mantel chi-square test is useful in comparing survival functions and may be applied to detect differences in the cumulative observed and expected numbers of second primary cancers for various treatment (exposure) subgroups. The log-rank chi-square test is designed particularly to infer the nature of differences in risks between groups that are consistent over time. In any such comparison, it is important to recognize and control for confounding variables, such as age, sex, race, and calendar period, that independently influence the rate of incidence of second primary cancers. In the log-rank test, a limited number of such confounding factors may be adjusted for in the analysis by stratification.[6,7,8]

The development of regression models for survival analysis and the availability of computer biostatistical software has made it possible to examine time-dependent, dose-response relationships and interactions among multiple causal factors. Regression models proposed for survival functions generally involve the assumption of proportional hazard. One such model introduced by Cox[9] has had wide application to the analysis of survival data. The assumption of proportional hazard implies that the probability of fatality or some end point for an individual, after adjusting for major prognostic characteristics (i.e., age, sex, stage of disease, treatment, etc.), is a constant multiple of a baseline risk level at all times. Thus, although the instantaneous risk may change with time, the ratio of risks or relative risk is assumed to be constant. The proportional hazards regression model is able to accommodate many clinical problems applicable to the analysis of time-dependent events and different levels of exposure or modes of therapy; it also can control simultaneously for the effects of confounding variables.

ILLUSTRATIVE PROBLEM

Comparison of crude cumulative probabilities of second primary cancers for different subgroups of Hodgkin's disease patients can often be misleading. We offer the following illustrative example:

Life tables were constructed, beginning six months after initiation of first treatment, to determine the cumulative probabilities of second primary cancers in Hodgkin's disease patients treated at the Memorial Sloan-Kettering Cancer Center during the years 1950 to 1954, 1960 to 1964, and 1968 to 1972. Five years after the first treatment, the cumulative probabilities were 1.26%, 1.22%, and 4.05%, respectively (Table 1–1).

Table 1–2 summarizes the analyses of relative risk, before and after age adjustment, for the various cohorts. In the comparison between 1960 to 1964 and 1968 to 1972, the 1960 to 1964 cohort was assumed to have a relative risk of 1.0. In the comparison for each unit interval of time, the log-rank chi-square test of statistical significance was employed. The Mantel-Haenszel summary chi-square test was used in all other two-way comparisons of risk.

Table 1–1. Ninety-Five Percent Confidence Intervals (CI) for the Cumulative Probabilities of Second Primary Cancers (SPC) Developing 5 and 10 Years After First Treatment for Hodgkin's Disease

Cohort	Five-Year Cumulative Probability of SPC	Ninety-Five Percent CI	Ten-Year Cumulative Probability of SPC	Ninety-Five Percent CI
1950–1954	1.27	1.25–1.28	2.63	2.55–2.71
1960–1964	1.22	1.20–1.24	7.67	7.24–8.10
1968–1972	4.05	3.93–4.18	—	—

The results of the log-rank chi-square test suggested that there were no significant differences, before age adjustment, in the numbers of subsequent primary cancers that developed 1 to 5 years after first treatment for the three cohorts. The other paired comparisons, before age adjustment, are also listed in Table 1–2.

We reported previously[10] on the development of second primary cancers in two male and two female Hodgkin's disease patients who were under 40 years of age when their second primary cancers developed. We also reported on the significant excess of second primary cancers among males and females during the interval 6 to 10 years following treatment. The excesses were interpreted on the basis of age-, sex-, and calendar period-specific incidence rates from the Connecticut Tumor Registry. These observations led us to compute the average annual incidence rates for the three cohorts stratified according to age at first treatment.

The comparison of average annual incidence rates, in the first five years post-therapy, for the groups under 40 years of age and those 40 years and over at first treatment were unremarkable for the 1950 to 1954 and 1960 to 1964 cohorts, but in the 1968 to 1972 cohort[2] the average annual incidence rate was 4 to 5 times higher among the older subgroup of patients.

The percent distributions of patients by five-year "age at first treatment" strata in each cohort were compared. No differences were observed. The estimations of relative risk were higher for nearly all of the comparisons, after controlling for the confounding effect of age. Stratification by age has the effect of increasing the magnitude of both the log-rank chi-square and the Mantel-Haenszel summary chi-square statistics (Table 1–2).

When computation of the adjusted relative risk was based on a standard comprised of the pooled experiences of all three cohorts 1 to 5 years post-therapy, the estimate of risk for the 1968 to 1972 cohort relative to the 1950 to 1954 cohort was 4.18, compared with 2.94 derived without age adjustment. An adjusted relative risk of 4.07 was derived for the 1968 to 1972 cohort based on a standard population comprised of the 1950 to 1954 and the 1968 to 1972 cohorts. A crude relative risk of 2.74 was determined previously for the 1968 to 1972 cohort.

POWER AND SAMPLE SIZE

The requirement of sufficient power, or the probability of finding a significantly increased risk that does in fact exist, influences the projected number of patients needed for a cohort study. However, the sample size or cumulative person-years of observation that is optimal for detecting or ruling out important sequelae of treatment may be inadequate in published studies of second primary cancers in patients with Hodgkin's disease.

Table 1–3 outlines the sample sizes required for a study and comparison or control group to establish or rule out relative risks of various magnitudes over and above the rate at which the event of interest is postulated to occur. In Table 1–3, the average annual incidence of second primary cancers is considered to be 0.008 (8 per 1000). The sample sizes required to study the occurrences of second primary cancers are influenced by the specified levels of types 1 and 2 errors, the expected incidence of site-specific second primary cancers, and the relative risk that one regards as important to detect. The limited experience of any single institution may constrain the precision of estimates of relative risk. A multi-institutional

Table 1-2. Tests for Statistical Significance of the Number of Second Primary Cancers Developing Within 1–5 and 6–10 Year Intervals Following First Treatment With and Without Control for Age at First Treatment

	Without Controlling for Age at First Treatment				Controlling for Age at First Treatment			
Cohort	Interval After Treatment (Year)	Relative Risk	X^2	Cohort	Interval After Treatment (Year)	Standardized Relative Risk	X^2
1950–1954		1.00		1950–1954		1.00	
1960–1964	1–5	1.42	5.41*	1960–1964	1–5	0.96	7.70*
1968–1972		2.94		1968–1972		4.18	
		$(0.05 < p < 0.10)$				$(0.01 < p < 0.025)$	
1950–1954	1–5	1.00	0.001†	1950–1954	1–5	1.00	0.16†
1960–1964		0.68		1960–1964		1.05	
		$(0.95 < p < 0.975)$				$(p = 0.20)$	
1950–1954	6–10	1.00	1.98†	1950–1954	6–10	1.00	2.05†
1960–1964		5.65		1960–1964		7.09	
		$(0.10 < p < 0.20)$				$(0.10 < p < 0.20)$	
1950–1954	1–5	1.00	1.62†	1950–1954	1–5	1.00	3.38†
1968–1972		2.74		1968–1972		4.07	
		$(0.20 < p < 0.30)$				$(0.05 < p < 0.10)$	
1960–1964	1–5	1.00	3.15†	1960–1964	1–5	1.00	3.42†
1968–1972		5.35		1968–1972		5.92	
		$(0.05 < p < 0.10)$				$(0.05 < p < 0.10)$	

*Log-rank chi-square test
†Mantel-Haenszel summary chi-square test

Table 1–3. Number of Person-Years Required to Detect Relative Risks for Equal Sample Sizes in Both Groups ($n_1 = n_2$)*

Relative Risk (P_1/P_2†)	P_1	n_1	n_2	Total Person-Years
2.0	0.016	3,062	3,062	7,124
2.5	0.020	1,421	1,421	2,842
3.0	0.024	918	918	1,836
4.0	0.032	628	628	1,256
4.5	0.036	390	390	780
5.0	0.040	340	340	680

*From Cohen, assuming event of interest is binomially distributed. Type 1 = 0.05 (two-sided); type 2 = 0.20.

†When the proportions of patients developing some event of interest in a study population (P_1) and a control population (P_2) are compared, the type 1 error is the probability of declaring a significant difference between the groups when in fact it does not exist. The type 2 error is associated with the probability that an investigator will conclude that there is no difference between the two study groups when in fact a difference does exist. $P_2 = 0.008$.

approach may be required, but it may be difficult to find sufficiently large groups of similarly classified patients with uniform and comprehensive characterization of risk factors and follow-up.

CASE-CONTROL WITHIN COHORT STUDY DESIGN

The use of a case-control design that is "nested" within a cohort study may provide an economical and efficient method of testing a hypothesis concerning the adverse effects of previous treatment on outcomes such as second primary cancers. For example, in such a design, assuming that one has a sufficiently large cohort with an optimal interval of follow-up, cases with second primary cancers are compared with a sample of age-, sex-, race-matched control patients with Hodgkin's disease from the same cohort who did not develop second primary cancers during the same interval of follow-up. In the traditional cohort method, all of the essential epidemiologic information is recorded for all subjects. In the example of a case-control design based within a cohort, detailed epidemiologic information is obtained only for the cases and controls or for a small fraction of the cohort population. The cohort, however, must be large enough to provide an adequate number of cases of a specific type of cancer to enable investigation of suspected etiologic factors (Table 1–4).[11]

NEOPLASTIC SEQUELAE OF THERAPY

During the late 1960s, treatment for Hodgkin's disease changed substantially with the introduction of extended field or total nodal radiotherapy and combination chemotherapy. In 1972, Arseneau et al.[12] described 425 patients with Hodgkin's disease, 12 of whom developed metachronous second primary cancers that were either carcinomas or sarcomas. The population studied included all patients with Hodgkin's disease who were evaluated and treated at the National Cancer Institute (United States) between 1953 and 1971 (with follow-up through 1971). The patients were classified as to the intensity of radiotherapy and chemotherapy received. Intensive radiotherapy was defined as total-nodal or extended-field irradiation given as a

Table 1–4. Number of Cases (n_1) and Controls (n_2) Required to Detect Relative Risks Where $n_1 = n_2$*

Relative Risk†	n_1	n_2
1.5	387	387
2.0	132	132
2.5	76	76

*From Schlesselman, Biometry Branch, National Institute of Child Health and Human Development. Type 1 = 0.05 (two sided); type 2 = 0.20

†Proportion of controls (Hodgkin's disease patients without second primary cancers) who had received intensive chemotherapy as primary treatment was assumed to be 0.40. This estimate was based on the publication by Curtis et al.[65]

unified course of therapy. Intensive chemotherapy was defined as the administration of a combination of four drugs used cyclically in a coordinated regimen for six monthly cycles. The four drugs used were nitrogen mustard or cyclophosphamide, vincristine, procarbazine, and prednisone. The period at risk (i.e., person-years) for the second primary cancer was considered to begin at diagnosis of Hodgkin's disease and to terminate at diagnosis of the second primary cancer, date of death, or date of most recent follow-up examination. The relative risk of second primary cancers was defined as the ratio of the observed to the expected numbers, whereby the expected numbers were based upon the site-specific general population cancer incidence rates of the Third National Cancer Survey (1969 to 1971).

The relative risk for 131 patients not receiving any intensive radiation therapy or combination chemotherapy (1.6) was not increased significantly. However, the relative risks for 149 patients who received intensive radiation therapy with or without nonintensive chemotherapy (3.8) or for 110 patients who received intensive chemotherapy with or without nonintensive radiation therapy (3.2) were increased more substantially than the risk exhibited by patients who did not receive any intensive level of exposure to any treatment modality. The most striking increase in risk was observed in 35 patients who were exposed to both intensive radiation therapy and chemotherapy (29.0). This particular subgroup of patients treated with both intensive radiation therapy and chemotherapy was then enlarged to 65 patients, and their follow-up surveillance revealed a total of eight second primary cancers. These included three patients with acute myelocytic leukemia and one with chronic myelocytic leukemia.[13] In an interim report by Canellos et al.,[14] a similar pattern was noted after patients treated at the National Cancer Institute received intensive therapy. The relative risk of second primary cancers in patients treated with both intensive radiotherapy and chemotherapy was 14.5, and in the total cohort of 452 patients, the relative risk of 4.3 reflected a statistically significant increase.

The experience at the Memorial Sloan-Kettering Cancer Center[10] indicated that the cumulative percent of Hodgkin's disease patients who developed second primary cancers of all sites and tissues five years after completion of their first treatment was 1.3% in patients treated between the years 1950 and 1954; the five-year cumulative percent remained at 1.2% for the cohort first treated between 1960 and 1964, but was observed to increase significantly to 4.1% in the cohort first treated between 1968 and 1972 (Fig. 1–1). Concurrently, the observed five-year survival rate increased from 40% (1950 to 1954) to 76% (1968 to 1972). Based on the cohort of patients first treated between 1960 and 1964, the cumulative probability of metachronous primary cancers of all sites and tissues at ten years increased to 7.7%, compared with 2.6% recorded for the 1950 to 1954 cohort. In a more recent publication, Coleman[15] estimated that the overall 10-year actuarial risk of developing second primary cancers was about 10%.

Following the publications from the National Cancer Institute and the published proceedings of a workshop on multiple primary cancers held at the Memorial Sloan-Kettering Cancer Center in 1976,[16] reports of increased incidence of second primary cancers in Hodgkin's disease patients have been issued from cancer referral centers and cooperative study groups. Various sources have described the increased risk of acute leukemias, non-Hodgkin's lymphomas, sarcomas, and carcinomas. The pathogenesis of these specific tumor types reflects the influence of treatment factors, predisposing host factors, and unique tissue susceptibilities.

ACUTE LEUKEMIA

In comparison with the clinical reports of Hodgkin's disease patients treated and evaluated before 1970,[17] the relative risk or cumulative actuarial risk of leukemia has been observed to increase significantly in cohorts studied during the past 20 years. Whereas less than 20 case reports were recorded before 1970, there are now reports of over 300 patients who have developed acute leukemia following chemotherapy alone, or more commonly, in conjunction with radiotherapy.[18] The results of ten major studies, published

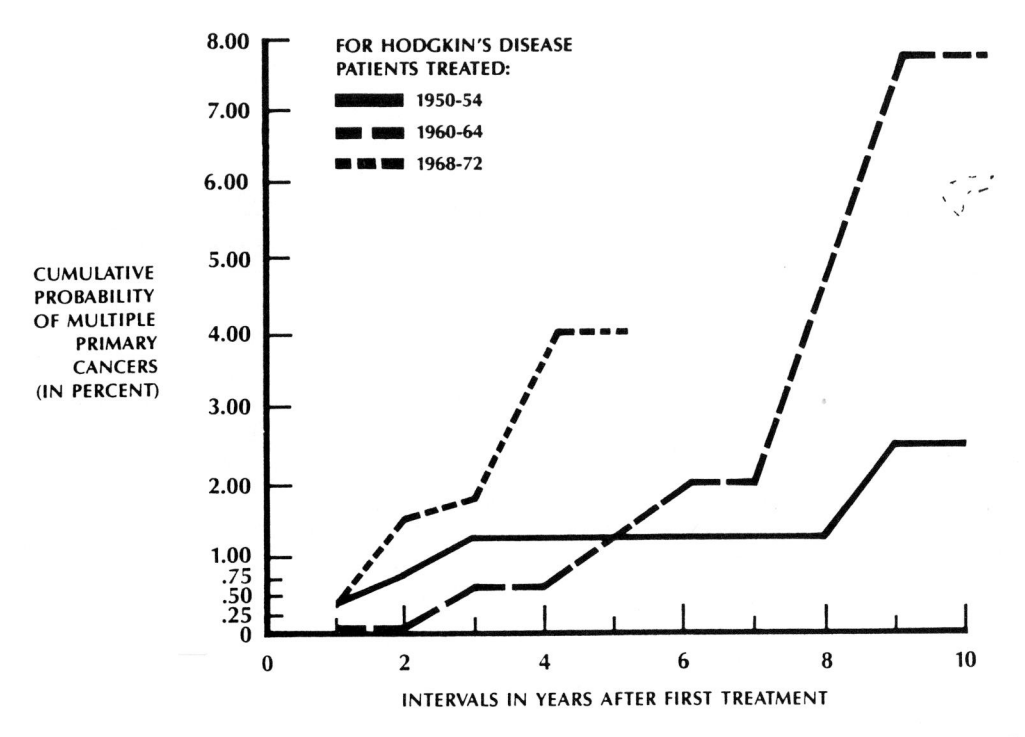

Fig. 1–1. Cumulative probability of multiple primary cancers by yearly interval after therapy. (From Brody, R.S. and Schottenfeld, D. Multiple primary cancers in Hodgkin's disease. Semin. Oncol. 7:187–201, 1980.)

since 1982, of leukemogenesis in 7274 patients with Hodgkin's disease are summarized in Table 1–5.[15,19-28]

The studies of Coleman[15,19] and Tester et al.[27] estimated that, overall, 3.5% of patients developed leukemia within 10 years. In most of the studies, few or no leukemias were observed among patients who received radiotherapy alone. The risk of leukemia was highest after prolonged, intensive, combination chemotherapy (about 6% at 10 years), which was generally administered with intensive radiotherapy, either as primary treatment or as salvage therapy.

Several studies reported, after controlling for interval of follow-up, an especially elevated risk in older patients (over 40 years of age) when compared with younger adults who received combined modality therapy. In an international study reviewed by Miké et al.,[29] children (15 years and younger) treated for Hodgkin's disease from 1950 to 1970 had a 14-fold increase in the observed to expected number of second primary cancers in the first 15 years after diagnosis. In 688 children, 20 second primary cancers, including six with acute myelocytic leukemia, were present.

Donaldson and Kaplan[30] and Meadows et al.[31] showed that the risk of acute myelocytic leukemia was increased in the subgroup of children with Hodgkin's disease who received intensive chemotherapy for relapse after irradiation. The cumulative risk of leukemia was about 1.5% at 10 years and 4% at 20 years.

An elevated risk of acute nonlymphocytic leukemia and related myelodysplastic disorders has been described in patients treated with alkylating agents for ovarian cancer,[32,33] breast cancer,[34,35] small cell lung cancer,[36,37] polycythemia vera,[38] multiple myeloma,[39] nonHodgkin's lymphoma,[40,41] and non-neoplastic diseases (e.g., rheumatoid arthritis[42,43]), and in patients with gastrointestinal cancer after adjuvant treatment with methyl-CCNU.[44]

Characteristic clinical, morphologic, and cytogenetic features were observed in patients with treatment-induced leukemias. The treatment-related leukemias were acute nonlymphocytic and often preceded over a period of months by a refractory pancytopenia. Bone marrow examination demonstrated advanced dysmyelopoiesis in most patients who subsequently progressed to overt leukemia. Cytogenetic studies showed a predominance of hypodiploid cell lines, most commonly because of nonrandom deletion, rearrangement, or partial or total loss of chromosomes 5 and 7. Various morphologic forms of ANLL were not, however, consistently associated with specific chromosome abnormalities, nor was it clear whether the various aberrations were involved primarily in malignant transformation of cells. When acute leukemia developed, no evidence of residual Hodgkin's disease was present in over two-thirds of the patients.[45-48]

Ionizing radiation and alkylating agents are capable of damaging DNA and producing stable and unstable chromosome aberrations. Some of the alkylating agents have been characterized as radiomimetic because of the similarity of their cellular and molecular spectrum of activity to that of ionizing radiation. A large proportion of the patients receiving chemotherapy for Hodgkin's disease were exposed to combinations of 2, 3, and 4 or more drugs; consequently, quantitative estimates of the independent leukemogenic effects of individual drugs were not obtainable, although inferences were derived based on the regimen as a whole. Another feature obscuring assessment of leukemogenic or carcinogenic complications of exposure to antineoplastic agents was the latency period. Only patients who have survived at least one or two years were at risk of developing leukemia. The median duration of the latency period may vary in relation to the intensity or aggressiveness of therapy and host factors that may affect tissue susceptibility, immune surveillance, and pharmacokinetics.[49]

The chemotherapeutic activity and toxicity of the alkylating agents (e.g., nitrogen mustard, cyclophosphamide, chlorambucil, procarbazine, melphalan, and the nitrosoureas) are related to covalent binding of an electrophilic constituent of the compound to relatively negatively charged nucleophilic purine or pyrimidine residues of DNA. The alkylating agents have been characterized as cytotoxic, mutagenic, teratogenic, immunosuppressive, and clastogenic. Electrophilic reactivity is correlated with mutagenic and/or carcinogenic potency. Cyclophosphamide and procarbazine must undergo chemical or metabolic activation to alkylating and/or free radical intermediates before exhibiting cytotoxic or mutagenic properties. The important pharmacologic actions of the alkylating agents are mediated through perturbation of the fundamental mechanisms concerned with cell growth and differentiation. The capacity of these agents to alter normal mitosis and cellular function and survival provides the basis for therapeutic efficacy, cytotoxicity, and potential carcinogenicity.[50,51]

The biologic effects of radiation are influenced by the energy of the radiation, the volume irradiated, the total dose delivered, fractionation, and the dose rate or absorbed dose delivered per unit time. The mechanism by which ionizing radiation induces cancer is associated with the quantity of energy absorbed within cells and is proportional to the number of ionizations produced in the exposed tissue. This impact of photons of radiant energy gives rise to ions and reactive chemical radicals that may disrupt chemical bonds, damage DNA, and alter the number and structure of chromosomes. Practically all human tissues are susceptible to the tumorigenic effects of ionizing radiation. The most radiosensitive tissues are the female breast, thyroid, and hematopoietic tissues, although modifying factors, such as age and sex of the host, the metabolic state of the organ or tissue at the time of exposure, associated diseases, and the capacity for DNA repair, must be considered.[52,53]

In the radiation therapy of patients with Hodgkin's disease, relatively large fractions and cumulative tissue doses are administered over a short period of time. As suggested by an epidemiologic study of patients with cancer of the uterine cervix, ionizing energy delivered in this manner may have a lethal or sterilizing effect on bone marrow stem cells.[54] As described previously, the induction of leukemia in patients with Hodgkin's disease was largely restricted to patients receiving chemotherapy. The inference of statistical significance depends on the observed number of leukemia cases and the apparent size of the excess relative to the baseline or expected risk. Conceivably, an independent leukemogenic effect of radiotherapy may be overlooked because the population at risk is too

Table 1–5. Summary of Epidemiologic Studies of Acute Leukemias Secondary to Therapy in Hodgkin's Disease

Author(s)	Year of Publication	Total Number of Patients	Number and Type of Leukemia Cases	Crude Incidence per 1,000 Patients/Year
Coleman[15]	1982	1160 Stanford University	18—acute nonlymphocytic (ANLL)	Not reported
Coltman et al.[20]	1982	659 Southwest Oncology Group (SWOG)	21—12 Acute myelocytic, M1 and M2; 7 acute myelomonocytic; 1 erythroleukemia; 1 undifferentiated	Not reported
Glicksman et al.[21]	1982	798 Cancer & Leukemia Group B (CALGB) 1332 patients were evaluated, of whom 798 achieved complete remission	10—acute myelocytic	Not reported
Pedersen-Bjergaard et al.[22]	1982	391 Finsen Institute, Copenhagen	10—ANLL In addition, 7 cases of preleukemia or acute myeloproliferative syndrome	5.8/1,000. Relative risk = 167
Aisenberg[23]	1983	408 Massachusetts General Hospital	8—ANLL	Not reported

Table 1-5. Summary of Epidemiologic Studies of Acute Leukemias Secondary to Therapy in Hodgkin's Disease *(Continued)*

Cumulative Actuarial Risk in % (Interval of Follow-up)	Number of Leukemia Cases Radiotherapy Only (Total Number Treated)	Number of Leukemia Cases Chemotherapy Only (Total Number Treated)	Number of Leukemia Cases Radiotherapy & Chemotherapy (Total Number Treated)	Commentary
3.6% (9 years)	0 (448)	2 (40)	16 (672)	Median interval from diagnosis to leukemia was 4 years (range 1.3–8.8 years). Compared with radiation therapy only group, all other treatment groups had significantly greater risk of developing leukemia.
For patients starting treatment for HD under age 40, the risk was 2.7% at 7 years, compared with 20.7% (8.5–32.9%; 95% confidence limits) for patients first treated at 40 years of age and older	0 (95)	3 (102)	18 (462)	For chemotherapy only patients (102), the 7-year actuarial risk was 6.2%; for patients treated initially with combined modalities, the 7-year actuarial risk was 6.4%.
With mean follow-up of 3.8 years, overall risk was 5.6%. At ages <40: 2.9% (4 years), 40–59: 11.8% (3.5 years), 60+ : 6.4% (3.2 years)	0 (0)	6 (369)	4 (429)	Induction chemotherapy with mechlorethamine-containing regimen, followed by chlorambucil maintenance was associated with actuarial risk of 26.2%. Addition of radiotherapy to various protocols of combination induction chemotherapy, with or without maintenance chemotherapy, did not increase significantly the relative risk evidenced by chemotherapy alone.
At ages <40; 8.6% (9 years), 40+ : 39.5% (9 years)	0 (79)	4 (75)	6 (237)	The cumulative risk of ANLL, preleukemia, and acute myeloproliferative syndrome was estimated at 3.9% at 5 years and 9.9% at 9 years. Secondary ANLL accounted for 8% of all deaths. No difference in incidence of ANLL was observed between patients treated exclusively with chemotherapy and patients treated with combined modality therapy. Risk of leukemia enhanced with reinduction combination chemotherapy, or maintenance chemotherapy with alkylating agent.
4.9% (12 years)	0 (188)	1 (6)	7 (214)	In MOPP-treated patients, with or without radiation therapy, the cumulative actuarial risk was: 0% (3 years); 2.5% (6 years); 4.2% (9 years); 9.1% (12 years). Significantly increased risk of leukemia noted in patients over age 40 years treated with MOPP, when compared with younger patients. While no leukemias were observed in 78 patients whose treatment was limited to 6 cycles of MOPP plus extended field irradiation, the subgroup at highest risk included patients who relapsed after the conventional 6 cycles of MOPP.

Table 1–5. Summary of Epidemiologic Studies of Acute Leukemias Secondary to Therapy in Hodgkin's Disease *(Continued)*

Author(s)	Year of Publication	Total Number of Patients	Number and Type of Leukemia Cases	Crude Incidence per 1,000 Patients/Year
Henry-Amar[24]	1983	334 Clinical stages I and II European Organization for Research and Treatment of Cancer	4—3 ANLL and 1 chronic myelomonocytic	Not reported
Boivin et al.[25]	1984	2591 Boston, Montreal, and New York City hospitals	21—Except for one acute lymphocytic and one acute stem cell, remainder ANLL	1.8/1,000
Hutchison et al.[26]	1984	460 Clinical stages I and II. 22 collaborating clinical centers in the United States and Canada; patients were randomly assigned to involved field or extended field radiotherapy	6 (type not specified)	1.7/1,000 (based on the 460 patients)
Tester et al.[27]	1984	473 National Cancer Institute (USA) Excludes patients treated prior to 1964, or who received any therapy before referral	9—8 ANLL and one CML (Philadelphia chromosome positive). In addition, there were 5 cases of "preleukemia" or with refractory cytopenias	Not reported
Blayney et al.[28]	1987	192 Cohort treated between 1964 and 1975 at National Cancer Institute	5 ANLL, 1 CML, 1 erythroleukemia, 5 myelodysplastic syndrome	Not reported

Table 1–5. Summary of Epidemiologic Studies of Acute Leukemias Secondary to Therapy in Hodgkin's Disease *(Continued)*

Cumulative Actuarial Risk in % (Interval of Follow-up)	Number of Leukemia Cases Radiotherapy Only (Total Number Treated)	Number of Leukemia Cases Chemotherapy Only (Total Number Treated)	Number of Leukemia Cases Radiotherapy & Chemotherapy (Total Number Treated)	Commentary
0% (5 years), 0.8% (10 years), 2.8% (15 years)	1 (280) An unspecified proportion received vinblastine alone in conjunction with radiotherapy. The one leukemia, chronic myelomonocytic, was in patient who received only mantle field irradiation	0 (0)	3 (54) Combination chemotherapy and extended field irradiation. Observed to expected ratio was 300 (62-877; 95% confidence limits). The leukemias were diagnosed 5, 6, and 10 years after MOPP therapy for relapse	Highest risk group consisted of patients who relapsed and then received combination chemotherapy: 0% (5 years), 2.7% (10 years), 13.7% (15 years). Using the Cox regression model, significant relative risks for variables over age 40 years, and combination chemotherapy.
Not reported	2 (5736 person-years) Extended field radiotherapy, but without combination chemotherapy; may have received single agent chemotherapy	0 (737 person-years)	19 (4973 person-years) Combination chemotherapy with extended field irradiation, either as initial or subsequent treatment, was associated with 13 leukemias, or a relative risk of 163	20 patients with secondary leukemias received chemotherapy, 19 classified as intensive, cyclical combination. Relative risk of leukemia after intensive chemotherapy with or without radiotherapy, was 136. For patients treated with radiotherapy, but without intensive chemotherapy, relative risk was 3, which was not significantly elevated. The relative risk of leukemia for intensive chemotherapy, relative to non-intensive chemotherapy, was 30
Not Reported	0 (293)	0 (0)	6 (167) Chemotherapy administered for recurrent disease after initial radiotherapy	Average annual leukemia incidence following chemotherapy was 8.1 per 1,000 per year, or more than 200 times the expected incidence in the general population.
3.6% (10 years)	0 (146)	1 (144)	8 (183) 4 of 5 cases of "pre-leukemia"	Median latency from initial treatment was 67 months, with range of 36–139 months. The cumulative actuarial risk at 10 years by method of treatment was: chemotherapy only: 2%; initial combined modality therapy: 6%; salvage combined modality therapy: 9%.
3.0% (5 years), 10.0% (10 years); cumulative risk for all leukemias and related complications (i.e., ANLL, myelodysplastic syndrome, refractory pancytopenia)	0 (?)	1 (63)	11 (52) (within 2 to 12 years after first treatment)	Use of combined radiation and MOPP chemotherapy was associated with greater risk of leukemia than radiation or chemotherapy alone. Patients beginning treatment after age 40 were at higher risk for acute leukemia after combined treatment with radiation and chemotherapy than younger patients in same stage of disease.

limited to exclude such a possibility. For example, in a collaborative study evaluating patients with stages I and II Hodgkin's disease,[26] the incidence of leukemia (8.1 per 1000 person-years) following combined modality therapy in 167 patients (739 person-years) was increased more than 200-fold over general population rates. No cases of leukemia were observed in the 293 patients (2837 person-years) who were treated only with radiotherapy. The upper 95% confidence limit for the observed number, however, did not exclude the possibility of an increase of about 25-fold. Little is known about the influence of various chemical agents on radiation-induced leukemia in man; however, the epidemiologic studies of Hodgkin's disease patients who received combined modality treatment were not always consistent with a synergistic relationship.

NONHODGKIN'S LYMPHOMA

The nonHodgkin's lymphomas are histopathologically distinct from Hodgkin's disease, and they are comprised of a heterogeneous group of malignant neoplasms that arise from lymphoid components of the immune system. At least 30 patients have been reported with lymphoproliferative neoplasms following treatment for Hodgkin's disease. Cell surface marker studies in these patients have identified lymphoid malignant neoplasms of either B-cell or T-cell origin. The histopathologic features of the secondary lymphoid neoplasms were not of a single type, although most commonly were described as diffuse large cell or poorly differentiated lymphomas.[55–59]

Coleman et al.[19] reported that the overall actuarial risk at 10 years was estimated to be 0.5%. The majority of secondary lymphoid neoplasms were observed in the patients who either received chemotherapy or combined modality treatment. In an analysis of pooled data from 10 published studies based on a total of 36,942 person-years, there were 14 observed cases of nonHodgkin's lymphoma.[60] The expected number, 1.8, was determined from the general population cancer incidence data of the Third National Cancer Survey. The observed-to-expected ratio was 7.8 ($p < 0.05$).

Currently, there has not been a sufficient number of patients with nonHodgkin's lymphoma following the diagnosis and treatment of Hodgkin's disease to enable a reliable assessment of risk in relation to modality of treatment and interval of follow-up.

NONHEMATOPOIETIC SOLID TUMORS

No clear pattern of risk of sarcomas and carcinomas after treatment in Hodgkin's disease patients has appeared in published cohort studies. An important limitation has been the concentration of person-years during the initial 10-year period of follow-up. Follow-up over longer intervals is necessary before reliable estimates of risk for various solid tumors can be derived. While individual case reports of relatively rare sarcomas occurring within or adjacent to heavily irradiated areas may be assumed to be the result of previous treatment exposure, the judgment of probable cause should be guided by observations in a population of patients and considerations of type and amount of exposure and latency.[61,62] For example, bone sarcomas have appeared in excess within five years after irradiation, and the distribution of the time-to-response pattern was similar to that of leukemia; for the malignant epithelial tumors, the minimal latency period has been about 10 years, and the occurrence of excess cancers has tended to follow the normal age-specific incidence patterns. Thus, in irradiated populations, an excess risk of breast or lung cancer may not be apparent until exposed individuals have reached ages at which these cancers usually occur, which suggests the net effect of a multistage process requiring other time-dependent etiologic factors.[63,64]

In a study by Boivin et al.,[25] the relative risk of all cancers, other than leukemia, was not significantly increased during the first decade after treatment; their data was based on 10,195 person-years of observation. They observed, however, a significantly increased relative risk (about twentyfold) for the occurrence of solid tumors in the small subgroup of patients who were followed beyond 10 years after receiving intensive radiotherapy; these patients had not received prior intensive, combination chemotherapy. This relative risk was based on only five observed second primary cancers. Because intensive chemotherapy was significantly associated with the risk of leukemia, it is conceivable that chemotherapy, with or without radiotherapy, may exhibit more general carcinogenic effects after a sufficient period of follow-up.[65]

REFERENCES

1. DeVita, V.T. Jr., Hubbard, S.M., and Moxley, J.H. The cure of Hodgkin's disease with drugs. Adv. Int. Med. 28:277–302, 1983.
2. Schottenfeld, D. Multiple primary cancers. In Cancer Epidemiology and Prevention. Edited by D. Schottenfeld and J.F. Fraumeni, Jr. Philadelphia, WB Saunders, 1982, pp 1025–1035.
3. Sheps, M. On the person years concept in epidemiology and demography. Millbank Mem. Fund Q. 44:69–91, 1966.
4. Mantel, N. and Byar, D.P. Evaluation of response-time data involving transient states: An illustration using heart transplant data. J. Am. Stat Assoc. 69:81–86, 1974.
5. Kaplan, E.L. and Meier, P. Nonparametric estimation from incomplete observations. J. Am. Stat. Assoc. 53:457–481, 1958.
6. Mantel, N. Evaluation of survival data and two rank order statistics arising in its consideration. Cancer Chemother. Rep. 50:163–170, 1966.
7. Peto, R. and Pike, M.C. Conservation of the approximation $\Sigma(O-E)^2/E$ in the Logrank test for survival data or tumor incidence data. Biometrics. 29:579–584, 1973.
8. Matthews, D.E. and Farewell, V. Using and Understanding Medical Statistics. Basel, S. Karger, 1988.
9. Cox, D.R. Regression models and life-tables. J. R. Stat. Soc., Series B, 34:187–220, 1972.
10. Brody, R.S. and Schottenfeld, D. Multiple primary cancers in Hodgkin's disease. Sem. Oncology. 7:187–201, 1980.
11. Schlesselman, J.J. Case-control studies. Design, Conduct, Analysis. New York, Oxford, 1982.
12. Arseneau, J.C., Sponzo, R.W., Levin, D.L. et al. Non-lymphomatous malignant tumors complicating Hodgkin's disease—possible association with intensive therapy. N. Eng. J. Med. 287:1119–1122, 1972.
13. Arseneau, J.C., Canellos, G.P., Johnson, R. et al. Risk of new cancers in patients with Hodgkin's disease. Cancer. 40:1912–1916, 1977.
14. Canellos, G.P., DeVita, V.T., Arseneau, J.C. et al. Second malignancies complicating Hodgkin's disease in remission. Lancet 1:947–949, 1975.
15. Coleman, C.N. Secondary neoplasms in patients treated for cancer: Etiology and perspective. Radiat. Res. 92:188–200, 1982.
16. Schottenfeld, D., Cahan, W.G. and Moertel, C.G. Proceedings of the International workshop on Multiple Primary Cancers. Cancer (Supplement). 40:(4), 1977.
17. Berg, J.W. The incidence of multiple primary cancers. I. Development of further cancers in patients with lymphomas, leukemias, and myeloma. J.N.C.I. 38:741–752, 1967.
18. Rosner, F. and Grunwald, H.W. Multiple hemolymphatic cancers. In Risk Factors and Multiple Cancer. Edited by B.A. Stoll, New York, John Wiley & Sons, 1984.
19. Coleman, C.N. Secondary malignancy after treatment of Hodgkin's disease: An evolving picture. J. Clin. Oncol. 4:821–824, 1986.
20. Coltman, C.A. and Dixon, D.O. Second malignancies complicating Hodgkin's disease: A Southwest Oncology Group 10-year followup. Cancer Treat. Rep. 66:1023–1033, 1982.
21. Glicksman, A.S. et al. Second malignant neoplasms in patients successfully treated for Hodgkin's disease: A Cancer and Leukemia Group B study. Cancer Treat Rep. 66(4):1035–1044, 1982.
22. Pedersen-Bjergaard, J. and Larsen, S.O. Incidence of acute nonlymphocytic leukemia, preleukemia, and acute myeloproliferative syndrome up to 10 years after treatment of Hodgkin's disease. N. Engl. J. Med. 307:965–971, 1982.
23. Aisenberg, A.C. Acute nonlymphocytic leukemia after treatment for Hodgkin's disease. Am. J. Med. 75:449–454, 1983.
24. Henry-Amar, M. Second cancers after radiotherapy and chemotherapy for early stages of Hodgkin's dsease. J.N.C.I. 71(5):911–916, 1983.
25. Boivin, J.-F., Hutchison, G.B., Lyden, M. et al. Second primary cancers following treatment of Hodgkin's disease. J.N.C.I. 72(2):233–241, 1984.
26. Hutchison, G.B. et al. Radiotherapy of Stage I and II Hodgkin's disease. Cancer. 54:1928–1942, 1984.
27. Tester, W.J., Kinsella, T.J., Waller, B. et al. Second malignant neoplasms complicating Hodgkin's disease: The National Cancer Institute experience. J. Clin. Oncol. 2(7):762–769, 1984.
28. Blayney, D.W., Longo, D.L., Young, R.C. et al. Decreasing risk of leukemia with prolonged follow-up after chemotherapy and radiotherapy for Hodgkin's disease. N. Engl. J. Med. 316:710–714, 1987.
29. Miké, B., Meadows, A.T. and D'Angio, G.J. Incidence of second malignant neoplasms in children: results of an international study. Lancet 2:1328–1331, 1982.
30. Donaldson, S.S. and Kaplan, H.S. Complications of treatment of Hodgkin's disease in children. Cancer Treat. Rep. 66:977, 1982.
31. Meadows, A.T., Baum, E., Fossati-Bellani, F. et al. Second malignant neoplasms in children: An update from the Late Effects Study Group. J. Clin. Oncol. 3:532–538, 1985.
32. Reimer, R.R., Hoover, R., Fraumeni, J.F. Jr. et al. Acute leukemia after alkylating-agent therapy of ovarian cancer. N. Engl. J. Med. 297:177–181, 1977.
33. Kapadia, S.B. and Kruse, J.R. Ovarian carcinoma terminating in acute nonlymphocytic leukemia follow-

ing alkylating agent therapy. Cancer. 41:1676–1679, 1978.
34. Rosner, F., Carey, R.W. and Zarrabi M.H. Breast cancer and acute leukemia: Report of 24 cases and review of the literature. Am. J. Hematol. 4:151–168, 1978.
35. Ershler, W.B. et al. Emergence of acute nonlymphocytic leukemia in breast cancer patients. Am. J. Med. Sci. 284:284, 1982.
36. May, H.T., Hsu, S.D. and Costanzi, J.J. Acute leukemia following combination chemotherapy for cancer of the lung. Oncology. 38:134–137, 1981.
37. Shimp, W. and Belzer, M.G. Acute leukemia after treatment of small cell carcinoma of the lung. N. Engl. J. Med. 304:845–846, 1981.
38. Berk, P.D. et al. Increased incidence of acute leukemia in polycythemia vera associated with chlorambucil therapy. N. Engl. J. Med. 304:441–447, 1981.
39. Rosner, F. and Grunwald, H. Multiple myeloma terminating in acute leukemia: Report of 12 cases and review of the literature. Am. J. Med. 57:927–939, 1974.
40. Zarrabi, M.H., Rosner, F. and Bennett, J.M. Non-Hodgkin's lymphoma and acute myeloblastic leukemia—a report of 12 cases and a review of the literature. Cancer. 44:1070–1080, 1979.
41. Greene, M.H., Young, R.C., Merrill, J.M. et al. Evidence of a treatment dose response in acute nonlymphocytic leukemias which occur after therapy of non-Hodgkin's lymphoma. Cancer Res. 43:1891–1898, 1983.
42. Love, R.R. and Sowa, J.M. Myelomonocytic leukemia following cyclophosphamide therapy of rheumatoid disease. Ann. Rheum. Dis. 34:534–535, 1975.
43. Hazleman, B. Incidence of neoplasms in patients with rheumatoid arthritis exposed to different treatment regimens. Am. J. Med. (Supplement 1A), 78:39–43, 1985.
44. Boice, J.D. et al. Leukemia and preleukemia after adjuvant treatment of gastrointestinal cancer with semustine (methyl-CCNU). N. Engl. J. Med. 309:1079–1084, 1983.
45. Yahalom, J. et al. Secondary leukemia following treatment of Hodgkin's disease: Ultrastructural and cytogenetic data in two cases with a review of the literature. Am. J. Clin. Pathol. 80:231–236, 1983.
46. Whang-Peng, J. and Sieber, S.M. Chromosomal damage by radiation and antitumor agents. In Risk Factors and Multiple Cancer. Edited by B.A. Stoll. New York, John Wiley & Sons, 1984.
47. Knapp, R.H., Dewald, G.W. and Pierre, R.V. Cytogenetic studies in 174 consecutive patients with preleukemic or myelodysplastic syndromes. Mayo Clin. Proc. 60:507–516, 1985.
48. Michels, V.V. and Hoagland, H.C. Chromosome abnormalities in preleukemic or myelodysplastic syndromes (Editorial). Mayo Clin. Proc. 60:555–556, 1985.
49. Borum, K. Increasing frequency of acute myeloid leukemia complicating Hodgkin's disease: A review. Cancer. 46:1247–1252, 1980.
50. Sieber, S.M. and Adamson, R.H. Toxicity of antineoplastic agents in man: chromosomal aberrations, antifertility effects, congenital malformations, and carcinogenic potential. Adv. Cancer Res. 22:57–155, 1975.
51. Weisburger. E.K. Bioassay program for carcinogenic hazards of cancer chemotherapeutic agents. Cancer (Supplement). 40:1935–1949, 1977.
52. Kohn, H.I. and Fry, R.J.M. Radiation carcinogenesis. N. Engl. J. Med. 310:504–511, 1984.
53. Mossman, K.L. Ionizing radiation and cancer. Cancer Invest. 2:301–310, 1984.
54. Boice, J.D. and Hutchison, G.B. Leukemia in women following radiotherapy for cervical cancer. Ten-year follow-up of an international study. J.N.C.I. 65:115–129, 1980.
55. Krikorian, J.G., Burke, J.S., Rosenberg, S.A. et al. Occurrence of non-Hodgkin's lymphoma after therapy for Hodgkin's disease. N. Engl. J. Med. 300:452–458, 1979.
56. Armitage, J.O., Dick, F.R., Goehen, J.A. et al. Second lymphoid malignant neoplasms occurring in patients treated for Hodgkin's disease. Arch. Intern. Med. 143:445–450, 1983.
57. Jacquillat, C., Khayat, D., Desprez-Curley, J.P. et al. Non-Hodgkin's lymphoma occurring after Hodgkin's disease. Four new cases and a review of the literature. Cancer. 53:459–462, 1984.
58. Caya, J.G. et al. Hodgkin's disease followed by mycosis fungoides in the same patient. Case report and literature review. Cancer. 53:463–467, 1984.
59. Gowitt, G.T. et al. T-cell lymphoma following Hodgkin's disease. Cancer. 56:1191–1196, 1985.
60. Boivin, J.F. Jr. Personal communication.
61. Halperin, E.C., Greenberg, M.S. and Suit, H.D. Sarcoma of bone and soft tissue following treatment of Hodgkin's disease. Cancer. 53:232–236, 1984.
62. Kim, J.H., Chu, E.C.H., Woodward, H.O. et al. Radiation induced sarcomas of bone following therapeutic radiation. J. Radiat. Oncol. Biol. Physiol. 9:107–110, 1983.
63. Schottenfeld, D. Radiation as a risk factor in the natural history of colorectal cancer. Gastroenterology (Editorial). 84:186–190, 1983.
64. Boice, J.D. and Land, C.E. Ionizing radiation. In Cancer Epidemiology and Prevention. Edited by D. Schottenfeld and J.F. Fraumeni, Jr. Philadelphia, WB Saunders, 1982, pp 231–253.
65. Curtis, R.E., Hankey, B.F., Myers, M.H. et al. Risk of leukemia associated with the first course of cancer treatment: An analysis of the Surveillance, Epidemiology, and End Results Program experience. J.N.C.I. 72:531–544, 1984.

CHAPTER 2

Late Effects of Radiation Therapy in the Treatment of Hodgkin's Disease

JAY S. LOEFFLER
PETER MAUCH
SAMUEL HELLMAN

In 1902, only a few years after the discovery of roentgenograms, Pusey[1] described what is considered the first attempt to treat Hodgkin's disease with radiation. It became obvious from this and from other early reports that Hodgkin's disease responded to lower doses of radiation than were found effective with other tumors. During the last 80 years, radiation therapy techniques have undergone significant changes. Technology resulting in the availability of higher energy treatment machines, the ability to perform accurate measurements of dose distribution in both tumors and normal tissue, and improved physical techniques for precise beam alignment have permitted safe and effective treatment of many disorders. Accompanying these technological changes has come a better understanding of the natural history of Hodgkin's disease.[2-4] The availability of high energy machines has enabled us to use large fields, which include the sites of disease as well as adjacent sites, and to use high doses with minimal toxicity to achieve permanent tumor control.

Radiation plays a significant role in the curative management of Hodgkin's disease. In early stage disease (stage IA,IIA,IB,IIB) radiation is often the only form of treatment employed. In patients with more advanced disease, radiation therapy may be integrated with systemic chemotherapy in a combined modality approach. Whereas patients with Hodgkin's disease faced a poor prognosis in the 1960s, nearly all patients with early and intermediate stage disease can be cured. This success has followed the development of new concepts in the natural history and staging of Hodgkin's disease and advances in treatment techniques.[5]

A major future goal in the treatment of Hodgkin's disease will be to maintain or improve the cure rate while minimizing or decreasing the potential risks for complications. The concept of a "complication-free cure rate" has become increasingly important. The basis for achieving this goal is to better understand the long-term tolerance of normal tissues to radiation therapy and chemotherapy. In some situations, the combined use of radiation therapy and chemotherapy may allow less intensive treatment of each individual modality, theoretically improving the patient's chance of having a relapse-free survival and a lower complication risk. The risks of complications with radiation therapy alone depend on such factors as the nature of the irradiated tissue, the volume of normal tissue irradiated, and the various time-dose features comprised in the treatment program. The radiotherapist must be aware of the tolerance of normal tissues when designing the large radiation fields that are used in Hodgkin's disease. In certain specific clinical situations (i.e., patients with large mediastinal masses) optimal radiation therapy is often limited by the estimated risk of significant radiation damage of normal tissues.

Risk-benefit considerations underly all patient management decisions and pose a complex theoretical and practical problem. Theoretical curves can be drawn describing the probability of tumor control and the risk of developing major complications as plotted as a function of the dose of radiation (Fig. 2–1). Both curves follow a sigmoid distribution with the separation between them representing the therapeutic gain.[6–8] The clinician's goal is to treat with doses that allow the highest probability for survival with the lowest risk for complications. In figure 2–1, two theoretical treatment programs (A and B) are illustrated. The difference between treatment programs A and B is an improvement with tumor control with program B, but with a substantially higher risk of complications. The simple graphics, however, do not fully describe the therapeutic problem. The physician must consider, in addition to the risk of major complications, the probability of effectively treating the complications. For example, if a recurrence after radiation therapy cannot be salvaged by retreatment (chemotherapy or surgery), the dose that will maximize tumor control must be used and the higher complication rate accepted. Conversely, in Hodgkin's disease with excellent salvage therapy (chemotherapy), one accepts a diminished probability of tumor control while minimizing the risk of complications that might be untreatable and life threatening.

Radiation toxicity is manifested by both early and late effects; however, late effects represent the dose-limiting factor for radiation therapy. Acute effects occur during treatment and continue weeks to a few months following radiation. These acute effects are caused by toxicity to the cell renewal tissues, such as skin, small intestine, rectum, bladder mucosa, and oropharyngeal mucosa. These cell renewal tissues are rapidly proliferating. As they are confronted with fractionated radiation, the process of repair, repopulation, and recruitment begins. Generally, the acute effects of radiation on normal tissue are both transient and reversible. Although occasionally severe enough to warrant a treatment break, acute effects should not be used as a criteria for terminating treatment. A 10% reduction in daily dose from 200 to 180 cGy a day is often all that is needed for patients to continue treatment. Such a reduction often eliminates excessive mucosal reaction and unacceptable gastrointestinal symptoms. An excellent example of reversible acute effects is illustrated by the esophagitis that accompanies mantle-field treatment. This syndrome usually begins during the third or fourth week of treatment and is completely resolved 1 to 2 weeks following treatment.

Late effects occur from several months to several years after the completion of radiation treatment. The exact underlying mechanism

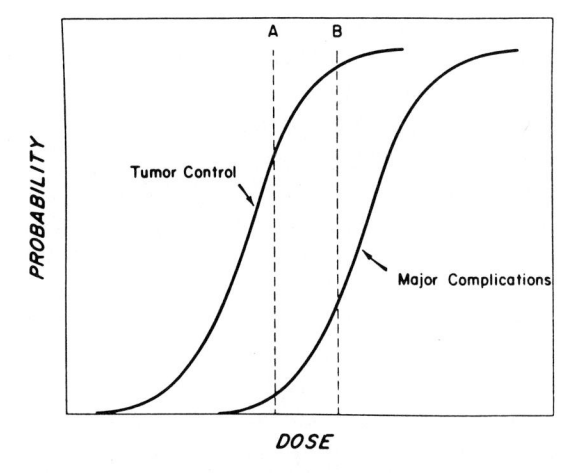

Fig. 2–1. Theoretical sigmoid curves describing the probabilities of achieving tumor control and the development of major complications as a function of the radiation dose delivered. A and B represent two separate treatment programs.

of late injury to normal tissue by radiation is not completely understood. Two major hypotheses for the pathogenesis of late effects are often discussed. One major theory holds that late effects are the result of damage caused by vasculoconnective tissue stroma. Since vasculoconnective stroma is ubiquitous, this theory would explain the mechanism for late effects anywhere in the body.[9] A variation on this hypothesis is that endothelial cell damage determines and predicts late effects.[10] The second major hypothesis suggests that the late effects of radiation are caused by cell depletion of major target cell renewal systems. This hypothesis depends on the belief that certain stem cells have only a limited proliferative capacity.[11] Compensation for extensive or repeated cell killing may exhaust this capacity, resulting in eventual tissue failure. It is important to note that acute effects of radiation do not necessarily predict late effects.

Hodgkin's disease is particularly suitable for the study of late effects of radiation therapy for many reasons: (1) the long-term observation of the disease, with improved diagnostic techniques, has created a clear picture of its clinical and histologic characteristics and has made standardization of treatment possible, which is an important prerequisite for comparative investigation. (2) The development of extended-field or total nodal irradiation as the primary treatment for early-stage Hodgkin's disease has allowed information to accumulate regarding the long-term risks of large-field irradiation. (3) Long-term survival is a prerequisite for studying the long-term consequences of irradiation.

PHYSICAL AND TECHNICAL CONSIDERATIONS

A basic understanding of the physical and technical aspects of radiation therapy in Hodgkin's disease is essential in determining potential late-radiation damage to normal tissue. The parameters that have to be considered in understanding late-radiation effects include, the total dose, the dose rate, and the fractionation schedule used. Technical considerations include the energy of the radiation beam, the distance between the radiation source and the patient, the distribution, shape, and alignment of the radiation beam, and the volume of normal tissue or organ included within the treatment field.

The radiation doses and field sizes recommended for treating Hodgkin's disease were established when clinical data demonstrated that doses high enough to be maximally effective against Hodgkin's disease were also low enough to cause little or no lasting radiation damage to normal tissues. In general, patients with early stage (I to IIIA) Hodgkin's disease are treated by radiation alone, with 3600 to 4400 cGy over a 4 to 5 week period. The evidence for this tumor dose is determined by calculations of the recurrence rate in previously treated lymph node areas at different doses.[12] In a retrospective review of the world literature and data from Stanford University Medical Center, Kaplan demonstrated a true recurrence rate as a function of radiation therapy.[13] Composite data (Fig. 2–2) indicate that the recurrence rate is inversely related to dose, falling from a level of 60 to 80% with dose of 1000 cGy or less, to a rate of only 4.4% with a dose range from 3500 to 4400 cGy.

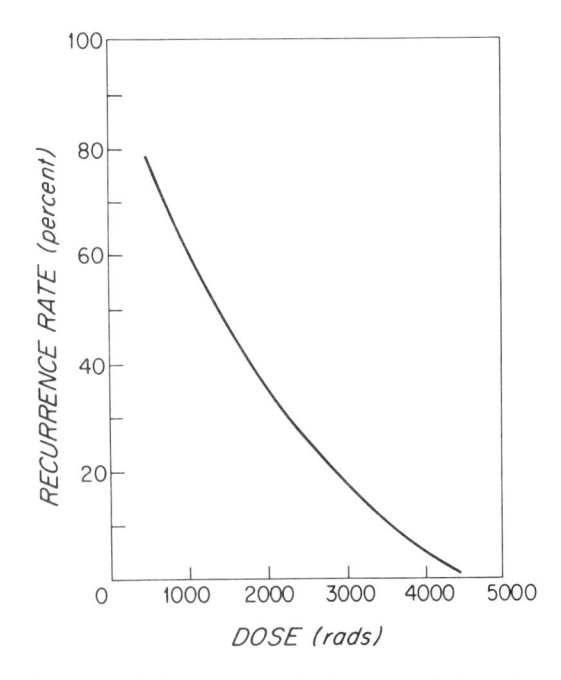

Fig. 2–2. Influence of radiation dose delivered on the recurrence rate in Hodgkin's disease.

At the dose level of 4400 cGy delivered in 4 to 4½ weeks, a true recurrence of only 1.3% was found.

The dose of radiation needed to control massive lymphadenopathy is greater than in the prophylactic treatment of apparently uninvolved nodes. Carmel and Kaplan[14] analyzed data on intrathoracic recurrence and relapse rates as a function of mediastinal tumor size. They found an overall recurrence rate in patients with massive mediastinal adenopathy of 24%, whereas the rate was only 7% in patients with minimal mediastinal involvement. These findings have been confirmed by similar reviews from the Joint Center for Radiation Therapy (JCRT)[15] and the University of Florida.[16] For this reason, many centers have adopted a policy of "boosting" the dose to the mediastinum for bulky or massive mediastinal adenopathy to a total dose of approximately 4400 cGy. The same augmented dose is used for other sites of massive lymphadenopathy, such as in the axillary or cervical regions. When boosting regions away from the central axis, however, care must be taken not to overdose. This often requires sophisticated treatment planning and dose-verification devices.

Combined modality treatment may allow lower doses of radiation to be used to control Hodgkin's disease. Excellent results have been obtained when radiation doses were reduced to levels as low as 1500 to 2500 cGy when supplemented with adjuvant combination chemotherapy in pediatric patients and patients with stage III and IV disease.[17,18] Further trials, however, are needed before these doses can be recommended on a routine basis for all patients.

The concept of fractionation of radiation doses has been fundamental in allowing radiotherapists to reduce complications of normal tissue while still achieving tumor control. For a given level of acute reaction, the late reactions are more severe when large fractionated doses of radiation are used. Thus, while acute reactions may be less when the dose is given in a few large fractions, late-radiation effects on normal tissue are worse. The influence of time and dose fractionation on the control of Hodgkin's disease has been examined by many investigators.[19-21] These various studies have used similar methods, which involve plotting the observed local control of Hodgkin's disease relative to a specific total dose given over a specific time interval. The results from these studies indicate an equal (essentially 100%) probability of local control of Hodgkin's disease with doses of 2500 cGy given in 10 days, 2900 to 3000 cGy in 30 days, or 4000 cGy in 40 days. The various dose fractionation schemes used in the treatment of Hodgkin's disease have also been evaluated for their influence on acute and long-term normal tissue tolerance. In a study of patients with stage I and II disease, Le-Bourgeois and associates found that complications rates were much higher from a dose of 4000 cGy, which was given in total fractions of 330 cGy each, three times a week for 4 weeks, as compared to giving the same total dose of 4000 cGy given at 200-cGy fractions five times a week for 4 weeks.[22] In general, most centers currently recommend that patients with Hodgkin's disease treated by radiation alone receive 3600 to 4400 cGy over a 4 to 5 week period. This dose-fractionation schedule provides excellent local control while minimizing normal tissue radiation effects.

The present treatment of Hodgkin's disease involves the use of megavoltage (4 to 8 MEV) energy x rays generated by linear accelerators. In contrast to orthovoltage x rays (usually 250 KV), megavoltage x rays have "skin sparing" qualities; the maximum dose is delivered at least 0.4 cm into the subcutaneous tissue. This "skin sparing" property of megavoltage therapy is essential since tumoricidal doses of radiation can be delivered to the lymph node chains, particularly those in the mediastinum and para-aortic regions, without seeing the accompanying severe cutaneous reactions (i.e., moist exudative erythema) and late subcutaneous reactions such as fibrosis, cutaneous atrophy, and telangiectasia—which were seen following irradiation by orthovoltage equipment. Acute and long-term cutaneous reactions associated with orthovoltage therapy were often the limiting factor in delivering the desired dose in Hodgkin's disease. In addition to depth-dose considerations, another advantage of megavoltage therapy is the sharp edges that are characteristic of its well collimated beams. This allows the dose to be delivered to the lymph nodes while minimizing lateral scatter to vital structures (kidney, lung, heart). This precision of the beam edge is in contrast to the large penumbra found with cobalt irradiation. This penumbra may add somewhat to the hazard of treating lymph nodes adjacent to vital structures. In contrast, the use of higher energy machines beyond 8 MEV may allow too much skin sparing and can underdose superficial nodes while adding little to sharp beam edges.

The initial localization and planning procedures used in the treatment of Hodgkin's disease with radiation should be carried out on a simulator in which a diagnostic x-ray tube occupies a position similar to that of the target of the linear accelerator. The simulators geometric and mechanical motions are designed to reproduce those of the corresponding treatment machine. If the facility lacks a simulator, I believe patients with Hodgkin's are best served by referring them to an institution that has such beneficial machinery. The dosimetric calculations, beam alignment procedures, patient positioning, and all subsequent treatment planning are done on the simulator. The radiotherapist uses the films derived from the simulation to outline necessary shielding needed to protect vital normal structures (Fig. 2-3). Once treatment starts, a new set of radiographs is made using the linear accelerator x-ray beam (port film) (Fig. 2-4). These port films are taken with shielding blocks in place and allow any fine adjustments to be made before treatment begins. The port film should be taken during each week of therapy and for every field used. The frequent use of port verification films is useful in detecting errors in shielding block placements; thus insuring that tumoricidal doses are being delivered to desired sites, while minimizing the dose to normal tissue.

As discussed earlier in this chapter, the philosophy of radiation therapy in the treatment of Hodgkin's disease involves treating multiple lymph node areas in continuity with as few fields as possible. Few fields are desirable because the symmetry in the vicinity of junctions between fields is complex, often resulting in errors of dose calculations. If the junction is too large, an inadequate dose is delivered to each structure in the plane of the junction. Theoretically, this could result in a correspondingly increased likelihood of recurrence in these undertreated regions. On the other hand, if errors are made at the junction resulting in overlapping a dose from adjacent fields, "hot spots" are created. These hot spots could potentially produce serious radiation damage to normal structures located in the plane of the junction. In order to encompass all the major lymph node chains above the diaphragm in a "mantle field," actual source to skin distances as great as 100 to 130 cm are necessary. The lymph nodes below the diaphragm may be treated with one field. This subdiaphragmatic field is either a para-aortic-splenic pedicle field or an extensive field that includes pelvic nodes in an "inverted Y" field. Thus, only one junction is required to treat nodes on both sides of the diaphragm. If the pelvic nodes are to be treated, however, usually two separate fields with a match at the bottom of L4 are preferable because of potential increased bowel and marrow toxicity seen with the single field. The inferior border of the mantle field should be at the bottom of T8 or T9 unless there is subcarinal, paricardial, or pericardial involvement in which the field must be extended lower. A T8–T9 inferior border allows the spleen or splenic pedicle to be included in the para-aortic field. Some have treated the mantle and upper para-aortic nodes (to the bottom of L2) in a single extended mantle field so as to avoid matching fields in early stage Hodgkin's disease patients.

The importance of precise matching of the mantle and para-aortic fields cannot be overemphasized. It is perhaps the most important technical aspect of radiotherapeutic management of patients with Hodgkin's disease. If excessive doses are given to the spinal cord because of an overlap between mantle and para-aortic fields, tragic neurologic consequences can result. Sophisticated treatment planning is needed to deliver an adequate dose of radiation to lymph nodes while preventing a high dose to the spinal cord. When planning the para-aortic field, a calculated skin gap based on the source to skin distance allows for divergence of the radiation beam

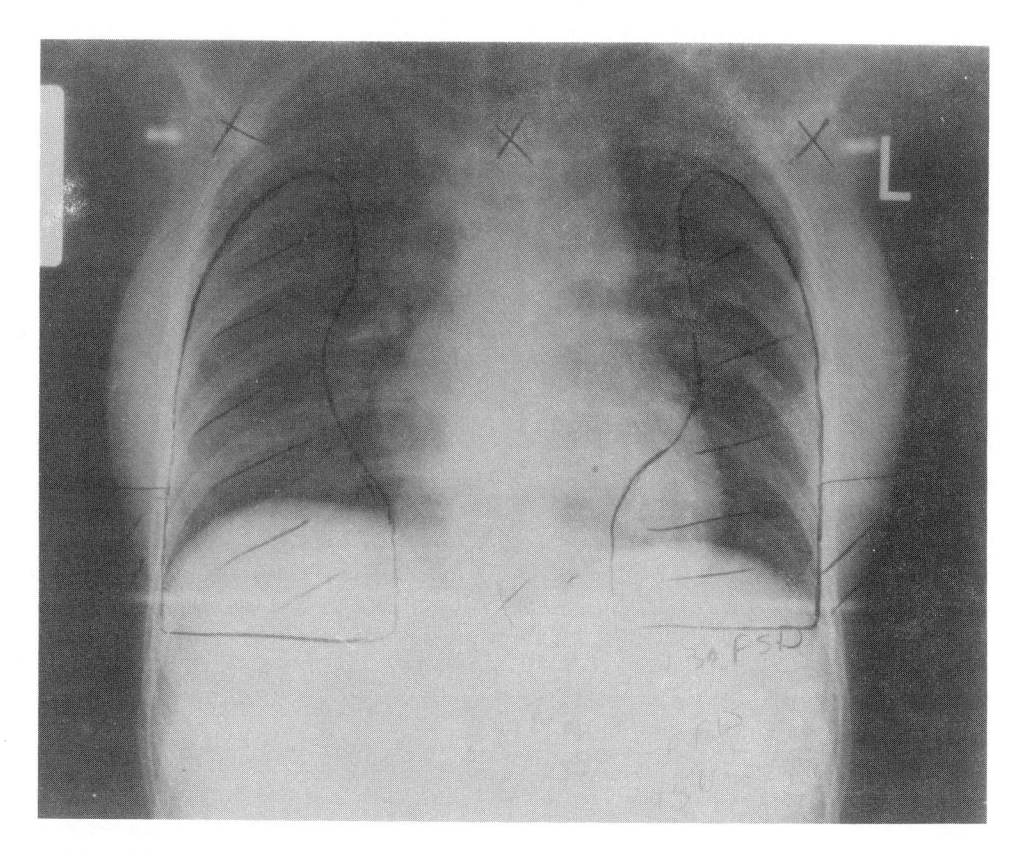

Fig. 2–3. Anterior simulator film outlining fields for mantle irradiation. Areas marked are used as a guide for making protective blocks to spare normal heart and lung.

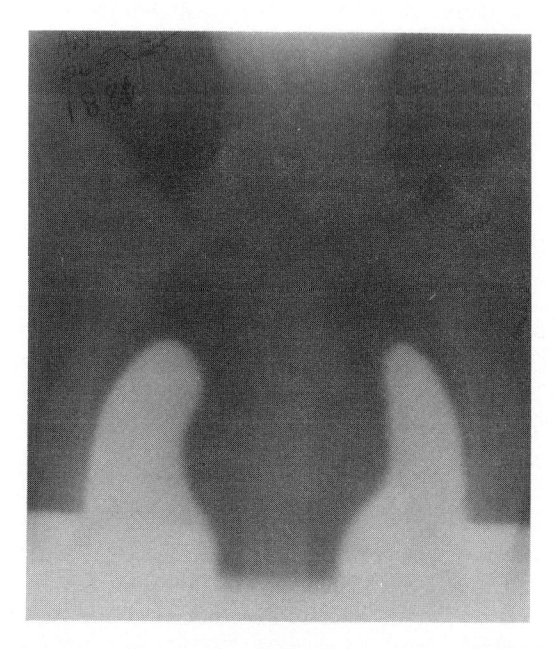

Fig. 2–4. Portal film showing protective blocks in place.

and is used to match with the lower border of the mantle field at midplane.[23] Permanent tatoos marking the bottom of the mantle and top of the para-aortic fields should be used. While preparing the mantle and para-aortic fields, special films that carefully visualize the vertebral bodies should be obtained. The divergent edge of the lower border of the anterior mantle field should match the divergent edge of the upper border of the posterior para-aortic field at the vertebral body. Similarly, the posterior mantle and anterior para-aortic fields should match. We also recommend placement of a half-value layer block on the posterior mantle and posterior para-aortic fields to protect the lower and upper 1 cm of the spinal cord within the two fields respectively.[24]

The large fields used in the treatment of Hodgkin's disease must contain blocks to protect normal heart and lung. These blocks must be shaped so that the individual lymph node areas that need to be treated are included within the radiation therapy portal. Individually contoured divergent blocks are constructed with lead block, an alloy with a low melting point.[25,26] The blocks are made with a specific device, mounted on a tray, and placed into the head of the linear accelerator to protect the desired portions of normal tissue from the radiation field. In addition, special blocks may be used in the treatment of large volumes of lung. These allow approximately 35% of the prescribed fractionated dose of radiation to reach the entire lung of patients with unilateral or bilateral hilar lymphadenopathy. The advantage of these transmission blocks is that the daily dose to the lungs is reduced while still achieving the same total dose desired.[23] Another technique treats the entire mantle at 150 cGy a day for 10 fractions before adding full thickness blocks.[15] These techniques are preferred over treating the entire lung volume with standard fractionation and then blocking the appropriate lung volume after the desired dose is achieved. As will be discussed later, the risk of late pulmonary complications is sharply decreased when smaller daily fractions are employed. Special subcarinal, pericardial, laryngeal, posterior spine, and gonadal blocks have been designed in order to protect as much normal tissue as possible without compromising the ability to deliver tumoricidal doses to desired lymphatic areas.

The use of the "shrinking-field technique" has been developed for clinical situations when large volumes of disease are located near other structures that cannot tolerate tumoricidal doses of radiation. Initial doses as low as 1500 cGy delivered in 150-cGy fractions are used followed by a treatment interruption for several days to one week during which time one often observes shrinkage of the nodes such that larger size blocks can then be used. Often the shrinking-field process may be repeated after a dose of 2500 to 3000 cGy, thereby permitting even further protection of normal tissue. The shrinking-field technique is most often employed in patients with large mediastinal nodes. In some situations chemotherapy may be used initially for patients with large mediastinal adenopathy, especially when it is felt that even with the "shrinking-field technique," treatment with radiation therapy alone will not adequately protect the heart and lung. In this situation, radiation therapy can be given to sites of residual disease following completion of chemotherapy, thus allowing smaller fields to be used.

Patients should be treated with equally weighted opposing fields. This technique provides a homogeneous dose distribution throughout the treatment volume and reduces the risk of normal tissue damage. All the standard treatment fields employed for Hodgkin's disease use opposed anterior and posterior techniques. It is desirable to treat both the anterior and posterior fields each day in order to deliver half the prescribed daily dose from each field. The use of both fields daily may reduce the risk of complications as compared to the use of a single daily alternating field.[27] A 2 to 3 week break between mantle and para-aortic fields is recommended and may reduce the acute effects of treatment.[28,29] Patients consistently recover their appetite, taste, strength, and a sense of well being during these rest periods.

LATE EFFECTS-SPECIFIC ORGANS

While the acute effects of radiation therapy in the treatment of Hodgkin's disease are usually reversible and transient, late effects resulting from impaired function of radiation-induced injury of normal tissues are not. Fortunately, the vast majority of late effects are not severe, and only a small proportion of patients develop major complications leading to permanent disability or death. Complication rates have been sharply reduced by the technical features discussed earlier.

HEART

Prior to the 1960s, cardiac complications resulting from thoracic irradiation were considered rare and unimportant events in clinical radiotherapy. While there are isolated reports of functional changes in cardiac rhythm—and occasional instances of pericarditis, myocardial fibrosis, and myocardial infarction—the reports are rare relative to the number of patients receiving thoracic irradiation; thus, it has been concluded that the heart is a radioresistant organ.[30] However, with the use of higher doses and larger fields, which have been available with megavoltage equipment and with longer patient survival, a re-exploration of the threshold levels of radiation for heart damage has occurred.

The late effects of radiation-induced heart dysfunction in Hodgkin's disease are related to the mantle field. At least six separate clinical syndromes, which follow mantle-field irradiation, have been described. Most commonly, patients will develop asymptomatic pericardial thickening, valvular thickening, and occasionally a decrease in left ventricular volume. Less frequently, asymptomatic pericardial effusions may be found on chest radiographs 1 to 2 years following the completion of radiation treatment.[31] Enlargement of the cardiac silhouette is often confused with recurrent Hodgkin's disease. A baseline echocardiogram is advised to both document the presence of a pericardial effusion and to monitor further progression. Rarely, patients require pericardiocentesis or the establishment of a pericardial window. The examination of pericardial fluid reveals a high protein level and few white or red blood cells. Cytology should also be performed to rule out the possibility of recurrent Hodgkin's disease, although the finding of Hodgkin's disease in pericardial fluid is extremely rare.

Constrictive pericarditis may be seen when large doses of irradiation are delivered to the heart. This occurs when anterior weighted fields are used and has been reported in patients receiving greater than 4500 cGy midcardiac dose and 5500 to 6000 cGy anterior cardiac dose.[32] This condition often is accompanied by cardiac tamponade and may require emergency medical attention. In the gross pathologic examination of the heart, the pericardium is thickened and has a fibrinous exudate that involves both parietal and visceral layers. The myocardium may also be damaged showing histologic evidence of dense collagen bands interspersed between muscle fibers.[33] This myocardial damage may be severe enough to cause significant changes in contractility and the subsequent development of congestive heart failure.[34]

Nonconstrictive pericarditis may be seen following mantle irradiation and may occur as late as 5 years after irradiation. It may be viral in origin in some instances. It is usually self-limited, occurs in 1 to 2% of patients, and is effectively treated with aspirin or indomethacin.[35]

Some evidence, although it is fragmentary, suggests that radiation can cause coronary artery injury. Development of coronary artery disease with precocious myocardial infarction has been reported several times.[36,37] In a recent review from the National Institute of Health on 16 young patients who received up to 6000 cGy to the anterior pericardium, Brosius et al.[38] provide detailed information regarding pathologic radiation damage to the coronary arteries. From this study, it is clear that high-dose irradiation can cause damage to the coronary arteries and allow intimal proliferation of fibrous tissue to produce luminal narrowing. Of 16 patients, 16 of their 64 major coronary arteries were narrowed greater than 75% in cross sectional area by fibrous plaques. Little lipid was present in these atherosclerotic plaques, as is seen in coronary artery disease unrelated to radiation. In contrast, one epidemiologic study failed to demonstrate that patients treated with mantle irradiation with conventional doses had a risk of coronary artery disease that was any greater than that of the normal expected incidence.[39]

Total dose, volume of heart treated, fraction size, and radiation techniques are all important factors in the development of late radiation complications to the heart as a consequence of mantle-field treatment. The risk of developing radiation pericarditis is a function of the dose delivered. Carmel and Kaplan[14] reported on 240 patients who had the entire pericardium treated at Stanford University Medical Center. When the whole heart was treated with 1500 cGy, pericarditis occurred in 7.9% of patients and required medical treatment in 2.9% of patients; whereas, with doses ranging from 1501 to 3000 cGy, 21.9% of patients developed pericarditis, and 9.5% of patients required medical treatment.

The daily fraction size of radiation is also important in determining the risk of radiation-induced heart damage following mantle-field treatment. Steward and Fajardo[40] plotted the incidence of pericarditis for varying fractionation schemes with the total dose to the heart held constant. They found that virtually all documented cases were associated with doses of greater than 3500 cGy delivered at the rate of 1000 to 1100 cGy a week (four treatments a week). Alternatively, the incidence of radiation pericarditis has been dramatically reduced when five treatments a week were used without altering the total dose given.

The technique of mantle-field irradiation is another important variable in predicting the probability of late radiation damage. Kinsella et al.[41] plotted the isodose curves for mantle-field irradiation using three different radiation techniques: equally weighted anterior posterior–posterior anterior (AP–PA) fields with a 6-MEV linear accelerator, 2 to 1 weighted AP–PA fields, and a single AP field with cobalt 60. The dose to the anterior pericardium compared to the midplane dose was 110%, 125%, or 150% respectively. Thus, for a prescribed dose of 4000 cGy to the midplane, the anterior pericardium would receive 6000 cGy from a single filled cobalt treatment arrangement. The use of equally weighted anterior and posterior fields dramatically reduces the risk of radiation damage to the heart as compared to using 2 to 1 AP–PA weighting or simply using the anterior field technique alone. Thus, it is not surprising that a higher incidence of pericarditis (25%) was found at the National Cancer Institute when a single course was delivered entirely by an anterior field.[42] A recent noninvasive study reports on different functional abnormalities of the heart including depression of left ventricular function in a group of patients who were studied by echocardiography and radionuclide angiocardiography 5 to 15 years after radiation by the single anterior field radiation technique.[43] In a separate evaluation of 38 patients treated by anterior weighted fields, constrictive or occult constrictive pericarditis was seen in 24 patients; abnormal hemodynamic response to fluid challenge was seen in 14 patients; coronary artery disease was seen in six patients; and two patients had left ventricular dysfunction.[44] Others have found an increased risk of constrictive pericarditis with anterior weighting.[45,46] Needless to say, anterior weighting is not currently an acceptable radiotherapeutic technique for mantle irradiation.

Simple technical modifications of blocking can reduce the probability of late radiation damage by further limiting the dose and the volume of the heart that is irradiated. In patients with no evidence of subcarinal or pericardial disease, the cardiac apex can be blocked throughout the entire mantle course. Some also advocate placement of a subcarinal block after delivering 3000 cGy in patients without mediastinal disease. In the first 400 patients treated at Stanford University Medical Center with the subcarinal block technique, only two patients developed radiation pericarditis.[14]

A recent study found that of 206 patients who had undergone mantle-field radiation at a dose of 3600 to 400 cGy (150 to 200 cGy a day, five days a week), with equally weighted AP–PA fields and with the left ventricle blocked, only three patients developed symptomatic pericarditis and none developed constrictive pericarditis.[35] Another study reported only one of 69 patients developed symptomatic radiation-induced heart disease following the sophisticated mantle irradiation techniques described.[47] In general, cardiac dysfunction is an infrequent sequela of mediastinal irradiation following treatment using an equally weighted AP–PA technique.[48]

The concomitant or sequential use of doxorubicin with mediastinal radiation may be associated with an increased risk of treatment-induced cardiomyopathy.[49] This consistent clinical observation of cardiomyopathy is seen with significantly lower doses of doxorubicin in previously or concurrently irradiated patients than is seen in patients without prior irradiation.[50] Rabbits treated with a single dose of 1000 cGy and a dose of doxorubicin of 167 mg per meter square develop cardiac damage comparable to that seen in animals receiving a doxorubicin dose of 255 mg per meter square.[51] Clinically, when both modalities have been employed, total dose of doxorubicin should probably be kept below 300 mg per meter square to reduce the risk of myocardial damage.

LUNG

Radiation damage to the lung may occur as early as 1 to 3 months following mantle-field treatment. Chronic radiation lung damage is manifested by prominent vascular changes, fibrosis of alveolar walls, and collagen necrosis.[34] Early signs of radiation damage include congestion and intra-alveolar edema with minimal cellular exudate. Within the lung, hyperplasia of the alveoli and cells with hypochromatic nuclei are found.[33] Radiation pneumonitis commonly occurs 2 to 6 months after radiation therapy and is considered an acute effect of treatment. The risk of developing radiation pneumonitis increases as the volume of lung in the treatment field increases, as the dose rate and the total dose increases, and as the number of fractions a week decreases.

Clinically, radiation pneumonitis is characterized by the often insidious onset of a mild nonproductive cough, a low-grade fever, and dyspnea on mild to moderate exertion. Some receiving mantle-field irradiation may develop signs and symptoms of radiation pneumonitis; however, the vast majority of these patients require no treatment because of spontaneous resolution of all symptoms.[14] Chest radiographs are essential in the diagnosis and treatment of radiation pneumonitis. Progressive interstitial markings that correspond to the mantle field are evident and help differentiate radiation pneumonitis from opportunistic infections or recurrent tumors (Fig. 2–5). Generally, if infiltrates are seen outside the radiation field or if they do not conform to the entire radiation portal, the diagnosis of infection is more likely than radiation pneumonitis.

The volume treated is the most significant factor in determining the clinical pattern of events. Huge doses to small segments of lung are clinically well tolerated, despite the resultant pathologic alteration.[34] Cases of radiation pneumonitis are only of clinical significance when large mediastinal masses are irradiated because treatment of the entire tumor often requires irradiation of large volumes of heart and lung. When hilar lymphadenopathy is present, the prophylactic irradiation of the entire lung is also associated with an increased risk of radiation pneumonitis. Dose rate and total dose are important in assessing the risk of radiation pneumonitis from whole lung irradiation. In the Stanford study, patients with one or both lungs treated were at greater risk for developing pulmonary complications.[14] Significant radiation pneumonitis developed in 23 of 69 patients (33%) who received whole lung irradiation at a dose of approximately 1500 cGy at dose rates of 200 cGy or more a day. The risk of fatal pneumonitis was less than 1% without whole lung irradiation, but it occurred in 5% of patients treated with 600 cGy or greater to one or both lungs. The introduction of "thin lung blocks" and lower daily dose rates has led to a significant decrease in symptomatic radiation pneumonitis as compared with patients treated for the whole lung at 200 cGy a day or greater.[14]

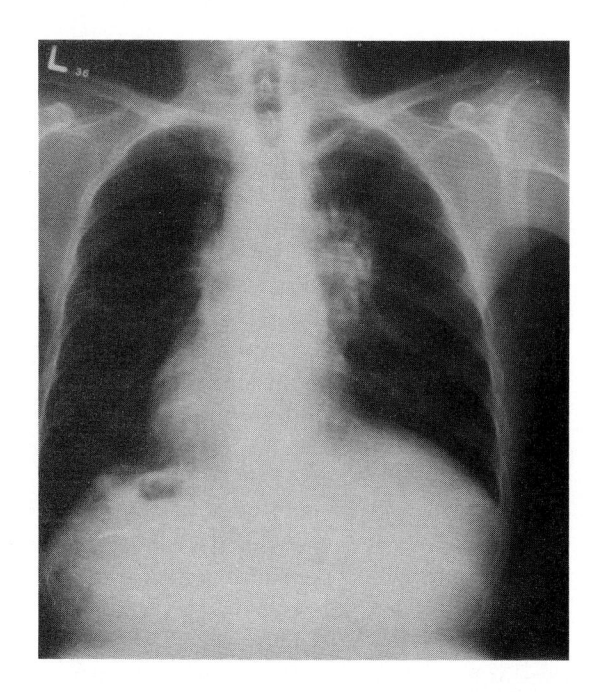

Fig. 2–5. Radiation pneumonitis in a patient 2 months following completion of mantle irradiation. Note the paramediastinal and bilateral upper-lung infiltrates that outline the areas of the irradiated lung.

The acute clinical course of severe radiation pneumonitis is characterized by progressive dyspnea, fever, and cough, which often necessitate hospitalization. Although most patients with this clinical course show gradual recovery, in approximately 10% of these severe cases, acute radiation pneumonitis may progress to chronic insufficiency with significant impairment of pulmonary ventilatory capacity.[52] In order to decrease the volume of the normal lung treated and thus potentially reduce the incidence of pneumonitis, patients with large mediastinal masses may require a modification of the standard mantle technique.[53] In the prone or supine position, the transverse diameter of the mediastinal mass is exaggerated and it is often impossible to place adequate lung blocks. However, by using the previously described "shrinking-field" technique and by modifying the fractionation schedule, an effective dose of radiation may be delivered without excessive pulmonary toxicity. Initially, patients may be treated while sitting up, if it is technically possible. This reduces the amount of lung required in the irradiated volume. Because the mantle-para-aortic match is made more difficult by treatment in the sitting position, this technique should not be used for more than half the mantle-field treatment. The use of CT scanning in patients with large mediastinal adenopathy may help tailor the radiation ports and minimize the dose delivered to the lung. Data from thoracic CT scans have allowed stage and treatment modifications in some patients with mediastinal Hodgkin's disease.[54-56] In addition, the CT scan may identify those patients who may be suitable for combined radiation therapy and chemotherapy. Initial chemotherapy may cause initial tumor shrinkage and thus decrease the amount of normal lung volume irradiated in the subsequent mantle field. Radiation therapy may be integrated with chemotherapy or used following the completion of chemotherapy. Care should be taken, however, since radiation pneumonitis following sudden cessation of steroid therapy has been observed in patients previously treated with radiation.[57]

The risk of significant radiation pneumonitis depends not only on the volume of lung treated, but also on the total radiation dose and the dose delivered each week.[58-60] Pneumonitis is more common when moderate lung volumes are treated with doses of 1000 cGy a week rather than 700 cGy a week.[61] In a retrospective analysis of 377 mantle-field-treated patients, Carmel and Kaplan[14] found that symptomatic radiation pneumonitis occurred in 16% of patients whose lungs were shielded throughout treatment. These patients, however, received five weekly fractions of 220 cGy each, so their overall incidence figure may be higher than seen in other studies with lower daily fractions. If patients received whole lung irradiation greater than 600 cGy, the risk of developing symptomatic radiation pneumonitis increased to 29%. The risk of radiation pneumonitis increases sharply when the mediastinum has to be retreated. Kaplan and Stewart showed that 16 of 238 patients (6.4%) who received treatment to the mediastinum at a dose between 4000 and 4400 cGy over a 4 week period developed pneumonitis; the rate more than doubled when the mediastinum had to be retreated for recurrent disease.[62]

Perimediastinal and perihilar pulmonary fibrosis may be seen radiographically as early as 6 months following mantle irradiation. These changes are not usually associated with any symptoms but can be confused with possible recurrence if prior films are not reviewed. Slanina and associates[52] observed that 85% of patients who received treatment to the mediastinum developed some radiographic evidence of fibrosis. The frequency of fibrosis was related to the dose delivered and quality of radiation. Those patients treated with kilovoltage therapy had a higher incidence of fibrosis than those patients treated with cobalt irradiation.

The role of corticosteroids in the treatment of radiation pneumonitis remains rather controversial.[60] Steroids appear to help ameliorate the symptomalogy of radiation pneumonitis, but do not appear to influence the overall treatment course. Steroids themselves may precipitate pneumonitis. Severe respiratory distress, characterized by dyspnea, severe cough, cyanosis, and a diffuse, dense flocculent infiltrate in one or more layers of lung can occur within 1 to 3 days following the last dose of steroids. The chest roentgenogram shows an infiltrate that corresponds to the previous radiation-treatment field, but can even extend out into segments of lung that were not irradiated. It is essential to gradually taper steroid use once they have been initiated. Physicians using prednisone as part of the MOPP regime should be cognizant of these risks when chemotherapy is used in conjunction with radiation.

The use of chemotherapeutic agents such as bleomycin, cyclophosphamide, and doxorubicin may enhance radiation pneumonitis and the development of radiation fibrosis. Doxorubicin, either alone or in conjunction with other drugs, may cause a "recall" radiation reaction in the lung.[57] There have been several reports of fatal pulmonary toxic reactions in patients who have received both radiation therapy and bleomycin to their lungs.[64,65] Patients who are receiving bleomycin should be monitored closely, with respect to pulmonary symptoms and physical findings. Routine chest radiographs should be obtained and pulmonary function studies should be performed if signs or symptoms of bleomycin toxicity occur. Careful attention to minimizing the volume of lung irradiated is important if prior bleomycin therapy has been used. Some have suggested that the total dose of bleomycin be reduced in patients who have or will receive mantle-field irradiation.

THYROID

Historically, the thyroid gland was considered radioresistant to external beam radiation. This belief was held despite the knowledge that hypothyroidism has been recognized as a relatively frequent complication of ^{131}I-iodide therapy for hyperthyroidism.[66] Until the early 1970s, there were few reports of thyroid dysfunction following radiation to the neck in the treatment of a variety of neoplasms.

Except for a small amount of midline shielding that is achieved with the anterior larynx and posterior spine blocks, it is not possible to shield the thyroid during mantle irradiation in Hodgkin's disease. Careful dosimetric monitoring is important during mantle irradiation. Because of decreased separation the thyroid may receive as much as 115% of the prescribed mantle dose; correction for this should be made at the end of the treatment course. The recognized clinical spectra of late radiation-induced thyroid dysfunction include: (1) elevated thyroid stimulating hormone (TSH) with normal thyroid hormone levels (compensated hypothyroidism); (2) clinical hypothyroidism; (3) Graves' ophthalmopathy and/or Graves' disease; (4) benign and malignant thyroid nodules. Based on pretreatment evaluation of thyroid function in Hodgkin's patients, it appears that this disease alone is not associated with an increased incidence of thyroid dysfunction.[67] Thus, most thyroid experts believe that the high incidence of thyroid abnormalities is a consequence of the radiation treatment, possibly in combination with the iodine load following bipedal lymphangiography.

Potential risks for the development of thyroid dysfunction following mantle-field radiation include the dose of radiation delivered, the volume of the thyroid gland irradiated, the use of lymphangiogram prior to radiation, and the age of the patient. The most common syndrome is elevated TSH with normal T3 and T4 levels (compensated hypothyroidism). The incidence of this disorder varies, but most studies report an incidence of approximately 20 to 50%.[68–73] The majority of patients demonstrate thyroid dysfunction within 5 years of treatment, with little change in incidence after that time. Overt clinical myxedema is uncommon (<5%). Approximately 20% of patients have decreased serum T3 and T4 levels with elevated TSH and only minimal signs or symptoms suggestive of hypothyroidism. Prophylactic levothyroxine (Synthroid) at that time may prevent eventual development of clinical hypothyroidism. Thyroid hormone replacement is also recommended based on experimental data showing an increased risk of thyroid cancer induction by chronic TSH stimulation.[74]

Graves' ophthalmopathy and/or Graves' disease following thyroid irradiation in Hodgkin's disease are uncommon and poorly understood entities. There have been scattered case reports over the last 10 years describing the clinical syndrome.[75–77] It has been postulated that radiation might damage the thyroid and cause the release of thyroid antigens, which could stimulate formation of autoantibodies commonly associated with Graves' disease. One study[78] reviewed the thyroid function in 437 patients receiving mantle-field irradiation between 1969 and 1980 and found seven cases of Graves' disease. This represents a 3.3% and 1% actuarial risk at 10 years for women and men respectively. This observed risk significantly exceeded that seen in the general population. All seven of these patients had elevated levels of antithyroidglobulin and antimicrosomal titers. In a small series of patients previously irradiated for Hodgkin's disease who underwent thyroid surgery for palpable thyroid nodules, Hürthle cell nodules and lymphocyte infiltration have been described.[79] These histologic findings are consistent with the diagnosis of Hashimoto's thyroiditis.

It is difficult to evaluate the relationship between the radiation dose and the incidence of thyroid dysfunction because the majority of clinical reviews are of patients treated with a narrow range of doses (3000 to 5000 cGy). Glatstein et al.[67] found that 77 of 174 patients treated with between 4000 and 4400 cGy had elevated serum TSH levels, while none of the four patients treated with 1500 cGy were found to have elevated TSH levels. Kaplan et al.[80] found that the fraction of patients with elevated TSH levels increased significantly when the thyroidal dose rose above 3000 cGy. Six of 41 patients (15%) treated with less than 3000 cGy had elevated TSH levels compared to 34 of 50 patients (68%) treated with greater than 3000 cGy. It must be noted, however, that these patients were children and not all were treated for Hodgkin's disease. In a recent study from Stanford University Medical Center, of 119 children treated for Hodgkin's disease, 4 of the 24 children (17%) who had received 2600 cGy or less had elevated levels of TSH versus 74 of 95 patients (78%) who had received greater than 2600 cGy.[81] Thus, evidence from these various reviews suggests that the dose delivered to the thyroid is an important determinant in the incidence of thyroid dysfunction.

The volume of the thyroid included within the treatment field is also an important factor in the development of thyroid dysfunction. The Stanford experience demonstrated that the incidence of compensated hypothyroidism dropped from 79% (when both sides of the neck were treated) to 16% (when only one side of the neck was included in the mantle field).[67] Both groups of patients received between 4000 and 4500 cGy over a 4 to 5 week period.

The use of Ethiodol in lymphangiography prior to mantle-field irradiation may contribute to the expression of radiation-induced hypothyroidism, particularly in young patients (<20 years old).[68,69] Ethiodol is a fat soluble organic iodide that is slowly and constantly released from lymph node deposits into the lymph; it travels through the thoracic duct into the bloodstream producing a prolonged iodide load. It has been estimated that the amount of iodide deposited in the body following lymphangiography may be sufficient to induce hypothyroidism. Fuks and associates[68] found thyroid dysfunction in 150 of 235 patients (64%) treated with mantle-field irradiation, with prior lymphangiography, at doses of 4000 to 5000 cGy, as compared to only 20 of 52 patients (38%) treated for various head and neck malignancies at higher doses of 5000 to 6500 cGy, but with no prior lymphangiogram. Other investigators have not only confirmed the association between lymphangiography and increased incidence of thyroid dysfunction, but they have also found that this relationship is time dependent, with the severity of dysfunction being inversely proportional to the lymphangiography-irradiation interval.[70,81] A possible explanation for this association is that the iodide released from the contrast material could inhibit thyroid biosynthesis and secretion within a few days, causing increased TSH secretion and consequent stimulation of thyroid cell division at the time of radiation. Also, a thyroid gland damaged by radiation may lose its ability to escape from the inhibiting effects of iodide, which is released for years from the lymphangiogram dye retained in the body.

Thyroid cancer following high-dose irradiation for Hodgkin's disease appears to be uncommon.[79,82] In fact, the induction of thyroid cancer following high-dose irradiation for Hodgkin's appears to be much less common than that reported for patients receiving low-dose irradiation (<1500 cGy). A proposed explanation is that high-dose radiation causes sufficient damage to the thyroid follicular cells to prevent subsequent cell division and mutagenesis, therefore reducing the risk of cancer induction. McDougall and others[79] reported only three cases of well differentiated thyroid carcinoma in 544 patients treated for Hodgkin's disease at Stanford. The experience at the National Cancer Institute is similar, with only two cases in over 150 patients treated.[82] Thyroid cancer usually first appears as an asymptomatic nodule or nodules without neck involvement. These nodules usually appear from 3 to over 20 years following irradiation, emphasizing the need for close follow-up of treated patients.

NERVOUS SYSTEM

The spinal cord is at particular risk for late radiation damage following treatment for Hodgkin's disease. The most common neurologic toxicity is Lhermitte's syndrome, which occurs in approximately 15% of patients.[14] It usually occurs within a few months following radiation therapy, but occasionally its onset has occurred years following therapy. Patients complain of numbness, tingling, or "electric" sensations in the upper and/or lower extremities, which may be present more or less continuously, but which are sharply exacerbated by flexion of the head and neck. The syndrome usually resolves over a 2 to 6 month period and no specific treatment is needed. Temporary, reversible demyelination of central neurons within the irradiated segment of the spinal cord is believed to be responsible for the clinical findings. No correlation between this syndrome and serious irreversible injury to the spinal cord has been demonstrated.

The development of radiation-induced transverse myelitis is a devastating late effect of treatment and should not occur in centers where careful treatment planning is available. Symptoms usually begin from 9 months to several years following irradiation. Patients usually present with lower extremity weakness, which is progressive and associated with loss of bowel and body function, proceeding to flaccid paralysis. Radiation fields should be carefully reviewed and an estimation of the spinal cord dose should be made. A myelogram, CSF analysis, and CT and plain films should be obtained in order to rule out recurrent interspinal Hodgkin's disease, multiple sclerosis, paraneoplastic syndrome, and other nonmalignant causes of myelitis. Unfortunately, no effective treatment for this dreaded complication exists, and most instances are traceable to errors in radiotherapeutic techniques.

While the tolerance of the spinal cord varies somewhat based on the irradiated segment, radiation myelitis is extremely rare when doses of less than 4500 to 5000 cGy are delivered at conventional fractionation (180 to 200 cGy a day).[83] Castaigne et al.[84] described the clinical and histopathologic features of four cases occurring after radiotherapy of Hodgkin's disease, all of which were the result of improper matching of mantle and para-aortic fields. The potential for radiation myelitis may increase when long segments of the spinal cord are irradiated, as in Hodgkin's disease treatment. Part of this is related to differences in the amount of radiation the patient receives at different levels of the spinal cord within the same field; some areas, like the neck, may receive a 10 to 15% higher dose than that prescribed for the mantle field. In order to minimize the risk of spinal cord injury, some centers use a posterior cervical spine midline block from the start of irradiation and extend it to include the thoracic cord after 2000 to 2500 cGy. At the JCRT, we add a posterior cervical spine midline block after 3000 cGy. As described in the physical and technical considerations section of this chapter, the calculated skin gap in the match of the mantle and para-aortic field is critical and is perhaps the most important technical part of radiotherapeutic management in patients with Hodgkin's disease.

Long-term radiation injury to the peripheral nervous system is uncommon and usually occurs when more than one course of treatment has been given to previously treated areas. While the radiation tolerance of peripheral nerves is much greater than that of the spinal cord, an occasional patient may develop neuropathy of the brachial or lumbarsacral plexus within 1 to 5 years from completion of radiation therapy.[52] We have witnessed brachial plexus neuritis following conventional doses and fractionation in nonoverlapped areas.[85] It is usually self-limiting, but may take up to one year to resolve. It may be viral related. With retreatment of nodal areas, so that high total doses of radiation have been delivered to peripheral nerves, the development of malignant schwannomas has also occasionally occurred.

KIDNEY

Radiation damage to the kidney is a well established hazard in subdiaphragmatic treatment of Hodgkin's disease. Radiation nephritis occurs when radiation doses to all or both kidneys exceed 2300 to 2500 cGy, delivered at a rate of approximately 1000 cGy a week.[86] The clinical manifestations of radiation nephritis usually occur insidiously over many years. The patients often present with protein urea and mild hypertension.

Post-mortem examination of patients with radiation nephritis reveals diffuse histologic abnormalities of glomeruli, tubules, and the microvasculature.[34] Although the underlying mechanism for radiation damage to the kidney is not understood completely, it is believed to be related to damage to the small arteries and to primary glomerular insult.[87] The severity of hypertension is directly proportional to the severity of small artery changes.

Megavoltage radiotherapy, with sharply columnated beams, can encompass minimal to moderate amounts of para-aortic lymphadenopathy while sparing all of the right kidney and all but the upper pole of the left kidney. In patients with an intact spleen, a larger amount of the left kidney receives the full radiation dose. An intravenous pyelogram or preferably an abdominal CT scan is important because it outlines the anatomic location of the kidneys. This study is useful if splenic irradiation is considered and also rules out the possibility of a single horseshoe kidney that would normally be within the radiation therapy portal. Birkhead and associates[88] performed renal function studies on 17 patients at least 5 years following para-aortic treatment. While all of these patients had a minimum of one third of their left kidney irradiated, none showed significant abnormalities in renal function (i.e., normal blood-urea nitrogen [BUN] and creatinine); only one patient demonstrated mild hypertension, which was readily controlled with medical management.

Among patients with massive lymphadenopathy in the upper abdomen that extends laterally to the kidneys, it is sometimes possible to use the shrinking-field technique described earlier in this chapter. Approximately 1500 to 2000 cGy can be delivered to a large field and then the treatment can be interrupted for 1 or 2 weeks to allow shrinkage of the lymphadenopathy. Once regression has occurred, the kidney can be blocked and the lymph nodes can be treated to full dose. If the lymphadenopathy remains too wide for shielding of the kidney from the anterior and posterior fields, opposed lateral fields can be employed with the kidney almost entirely blocked posteriorly.[89] No instances of radiation nephritis have occurred in the over 1200 patients with Hodgkin's disease treated with this modified para-aortic treatment.[5]

If it becomes impossible to block an entire kidney from high-dose irradiation, maximal effort should be employed to limit the dose to the opposite kidney to less than 2000 cGy. The kidney that receives high-dose irradiation demonstrates functional abnormalities by renal scans, and up to one-third of these patients become hypertensive.[90] If the unilateral radiation nephritis causes severe hypertension, nephrectomy may be required if medical management does not suffice.[91]

REPRODUCTIVE SYSTEM

Testis

Radiation injury to the testes in Hodgkin's disease results from the external and internal scatter that results when the pelvic nodal field is employed. The major variables that influence the amount of scatter dose are the field size, the dose delivered to the pelvic nodes, and the field shape and distance from the field edge to the testis. Although a low amount of scatter occurs from the mantle and para-aortic fields, no evidence suggests that sterility results from the scatter of these two fields alone.[92] Using serial measurements by thermoluminescent dosimetry with a 0.2 cm build-up attached to the scrotum, Kinsella and associates[41] of the National Cancer Institute have determined the scatter dose to an unshielded testis (from separate mantle and para-aortic fields using a 6-MEV linear accelerator) to be 0.2 to 0.5% and 0.25 to 1% of a midline dose of 4000 cGy, respectively. When a pelvic field is included in the treatment, an estimated testicular dose of 140 to 300 cGy is found.[93] If a scrotal shield of two half value layers is used, the testicular dose can be reduced to less than 100 cGy in some instances. The scatter dose, however, is largely from internal scatter and when it is necessary to treat the femoral nodes (such as in a patient with a subdiaphragmatic presentation) the dose to the testes is higher.

Transient aspermia or oligospermia is found in the majority of male patients who receive treatment to the pelvic field. While a single dose of 100 cGy to the testis allows recovery of the sperm count within 1 to 2 years,[94] fractionated low-dose radiation to the testis, as in Hodgkin's disease, is associated with a much higher incidence of sterility.[93] In a review of patients with total nodal irradiation and no chemotherapy, only one patient was able to father children.[92] Sperm counts were obtained in four patients, with oligospermia noted in three patients and azospermia noted in one patient; samples were taken up to 7 years following radiation.[91] Others have found slightly more optimistic results: three of seven patients and five of 11 patients in two separate studies were able to father children.[95,96] There appears to be no increased incidence of abnormal children in patients regaining adequate sperm counts.[97] Because pelvic irradiation is rarely used in patients with early-stage subdiaphragmatic Hodgkin's disease (stage IA to IIB), the risk of sterility from radiation therapy in these patients is largely eliminated.

Ovary

The threshold for radiation damage to the ovary is not as clearly defined and understood as it is for the testis. It is known, however, that if the ovaries receive 3500 cGy, sterility and amenorrhea occurs in 100% of females. If fact, ovarian function is usually permanently abolished, in the majority of women, with doses in excess of 500 to 800 cGy delivered to both ovaries. If pelvic-field irradiation is indicated, maximal effort is needed to limit the scatter dose to the ovaries. An oophoropexy formed at the time of staging laparotomy is recommended if the pelvis is included in the treatment field.[98] In this procedure, both ovaries together with intact vascular pedicles and tubes are moved to the midline and pelvis and sutured low on the uterus; one ovary is placed anteriorly and the other placed posteriorly. The surgeon places metallic clips at the suture sites to help localize the ovaries during simulation. To further reduce the dose to the ovaries, double thickness blocks are used in order to provide maximal protection to the midvaginal point. With this technique, less than 250 cGy are delivered to the ovaries in the majority of patients. More than 70% of the female patients subjected to oophoropexy and radiotherapy to the pelvis, by this technique, continue to have or have resumed normal menstrual function. Twenty-one of these patients later proved fertile and 15 were able to carry one or more pregnancies to term.[99] No cases of congenital abnormalities appeared in their offspring. Oophoropexy should, however, not be routinely done at staging laparotomy if pelvic irradiation is not contemplated.

The most important factor in predicting the probability of return of menstrual function is the age at the time of treatment.[99] Most patients receiving total-nodal irradiation prior to age 20 regain normal menses, but this probability decreases after the age of 20 and approaches zero by the age of 35. It should be pointed out, however, that temporary amenorrhea may persist for several months to several years following treatment in some of these patients.

SECOND CANCERS

Survivors of Hodgkin' disease treated with radiation therapy are at an increased risk of second primary cancers. Recent studies have shown a twentyfold increased risk of all solid tumors 10 or more years after the diagnosis of Hodgkin's disease.[100,101] At Stanford University Medical Center, after 10 years of observation, the actuarial risk of second cancer was 9.9% (3.5% for leukemia, 0.5% for nonHodgkin's lymphoma, and 5.9% for solid tumors).[100] It appears from this data that the risk for solid tumors continues to increase with time.

In the Stanford study, most of the solid tumors were lung cancers in almost all of the patients who were smokers.[100,102] Cancers of the stomach, bone, and soft tissue, however, also arose within the field of radiation in a temporal pattern consistent with a radiogenic effect.[103] The risk of breast cancer (mainly inner-quadrant tumors) appeared almost exclusively among women treated at young ages.

The significant risk of solid tumors may not be strictly related to radiation therapy. It appears that the immunosuppression that accompanies the diagnosis and persists even after treatment is complete and the addition of adjuvant chemotherapy may interact with radiation. This interaction may elevate the risk of certain solid tumors, which has been observed in cases of bone sarcoma after treatment in childhood cancers; this interaction has also been seen in recipients of renal transplants and in other immunosuppressed populations.[103,104]

These studies underscore the importance of continued monitoring of patients who received treatment for Hodgkin's disease, even if they no longer have evidence of the disease. All medical symptoms should be carefully evaluated.

The use of modern radiotherapy alone or in combination with chemotherapy has led to the cure of Hodgkin's disease in the vast majority of patients. Attention now has to be directed to the understanding and prevention of long-term normal tissue effects from our successful treatment programs. Since approximately one half of patients with Hodgkin's disease are under the age of 25 at the time of treatment and have a near normal life expectancy, we can expect to see potential long-term complications at long-time intervals following initial therapy. It is clear from the clinical reviews presented in this chapter that radiation complications are directly related to the dose, fractionation schedule, volume of tissue treated, and technique used. Oncologists treating patients with Hodgkin's disease should not only be concerned with the best treatment modality available for a particular patient, but they should also be concerned with the way in which this therapy is administered. Radiotherapists, in particular, should be as meticulous and disciplined as possible in delivering well conceived radiation treatment. An understanding of normal tissue response to radiation is critical, and the involved physician should be cognizant of the potential long-term complications in the treated Hodgkin's disease patient.

REFERENCES

1. Pusey, W.A. Cases of sarcoma and of Hodgkin's disease treated by exposure to x-rays: a preliminary report. J.A.M.A. 38:166–169, 1902.
2. Gilbert, R. Radiotherapy in Hodgkin's disease (malignant granulomatosis): anatomic and clinical foundation: governing principles: results. Am. J. Roentgenol. 41:198–241, 1939.
3. Peters, M.V. Prophylactic treatment of adjacent areas in Hodgkin's disease. Cancer Res. 26:1232–1243, 1966.
4. Kaplan, H.S. The radical radiotherapy of regionally localized Hodgkin's disease. Radiology 78:553–561, 1962.
5. Kaplan, H.S. Hodgkin's Disease. Cambridge, Harvard University Press, 1972.
6. Holthusen, H. Erfahrungen uber die Vertraglichkeitsgrenze fur Rontgenstrahlen und deren Nutzanwendung zur Verhutung von Schaden. Strahlentherapie[Sonderb] 57:254–269, 1936.
7. Hellman, S. Cell kinetics, models, and cancer treatment—some principles for the radiation oncologist. Radiology 114:219–223, 1975.
8. Hellman, S. Improving the therapeutic index in breast cancer treatment. Cancer Res. 40:4335–4342, 1980.
9. Rubin, P. and Casarett, G.W. Clinical Radiation Pathology, vol. 1. Philadelphia, WB Saunders, 1968.
10. Reinhold, H.S. and Buisman, G.H. Radiosensitivity of capillary endothelium. Br. J. Radiol. 46:54–57, 1973.
11. Hellman, S. and Botnick, L.E. Stem cell depletion: an explanation of the late effects of cytoxins. Int. J. Radiat. Oncol. Biol. Phys. 2:181–184, 1977.
12. Kaplan, H.S. Evidence for tumorcidal dose level in radiotherapy of Hodgkin's disease. Cancer Res. 26:1250–1252, 1966.
13. Kaplan, H.S. On the natural history, treatment and progress of Hodgkin's disease. Harvey Lectures 1968–1969. New York, Academic Press, 1970, pp. 215–259.
14. Carmel, R.J. and Kaplan, H.S. Mantle irradiation in Hodgkin's disease. Cancer 37:2813–2825, 1976.
15. Mauch, P., Goodman, R. and Hellman, S. The significance of mediastinal involvement in early stage Hodgkin's disease. Cancer 42:1039–1045, 1978.
16. Thar, T.L., Million, R.R., Hausner, R.J. et al. Hodgkin's disease Stage I and II: relationship of recur-

rence to size of disease, radiation dose and number of sites involved. Cancer 43:1101–1105, 1979.
17. Prosnitz, I.R., Farber, L.R., Fischer, J.J. et al. Long term remissions with combined modality therapy for advanced Hodgkin's disease. Cancer 37:2826–2833, 1976.
18. Donaldson, S.S. and Kaplan, H.S. A survey of pediatric Hodgkin's disease at Stanford. Results of therapy and quality of survival. In Advances in Malignant Lymphomas. Edited by H.S. Kaplan and S.A. Rosenberg. New York, Academic Press, 1982, pp. 571–590.
19. Scott, R.M. and Brizel, H.E. Time-dose relationship in Hodgkin's disease. Radiology 82:1043–1049, 1963.
20. Seydel, H.G., Bloedorn, F.G., Wizenberg, M.J. Time-dose-volume relationship in Hodgkin's disease. Radiology 89:919–922, 1967.
21. Friedman, M. Pearlman, A.W., and Turgeon, L. Hodgkin's disease: tumor lethal dose and iso-effect recovery curve. Am. J. Roentgenol. 99:843–850, 1967.
22. LeBourgeris, J.P. and Bouhnik, H. The importance of fractionation in radiotherapy for Hodgkin's disease. J. Radiol. Electrol. Med. Nucl. 57:828–830, 1976.
23. Page, V., Gardner, A. and Karzmark, C.J. Physical and dosimetric aspects of radiotherapy of malignant lymphomas II. The inverted-Y technique. Radiology 96:619–626, 1970.
24. Lutz, W. and Larsen, R.D. Technique to match mantle and para-aortic fields. Int. J. Radiat. Oncol. Biol. Phys. 5(suppl. 2):159, 1979.
25. Powers, W.F., Kinzie, J.J., Demidecke, A.J. et al. A new system of field shaping for external beam radiation therapy. Radiology 108:407–411, 1977.
26. Paliwal, B.R. and Asp, L. A new technique to evaluate styrotoon cutouts used in irregular field shaping. Int. J. Rad. Oncol. Biol. Phys. 1:791–793, 1976.
27. Marks, R.D., Agarwal, S.K. and Constable, W.C. Increased rate of complications as a result of treating only one prescribed field daily. Radiology 107:615–619, 1973.
28. Landerg, T., Liden, K. and Forslo, H. Split-course radiation therapy of mediastinal Hodgkin's disease. TSD and CRE concepts. Acta. Radiol. 12:33–39, 1973.
29. Johnson, R.E., Ruhl, R., Johnson, S.K. et al. Split-course radiotherapy of Hodgkin's disease. Local tumor control and normal tissue reactions. Cancer 37:1713–1717, 1976.
30. Leach, J.E. Effects of roentgen therapy on the heart. Arch. Intern. Med. 72:715–745, 1943.
31. Cohn, K.E., Stewart, J.J., Fajardo, L.F. et al. Heart Disease following radiation. Medicine 46:281–298, 1967.
32. Appelfeld, M.M., Slawson, R.G., Spicer, K.M. et al. Long term cardiovascular evaluation of patients with Hodgkin's disease treated by thoracic mantle radiation therapy. Cancer Treat. Rep. 66:1003–1013, 1982.
33. Fajardo, L.F. and Berthrong, M. Radiation injury in surgical pathology. Am. J. Surg. Pathol. 2:159–199, 1978.
34. Rubin, P. and Casarett, G.W. Clinical Radiation Pathology. vol. II. Philadelphia, WB Saunders, 1968.
35. Mauch, P., Lewin, A., and Hellman, S. The role of radiation therapy in the treatment of Stage I and Stage II Hodgkin's disease. In Malignant Lymphomas. New York, Academic Press, 1982, 552–567.
36. Ali, M.K., Khalil, K.G., Fuller, L.M. et al. Radiation-related myocardial injury. Management of two cases. Cancer 38:1941–1946, 1976.
37. McReynolds, R.A., Gold, G.I., and Roberts, W.C. Coronary heart disease after mediastinal irradiation for Hodgkin's disease. Am. J. Med. 60:39–45, 1976.
38. Brosius, F.C., Waller, B.F., and Roberts, W.C. Radiation heart disease. Am. J. Med. 70:519–530, 1981.
39. Boivin, J.-F. and Hutchison, G.B. Coronary heart disease mortality after irradiation for Hodgkin's disease. Cancer 49:2470–2475, 1982.
40. Stewart, J.R. and Farjardo, L.F. Radiation-induced heart disease. Front. Radiat. Ther. Oncol. 6:274–288, 1972.
41. Kinsella, T.J., Fraass, B.A., and Glatstein, E. Late effects of radiation therapy in the treatment of Hodgkin's disease. Cancer Treat. Rep. 66:991–1001, 1982.
42. Pierce R.H., Haferman, M.D., and Kagan, A.R. Changes in transverse cardiac diameter following mediastinal irradiation for Hodgkin's disease. Radiology 93:619–624, 1969.
43. Gottdiener, J.S., Katin, M.J., Borere, J.S. et al. Late cardiac effects of therapeutic mediastinal irradiation: assessment by echocardiography and radionuclide angiography. N. Engl. J. Med. 308:569–572, 1983.
44. Applefield, M.M. and Wiernik, P.H. Cardiac disease after radiation therapy for Hodgkin's disease: Analysis of 48 patients. Am. J. Cardiol. 51:1679–1681, 1983.
45. Byhardt, R., Brace, K., Rouckpeschet et al. Dose and treatment factors in radiation-related pericardial effusion associated with mantle technique for Hodgkin's disease. Cancer 35:795–802, 1975.
46. Kagan, A.R., Moiton, D.L., Haferman, M.D. et al. Evaluation and management of radiation-induced pericardial effusion. Radiology 92:632–634, 1969.
47. Marks, R.D., Agarwal, S.K., and Constable, W.C. Radiation induced pericarditis in Hodgkin's disease. Acta. Radiol. 12:305–312, 1973.
48. Green, D., Gingell, R.L., Pearce, J. et al. The effect of mediastinal irradiation on cardiac function of patients treated during childhood and adolescence for Hodgkin's disease. J. Clin. Oncol. 5:239–245, 1987.
49. Fajardo, L.F., Eltringham, J.R., and Steward, J.R. Combined cardiotoxicity of adriamycin and irradiation. Lab. Invest. 34:86–96, 1976.
50. Phillips, T.L. and Fu, K.K. Quantification of combined radiation therapy and chemotherapy effects on critical normal tissues. Cancer 37:1186–1200, 1976.
51. Eltringham, J.R., Fajardo, L.F., and Stewart, J.R. Adriamycin cardiomyopathy: enhanced cardiac

52. Slanina, J., Musshoff, K., Rahner, T. et al. Long term side effects in irradiated patients with Hodgkin's disease. Int. J. Radiat. Oncol, Biol. Phys. 2:1–19, 1977.
53. Hoppe, R.T. Radiation therapy in the treatment of Hodgkin's disease. Semin. Oncol. 7:144–154, 1980.
54. Rostock, R.A., Giangreco, A., Wharam, M.D. et al. CT scan modification in the treatment of mediastinal Hodgkin's disease. Cancer 49:2267–2275, 1982.
55. Jochelson, M.S., Balikian, J.P., Mauch, P. et al. Peri- and paracardial involvement in lymphoma: a radiographic study in 11 cases. Am. J. Roentgenol. 140:483–488, 1983.
56. Pilepich, M.V., Rene, J.B., Munzenrider, J.E. et al. Contribution of CT to the treatment of lymphomas. Am. J. Roentgenol. 131:69–73, 1978.
57. Castellino, R.A., Glatstein, E., Turbow, M.M. et al. Latent radiation injury of lungs and heart activated by steroid withdraw. Ann. Intern. Med. 80:593–599, 1974.
58. Jennings, F.L. and Arden, A. Development of radiation pneumonitis. Time and dose factors. Arch. Pathol. 74:351–360, 1962.
59. Phillips, T.L. and Margolis, L. Radiation pathology and the clinical response of lung and esophagus. Front. Rad. Ther. Oncol. 6:254–273, 1972.
60. Wara, W.M., Phillips, T.L., Margolis, L. et al. Radiation pneumonitis: a new approach to determination of time-dose factors. Cancer 32:547–552, 1972.
61. Holt, J.A. The acute radiation pneumonitis syndrome. J. Coll. Radiol. Australas. 26:595–598, 1953.
62. Kaplan, H.S., Stewart, J.R., and Bissinger, P.A. Complications of intensive megavoltage radiotherapy for Hodgkin's disease. N.C.I. Monogr. 36:439–444, 1973.
63. Moss, W.T., Haddy, F.S., and Sweany, S.K. Some factors altering the severity of acute radiation pneumonitis: variation with cortisone, heparin, and antibiotics. Radiology 75:50–54, 1960.
64. Bonadonna, G., Dehena, M., Manfardini, S. et al. Clinical trials with bleomycin in lymphomas and in solid tumors. Eur. J. Cancer. 8:205–215, 1972.
65. Iacovino, J.R., Leitner, J., Abbas, A.K. et al. Fatal pulmonary reaction from low doses of bleomycin. An idiosyncratic tissue response. JAMA 235:1253–1255, 1976.
66. Dunn, J.T. and Chapman, E.M. Hypothyroidism following I^{131}-iodide therapy. N. Engl. J. Med. 271:1037, 1964.
67. Glatstein, E., McHardy-Young, S., Brast, N. et al. Alterations in serum thyrotropin (TSH) and thyroid function following radiotherapy in patients with malignant lymphoma. J. Clin. Endocrinol. 32:833–841, 1971.
68. Fuks, Z., Glatstein, E., Marsa, G.W. et al. Long-term effects of external radiation in the pituitary and thyroid glands. Cancer 37:1152–1161, 1976.
69. Shalet, S.M., Rosenstock, J.D., Beardwell, C.G. et al. Thyroid dysfunction following external irradiation to the neck for Hodgkin's disease in childhood. Radiology 28:511–515, 1977.
70. Smith, R.E., Alder, R.A., Clark, P. et al. Thyroid dysfunction after mantle irradiation in Hodgkin's disease. JAMA 245:46–49, 1981.
71. Nelson, D.F., Reddy, K.V., O'Mara, M. et al. Thyroid abnormalities following neck irradiation in Hodgkin's disease. Cancer 42:2553–2562, 1978.
72. Schimpff, S.C., Diggs, C.H., Wiswell, J.G. et al. Radiation-related thyroid dysfunction: Implications for the treatment of Hodgkin's disease. Ann. Intern. Med. 92:91–98, 1980.
73. Mauch, P.M., Weinstein, H., Botnick, L. et al. An evaluation of long term survival and treatment complications in children with Hodgkin's disease. Cancer 51:925–932, 1983.
74. Lindsay, S., Nichols, C.W., and Chaikoff, I.L. Induction of benign and malignant thyroid neoplasms in the rat. Arch. Pathol. 81:308–316, 1966.
75. Wasnich, R.D., Grumet, T.C., Payne, R.O. et al. Graves' ophthalmopathy following external neck irradiation for non-thyroidal neoplastic disease. J. Clin. Endocrinol. Metab. 37:703–713, 1973.
76. Jackson, R., Rosenberg, C., Kleinman et al. Ophthalmopathy after neck irradiation in Hodgkin's disease. Cancer Treat. Rep. 63:1393–1395, 1979.
77. Pilepich, M.V., Jackson, I., Munzenrider, J.E. et al. Graves' disease following irradiation for Hodgkin's disease. JAMA 240:1381–1382, 1978.
78. Loeffler, J.S., Tarbell, N.J., Garber, J.R., and Mauch, P. The development of Graves' disease following radiation therapy for Hodgkin's disease. Int. J. Radiat. Oncol. Biol. Phys. 14:175–178, 1988.
79. McDougall, I.R., Coleman, C.N., Burke, J. et al. Thyroid carcinoma after high-dose external radiotherapy for Hodgkin's disease. Cancer 45:2056–2060, 1980.
80. Kaplan, M.M., Garnick, M.B., Gelber, R. et al. Risk factors for thyroid abnormalities after neck irradiation for childhood cancer. Am. J. Med. 74:272–280, 1983.
81. Constine, L.S., Donaldson, S.S., McDougall, I.R. et al. Thyroid dysfunction after radiotherapy in children with Hodgkin's disease. Cancer 53:878–883, 1984.
82. Pretorius, H.T., Katikineni, M., Kinsella, T.J. et al. Thyroid nodules after high-dose radiotherapy. Fine aspiration cytology in diagnosis and management. JAMA 247:3217, 1982.
83. Wara, W.M., Phillips, T.L., Sheline, G.E. et al. Radiation tolerance of the spinal cord. Cancer 35:1558–1565, 1975.
84. Castaigne, P., Cambier, J., Escourolle, R. et al. Les myelopathies post-radiotherapiques au cours de la maladie de Hodgkin. A propos de 4 observations. Rev. Neurol. 123:369–386, 1970.
85. Salner, A.I., Botnick, L.F., Herzog, A.G. et al. Reversible brachial plexopathy following radiation for breast cancer. Cancer Treat. Rep. 65:9–10, 1981.
86. Luxton, R. Radiation nephritis. Q. J. Med. 22:215–242, 1953.

87. Glatstein, E., Fajardo, L.F., and Brown, J.M. Radiation injury in the mouse kidney. Int. J. Radiat. Oncol. Biol. Phys. 2:933–943, 1977.
88. Birkhead, B.M., Dobbs, C.E., Beard, M.F. et al. Assessment of renal function following irradiation of the intact spleen for Hodgkin's disease. Radiology 130:473–475, 1979.
89. Goffinet, D.R., Glatstein, E., Fuks, Z. et al. Abdominal irradiation in non-Hodgkin's lymphomas. Cancer 37:2797–2805, 1976.
90. Kim, T.H., Freeman, C.R., and Webster, J.H. The significance of unilateral radiation nephropathy. Int. J. Radiat. Oncol. Biol. Phys. 6:1567–1571, 1980.
91. Crummy, A.B., Hellman, S., Stansel, H.C. et al. Renal hypertension secondary to unilateral radiation damage relieved by nephrectomy. Radiology 84:108–111, 1965.
92. Cunningham, J., Mauch, P.M., Rosenthal, D., et al. Long-term complications of MOPP chemotherapy in patients with Hodgkin's disease. Cancer Treat. Rep. 66:1015–1022, 1982.
93. Speiser, B., Rubin, P., and Casarrett, G. Aspermia following lower truncal irradiation of Hodgkin's disease. Cancer 32:692–698, 1973.
94. Rowly, M.J., Leich, O.R., Warner, G.A. et al. Effects of gradual doses of ionizing radiation on the human testes. Radiat. Res. 59:665–678, 1974.
95. Asbjornsen, G., Molne, K., Klepp, O. et al. Testicular function after radiotherapy to inverted "Y" field for malignant lymphoma. Scand. J. Haematol. 17:96–100, 1976.
96. Hahn, E.W., Feingold, S.M., and Nisce, L. Aspermia and recovery of spermatogenesis in cancer patients following incidental gonadal irradiation during treatment: a progress report. Radiology 119:223–225, 1976.
97. Holmes, G.E. and Holmes, F.F. Pregnancy outcome of patients treated for Hodgkin's disease: a controlled study. Cancer 41:1317–1322, 1978.
98. Ray, G.R., Trueblood, H.W., Enright, L.P. et al. Oophoropexy: a means of preserving ovarian function following pelvic megavoltage radiotherapy for Hodgkin's disease. Radiology 96:175–180, 1970.
99. Horning, J.S., Hoppe, R.T., Kaplan, H.S., et al. Female reproductive potential after treatment for Hodgkin's disease. N. Engl. J. Med. 304:1377–1382, 1981.
100. Tucker, M.A., Coleman, C.N., Cox, R.S. et al. Risk of second cancers after treatment for Hodgkin's disease. N. Engl. J. Med. 318:76–81, 1988.
101. Boivin, J., Hutchison, G.B., Lyden, M. et al. Second primary cancer following treatment for Hodgkin's disease. J.N.C.I. 72:233–241, 1984.
102. List, A.F., Doll, D.C., and Greco, F.D. Lung cancer in Hodgkin's disease: association with previous radiotherapy. J. Clin. Oncol. 3:215–221, 1985.
103. Tucker, M.A., D'Angio, G.J., Boice, J.D. et al. Bone sarcomas linked to radiotherapy and chemotherapy in children. N. Engl. J. Med. 317:588–593, 1987.
104. Blattner, W.A. and Hoover, A.N. Cancer in the immunosuppressed host. *In* Cancer: Principles and Practice of Oncology. 2nd Ed. Edited by V.T. DeVita, S. Hellman, and S.A. Rosenberg. Philadelphia, JB Lippincott, 1985, 1990–2006.

CHAPTER 3

Late Effects of Chemotherapeutic Agents

BRIAN LEYLAND-JONES
PETER O'DWYER
TERESA ALONSO

The first suggestion of successful chemotherapy in Hodgkin's disease was reported by De Vita in 1965.[1] Today, between 60 and 80% of patients with advanced (Stages III and IV) Hodgkin's disease achieve complete remission with MOPP or an equivalent combination.[2,3] Half of these patients will become long-term survivors,[4] compared with an approximate 80% cure rate for Hodgkin's disease patients overall.[5]

These cure rates have only been achieved by treatment involving extensive radiotherapy, aggressive chemotherapy, or both.[5] Indeed, the importance of dose intensity was emphasized in a 1986 address by De Vita.[6] Intensive chemotherapy has immediate toxicities, which include leucopenia and thrombocytopenia, lethargy and malaise, nausea and vomiting, mucositis, diarrhea and constipation, phlebitis, alopecia, skin reactions, neuropathy, xerostomia, and the acute effects of corticosteroids. Fortunately these toxicities, although extremely unpleasant for the patient, usually are resolved promptly. Chemotherapeutic drugs, however, also lead to long-term complications, which span the range from subtle to fatal.[5,7] This chapter describes these late complications; the late effects of radiotherapy are only mentioned when radiotherapy interacts with chemotherapy, possibly potentiating these late complications. Moreover, the long-term cardiac, pulmonary, neurologic, and dermatologic complications of Hodgkin's disease are only mentioned when they pertain directly to cytotoxic chemotherapy.

SECOND MALIGNANCIES

In the 1950s, Moertel[8] and Razis[9] postulated that the finding of second tumors in patients previously treated for malignancies might relate to the treatment of cancer with radiotherapy or chemotherapy. Reports of late malignancies in patients treated for Hodgkin's disease appeared in the early 1970s,[10–14] but the sporadic nature of the cases, culled from diverse sources, did not allow definition of the incidence of the complication. The first reports on a consecutive series of 452 patients treated at a single clinic with a uniform group of treatment regimens came from the National Cancer Institute (NCI) in 1975.[13,40] The subsequent updating of this study,[41] and the publication of larger series from other major centers,[16-25] has established secondary malignancies as the major late effect of successful treatment of Hodgkin's disease. While early studies suggested an increased incidence of solid tumors, recent analyses[41,17] show that the major actuarial risk is for the development of hematologic malignancies, principally acute nonlymphocytic leukemia (ANLL).

The risk of a patient cured of Hodgkin's disease developing ANLL cannot be estimated with certainty. As median follow-up on the major studies enters a second decade, the actuarial risk continues to rise, and subgroups with especially high-risk ratios may be identified. In most groups comprising unselected patients, the actuarial risk of ANLL at 5 years is approximately 2%. With increasing follow-up to 10 years and beyond, it is clear that the development of ANLL represents the major threat to the long-term survival of patients cured of Hodgkin's disease.

Tester has compared data from four large studies (Table 3–1). It is clear that treatment with radiotherapy alone does not measurably increase one's risk of developing ANLL. Combined treatment with radiotherapy and chemotherapy, on the other hand, results in an actuarial risk several orders of magnitude higher than that of the general population. In a recent article by Valagussa, the 12-year estimate of leukemia by treatment was as follows: chemotherapy only, 1.4% ± 3%; radiation plus MOPP, 10.2% ± 5.2%; radiation plus ABVD, 0; and radiation plus other drug regimens, 4.8% ± 1.6%. With a median follow-up of 9.5 years for the overall population, the actuarial risk in this study at 12 years was 3.6% for acute nonlymphocytic leukemia.[40] Results are conflicting concerning differences in the risks attributable to timing of the combined modality studies; however, treatment with combined modality therapy at initial diagnosis does not appear to confer a higher risk than initial treatment with one modality followed by salvage with the other. Again, the Valagussa study notes an exception to this, in that the risk of leukemia was particularly high (15.5% ± 7.4%) in patients who received salvage MOPP after radiation failure.[41] Finally, the variability of risk in patients treated with chemotherapy alone should be noted. While the incidence of ANLL in this group is clearly higher than that in the general population, two factors are important. First, treatment centers generally agree on strategies for the therapy of Hodgkin's disease at a specific stage; thus, the combined modality data are comparable. Chemotherapy regimens vary considerably, however, and the low mutagenicity of the constituents of ABVD, as used in Milan, may translate into a lower risk of leukemogenesis than that associated with alkylator-containing regimens. Second, the smaller numbers of this subgroup account for some of the observed variability.

In addition to therapy-specific risk, age appears to be another important factor. Four studies demonstrate that age ≥40 or ≥50 at time of onset of treatment confers a greater risk of secondary ANLL.[15,18,19,40] In the SWOG study,[11] patients age 40 or greater had a 20.7% actuarial risk of ANLL at the 7 year follow-up. Among this group, the risk of those treated with combined modality was 32.5% in the same period. Pederson-Bjergaard and Larsen[19] reported on 391 patients; in the group age 40 or over the cumulative risk of leukemia complications (ANLL, preleukemia, or myeloproliferative disease) was 39.5%. In the NCI study,[15] on the other hand, age was not a significant risk factor.

It seems evident that patients with Hodgkin's disease who are not cured by radiotherapy alone have a significantly increased risk of ANLL. In subgroups of even higher risk, the impact of curative therapy is diminished by this late complication. Further analysis of these data, possibly by pooling information from the major studies, is indicated to select patient groups that may benefit from more specific therapeutic guidelines.

The characteristics of the syndrome of secondary leukemia have been reviewed.[12] Latent periods of 1 to 10 years are characteristic; the medians may increase with longer follow-up, but 4 to 6 years is usual.[12,15,19] A preleukemic syndrome is characterized by detectable cytogenetic abnormalities; a characteristic translocation has been described. Over-represented morphologic subtypes include monocytic and myelomonocytic variants. The major feature of these leukemias, however, is

Table 3-1. Studies Using RT Alone

Reference	Number of Patients	Number of Malignancies	Type	Latent Period	Comments
Limited					
Moertel et al.[8]	2340	17	Skin; ST	1.25 to 13 years	Review confirmed Grunwald, Rosner[37]
Razis et al.[9]	(1102)	(24)	Skin; ST		
Cadman et al.[26]	10	10 ANLL	ANLL		
Arseneau et al.[27]	149	457			
Coleman et al.[16]	26	0 ANLL			Median follow-up 5 years
Cavallin-Stahl et al.[28]	6	0 ANLL			Follow-up not specified
Gomaz et al.[29]	45	0 ANLL			Median follow-up 6.3 years
Nelson et al.[30]	67	6 ST	2 melanoma, cervix, glioblastoma, 2 colon	1.3 to 12.9 years	1 of 6 with fold
Larsen et al.[31]	40	0 ANLL			Median follow-up 4 years
Brusamolino et al.[32]	4	0 ANLL		Blank	
Coleman et al.[16]	294	0 ANLL		Blank	Median follow-up 5 years
Nelson et al.[30]	41	0			Median follow-up 5.8 years
Larsen et al.[31]	31	1	ANLL	2 years	
Gomaz et al.[29]	42	0	0		Median follow-up 6.3 years
Brusamolino et al.[32]	14	0 ANLL	0		Median follow-up 4 years
Cadman et al.[26]	64	6 ANLL	ANLL	1.25–13 years	
Bartolucci et al.[20]		0 ANLL 0 ST			Follow-up 3.7 years
Valagussa et al.[33]	236	0 ANLL 5 ST	Melanoma, lung, thyroid, stomach, leiomyox	2.3–8.6 years	Non-skin cancers (3 of 5 in irradiation area)
Baccarani et al.[34]	117	0 ANLL			Follow-up 2–10 years
Pederson-Bjergaard et al.[19]	79	0 ANLL			
Valagussa et al.[17]	272	0 ANLL 9 ST			Follow-up 3–4 years
Coltman et al.[18]	95	0 ANLL 1 ST	Not specified		
Aisenberg[23]	188	0 ANLL			Median follow-up 7.5 years
Tester et al.[15]	146	0 ANLL 0 ST			Median follow-up 12 years
Armitage et al.[35]	242	2 NHL	NHL	13, 26 months	

Table 3–2. Studies Using Chemotherapy Alone

Reference	Number of Patients	Number of Malignancies	Type	Latent Period	Comments
ABVD					
Valagussa et al.[17]	20	0			Follow-up 4.3 years
Cadman et al.[26]		1	ANLL	10 months	
		1	ANLL	38 months	
		1	ANLL	20 months	
Pederson-Bjergaard et al.[19]	312	6	3 ANLL	40,46,84 85,108,120	Follow-up 10 years
Bartolucci et al.[20]	209	6	ANLL		54.3 months in 4 of 6 patients
Grünwald et al.[37]		33	ANLL		
Glicksman et al.[21]	613	12	6 ANLL		
Auclerc et al.[22]	300	9	ANLL		
MOPP					
Tester et al.[15]	44	2 ANLL 0 ST			Follow-up 10 years
Cadman et al.[26]	236	1 ANLL		6 months	
Brusamolino et al.[32]	MOPP + ABVD, CCNU	0 ANLL			
Baccarini et al.[34]	152	2 ANLL 1 ST		12, 59 months	2% at 5–7 years

LATE EFFECTS OF CHEMOTHERAPEUTIC AGENTS 51

Table 3–3. Studies Using Combined Modality

Reference	Number of Patients	Number of Malignancies	Type	Latent Period	Comments
RT → Chemotherapy					
Moertel et al.[8]	147	3	1 ANLL (1.6%) 2 ST (2.9%)		Follow-up 10 years
Burns et al.[10]	191	1.2	ANLL (5.2)		MOPP 6.5% ABVD 0%
Larsen et al.[31]	107	6 ANLL	5 ST (9%, 9%)		Follow-up 10 years
Weiden et al.[11]	179	7 ANLL	3 ST (7.7%, 2.6%)		Higher in patients >40 year
Pederson-Bjergaard et al.[19]		35	ANLL	7 years	
Boivin et al.[24]	41	2 ANLL		6, 9 years	
Rosner et al.[12]	312	1 preleukemic		120 months	Follow-up 10 years
Nelson et al.[30]		67	ANLL		
Brusamolino et al.[32]	174	5	2 ANLL; 3 ST	57.8 months	44.3 months
Initial Combined Modality					
Tester et al.[15]	525	25	16 ANLL (6.1%) 9 ST (5.6%)		Follow-up 10 years
Valagussa et al.[17]	499	1.2	ANLL		MOPP 6.5 ABVD 0
National Cancer Institute[38]	76	2 ANLL	3 ST (6%, 7%)		Follow-up 10 years
Coltman et al.[18]	283	11 ANLL	5 ST (6.4%, 3.0%)		Follow-up 7 years
Cadman et al.[26]		14	ANLL	5 years	
Gomaz et al.[29]	36	4 ANLL		17–91 months	19% actuarial risk at 91 months
Pederson-Bjergaard et al.[19]	312	10	6 ANLL, 4 pre- or myeloprolif	13,18,18,31,40,43, 50,63,64,74	Follow-up 10 years
Grünwald et al.[37]		49	ANLL		
Glicksman et al.[21]	719	15	4 ANLL; 11 ST		
Auclerc et al.[22]	400	7	ANLL		
Not Specified					
Aisenberg[23] (MOPP/XRT)	220	8 ANLL (9.1%)			12 year actuarial follow-up greatest in >40, stage IV, recurrence with MOPP
Brusamolino et al.[32]	163	6 ANLL (5.8%)		30–90 months	Actuarial follow-up 5 years
Baccarini et al.[34]	344	5 ANLL, 4 ST		29–83 months	Risk 2% at 7 years
Boivin et al.[24]	1553	6 ANLL, 21 ST		2–15 years	RR with RT + C
Papa et al.[25]	254	3 ANLL		3–7 years	Follow-up >2 years

Table 3–4. Effects of MOPP (or similar regimens) on Spermatogenesis in Patients Treated for Hodgkin's Disease

Investigator	Number of Patients	Time After MOPP (yr)	Number of Patients with Azoospermia (%)	Number of Patients with Oligozoospermia	Abnormal Motility
Sherins et al.[53]	11	0.2–7	7	2	NR*
Asbjornsen et al.[54]	8	1–2.4	7	1	+
Chapman et al.[55]	64	0.1–5.3	54	5	+
Chapman et al.[56]	14	0	14	0	NR
Andrieu et al.[57]	16	2+	10	4	NR
Whitehead et al.[58]	49	0.5–8	42	5	+
Cunningham et al.[59]	13	3.6–10	12	0	NR
Da Cunha et al.[62]	25	0.6–10	12	6	–

*NR = not reported
†Most patients were also treated with radiotherapy (mantle, inverted Y, or both).

their resistance to standard antileukemic therapy. Small studies indicate that remissions may be initially obtained by the use of nonstandard therapy. Preisler has shown that high-dose ara-C may have a role in this setting. It appears that the difficulty in treating secondary leukemia is achieving complete remission. The prognosis of complete responders is not significantly different from that of de novo ANLL patients of comparable age. Such inferences, however, are made on the basis of small numbers. Further studies are required to elucidate the optimal antileukemic therapy for these patients.

Finally, the question of other secondary malignancies in patients cured of Hodgkin's disease remains unsettled. NonHodgkin's lymphoma (NHL) has been reported most frequently: 3 of 473 patients at NCI, 5 of 579 at Stanford, 1 of 1032 at Milan, 0 of 659 at SWOG, and 11 additional cases in the literature. Aggressive histology, poor response to therapy, and short survival have been the rule in all these tumors.

Though the Stanford Group has suggested that the incidence of NHL is comparable to that of leukemia, this concern is not borne out by the data from other studies.

In terms of the future, a 1986 editorial by Coleman[41] delineates the importance of choice of treatment and that this choice should not merely be made based on the risk of developing a secondary neoplasm. Indeed, some researchers, who supported the tendency to give chemotherapy to children in earlier stages of the disease,[42] successfully lessened the acute side effects (especially nausea and vomiting) by substituting chlorambucil for nitrogen mustard; this practice, however, seems unlikely to prevent secondary tumors or disturbances of fertility.

Although alkylating agents and procarbazine were originally postulated to be the probable mutagenic agents, especially procarbazine because of its preclinical leukemogenic potential,[43] later studies have suggested that procarbazine is not the major offender. Both the Stanford PAVe trial (procarbazine, alkeran, vinblastine) and the recent trials by the European Organization on Research and Treatment of Cancer (EORTC) in which procarbazine is used as maintenance therapy[44] have reduced secondary malignancy rates; indeed, no secondary tumors have been seen in the Stanford study to date. The Stanford investigators suggested that the substitution of oral melphalan for intravenous nitrogen mustard was responsible for the change. Dr. Coleman[41] also addresses the enormous number of patients required in such trials to define small differences in the actuarial rates of these complications. The next few years should give some indication of whether, firstly, the use of chemotherapy for a limited number of cycles without radiation therapy is advisable for early stages of disease, and secondly, whether the use of alkylating agents, other than nitrogen mustard, in the initial regimen successfully reduces the incidence of secondary malignancies.

LONG-TERM GONADAL TOXICITY

Both of the major modalities used in the treatment of Hodgkin's disease—chemotherapy and radiotherapy—are toxic to the gonads. The relative youth of the majority of patients cured of their disease underlines the importance of impaired fertility in these patients. Observational studies in the past 10 years have indicated important prognostic factors for gonadal toxicity. The majority of males cured of Hodgkin's disease by current treatment regimens are likely to experience irreversible infertility. Females, on the other hand, are more likely to achieve normal childbearing potential following the cessation of therapy.

Single doses of radiation are toxic to the testes, but recovery of spermatogenesis occurs after an interval, depending on the dose.[45] After a dose of less than 100 cGy, sperm counts return to normal within 18 months, while five or more years may be required after doses up to 600 cGy.[45] The effect of fractionation and interactions with chemotherapy are unknown.

More information is available on the effects of cytotoxic drugs on the testes, with relevance to Hodgkin's disease treatment; both mechlorethamine and procarbazine exhibit dose-related cytotoxicity to stem cells in the normal tests.[46] These agents also decrease fertility in mice of both sexes and cause meiotic chromosomal abnormalities in the spermatocytes of treated animals.[47] Of concern is the observation that similar abnormalities were detected in the spermatocytes of the offspring of treated mice, but not in the progeny of untreated controls.[47] In the rat, both cyclophosphamide and procarbazine produce toxicity to spermatogenic cells, which is dose- and time-dependent.[48] Recovery of germinal elements does not occur following high doses of procarbazine.[48]

These results parallel the initial observations of gonadal toxicity following treatment with alkylating agents in man.[49-52] At 2 to 28 months following cyclophosphamide therapy, testicular biopsies showed an absence of germinal cells in six of eight males.[50] Several studies have shown decreased or absent spermatogenesis after treatment with alkylators, as single agents[49] or in combination.[53] After standard MOPP regimens (comprising about six cycles), with or without radiation therapy, azoospermia or oligozoospermia occurs in 0 to 54% of patients (Table 3–1). Whitehead et al.[58] documented the persistence of this infertility: of 11 patients who had sperm counts performed 6 to 8 years after chemotherapy, 10 were azoospermic. Hence, the prognosis for recovery is poor, though as Chapman[55,56] indicates, recovery in a small proportion of patients should be documented and provisions made for appropriate birth control. Consistent with the animal data, the incidence of azoospermia is proportional to dose. Dr. Da Cunha[46] found that of 14 patients who received three or fewer courses of MOPP, seven had normal sperm counts, five were oligozoospermic, and two were azoospermic. Of 11 patients who received six or more courses, 10 of 11 were azoospermic.

The evaluation of these data is limited by the relatively small number of patients studied and the short median follow-up. Retrospective studies of patient populations treated at the larger centers would provide a clearer guide to eventual prognosis. Prospective studies should evaluate the potential role of protective agents such as luteinizing hormone-releasing hormone stimulator (LH-RH) agonists, as suggested by the data of Glade et al.[60]

It is important, however, to note that subnormal sperm counts and testicular biopsy abnormalities are common in the Hodgkin's disease population before the institution of treatment.[56] Finally, comparative data on the incidence of sterility following other effective regimens are lacking. A brief report suggests that ABVD may be less toxic, based on sperm counts in seven patients,[51] and recovery from azoospermia in patients treated with doxorubicin has been reported.[62]

The hormonal functions of the testes are also affected. Sherins and De Vita[53] reported elevations of FSH in their azoospermic patients. Chapman et al. confirmed this in both retrospective[55] and prospective[56] studies. Luteinizing hormone and protection levels were also increased,[55,58] and testosterone levels have been reported as normal[55] or decreased.[58] These abnormalities, however, do not correlate with libido, which is uniformly depressed during treatment, but which returns to normal following therapy.[56] Hence, replacement hormonal therapy is not indicated.

The effect of treatment for Hodgkin's disease on the prepubertal testis is less clear. Despite initial reports that young males might be less susceptible to the gonadotoxic effects of chemotherapy (summarized by Shalet[63]), recent studies show persistent azoospermia in these patients.[64] Pubertal development, however, proceeds normally.

The late effects of chemotherapy and radiation on ovarian function are also poorly characterized. Over 50% of women become amenorrheic during the course of their treatment; hormonal findings are consistent with primary ovarian failure.[65-67] These patients experience menopausal symptoms, such as flushing and dyspareunia[67] as well as emotional distress and disruption of personal relationships.[68] The reversibility of this syndrome depends greatly on the age of the patient.[63,67] The experience of physicians at the Dana-Farber Cancer Institute[59] indicates the importance of the modality used in treatment: 18 of 20 patients who received mantle irradiation and 5 of 8 who received MOPP without pelvic irradiation conceived, while only one of ten who received both MOPP and total nodal irradiation (TNI) are amenorrheic, but only two of 22 patients who received MOPP with or without mantle irradiation have amenorrhea. These data suggest that recovery from the ovarian effects of chemotherapy may occur, but the combined insult of chemotherapy and radiation produces irreversible damage. Oophoropexy did not appear to protect patients in the combined MOPP/TNI group, but the number of patients was small.

Based on an analysis of ovarian biopsies before and after treatment, Chapman suggests that oral contraceptives administered during the course of MOPP may protect ovarian function.[69] This suggestion should be easily confirmed since many centers routinely administer hormonal agents to suppress menstruation during the course of myelosuppressive chemotherapy.

In summary, the successful treatment of Hodgkin's disease is complicated by disturbances of gonadal function in both men and women. Male infertility is usually irreversible, but in females amenorrhea during the course of chemotherapy may be followed by the resumption of normal ovulatory cycles except in patients treated with MOPP/TNI. In both sexes these long-term effects are an additional disruptive emotional burden. There is an urgent need for the evaluation of techniques that may protect the gonads, and thus lessen this serious disability.

MUTAGENIC EFFECTS OF TREATMENT

The significant increase in the incidence of leukemia and other malignancies in patients cured of Hodgkin's disease may be a consequence of a "neoplastic diathesis," which renders a patient with one tumor more susceptible to another. Alternatively, the disordered immune function noted prior to treatment of Hodgkin's disease, and known to persist in patients apparently cured of the disease, may render these patients more susceptible to second tumor formation by virtue of disordered tumor immunity. Finally, the possibility that the treatment itself is responsible has been examined in detail.

Historically, techniques of total-body irradiation and chemotherapy developed almost simultaneously. Hence, an analysis of leukemia risk, which shows a fifty- to hundredfold increase in Hodgkin's disease in patients from the mid-1960s,[70] cannot distinguish between the modalities as primary causative agents. Radiation was the earliest known mutagen. Its carcinogenic characteristics have been well described,[71] but as shown above, the addition of chemotherapy seems to be responsible for the majority of second tumors in Hodgkin's disease patients.

In the MOPP regimen, the major candidates for a causative role in oncogenesis are procarbazine and nitrogen mustard. Procarbazine is positive in all known mammalian tests of mutagenicity.[72]

In rodents, it induces lung and mammary carcinomas, sarcomas, and lymphoid leukemias.[73-76] In nonhuman primates, 13 of 50 monkeys treated with procarbazine for periods up to 14 years developed malignancies, of which 7 were ANLL.[70] It has been proposed that hepatic metabolism of procarbazine to one or more carcinogenic species occurs,[76-78] but the major mutagenic metabolite has not been identified. Nitrogen mustard has not been so extensively tested; however, it too is positive in tests of chromosomal aberrations[72] and unscheduled DNA synthesis.[79] The mutagenic effects of vincristine and prednisone are not well established, and these drugs are believed to be of secondary importance. Similarly, the mutagenicity of components of the ABVD regimen is not well described, but it is believed to be lower than that of procarbazine and nitrogen mustard.

IMMUNOLOGIC EFFECTS

The immune status of patients with Hodgkin's disease before treatment has been well documented;[80-85] in addition, the short-term effects of therapy on various aspects of immune function have been well documented.[85-87] The immune status of long-term survivors of Hodgkin's disease, however, has only been described since 1980.[88,89] Aisenberg[90] has documented the depression of cell-mediated immunity, which is a well recognized accompaniment of advanced disease. This contributes to the patient's susceptibility to viral opportunistic infections, especially herpes zoster, which occurs in about 20% of patients.[91] In terms of T-cell number and function, untreated patients have impaired delayed hypersensitivity skin tests,[80,83,92,93] impaired E-rosette formation,[81,94] and reduced mitogen-induced lymphocyte proliferation.[82,95] In addition, imbalances of functional and phenotypically defined T-cell sets between blood and tissues have been observed in children.[96,97]

After radiation therapy, reduced peripheral T lymphocytes and impaired lymphocyte responses to phytohemagglutinin, concanavalin A, and tetanus toxoid may persist for as long as 9 years.[98] Fisher has reported that persistent immunologic abnormalities occur following chemotherapy in the population of long-term survivors.[88] In vitro tests of T-cell number and function were significantly abnormal in patients as compared with controls. Both E-rosette and mitogen-induced lymphocyte proliferation were significantly reduced, and there was no tendency for these abnormalities to return to the normal range at increasing disease-free intervals. In this study, no abnormalities of B-cell number or function were detected. There was also a significant reduction in lymphocyte stimulation induced by phytohemagglutinin, concanavalin A, and poke-weed mitogen, as compared with controls ($P < 0.003$). Abnormalities of immune function in the group receiving radiation therapy did not differ statistically from those found in patients treated with MOPP alone. The authors questioned whether the depressed cellular immunity may be an inherent characteristic in the person who develops Hodgkin's disease.

Recovery of the phytohemagglutinin response has, however, occurred after successful treatment in children;[85] this appeared to be related both to modality of therapy and prognosis. In addition, in children, slight B lymphocytopenias were observed at all stages of the disease. Finally, it should be noted that in children, extent of lymphopenia does not correlate with advanced state of disease[85,99] as it does in adults.[100]

Neutrophil migration, phagocytic activity, candidacidal and bactericidal activity were studied in advanced Hodgkin's disease patients and appropriate control populations by Gandossini.[87] The majority of patients with advanced Hodgkin's disease or in remission had normal neutrophil function. A minority of patients on treatment had significant functional defects, especially in killing activity. These defects were partly cell-associated and partly plasma-related. The defects in neutrophil function might increase susceptibility to infection during chemotherapy for the disease.

Splenectomy increases the risk from infections caused by encapsulated bacteria, particularly *Streptococcus pneumoniae*, *Haemophilus influenzae* and *Neisseria meningitidis*, several years after treatment has been completed. Reductions in antibody response to *Haemophilus influenzae* type B[101] and pneumococcal vaccine,[102,103] and significantly reduced levels of IGM[103,104] have been demonstrated postsplenectomy. Vaccination with a pneumococcal antigen has been studied,[104,105] but its ability to protect is doubtful; it certainly does not protect against all pneumococcal serotypes. In order to reduce the risk of pneumococcal sepsis, however, vaccination is sufficiently nontoxic to justify vaccination in all patients prior to laparotomy staging.

Finally, the sheer variability of differing patient subsets and sample sizes may account for some discrepancies in the literature. Hancock[106] did not report an excess of infections in his splenectomy group, although the numbers studied were small. (At the same time, he confirmed higher lymphocyte and monocyte counts, but lower neutrophil counts in patients at five year remission rather than at presentation.)

Reports of the extent of lymphocytopenia and its duration vary among researchers.[107-111] In terms of prognostic value, Raileanu-Motoiu[112] found that the in vitro lymphocyte response to purified protein derivative (PPD) was the only test that correlated with the group of patients who showed good response to treatment. Spontanous lymphocyte transformation, as measured by tritiated thymidine incorporation by low-density lymphocytes, returns from an increased range to a normal one in patients in clinical remission but does not change in patients with residual disease.[113] Finally, diffuse thymic hyperplasia has been reported in patients with Hodgkin's disease and is most likely a favorable indicator of the host-immune system.[114]

OTHER LATE EFFECTS

Although these "consequences of survival" are dealt with at length in other chapters, we have chosen to briefly review those toxicities that appear to be directly drug related in this section.

PSYCHOSOCIAL AND PSYCHOSEXUAL SEQUELAE

Chapman and her colleagues have highlighted how combination chemotherapy with alkylating agents makes reproductive and psychosexual function vulnerable; this is a serious psychologic complication confronting the patient treated for Hodgkin's disease.[115-117] There is inconclusive evidence that regimens like ABVD, used in the absence of procarbazine, may be associated with a diminished risk of iatrogenic complications. The Cancer and Leukemia Group B is currently conducting a three arm study of MOPP alone, ABVD alone, and MOPP alternating with ABVD, to compare the differential psychologic liabilities of each treatment.

CARDIAC AND PULMONARY TOXICITY

In terms of doxorubicin-induced cardiac damage, the dose given with each cycle of therapy appears to be a risk factor. Weiss et al. first reported lower cardiac toxicity when doxorubicin was given at the rate of 20 mg/m^2 a week. Much of the research at Stanford and M.D. Anderson[119-123] has established some of the pathophysiologic and endomyocardial biopsy endpoints of anthracycline-induced cardiomyopathy. Continuous infusion and frequent intermittent bolus schedules of doxorubicin administration have indicated that greater doses of the drug can be given to patients with breast cancer before cardiotoxicity is reached. Trials are now under way to demonstrate whether this leads to a direct improvement in therapeutic index in breast cancer; as of the publication of this text, no such trials have been attempted in Hodgkin's disease.

The most clearly established risk factor increasing the incidence of doxorubicin cardiomyopathy is mediastinal radiation therapy.[121,124,125] Other risk factors include uncontrolled hypertension,[124] administration of individual doses greater than 50 mg/m^2,[118] and coadministration with either cyclophosphamide or mitomycin C.[126,127]

In terms of pulmonary toxicity, the incidence of bleomycin-induced damage is related to total dose, with an incidence in those who have received less than 450 mg/m^2 of about 5%.[128,129] It must be remembered, however, that at doses less than 100 mg/m^2, severe pulmonary fibrosis has occasionally been seen. This pulmonary toxicity is presumed to be caused by the formation of an iron chelate that, when bound to DNA, can react with tissue thiols and oxygen to produce reactive oxygen species.[130] Selectivity may be attributed both to the inability of lung tissue to inactivate the drug metabolically and to higher oxygen concentrations in the alveolar-lining cells.[131]

Pulmonary toxicity also appears to be associated with some of the more frequently used alkylating agents; incidences between 2 and 20% are quoted for busulphan and BCNU.[132,133] For the other alkylating agents the incidence is low enough that accurate figures are not available. Finally, procarbazine can lead to the development of pulmonary infiltrates as one of the manifestations of an allergic reaction.[134] This toxicity, however, usually subsides on discontinuation of therapy or corticosteroid treatment.

PATHOPHYSIOLOGY: A GUIDE TO THE FUTURE?

Ultimately, major advances in reducing late effects of chemotherapy would be expected to ensue from basic laboratory work. Rubin[135] has postulated that the differences between late effects of chemotherapy and radiation therapy are based upon pathophysiology. He believes that fundamental radiation effects are the result of parenchymal cellular hypoplasia of stem cells and alterations in the fine vasculature and fibroconnective tissues. In contrast, the late effects of chemotherapy largely spare the microcirculation and fibroconnective tissue stroma, and are predominantly the result of parenchymal cellular depletion of both noncycling and cycling cells.

Certainly, our views on chemotherapeutic cellular damage are changing: postmitotic cells previously thought to be impervious to cytotoxic drugs are now showing damage as a consequence of chemotherapy. The most obvious example are the postmitotic cells comprising normal cardiac muscle (myocytes) that are vulnerable to cumulative doses of doxorubicin. This is a result of direct cytotoxicity[136–140] as opposed to radiation, which alters the fine vasculoconnective stroma of the myocardium.[141–143] For anthracycline-induced damage, the myocyte shows loss of contractile elements (myofibrillar degeneration) or shows sacrotubular vascularization.[144] On the other hand, radiation induces a predictable and identifiable sequence of lesions in the myocardial microvasculature that is experimentally reproducible in rabbits and in some primates.[141,145,146] Precise dose-response information exists for both radiation and adriamycin.[138,147] In terms of the radiation "recall phenomenon," however, no true additive effect has been noted in preclinical models; this may be attributable to the differing pathophysiologic effects.

For bleomycin-induced lung damage, prominent lesions are seen in the nucleus of the alveolar type I cell, which in turn triggers proliferative activity in the "stem" type II alveolar cells.[148] Experimental work on mice has shown that this proliferative activity yields alveolar surfactant, which is used to detect later pneumonitis.[149,150]

Acute and late central nervous syndromes have been associated with an expanding number of chemotherapeutic agents, and the vinca alkaloids and alkylating agents are predominantly on these lists.[151–153] Again, chemotherapy has been shown to be directly cytotoxic and may act directly on the glial cells producing diffuse white matter necrosis.[144] Radiation effects on increased capillary permeability can lead to increased cerebral uptake of systemically administered methotrexate.

In terms of gastrointestinal effects, most experimental systems investigating intestinal mucosa have used the regenerating crypt-counting technique as an index of early mucosal damage; however, these readily quantifiable changes do not correlate with the severe, late intestinal effects following anticancer drugs.[156,157]

Hellman has studied the long-term toxicity of adjuvant chemotherapy on hematopoietic stem cells.[158] Tissues that appear normal following chemotherapeutic response have limited reserve only when challenged. Similarly, the use of alkylating agents leads to long-term defects in the proliferation capacity of bone marrow stem cells in mice.[159]

It is clear that more work needs to be done using drugs and radiation in animal model systems, especially to define differences in timing and sequence. In that way the differing pathophysiologic effects on both normal and malignant tissues may be studied in terms of additive biologic effect, altered membrane permeability, and modulation of therapeutic index. A dose-effect factor has been constructed to determine the radiation effect on a variety of murine tissues with and without drugs.[160] The next step would be to improve this model by incorporating pharmacokinetic interactions in larger animals. Ultimately, we are restricted by our limited molecular understanding of the cytotoxic versus the carcinogenic effects of anticancer agents and by our inability to introduce new agents in the clinic with greatly improved selectivity.

REFERENCES

1. De Vita, V.T. Jr., Moxley, J.H. III, Brace, K., et al. Intensive combination chemotherapy and X-irradiation in the treatment of Hodgkin's disease. Proc. Am. Assoc. Cancer Res. 6:15, 1965.
2. De Vita, V.T. Jr., Canellos, P., and Moxley, J.H. III. A decade of combination chemotherapy of advanced Hodgkin's disease. Cancer 30:1495–1504, 1972.
3. Santoro, A., Bonadonna, G., Bonfante, V. et al. Alternating drug combinations in the treatment of advanced Hodgkin's disease. N. Engl. J. Med. 307:770–775, 1982.
4. McVie, J.G. and Somers, R. Chemotherapy of Hodgkin's disease comes of age. Br. Med. J. 290:950–951, 1985.
5. Coleman, C.N. Hodgkin's disease: complications of treatment may occur many years later. Primary Care & Cancer 5(9):23–33, 1985.
6. De Vita, V.T. Jr. Chemotherapy of the lymphomas: looking back—moving forward. The Tenth Richard and Hilda Rosenthal Foundation Award Lecture. American Society of Clinical Oncology May 1986.
7. Tubiana, M., Henry-Amar, M., Hayat, M. et al. Prognostic significance of the number of involved areas in the early stages of Hodgkin's disease. Cancer 54:885–894, 1984.
8. Moertel, C.G. and Hagedorn, A.B. Leukemia or lymphoma and coexistent primary malignant lesions: a review of the literature and a study of 120 cases. Blood 12:788–803, 1957.
9. Razis, D.V., Diamond, H.D., and Craver, L.F. Hodgkin's disease associated with other malignant tumors and certain neo-plastic diseases. Am. J. Med. Sci. 238:327–335, 1959.
10. Burns, C.P., Sternholm, R.L., and Kellermeyer, R.W. Hodgkin's disease terminating in acute lymphosarcoma cell leukemia: a metabolic study. Cancer 27:806–811, 1971.
11. Weiden, P.L., Lerner, K.G., Gerdes, A., et al. Pancytopenia and leukemia in Hodgkin's report of three cases. Blood 42:571–577, 1973.
12. Rosner, F., and Grünwald, H. Hodgkin's disease and acute leukemia: report eight cases and review of the literature. Am. J. Med. 58:339–353, 1975.
13. Canellos, G.P., De Vita, V.T. Jr., Arseneau, J.C. et al. Second malignancies complicating Hodgkin's disease in remission. Lancet 1:947–949, 1975.
14. Canellos, G.P. Letter: second malignancies complicating Hodgkin's disease in remission. Lancet 1:1294, 1975.
15. Tester, W.J., Kinsella, T.J., Waller, B., et al. Second malignant neoplasms complicating Hodgkin's disease: The National Cancer Institute experience. J. Clin. Oncol. 2:762–769, 1984.
16. Coleman, C.N., Williams, C.J., Flint, A. et al. Hematologic neoplasia in patients treated with Hodgkin's disease. N. Engl. J. Med. 297:1249–1252, 1977.
17. Valagussa, P.A., Santoro, A., Fossati-Bellani, F. et al. Absence of treatment-induced second neoplasms after ABVD in Hodgkin's disease. Blood 59:488–494, 1982.
18. Coltman, C.A. Jr. and Dixon, D.O. Second malignancies complicating Hodgkin's disease: a Southwest Oncology Group 10-year followup. Cancer Treat. Rep. 66:1023–1033, 1982.
19. Pederson-Bjergaard, J. and Larsen, S.O. Incidence of acute nonlymphocitic leukemia, preleukemia, and acute myeloproliferative syndrome up to 10 years after treatment of Hodgkin's disease. N. Engl. J. Med. 307:966–971, 1982.
20. Bartolucci, A.A., Liu, C., Durant, J.R. et al. Acute myelogenous leukemia as a second malignant neoplasm following the successful treatment of advanced Hodgkin's disease. Cancer 52:2209–2213, 1983.
21. Glicksman, A.S., Pajak, T.F., Gottleib, A. et al. Second malignant tumors in patients successfully treated for Hodgkin's disease: a cancer and leukemia Group B study. Cancer Treat. Rep. 66:1035–1044, 1982.
22. Auclerc, G., Jacquillat, C., Auclerc, M.F. et al. Posttherapeutic acute leukemia. Cancer 44:2017–2025, 1979.
23. Aisenberg, A.C. Acute nonlymphocytic leukemia after treatment for Hodgkin's disease. Am. J. Med. 75:449–454, 1983.
24. Boivin, J.-F. and Hutchison, G.B. Leukemia and other cancers after radiotherapy and chemotherapy for Hodgkin's disease. J.N.C.I. 67:751–760, 1981.
25. Papa, G., Alimena, G., Annino, L. et al. Acute nonlymphoid leukaemia following Hodgkin's disease therapy. Acta. Haematol. 23:339–347, 1979.
26. Cadman, E.C., Capizzi, R.I., and Bertino, J.R. Acute nonlymphocytic leukemia. A delayed complication of Hodgkin's disease therapy: Analysis of 109 cases. Cancer 40:1280–1296, 1977.
27. Arseneau, J.C., Canellos, G.P., Johnson, R. et al.

Risk of new cancers in patients with Hodgkin's disease. Cancer 40:1912–1916, 1977.
28. Cavallin-Ståhl, E., Landberg, T., Ottow, Z. et al. Hodgkin's disease and acute leukemia. Scand. J. Haematol. 19:273–280, 1977.
29. Gomaz, G.A., Friedman, M., and Reese, P. Occurrence of acute nonlymphocytic disease. Am. J. Clin. Oncol. 6:319–324, 1983.
30. Nelson, D.F., Cooper, S., Weston, M.G. et al. Second malignant neoplasms in patients treated for Hodgkin's disease with radiotherapy or radiotherapy and chemotherapy. Cancer 48:2386–2393, 1981.
31. Larsen, J. and Brincker, H. The incidence and characteristics of acute myeloid leukaemia arising in Hodgkin's disease. Scand. J. Haematol. 18:197–206, 1977.
32. Brusamolino, E., Lazzarino, M., Salvaneschi, L. et al. Risk of leukemia in patients treated for Hodgkin's disease. Eur. J. Cancer Clin. Oncol. 18:237–242, 1982.
33. Valagussa, P.A., Santoro, A., Kenda, R. et al. Second malignancies in Hodgkin's disease: a complication of certain forms of treatment. Brit. Med. J. 20:216–219, 1980.
34. Baccarani, M., Bosi, A., and Papa, G. Second malignancy in patients treated for Hodgkin's disease. Cancer 46:1735–1740, 1980.
35. Armitage, J.O., Dick, F.R., Goeken, J.A. et al. Second lymphoid malignant neoplasms occurring in patients treated for Hodgkin's disease. Arch. Intern. Med. 143:445–450, 1983.
36. Coleman, C.N., Kaplan, H.S., Cox, R. et al. Leukemias, non-Hodgkin's lymphomas and solid tumors for patients treated for Hodgkin's disease. Cancer Surveys (in press).
37. Grünwald, H.W. and Rosner, F. Acute myeloid leukemia following treatment of Hodgkin's disease. Cancer 50:676–683, 1982.
38. Third National Cancer Survey: Incidence Data. Natl. Cancer Inst. Monogr. 41, 1985.
39. Neufeld, H., Weinerman, B.H., and Kemel, S. Secondary malignant neoplasms in patients with Hodgkin's disease. JAMA 239:2470–2471, 1978.
40. Valagussa, P.A., Santoro, A., Fossati-Bellani, F. et al. Second acute leukemia and other malignancies following treatment of Hodgkin's disease. J. Clin. Oncol. 4:830–837, 1986.
41. Coleman, C.N. Editorial—Secondary malignancies after treatment of Hodgkin's disease: an evolving picture. J. Clin. Oncol. 4:821–824, 1986.
42. Robinson, B., Kingston, J., Noguiera Costa, R. et al. Treatment of childhood Hodgkin's disease with chlorambucil, vinblastine, procarbazine and prednisolone (ChlVPP), and irradiation to sites of initial bulk disease. Arch. Dis. Child. 59:1162–1167, 1984.
43. Adamson, R.H. and Seiber, S.M. Studies on the oncogenicity of procarbazine and other compounds in nonhuman primates. In Malignant Lymphomas: Etiology, Immunology, Pathology, Treatment. Edited by S.A. Rosenberg and H.S. Kaplan. Orlando, Academic, 1982, pp. 239–257.
44. Henry-Amar, M. Second cancers after treatment in two successive cohorts of patients with early stages of Hodgkin's disease. In Malignant Lymphomas and Hodgkin's Disease: Experimental and Therapeutic Advances. Edited by F. Cavalli, G. Bonadonna, and M. Rozencweig. Boston, Martinus Nijhoff, 1985, pp. 417–428.
45. Rowley, M.J., Leach, D.R., Warner, G.A. et al. Effect of graded doses of ionizing radiation on the human testis. Radiat. Res. 59:665–678, 1974.
46. Da Cunha, M.F., Meistrich, M.L., Fuller, L.M. et al. Recovery of spermatogenesis after treatment for Hodgkin's disease: limiting dose of MOPP chemotherapy. J. Clin. Oncol. 2:571–577, 1984.
47. Cryssanthou, C.P., Wallach, R.C., and Atchison, M. Meiotic chromosomal changes and sterility produced by nitrogen mustard and procarbazine in mice. Fertil. Steril. 39:97–102, 1983.
48. Gould, S.F., Powell, D., Nett, T. et al. A rat model for chemotherapy-induced male infertility. Arch. Androl. 11:141–150, 1873.
49. Fairley, K.F., Barrie, J.U., and Johnson, W. Sterility and testicular atrophy related to cyclophosphamide therapy. Lancet 1:568–569, 1972.
50. Kumar, R., Biggart, J.D., McEvoy, J. et al. Sterility and testicular atrophy related to cyclophosphamide therapy. Lancet 1:1212–1214, 1972.
51. Richter, P., Calamera, J.C., Morgenfeld, M.C. et al. Effect of dilosaubicil on spermatogenesis in the human with malignant lymphoma. Lancet 15:1026–1030, 1970.
52. Miller, D.G. Alkylating agents and human spermatogenesis. JAMA 217:1662–1665, 1971.
53. Sherins, R.J. and De Vita, V.T. Jr. Effects of drug treatment for lymphoma on male reproductive capacity studies of men in remission after therapy. Ann. Intern. Med. 79:216–220, 1973.
54. Asbjornsen, G., Molne, K., Klepp, O. et al. Testicular function after combination chemotherapy for Hodgkin's disease. Scand. J. Hematol. 16:66–69, 1976.
55. Chapman, R.M., Sutcliffe, S.B., Rees, L.H. et al. Cyclical combination chemotherapy and gonadal function. Lancet 1:285–289, 1979.
56. Chapman, R.M., Sutcliffe, S.B., and Malpas, J.S. Male gonadal dysfunction in Hodgkin's disease. A prospective study. JAMA 245:1323–1328, 1981.
57. Andrieu, J.M., Masson, D., Fiet, J. et al. La fertilite des jeunes hommes atteints de la maladie de Hodgkin avant et apres chimiotherapie. Nouv. Presse. Med. 10:2085–2088, 1981.
58. Whitehead, E., Shalet, S.M., Blackledge G., et al. The effects of Hodgkin's disease and combination chemotherapy on gonadal function in the adult male. Cancer 49:418–422, 1982.
59. Cunningham, J., Mauch, P., Rosenthal, D.S. et al. Long-term complications of MOPP chemotherapy in patients with Hodgkin's disease. Cancer Treat. Rep. 66:1015–1022, 1982.
60. Glade, L.M., Robinson, J., and Gould, S.F. Protection from cyclophopshamide-induced testicular damage with an analogue of gonadotropin-releasing hormone. Lancet 1:1132–1134, 1981.

61. Ragui, G., Lombardi, C., Santero, A. et al. Male infertility caused by the chemotherapy of Hodgkin's disease: MOPP versus ABVD. Acta. Eur. Fertil. 14:221–222, 1983.
62. Da Cunha, M.F., Meistrich, M.L., Reid, H.L. et al. Active sperm production after cancer chemotherapy with doxorubicin. J. Urol. 130:927–930, 1983.
63. Shalet, S.M. Effects of cancer chemotherapy on gonadal function of patients. Cancer Treat. Rev. 7:141–152, 1980.
64. Whitehead, E., Shalet, S.M., Jones, P.H.M. et al. Gonadal function after combination chemotherapy for Hodgkin's disease in childhood. Arch. Dis. Child. 47:287–291, 1982.
65. Morgenfeld, M.C., Goldberg, V., Parisier, H. et al. Ovarian lesions due to cytostatic agents during the treatment of Hodgkin's disease. Surg. Gynecol. Obstet. 134:826–828, 1972.
66. Sherins, R., Winokur, S., De Vita, V.T. Jr. et al. Surprisingly high risk of functional castration in women receiving chemotherapy for lymphoma. Clin. Res. 23:343A, Abstract, 1975.
67. Chapman, R.M., Sutcliffe, S.B., and Malpas, J.S. Cytotoxic-induced ovarian failure in women with Hodgkin's disease: I. Hormone function. JAMA 242:1877–1881, 1979.
68. Chapman, R.M., Sutcliffe, S.B., and Malpas, J.S. Cytotoxic-induced ovarian failure in Hodgkin's disease. II. Effects on sexual function. JAMA 242:1882–1884, 1979.
69. Chapman, R.M., Sutcliffe, S.B. Protection of ovarian function by oral contraceptives in women receiving chemotherapy for Hodgkin's disease. Blood 58:849–851, 1981.
70. Adamson, R.H., Seiber, S.M. Chemically-induced leukemia in humans. Environ Health Perspect. 39:93–103, 1981.
71. Gray, L.H. Radiation biology and cancer. In Cellular Radiation Biology, 7–25. M.D. Anderson Hospital and Tumor Institute 18th Symposium on Fundamental Cancer Research. Baltimore, Williams & Wilkins, 1965.
72. Adler, I-D. Comparison of types of chemically-induced genetic changes in mammals. Mutat. Res. 115:293–321, 1983.
73. Kelly, M.G., O'Gara, R.W., Gadekar, K. et al. Carcinogenic activity of a new antitumor agent, N-isopropyl- -(methylhydrazine)-p-toluamide, hydrochloride (NSC77213). Can. Chemother. Rep. 39:77–80, 1964.
74. Kelly, M.G., O'Gara, R.W., Yancey, S.T. et al. Induction of tumors in rats with procarbazine hydrochloride. J. of the Natl. Cancer Inst. 40:1027–1051, 1968.
75. Weisberger, J.H., Griswold, J.P., Prejean, J.D. et al. The carcinogenic properties of some of the principal drugs used in cancer chemotherapy. Recent Results Cancer Res. 52:1–17, 1975.
76. Zbinden, G. and Maier, P. Single dose carcinogenicity of procarbazine in rats. Cancer Lett. 21:155–161, 1983.
77. Dunn, D.L., Lubet, R.A., and Prough, R.A. Oxidative metabolism of N-isopropyl- -(2)-methylhydrazino)-p-toluamide hydrochloride (Procarbazine) by rat liver microsomes. Cancer Res. 39:4555–4563, 1979.
78. Wiebkin, P. and Prough, R.A. Oxidative metabolism of N-isopropyl- -(2)methylazo)-p-toluamide (azoprocarbazine) by rodent liver microsomes. Cancer Res. 40:3524–3529, 1980.
79. Lieberman, M.W., Baney, R.N., Lee, R.E. et al. Studies on DNA repair in human lymphocytes treated with proximate carcinogens and alkylating agents. Cancer Res, 31:1297–1306, 1971.
80. Young, R.C., Corder, M.P., Haynes, H.A. et al. Delayed hypersensitivity in Hodgkin's disease: a study of 103 untreated patients. Am. J. Med. 52:63–72, 1972.
81. Holm, G., Mellstedt, H., Bjorkholm, M. et al. Lymphocyte abnormalities in untreated patients with Hodgkin's disease. Cancer 37:751–762, 1976.
82. Faguet, G.B. Quantitation of immunocompetence in Hodgkin's disease. J. Clin. Invest. 56:951–957, 1975.
83. Fisher, R.I. and Young, R.C. Immunology of Hodgkin's disease. In The Handbook of Cancer Immunology. Edited by H. Waters. New York, Garland STPM Press, 4B:1–28, 1978.
84. Walzer, P.D., Armstrong, D., Weisman, P. et al. Serum immunoglobulin levels in childhood Hodgkin's disease. Cancer 45:2084–2089, 1980.
85. Tan, C.T.C., De Sousa, M., and Good, R.A. Distinguishing features of the immunology of Hodgkin's disease in children. Cancer Treat. Rep. 66:969–975, 1982.
86. Van Rijswijk, R.E.N. Sybesma, J.P.H.B., and Kater, L. A prospective study of the changes in the immune status before, during, and after multiple-agent chemotherapy for Hodgkin's disease. Cancer 51:637–644, 1983.
87. Gandossini, M., Souhami, R.L., Babbage, J. et al. Neutrophil function during chemotherapy for Hodgkin's disease. Br. J. Cancer 44:863, 1981.
88. Fisher, R.I., De Vita, V.T. Jr., Bostick, F. et al. Persistent immunologic abnormalities in long-term survivors of advanced Hodgkin's disease. Ann. Intern. Med. 92:595–599, 1980.
89. Vanhaelen, C.P.L. and Fisher, R.I. Increased sensitivity of T cells to regulation by normal suppressor cells persists in long-term survivors with Hodgkin's disease. Am. J. of Med. 72:385, 1982.
90. Aisenberg, A.C. Hodgkin's disease. In Immunological Diseases. 2nd Ed. Edited by M Samter. Boston, Little Brown & Co., 1971, p. 571.
91. Kaplan, H.S. Hodgkin's disease: unfolding concepts concerning its nature, managment and prognosis. Cancer 45:2439–2474, 1980.
92. Eltringham, J.R., Kaplan, H.S. Impaired delayed-hypersensitivity responses in 154 patients with untreated Hodgkin's disease. Natl. Cancer Inst. Monogr. 36:107–115, 1973.
93. Case, D.C., Hansen, J.A., Corrales, E. et al. Comparison of multiple in vivo parameters in untreated

patients with Hodgkin's disease. Cancer 38:1807–1815, 1976.
94. Swain, A. and Trounce, J.R. Rosette formation in Hodgkin's disease. Oncology 30:449–457, 1976.
95. Young, R.C., Corder, M.P., Berard, C.W. et al. Immune alterations in Hodgkin's disease. Arch. Intern. Med. 131:446–454, 1973.
96. Gupta, S. and Tan, C. Subpopulations of human T lymphocytes. XIV. Abnormality of T-cell locomotion and of distribution of subpopulations of T and B lymphocytes in peripheral blood and spleen from children with untreated Hodgkin's disease. Clin. Immunol. Immunopathol. 15:133–143, 1980.
97. De Sousa, M., Smithyman, A., and Tan, C.T.C. Suggested models of ecotaxopathy in lymphoreticular malignancy. Am. J. Pathol. 90:497–520, 1978.
98. Steele, R. and Han, T. Effects of radiotherapy and splenectomy on cellular immunity in long-term survivors of Hodgkin's disease and non-Hodgkin's lymphoma. Cancer 42(1):133–139, 1978.
99. De Sousa, M., Tan, C.T.C., Siegal, F.P. et al. Immunologic parameters in childhood Hodgkin's disease II. T and B lymphocytes in the peripheral blood of normal children and in the spleen and peripheral blood of children with Hodgkin's disease. Pediatr. Res. 12:143–147, 1978.
100. Case, D.C., Hansen, J.A., Corrales, F. et al. Depressed in vitro lymphocyte responses to PHA in patients with Hodgkin's disease in continuous long remission. Blood 49:771–779, 1977.
101. Weitzman, S.A., Aisenberg, A.C., Silber, G.R. et al. Impaired humoral immunity in treated Hodgkin's disease. N. Engl. J. Med. 297:245–248, 1977.
102. Siber, G.R., Weitzman, S.A., Aisenberg, A.C. et al. Impaired antibody response to pneumococcal vaccine after treatment for Hodgkin's disease. N. Engl. J. Med. 299:442, 1978.
103. Minor, D.R., Schiffman, G., and McIntosh, L.S. Response of patients with Hodgkin's disease to pneumococcal vaccine. Ann. Intern. Med. 90:887–892, 1979.
104. Walzer, P.D., Armstrong, D., Weisman, P. et al. Serum immunoglobulin levels in childhood Hodgkin's disease: effect of splenectomy and long-term followup. Cancer 45:2084–2089, 1980.
105. Shildt, R.A., Boyd, J.F., McCracken, J.D. et al. Antibody response to pneumococcal vaccine in patients with solid tumors and lymphomas. Med. Pediatr. Oncol. 11:305–309, 1983.
106. Hancock, B.W., Bruce, L., Whitham, M.D. et al. Immunity in Hodgkin's disease: status after 5 years' remission. Br. J. Cancer 46:593–600, 1982.
107. Fuks, A., Strober, S., Bobrove, A.M. et al. Longterm effects of radiation on T and B lymphocytes in peripheral blood of patients with Hodgkin's disease. J. Clin. Invest. 58:803–814, 1976.
108. Van Rijswijk, R.E., Sybesma, J.P., and Kater, L. A prospective study of the changes in the immune status before, during and after multiple agent chemotherapy for Hodgkin's disease. Cancer 53(1):637–644, 1983.
109. Van Rijswijk, R.E., Sybesma, J.P., and Kater, L. A prospective study of the changes in immune status following radiotherapy for Hodgkin's disease. Cancer 53:62–69, 1984.
110. Posner, M.R., Reinherz, E., Lane, H. et al. Circulating lymphocyte populations in Hodgkin's disease after mantle and para-aortic irradiation. Blood 61:705–708, 1983.
111. Case, D.C., Hansen, J.A., Corrales, E. et al. Depressed in vitro lymphocyte responses to PHA in patients with Hodgkin's disease in continuous long remissions. Blood 49:771–778, 1977.
112. Raileanu-Motoiu, I., Dumitrescu, A., Costescu, M. et al. Changes of the cellular immunity tests during the evolution of Hodgkin's disease. Rev. Roum. Med. Int. 21:203–215, 1983.
113. De Pauw, B.E., De Mulder, P.H.M., Smeulders, J.B.J.M. et al. Spontaneous transformation of low density lymphocytes as parameter of activity in Hodgkin's disease. Scand. J. Haematol. 25:58–62, 1980.
114. Shin, M.S. and Ho, K.-J. Diffuse thymic hyperplasia following chemotherapy for nodular sclerosing Hodgkin's Disease. An immunologic rebound phenomenon? Cancer 51:30–33, 1983.
115. Chapman, R., Sutcliffe, S., and Malpas, J. Cytotoxic-induced ovarian failure in women with Hodgkin's disease I: hormone function. JAMA 242(17):1877–1881, 1979a.
116. Chapman, R., Sutcliffe, S., and Malpas, J. Cytotoxic-induced ovarian failure in women with Hodgkin's disease II: effects on sexual function. JAMA 242(17):1882–1889, 1979b.
117. Chapman, R., Sutcliffe, S., and Malpas, J. Male gonadal dysfunction in Hodgkin's Disease: a prospective study. JAMA 245(13):1323–1328, 1981.
118. Weiss, A.J. and Manthel, R.W. Experience with the use of Adriamycin in combination with other anticancer agents using a weekly schedule, with particular reference to lack of cardiac toxicity. Cancer 40:2041–2052, 1977.
119. Bristow, M.R., Mason, J.W., Billingham, M.E. et al. Adriamycin cardiomyopathy: evaluation by phonography, endomyocardial biopsy and cardiac catheterization. Ann. Intern. Med. 88:168–175, 1978.
120. Billingham, M.E., Mason, J.W., Bristow, M.A. et al. Anthracycline cardiomyopathy monitored by morphologic changes. Cancer Treat. Rep. 62:865–872, 1978.
121. Billingham, M.E., Bristow, M.R., Glatstein E. et al. Adriamycin cardiotoxicity: endomyocardial biopsy evidence of enhancement by irradiation. Am. J. Surg. Pathol. 1:17–23, 1977.
122. Bristow, M.R., Billingham, M.E., Daniels, J.R. Histamine and catecholamine mediate adriamycin cardiotoxicity. Proc. Am. Assoc. Cancer Res. 20:477, 1979.
123. Benjamin, R.S., Ewer, M.S., MacKay B. et al. Endomyocardial biopsy study of anthracycline-induced cardiomyopathy: detection, reversibility, and potential amelioration. Proc. Am. Soc. Clin. Oncol. 20:C-335, 1979.
124. Minow, R.A., Benjamin, R.S., Lee, E.T. et al. Adri-

amycin cardiomyopathy-risk factors. Cancer 39:1397–1402, 1977.
125. Deasis, D.N., Ali, K.M., Soto, A. et al. Acute toxicity of antineoplastic agents as the first manifestation of pheochromocytoma. Cancer 42:2005–2008, 1978.
126. Denine, E.P., Schmidt, L.M. Adriamycin-induced myopathies in the rhesus monkey with emphasis on cardiomyopathy. Toxicol. Appl. Pharmacol. 33:162, 1975.
127. Buzdar, A.O., Legha, S., Tashima, C.K. et al. Adriamycin and mitomycin C. Possible synergistic cardiotoxicity. Cancer Treat. Rep. 62:1005–1008, 1978.
128. DeLena, M., Guzzon, A., and Monfardini, S. Clinical, radiologic, and histopathologic studies on pulmonary toxicity induced by treatment with bleomycin. Cancer Chemother. Rep. 56:343–356, 1972.
129. Luna, M.A., Bedrossian, C.W., and Lichtiger, B. Interstitial pneumonitis associated with bleomycin therapy. Am. J. Clin. Pathol. 58:501–510, 1972.
130. Takita, T., Muraoka, Y., and Nakatani, T. Chemistry of bleomycin. XXI. Metal-complex and its implication for the mechanism of bleomycin action. J. Antibiot. (Tokyo) 31:1073–1077, 1978.
131. Lazo, J.S., and Humphreys, C.J. Lack of metabolism as the biochemical basis of bleomycin-induced pulmonary toxicity. Proc. Natl. Acad. Sci. USA. 80:3064–3068, 1983.
132. Pearl, M. Bisulfan lung. Am. J. Dis. Child. 131:650–652, 1977.
133. Durant, J.R. Norgard, M.J., and Murad, T.M. Pulmonary toxicity associated with bischoroethylnitrosurea. Ann. Intern. Med. 90:191–194, 1980.
134. Ecker, M.D., May, B., and Keohane, M.F. Procarbazine lung. Am. J. Radiol. 131:527–528, 1978.
135. Rubin, P. The Franz Buschke lecture: late effects of chemotherapy and radiation therapy: a new hypothesis. Int. J. Radiat. Oncol. Biol. Phys. 10(1):5–34, 1984.
136. Bristow, M.R., Mason, J.W., Billingham, M.E. et al. Doxorubicin cardiomyopathy: evaluations by phonocardiology, endomyocardial biopsy, and cardiac catheterization. Ann. Intern. Med. 88:168–175, 1978.
137. Billingham, M.E. Endocardial changes in anthracycline-treated patients with and without irradiation. Front. Radiat. Ther. Oncol. 13:67–81, 1979.
138. Eltringham, J.R. Cardiac response to combined modality therapy. Front. Radiat. Ther. Oncol. 13:161–174, 1979.
139. Von Hoff, D.D., Layard, M.W., Basa, P. et al. Risk factors for doxorubicin-induced congestive heart failure. Ann. Intern. Med. 91:710–717, 1979.
140. Von Hoff, D.D., Rozencweig, M., and Piccart, M. The cardiotoxicity of anticancer agents. Sem. Oncol. 9:23–33, 1982.
141. Fajardo, L.F. and Stewart J.R. Experimental radiation-induced heart disease. I. Light microscopic studies. Am. J. Pathol. 59:299–316, 1970.
142. Fajardo, L.F., Stewart, J.R., and Cohn, K.E. Morphology of radiation-induced heart disease. Arch. Pathol. Lab. Med. 86:512–519, 1968.
143. Stewart, J.R. and Fajardo, L.F. Radiation-induced heart disease. Clinical and experimental aspects. Radiol. Clin. North Am. IX(3):511–531, 1971.
144. Fajardo, L.F., Eltringham, J.R., and Stewart, J.R. Combined cardiotoxicity of adriamycin and x-radiation. Lab. Invest. 34:89–96, 1976.
145. Bieber, C.P., Jamieson, S., Raney, A., et al. Cardiac allograft survival in Rhesus primates treated with combined total lymphoid irradiation and rabbit antithymocyte globulin. Transplantation 28:347–350, 1979.
146. Stewart, J.R., Fajardo, L.F. Dose response in human and experimental radiation-induced heart disease. Radiology 99(2):403–408, 1971.
147. Eltringham, J.R., Fajardo, L.F., Stewart, J.R. et al. Investigation of cardiotoxicity in rabbits from adriamycin and fractionated cardiac irradiation: preliminary results. Front. Radiat. Ther. Oncol. 13:21–35, 1979.
148. Aso, Y., Yoneda, K., and Kikkawa, Y. Morphologic and biochemical study of pulmonary changes induced by bleomycin in mice. Lab. Invest. 35:558–568, 1976.
149. Penney, D.P., Shapiro, D.L., Rubin, P. et al. Effects of radiation on mouse lung and potential induction of radiation pneumonitis. Virchows Arch. (Cell Pathol.) 37:327–336, 1981.
150. Rubin, P., Shapiro, D.K., Finkelstein, J.N. et al. The early release of surfactant following lung irradiation of alveolar type II cells. Int. J. Radiat. Oncol. Biol. Phys. 6:75–77, 1980.
151. Burger, P.C., Kamenar, E., Schold, S.C. et al. Encephalomyelopathy following high-dose BCNU therapy. Cancer 48:1318–1327, 1981.
152. Evans, A., Bleyer, A., Kaplan, R.S. et al. Central nervous system workshop. Cancer Clin. Trials 4(Suppl):31–35, 1981.
153. Kaplan, R.S. and Wiernik, P.H. Neurotoxicity of antineoplastic drugs. Sem. Oncol. 9:103–130, 1982.
154. Rubin, P. and Casarett, G.W. Clinical Radiation Pathology, vols. I and II. Philadephia, W.B. Saunders, 1968.
155. Griffin, T.V., Rasey, J.S., and Bleyer, W.A. The effect of photon irradiation on blood-brain barrier permeability to methotrexate in mice. Cancer 40:1109–1111, 1977.
156. Dethlefsen, L.A. Cellular recovery kinetic studies relevant to combined modality research and therapy. Int. J. Radiat. Oncol. Biol. Phys. 5:1175–1184, 1979.
157. Schenken, L.L., Burdolt, D.R., and Kovacs, C.J. Adriamycin radiation induced combinations: drug induced delayed gastrointestinal radiosensitivity. Int. J. Radiat. Oncol. Biol. Phys. 5:1265–1270, 1979.
158. Hellman, S. and Botnik, L.E. Stem cell depletion: an explanation of the late effects of cytotoxins. Int. J. Radiat. Oncol. Biol. Phys. 2:181–184, 1977.
159. Keizer, M.J. Protection of hematopoietic stem cells during cytotoxic treatment. Rijswijk, Netherlands, Radiobiological Institute, 1976, p. 96.
160. Phillips, T.L. Tissue toxicity of radiation-drug interactions. In Radiation-Drug Interactions in the Treatment of Cancer. Edited by G.H. Sokal and R.P Maickel. Wiley Series in Diagnostic and Therapeutic Radiology. New York, John Wiley and Son, 1980, pp. 175–200.

CHAPTER 4

Late Hematologic Complications after Treatment of Hodgkin's Disease

SANFORD KEMPIN

The treatment of Hodgkin's disease exposes hematopoietic tissues to chemotherapy, radiation therapy, and infectious agents, resulting in a number of acute effects complicating the management of patients (Table 4–1). These effects are seen in all patients to a greater or lesser degree and occasionally result in significant morbidity and rarely mortality. As a result of these acute injuries, initially unapparent alterations in these tissues may lead to long-term sequelae, eventually resulting in a variety of post-treatment disorders (Table 4–2), some of which are amenable to treatment and others that result in the demise of the patient in spite of a cure of the underlying lymphoma. In order to understand these long-term effects, an initial description of normal hematopoiesis is necessary. This is followed by a review of the physiologic alterations induced by chemotherapy and radiation therapy and a discussion of late complications.

I wish to acknowledge Ms. Robie Lipperman and Mrs. Iris Kaplan for their excellent assistance in the preparation of this chapter.

Table 4–1. Acute Effects of Hodgkin's Disease Therapy on Hematopoietic Tissue

Inhibition of Hematopoiesis
- anemia
- thrombocytopenia
- neutropenia
- alterations in monocyte-macrophage number and function

Inhibition of Lymphopoiesis
- lymphopenia
- hypogammaglobulinemia
- "immune imbalance"

MODEL OF NORMAL HEMATOPOIESIS

The production of normal hematopoietic tissue depends on an adequate supply of hematopoietic stem cells (HSC), normal function of the bone marrow microenvironment, and the delivery of nutritional and stimulatory factors (Fig. 4–1). Each of these aspects may be altered by the treatment of Hodgkin's disease. HSCs are derived embryologically from mesodermal tissue and will ultimately

Table 4–2. Chronic Effects of Hodgkin's Disease Therapy on Hematopoietic Tissue

Decreased Reserve of Hematopoietic Tissue
- Pancytopenia
- Impaired response to hematopoietic stress after bleeding or infection (?)

Decreased Immunocompetence
- Susceptibility to infection (i.e., herpes zoster)
- Susceptibility to neoplasia

Altered Immunoregulation
- Autoimmune cytopenias
- Immune complex disease

Neoplastic Proliferation
- Leukemia
- NonHodgkin's lymphomas

give rise to all the circulating blood elements. Present initially in the yolk sac and later in hepatic and splenic tissue, the vast majority migrate toward the end of intrauterine life to the bone marrow, where a self-renewal and terminal differentiation capacity remains throughout life. It is still unclear whether this self-renewal capacity is limited[1,2] or unlimited.[3] Chromosomal studies of allogeneic marrow transfers suggest a more restricted or finite ability.[4] In vitro culture studies demonstrate a decline in self-renewal capacity with aging,[5] although in vivo serial passage studies show no age difference.[6] This self-renewal capacity and proliferative activity is heterogeneous within the stem cell compartment, with a hierarchy of self-regenerative potential ranging from the most primitive or "younger" stem cells to those possessing less regenerative capacity ("older" stem cells).[3,7–9] As more of a demand for differentiated cells occurs, there is an increasing loss of capacity for unlimited proliferation.[3] In general, less than 50% of normal stem cell progeny retain a self-renewal capacity. It has been estimated that 20 to 25 cell divisions represent the maximal cellular reserve.[10]

Because of the finite life span of blood cells, a constant renewal from a pluripotent stem cell compartment must occur. The HSC compartment is small relative to the number of hematopoietic cells.[11] The ability of hematopoietic tissue to expand during stress, however, illustrates the importance of this compartment from the standpoint of life-long homeostasis. This can be demonstrated in vi-

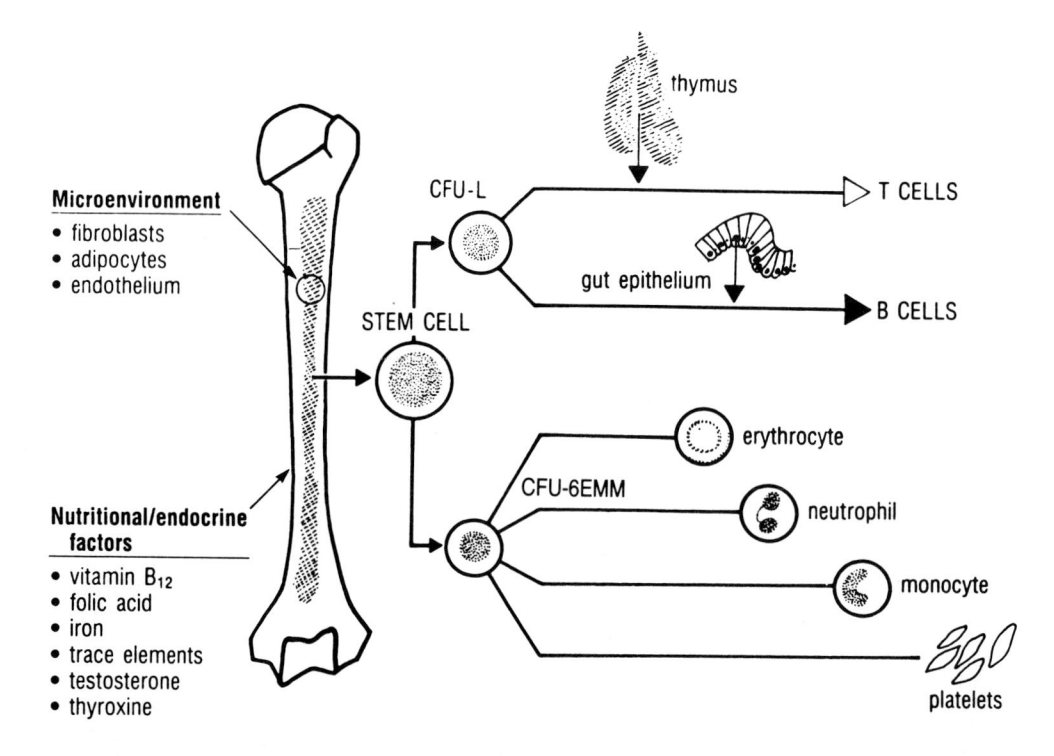

Fig. 4–1. Normal hematopoietic tissue depends on an adequate supply of stem cells, normal function of the bone-marrow microenvironment, and the delivery of nutritional and stimulatory factors.

tro after chemotherapeutic injury where a "pre-colony forming unit (pre-CFU-S)" population may play a prominent role in marrow repopulation.[7] Measurement of the total mass of stem cells is not possible at this time. Although it is assumed that hypoplastic marrow states caused by ionizing radiation or chemotherapy result in pancytopenia by depletion of stem cells, marrow stromal injury and injury to target organs responsible for feedback regulation may also play a significant role. Until recently, only animal models were available to study the HSC; however, with newer techniques of marrow cell culture,[11] and particularly in vitro long-term marrow culture,[12,13] the cells can be better defined and studied. Control mechanisms of HSC proliferation and differentiation are still poorly understood. In 1982, it was demonstrated that interleukin-3, a glycoprotein necessary for the growth of a variety of cell lines (thymic lymphoma, splenic lymphoma, erythroleukemia) plays a possible role in the proliferation of a pluripotent progenitor.[14] As certain long-term hematopoietic injuries may be irreversible, cryopreserving viable (and normal) stem cells early in therapy ("marrow banks" analogous to sperm banks) may be a resource for the future therapy of potentially life-threatening problems.

The progeny of stem cells are committed colony-forming cells, which are more easily recognized in semisolid and liquid cultures (CFU-C), and on which cellular and extracellular influences can be more easily measured. In the adult, colony-forming cells are predominantly found in the bone marrow, and in smaller numbers, in the spleen and blood. During hematopoietic stress, these cells (and presumably stem cells) are present in significant quantities in peripheral blood. The number of these cells in the bone marrow is low compared to other marrow elements (100 to 200/10^5 marrow cells for granulocyte-monocyte [CFU-GM] precursors and 10 to 20/10^5 marrow cells for eosinophil and megakaryocyte colony-forming cells). The mass of CFU-Cs in the normal and marrow-injured host has not been measured.

Committed stem cells proliferate and differentiate under the influence of colony stimulating factors (CSFs) secreted by hematopoietic and nonhematopoietic tissues. These glycoproteins are produced by numerous cells and are present in serum and urine. A number have been purified to homogeneity and biochemically and physiologically characterized. Among the cells producing CSFs are macrophages,[15] as well as a number of malignant cells,[16,17] including ALL-lymphoblasts.[18] In addition to humoral products, cell to cell interaction may be important in normal hematopoietic cell development (e.g., T-cells in erythropoiesis),[19] and alteration of these "helper" populations by chemotherapy and radiation therapy may have chronic effects, independent of the decrease in stem-cell mass.

Lymphocytes, when stimulated by mitogens or antigens, secrete a number of glycoproteins known as lymphokines. These function as regulatory hormones affecting both lymphocytopoiesis and hematopoiesis. Established T-cell lines, such as the Mo cell line from an HTLV-II infected T-cell variant of hairy-cell leukemia have permitted characterization of these molecules, which include interleukin-2, interleukin-3, and T-cell CSF.[20–24] Lymphokines from this cell line, as well as more recently described lymphokines (IL-4, IL-5, IL-6), influence progenitor cell proliferation and differentiation. Mature neutrophils and monocytes respond to other factors produced by these cells (neutrophil migration inhibition factor, macrophage migration inhibition factor), demonstrating their influence in the regulation of the inflammatory reaction.[24] Therefore, depletion of the normal counterpart of these T-cells by chemotherapy and radiation therapy may have subtle effects, which are not possible to quantify at this time.

The marrow stromal elements and microenvironment are being increasingly recognized for their central role in normal hematopoiesis (Table 4–3).[25–28] Fibroblasts[26] and endothelial cells[27,29] are sources of stimulatory (CSFs, CFU-mix hemopoietin) and inhibitory factors.[25] The role of adipocytes ("giant fat cells") is less clear.[12] Endothelial cell secretion of colony-stimulating activity (CSA) may be controlled or stimulated by monocytes.[27,30] The structural matrix allowing cell to cell interactions depends on fibroblasts and adipose

Table 4-3. Role of Marrow Stromal Elements

Fibroblasts
- CSF production
- Collagen-cell intermatrix

Adipocytes
- Source of nutrition (?)
- Support tissue

Vascular tissue (Endothelial cells)
- Source of CSF
- Control of cell release

tissue. Although fibronectin is formed as part of the extracellular matrix, predominantly by fibroblasts,[31] it is uncertain what its role may be in the regulation of hematopoiesis. An age-related decline in marrow function occurs and may be explained by the increased sensitivity of older individuals to stromal injury.[5]

Nutritional and endocrine factors necessary for normal hematopoiesis include vitamin B12, folic acid, iron, trace elements, thyroid hormones, testosterone, and erythropoietin. Vitamin B12 is absorbed in the terminal ileum, complexed to intrinsic factor. The latter is produced in the parietal cells of the gastric mucosa. Folic acid and iron are absorbed proximally; iron absorption depends on gastric acid secretion. Acute and chronic changes in gastrointestinal mucosa induced by surgical resection, chemotherapy, and radiation therapy may alter the absorption of vital nutrients, which may become depleted with time. Malnutrition may significantly alter granulocyte reserves.[32]

The in vitro effects of testosterone[33] and thyroid hormones[34] have been studied in cultures of hematopoietic cells, and the in vivo correlate of their effects includes an increased red-cell mass in males and chronic anemia in hypothyroidism. Hypothyroidism in dogs, induced by administration of radioiodine, causes a reduction in red-cell mass and a decrease in plasma iron turnover.[35] Administration of thyroid hormone increases hematocrit, total red-cell mass and red-cell synthesis—as measured by red cell iron turnover,[36] iron incorporation into red cells,[37] and globin chain synthesis.[38] The effects of thyroxine may in part be related to erythropoietin production, either by a direct anabolic effect, or as a result of increased oxygen consumption. Therefore, the ability of the individual to increase red-cell mass during hypoxic stress (bleeding, anema, high altitude) may be decreased by the absence of the thyroid hormone. Erythropoietin, produced in renal parenchymal cells, stimulates red-cell precursors to mature and proliferate normally. Renal failure results in a hypoplastic marrow state, which is at least partially responsive to exogenous erythropoietin stimulation.

ABNORMALITIES OF NORMAL HEMATOPOIESIS INDUCED BY THE PRESENCE OF HODGKIN'S DISEASE, CHEMOTHERAPY, RADIATION THERAPY, AND HORMONAL DEPRIVATION

The presence of tumor and inflammatory states influences hematopoiesis in numerous ways and results in a variety of abnormalities observed during periods of disease activity. The anemia of chronic inflammation is the most common abnormality. Ferrokinetic studies demonstrate sideropenia, normal to high serum ferritin levels,[39] and rapid iron clearance (but reduced reutilization as hemoglobin iron).[40] Erythropoiesis has been studied in untreated patients with Hodgkin's disease,[41,42] with worsening of the above abnormalities observed in more advanced stages or if systemic symptoms were present. When anemia is present, it is generally normocytic or microcytic. The endogenous leukocyte mediator, which is released from neutrophils or the monocyte-macrophage cells, stimulates the release of iron-binding proteins,[43,44] which direct iron to storage depots, making it unavailable for hemoglobin synthesis. Although not a manifestation of the treated and presumably cured Hodgkin's disease patient, the reappearance of this chronic anemia may be a manifestation of recurrent disease. Acquired sideroblastic anemia has been reported in Hodgkin's disease.[40,45,46] This abnormality of intracellular iron metabolism is either drug-induced (nitrogen mustard, melphalan)[46] or represents a premalignant change in hematopoietic stem cells.[47] Rarely, erythrocytosis has been reported.[48] Leukocytosis, predominantly neutrophilia, may be observed.[49] A leucoerythroblastic blood picture with immature marrow elements, however, is more likely a reflection of bone marrow involvement with tumor. Thrombocytosis is commonly observed during active disease.[49] Both leukocytosis and thrombocytosis are accompaniments of the postsplenectomy state and may persist for months to years and should not be confused with reactivation of the Hodgkin's disease.[50] The thrombocytosis rarely results in thromboembolic disease.[51]

All chemotherapy agents used in the treatment of Hodgkin's disease affect hematopoietic cell proliferation. The inhibition of hematopoiesis is a reflection of a decline in DNA synthesis, most often by alkylation of nucleic acids, as well as mitotic inhibition. Because the stem cell population is predominantly noncycling, antimetabolites, generally cycle-specific, are less likely to result in stem cell depletion than alkylating agents. The effects of corticosteroids are probably negligible, although their catabolic properties may play a modest role. The acute hematopoietic toxicity of both antimetabolites and alkylating agents has been well characterized,[52–54] and recovery of apparently normal hematopoiesis ensues in a cyclical fashion—once the acute exposure is terminated.[53] For certain agents (i.e., nitrosoureas, procarbazine), the acute toxic injury is prolonged, possibly by products of drug metabolism, and a more prolonged cytotoxic effect is observed.[53,55,56]

Several authors working with animal models have demonstrated a decrease in self-replicative capacity of hematopoietic stem cells after short-term drug administration.[57–60] Drugs used in these experiments included busulfan and melphalan; these results demonstrate the prolonged effects of these agents on stem-cell reserve. The depletion of the stem-cell compartment by chemotherapeutic agents may result in an imbalance in the "age" structure of this compartment with depletion of "young" stem cells and a subsequent decreased ability to respond to hematopoietic stress. This depends on the time frame of marrow exposure and the unique toxicities of each agent. Busulfan induces a chronic marrow failure related to depletion of pluripotent hematopoietic stem cells.[57,61,62] This chronic myelosuppressive effect appears more profound than other alkylating agents and may be demonstrated up to two years after the initial injury.[58,61] Other alkylating agents, such as melphalan and chlorambucil,[63] may likewise induce long-term hematopoietic stem cell failure after apparent short-term marrow recovery.[57,58,61,64,65] Cyclophosphamide induces cyclic oscillations in hematopoiesis, but does not appear to deplete stem cells.[61] The acute chemotherapeutic effects on the marrow stromal elements have been less well studied, and the long-term effects of marrow stromal injury induced by agents used in the treatment of Hodgkin's disease is not known. Busulfan stimulates fibrosis, both in marrow and other organs (i.e., lungs), and busulfan marrow injury may be profound, suggesting that other alkylating agents may induce similar but less significant injury. Chemotherapy agents are known to injure endothelial cells inducing a phlebitis, most often, in peripheral veins. It is not inconceivable, however, that marrow sinusoidal injury may result.

Although numerous animal model studies have been performed investigating the bone marrow reserve after the acute administration of chemotherapeutic agents, including nitrogen mustard,[66,67] cyclophosphamide,[67,68] and vinblastine,[32,66] few studies in humans have been undertaken to measure the hematopoietic reserves several years after chemotherapy has been administered.[69] Studies of granulopoietic reserves several years after chemotherapy has been administered are not available for patients treated for Hodgkin's disease. With increasingly effective chemotherapy and subsequently improved survival, however, a much larger population of patients is available for analysis, and studies addressing these questions are likely to appear. Because many patients have received radiation therapy, as well, the prolonged effects of chemotherapy alone are difficult to evaluate. Few studies are available that explore bone marrow hematopoiesis after exposure to radiation and chemotherapy.[70,71] The administration of adriamycin significantly impaired the stem cell reserves of irradiated mice,[72] suggesting that combined modality approaches may be associated with longer lasting defects in hematopoiesis.

Because of its systemic administration, chemotherapy is more myelosuppressive in the short term than radiation therapy, which most often is delivered only to a part of the hematopoietic tissue. The degree of marrow injury, however, for a given exposed marrow area is probably greater for radiotherapy than chemotherapy, because free radicals induce a more toxic cellular injury than alkylation.[73] The LD 100/30 for human bone marrow is about 1000 cGy.[74] Radiation induces both stromal[75] and stem cell compartment[76] injury; however, persistent clonogenic function (regenerative capacity) and recovery can be demonstrated in stem cell assays. Stromal alterations induced by radiation therapy were among the earliest observations in the hematology literature.[75,77] Fibrosis in the bone marrow may be seen after radiation-induced injury and may effect long-term hematopoiesis.[75] Radiation-induced changes in endothelium are common.[75] Recent information suggests that even modest dosages of radiation may alter this microenvironment.[78] The latter is particularly important because of reseeding of hematopoietic stem cells in irradiated regions by normal bone marrow. In a study of irradiated sternal bone marrow in breast cancer patients, only 2 of 33 patients demonstrated recovery after 4500 cGy up to 84 months after irradiation.[79,80] Repeat sternal bone marrows in patients treated with mantle ports have shown some regenerative capacity,[81] although others have found only minimal regeneration (96% either hypoplastic or aplastic).[82] In spite of normal peripheral blood parameters, iliac crest bone marrow studies used as a control specimen for "nonirradiated areas" demonstrated slight hypoplasia in 38% of patients,[82] suggesting a distant effect of radiation therapy, since no chemotherapy had been administered. Other studies have not confirmed this observation.[81]

Because most hematopoietic tissue in the adult is found in the axial skeleton,[83] nearly 75% of the bone marrow may be irradiated during extended-field irradiation for Hodgkin's disease.[84] The time frame of myelosuppression and recovery depends on the extent of the radiation port, dosage, and age of the patient.[74,79–81,85–88,397] Since the axial skeleton is most often irradiated, outerlying marrow regions become important for reconstitution of marrow reserves, and the loss of these outerlying regions with age will have a significant impact on these stores. Various methods of bone marrow scanning have been employed to study bone marrow regeneration after radiation therapy, including ^{99m}Tc-S scans[74]; ^{52}Fe scans[89]; ^{59}Fe scans[85]; and ^{111}InCl scans.[86] Using ^{99m}Tc-S scanning, a rough measure of marrow reserves, the recovery from total-nodal radiation may be followed with time.[74] Little in-field marrow regeneration is seen between 6 months to a year after treatment. Within two years, however, 85% of irradiated areas demonstrate regeneration with 55% of patients having apparently normal activity, even after 4,000 to 5,000 cGy exposure.[74] Prior chemotherapy does not appear to influence this regeneration.[74] Recovery of normal blood counts (not synonymous with normal reserves) after total irradiation generally occurs between 2 to 6 months after completion of therapy. Serial studies using ^{111}InCl demonstrate initial redistribution of marrow from axial to more peripheral locations (skull, femurs, humeri).[86] A year after radiotherapy, a gradual return to a more axial distribution may be noted. After 5 years, almost all patients irradiated for Hodgkin's disease do not demonstrate evidence of hematologic suppression.[90]

Although ferrokinetic studies are normal after mantle-field irradiation (hemoglobin level, radioiron red-cell utilization, and plasma iron turnover), only modest recovery is noted in the irradiated area utilizing ^{59}Fe scanning, even up to 13 years after irradiation.[85] This is in contrast to studies using ^{99m}Tc-S, which demonstrate significant recovery. Extension of bone marrow into distal bones, as well as extramedullary hematopoiesis, has been observed.[85] Ineffective erythropoiesis, with evidence of ferrokinetic abnormalities, is more commonly observed after extended-field irradiation.[85] The administration of chemotherapy did not appear to alter these observations. Granulopoietic reserve has been measured after radiation therapy.[91] Depending on the dose administered, either exhaustion with late marrow failure or decreased responsiveness to hematopoietic stress may result. The latter situation may be observed by the decreased tolerance to chemotherapy after radiation.[74] Although normal blood counts are observed in patients treated with chemotherapy and radiotherapy, when stressed during episodes of infection or bleeding, the normal responses, such as neutrophilia or reticulocytosis, may be impaired with a subsequent decreased ability to fight infection or compensate hemodynamically for blood loss. The occurrence of pancytopenia several years after radiation therapy generally signals the onset of a myelodysplastic syndrome, leukemia, or progressive Hodgkin's disease with bone-marrow involvement.

The long-term effects of chemotherapy agents on gonadal function in males relate to impaired spermatogenesis with tubular epithelial damage rather than decreased production of androgens.[92] Androgens remain at normal levels because Sertoli and Leydig cells remain histologically and functionally normal. Therefore, the effects of androgen deprivation on erythropoiesis, which have been known since 1941,[93] are not observed in male patients treated for Hodgkin's disease. Oligomenorrhea and amenorrhea with low urinary estrogens, high urinary gonadotrophins, high serum gonadotrophin and estradiol are common during and after chemotherapy for Hodgkin's disease.[94-96] Chronic administration of cyclophosphamide (10 to 39 months) results in a high frequency of amenorrhea and ovarian failure, with minimal return of ovarian function.[97] Although the inhibitory effect of synthetic estrogens on erythropoiesis has been demonstrated by the use of ^{59}Fe incorporation studies, there is no evidence that replacement therapy impairs hematopoiesis.

The incidence of treatment-related hypothyroidism in a large series of 235 Hodgkin's disease patients treated with neck irradiation is approximately 64%, with 44% compensated (elevated TSH, normal T_4) and 20% overtly hypothyroid (elevated TSH, decreased T_4).[98] Other series show a somewhat lesser incidence.[82] Although anemia may be present in as many as 50% of patients with "idiopathic" hypothyroidism,[99] only a minority (5%) are related to thyroxine deficiency alone, the rest being associated with iron deficiency and pernicious anemia. The blood smear in pure hypothyroid anemia is normochromic and normocytic, with occasional contracted erythrocytes noted in approximately 50% of patients.[100] The anemia is generally mild with normal red-cell survival. Because of the contracted plasma volume, anemia may be more severe than initially thought. Ferrikinetic studies and erythropoietin levels, which are useful in defining the anemia of the hypothyroid state, may not accurately reflect the role of thyroxine deficiency because of marrow injury in the treated patient and the associated dyserythropoiesis. Thyroid replacement corrects this deficiency in erythropoiesis. Disorders of hemostasis may be observed in the hypothyroid state, clinically manifested by excessive bleeding.[387] Decreased antihemophilic factor (factor VIII) and plasma thromboplastin antecedent (factor XI)[101] and an increase in blood fibrinolytic activity have been reported.[334,387]

BIOLOGY OF LEUKEMIC PROLIFERATION

Leukemic hematopoiesis results in the expansion of an abnormal stem cell population with a significant increase in self-renewal capacity and a decrease in terminal differentiation. This has been demonstrated in vitro by comparing normal granulocyte-macrophage progenitor cells to the WEHI-3B myelomonocytic leukemic cells.[102] This self-renewal capacity is influenced by at least one lymphokine (interleukin-3) reported to stimulate the pluripotent stem cell.[102] This lymphokine is produced by both normal and neoplastic cell lines (T cells, thymic lymphoma) and by leukemia cells themselves (WEHI-3B).[102] The appearance of a leukemic clone secreting these lymphokines results in a self-stimulatory process (autocrine-type secretion), which results in an obvious growth advantage over normal stem cells. Colony stimulating factors may also induce differentiation of leukemic cell lines, but sublines may be resistant to its effects (D-sublines).[103] A number of agents (e.g., cytotoxic agents, cortisone, phorbol esters),[104] including CSFs,[249,317] can induce leukemic cells to differentiate and lose this self-renewal capacity. Studies with such agents are presently undergoing clinical trials, which may result in novel approaches for the treatment of leukemic hematopoiesis.[104]

The phenotypic properties of leukemic cells are related to cytogenetic alterations. Chromosomal abnormalities are commonly observed in leukemic cells (see Table 4–10) and consist of gains, losses, and rearrangements.[313,340,354,390–393] A gain of chromosome 8 (+8) and a loss of parts of chromosome 7 (7q−) are the most commonly observed alterations. Frequent translocations and structural alterations include t9;22 (q34;q11) in chronic myelogenous leukemia, t8;21 [t(8q−;21q+)] in acute myelogenous leukemia (M2), t15;17 [t(15q+;17q−)] in acute promyelocytic leukemia (M3), and chromosome 11 rearrangements in acute monocytic leukemia (M5). Leukemias noted after treatment of another malignancy with cytotoxic agents or radiation therapy (S-ANLL) are manifested by cytogenetic abnormalities in almost all patients. Hypodiploidy with involvement of chromosomes 5 (−5) and 7 (−7) are the most common observations. An unusual chromosomal abnormality, a deletion of the short arm of chromosome 16 del (16)(q22), has been reported both in de novo ANLL,[106] as well as in a case of S-ANLL after treatment for a non-Hodgkin's lymphoma.[107]

Although the critical events in leukemogenesis are almost certainly related to these structural alterations, only recently, through oncogene research, has this relationship been clarified. RNA retroviruses are now recognized as the predominant carcinogenic viruses throughout the animal kingdom; they cause a variety of neoplasms, including carcinomas, sarcomas, leukemias, and lymphomas.[108–111] The presence of reverse transcriptase (pol gene product) permits synthesis of DNA from the RNA template, which allows viral genome incorporation in the host and viral replication.[112] Other proteins are transcribed from the gag (viral core protein) and env (protein envelope) genes. The incorporation of oncogenes within the genomic material of the virus allows rapid malignant change to occur when viruses enter the cell. Viruses that lack identifiable oncogenes induce malignant changes more slowly, necessitating a close interaction with a cellular oncogene.[113] The result of oncogene transcription is the production of oncoproteins. The latter function as phosphokinases, DNA-binding proteins, or growth factors, and induce in as yet an unknown fashion, neoplastic proliferation. Both quantitative and qualitative changes in oncogene expression have been described. It is likely that secondary cancers seen after therapy for Hodgkin's disease result from alterations in DNA induced by radiation or chemotherapy, and that these physical injuries occur near areas of oncogenes. Among the oncogenes involved in leukemic cell transformation are the myc oncogene on chromosome 8 (translocated to 14 in Burkitt's lymphoma) and the abl oncogene translocated to chromosome 22 in chronic myelocytic leukemia.[114]

It has been recognized for nearly a century that various physical agents induce leukemia in animals, including primates.[115] Myeloid, monocytic, and stem-cell leukemias have been observed in mice exposed to ionizing radiation, including isotopes such as ^{32}P.[116–118] Transplantation experiments using irradiated thymic issue[119] suggests the appearance of viruses from the donor tissue, which are capable of inducing leukemia. The mechanism by which radiation allows the appearance of such viruses in an oncogenic form is not known, but occurs in vitro as well.[120] The association of radiation exposure and leukemia in humans is based on the results of catastrophic events and the statistical increase in leukemia among individuals exposed to a spectrum of radiation dosages.[121–125] For individuals exposed to the Hiroshima bomb (0 to 3000 meters from the epicenter), there has been a greater than thirtyfold increase in leukemia when compared to the unexposed.[126] ALL, AML, and CML, but not CLL, were increased. The latency period varied from 9.3 to 12.6 years, depending on the age at the time of exposure. Morphologic abnormalities preceded the development of acute leukemia and included giant neutrophils and basophils, immature eosinophils, and binucleate and multiple lobulated megakaryocytes.[127] The earliest reports of an increase in leukemia in patients treated with radiation for a medical indication were those following irradiation for ankylosing spondylitis,[128] "thymic hypertrophy" in childhood,[124] and menometrorrhagia.[129] Occupational radiation exposure (i.e., radiologists) has likewise been associated with an increased risk.[122] Although environmental exposure and diagnostic radiologic examinations are unlikely to result in a significant risk of leukemia, doses received during therapeutic radiation may well be responsible for at least some leukemias after treatment. There is a significantly increased risk of secondary leukemia after ^{32}P treatment of polycythemia vera.[130] Radiation is known to induce breaks in DNA, and presumably, if excision repair mechanisms are faulty in sublethally irradiated cells, chromosomal abnormalities may persist. The biochemical mechanism by which such abnormalities are translated into leukemia is not known. Chromosomal abnormalities may be noted preceding leukemia in cases with anemia and in cases with no apparent hematologic disorders.

Numerous compounds have been recognized as lymphoma- or leukemia-inducing in rodents. These include organochemicals, such as methylcholanthrene,[131] as well as a number of chemotherapeutic agents, including procarbazine,[140] nitrosoureas,[132] and alkylating agents.[116,133,134] As with radiation in rodents, murine leukemia viruses (MULVs) have been isolated from chemically induced leukemias.[115] Chemical carcinogenesis results from a multistep process of initiation and promotion. The critical target for initiation are bases in nucleic acids. Both alkylating agents and nitrosoureas interact with such bases. It is conceivable, therefore, that throughout the course of chemotherapy, initiating steps in chemical carcinogenesis are occurring. Whether leukemia will ultimately result depends on cellular repair mechanisms, genetic factors, immunocompetence, and exposure of cells to sublethal physical injury (i.e., radiation). The fact that secondary leukemias are rare suggests that host protective factors are capable of controlling these carcinogenic changes in most patients. A number of chemicals, particularly benzene[135] and drugs such as chloramphenicol[136] and phenylbutazone,[137] have been implicated as causes of acute leukemia in humans. Each of these agents is associated with marrow injury and a period of myelosuppression preceding leukemic change. The appearance of acute leukemia has been observed after exposure to lithium.[138] Chemotherapeutic agents, particularly alkylating agents (cyclophosphamide, melphalan, chlorambucil), procarbazine, and nitrosoureas have all been implicated as leukemia-causing agents in primates and humans[139-143] because of their known leukemogenic and carcinogenic potential in animal models.[144] Disorders in which these agents have been used and in which leukemia has developed include multiple myeloma,[145-148] Waldenström's macroglobulinemia,[148] Hodgkin's disease,[149,150] non-Hodgkin's lymphoma,[145,151-154] chronic lymphocytic leukemia,[152,155,156] polycythemia vera,[130] and a variety of solid neoplasms and non-neoplastic disorders.[157-161]

Apart from physical and biologic agents, susceptibility to leukemia and lymphoma depends on both genetic and constitutional influences. Considering that only a small percentage of patients treated for Hodgkin's disease with combined modality approaches (likely to be most leukemogenic) develop second malignancies, these influences must play a significant role. Genetic influences are apparent in the high incidence of spontaneous thymic lymphoma in certain strains of mice (AKR)[162] and in the need for host genetic material, which determines a susceptibility for viral genomic leukemic transformation by endogenous murine leukemia virus (MuLV).[162] This latter agent does not appear to be responsible for the appearance of radiation or carcinogen-induced thymoma.[163] In young animals, both x-irradiation and chemically induced leukemias are frequently observed.[164] Sex and hormonal balance may also be important in leukemogenesis but are infrequently, if at all, considered etiologic factors.[165,166]

Immunocompetence is necessary in order to prevent neoplastic proliferation.[167] The development of Hodgkin's disease itself may at least be partially a reflection of impaired immunity. Immunologic defects have been observed in healthy siblings of patients with Hodgkin's disease, suggesting a possible constitutional propensity.[168] While the disease is present and after treatment, immunocompetence is compromised further, which may result in an increased susceptibility to neoplasia. In MuLV infected mice, radiation-induced immunosuppression may increase the incidence of spontaneous leukemia.[169] In humans immunosuppressive therapy for primary nonmalignant disease is associated with the development of leukemia and lymphoma.[157,170-173] Whereas drugs capable of injuring DNA (i.e., alkylating agents such as melphalan and chlorambucil) are directly responsible for the leukemias noted, antimetabolites that are less likely to irreversibly alter DNA (i.e., azathioprine, methotrexate) probably act indirectly through alterations in lymphocyte subpopulations. In certain constitutional immunocompromised states[174] and disorders manifested by abnormalities of immunoregulation,[173] the incidence of leukemia and lymphoma may be significantly higher; for example, as in the Wiskott-Aldrich syndrome.[174]

ABNORMALITIES OF LYMPHOPOIESIS AND IMMUNOREGULATION

Alterations in immune function are commonly observed in patients with Hodgkin's disease.[175] Disorders of both cell-mediated[175-177] and humoral immunity[178] have been described in newly diagnosed as well as treated patients in remission. Subtle changes in immune competence in siblings[179] suggest that impaired immunity may be one of the earliest markers of Hodgkin's disease. Lymphoid proliferation is considerably more difficult to study than myelopoiesis, and indirect methods of study (immunoglobulin levels, in vitro stimulation by mitogens and antigens, skin tests, etc.) have been used when studying the long-term effects of these agents. One of the earliest clinical observations demonstrating impaired cellular immunity was the observation of cutaneous anergy to tuberculin first described in 1902.[180] In more recent years, numerous reports have appeared demonstrating cutaneous anergy to a variety of skin test antigens[175,181,182] as well as abnormal in vitro responses to PHA.[181] The degree of anergy is clearly related to the extent of disease activity.[167] Lymphocyte depletion,[175] both of T and B lymphocytes,[183] is commonly observed, as are qualitative abnormalities demonstrated by in vitro hyporesponsiveness.[175] Not only are these changes seen in untreated patients, but abnormalities have been demonstrated in patients in apparent remission.[184] This suggests an underlying immunosuppressed state as well as a treatment effect. Humoral immunity remains well preserved in untreated Hodgkin's disease patients in spite of B lymphocyte depletion,[185] although subtle abnormalities have been described.[178] Normal levels of immunoglobulins are generally observed,[185] even after total nodal or extended-field irradiation;[90] only rarely has hypogammaglobulinemia been reported.[178] Recently, it has been recognized that the immunosuppressed patient may be susceptible to graft versus host disease, which complicates blood product administration. This disorder, a result of the immunoreactivity of donor lymphocytes, is a common accompaniment of bone marrow transplantation and was described in a patient in remission from Hodgkin's disease in 1980.[186] Although a rare occurrence, this devastating complication may be prevented by administering only irradiated blood products.

Lymphopoiesis is inhibited by chemotherapy[58] and radiation therapy.[82] These alterations are probably longer lasting and more profound than the inhibitory effects on the production of myeloid tissue, and there is a striking depletion of lymphoid tissue after total nodal irradiation; the long-term effects of this may not be evident for many years. Although unproven, erythropoiesis, being partially mediated by T-cell proliferation, may not be completely normal after such therapy until immunocompetence is restored. Prolonged immune suppression, occurring after alkylating agent administration has been studied, and using a plaque-forming cell assay demonstrates immune stem-cell depletion.[58]

The long-term effects of inhibited lymphoid proliferation may play a permissive role in allowing the appearance and subsequent growth advantage of abnormal clones of cells induced by either chemotherapy, radiation therapy, or viruses. The increasing incidence of lymphoproliferative and endothelial (Kaposi's sarcoma) malignancy in patients with acquired immunodeficiency syndrome (AIDS) underscores the important role of normal lymphopoiesis and the consequence of injury to or destruction of tissues and cells involved in this process or their use as a reservoir for infectious agents.[187] In 1985, Hodgkin's disease itself was reported to be a complication of this syndrome.[187] In fact, non-Hodgkin's lymphomas are observed in Hodgkin's disease patients, either as a long-term consequence of therapy or as a reflection of a constitutionally immunocompromised host.

Although impaired immunocompetence is a feature present in most patients with Hodgkin's disease, evidence of immune activation is present as well. Both T[188] and B[189] lymphocytes appear to show evidence of in vivo activation. Reactive splenomegaly, noncaseating granulomas,[177] increased serum migration inhibition factor (MIF),[190] increased bone marrow plasmacytosis and eosinophilia,[191] increased splenic lymphocyte immunoglobulin production,[189] increased monocyte-mediated antibody-dependent cellular cytotoxicity (MD-ADCC),[192] increased number of T cells and Ia+, ANAE-, E-rosette forming cells (activated T cells) in involved lymph nodes,[193,194] increased T_4/T_8 ratio in lymph nodes,[194-196] immune complex disease[197] and injury to lymphoid cells[198] are all manifestations of this hyperreactivity. These alterations suggest that imbalances in cell populations, particularly of T cells, result in both compromised immunity and at the same time, hyperreactivity. Alternatively, regional hyperreactivity in an organ system (i.e., monocyte-macrophages in the spleen),[199] with progressive sparing of suppressor lymphocytes during lymphocyte depletion, may be responsible for this dysimmunoregulation. Increased macrophage activity, as reflected in increased lysozyme levels, has been observed.[200]

Antibodies directed against circulating blood cells, although unusual, are observed in Hodgkin's disease as in other lymphoproliferative disorders. These "auto"-antibodies are directed against red-blood cells, platelets, neutrophils, and lymphocytes, resulting in immunohemolytic anemia, immune thrombocytopenic purpura, autoimmune neutropenia, and lymphopenia. Antibodies directed against monocytes have not been described. These antibodies may be specific and directed against antigenic determinants on the surface of the cell, against antigens shared in common between the tumor and cell, or nonspecific in the form of immune complexes deposited on the surface of the cell. The presence of antibodies on the surface of cells results in rapid clearance of cells through the monocyte-macrophage system.

Immunohemolytic anemia (AIHA) has been recognized as a complication of Hodgkin's disease for a number of years.[201-224] This syndrome may antedate the diagnosis, occur simultaneously with its appearance, or appear several years after treatment, at which time it may or may not be a harbinger of relapse (Table 4-4; Fig. 4-2). The reported incidence of a positive direct Coombs' test in patients with Hodgkin's disease ranges from 2.7 to 24%.[210,214,215] The incidence of overt hemolytic anemia is less, however, ranging from 3 to 10%.[210,214] Most patients with Hodgkin's disease do not have a Coombs' test performed as part of a routine screening or staging workup, suggesting that there is patient selection in reports of the incidence of Coombs' positivity in Hodgkin's disease, and the actual incidence of this observation may be somewhat less. In the largest series of patients with Hodgkin's disease studied,[210] 8 of 10 patients with a positive direct Coombs' test had one or more episodes of overt hemolytic anemia. Immune thrombocytopenia was noted in two of these patients. In a large series of patients with malignant lymphoma, five patients with Hodgkin's disease had AIHA (5 of 109 or 4.5%), and this represented 35% of the AIHAs seen in this group of diseases.[217] In a series of 104 patients with AIHA, 8% had Hodgkin's disease.[223] The antibody is, in general, an IgG antibody of warm-reacting type; it demonstrates its affinity for a red-cell membrane antigen at 37°C. The antibody is probably di-

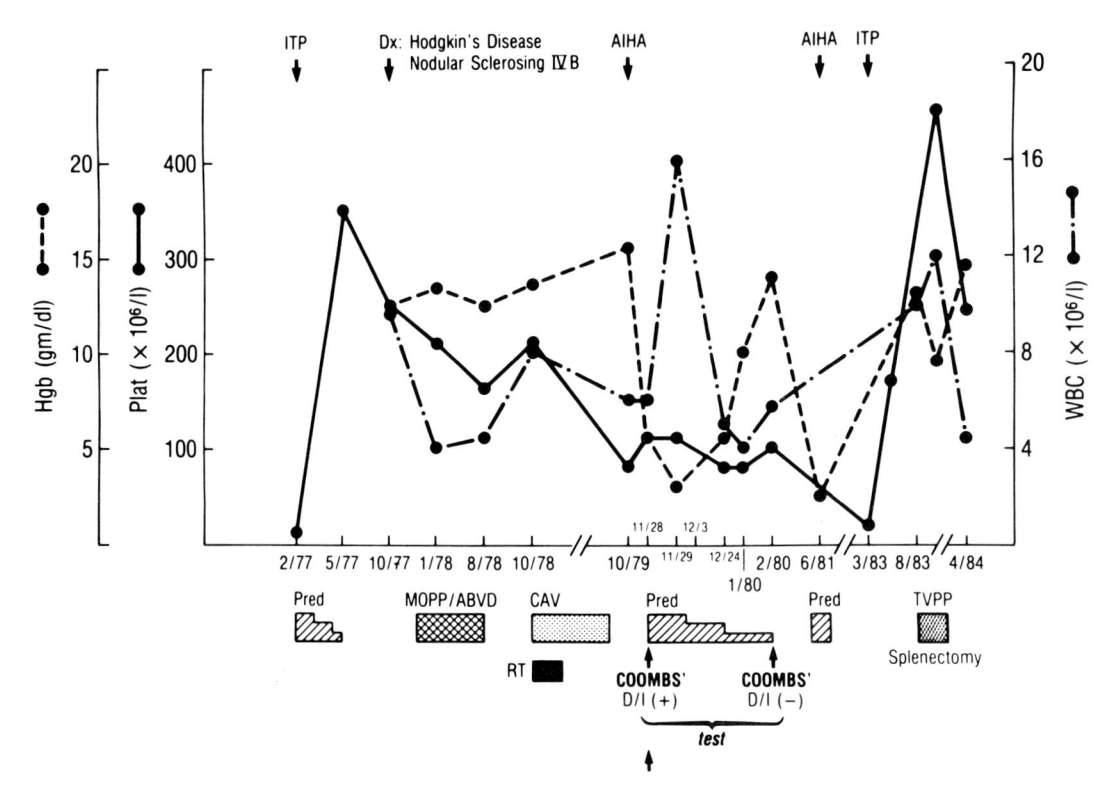

Fig. 4–2. Male patient, age 31, with autoimmune hemolytic anemia and idiopathic thrombocytopenic purpura (ITP) in Hodgkin's disease.

rected against a glycoprotein of the Rh system of membrane proteins, although the exact antigenic determinant in most cases has not been demonstrated. Antibodies with specificity against the I+ antigen[225] as well as the e antigen[207] have been described. It is not known if the Hodgkin's disease cell shares a similar determinant and therefore if the pathogenesis is related to an immune reaction directed against the Hodgkin's disease. In view of the appearance of the antibody and the similar clinical presentation in patients apparently "cured" of the disease, dysimmunoregulation rather than a tumor-specific antigen-antibody reaction is likely to be the pathogenesis. Therapy itself, by altering immunoregulation, may be responsible for the appearance of "auto-immune" states, as has been observed in CLL after the use of radiation and chemotherapy.[226] There are no reports of an IgA antibody responsible for the hemolytic anemia, as for example, in other lymphoproliferative diseases. IgM antibodies are rare, and the syndrome of cold agglutinin disease has not been reported.[210] Once the antibody is present on the surface of the red blood cell, Fc receptors, present on monocytes and macrophages, are responsible for their sequestration in environmentally unfavorable locations (spleen, liver); cell death eventually results.

The clinical picture of immunohemolytic anemia in Hodgkin's disease does not differ from that seen with other disorders. In general, a profound and sudden drop in red-blood-cell count is manifested by pallor, weakness, and dyspnea on exertion. As heme is degraded to bilirubin, acholuric jaundice results with an increase in unconjugated (indirect) bilirubin. Pruritis, unless present as a paraneoplastic syndrome, is absent and the stool is normally colored. Examination of the blood smear discloses anisopoikilocytosis, spherocytosis, schistocytes, polychromasia, and an increase in reticulocytes. The latter, however, may not be observed in a marrow-compromised patient. Such changes must be differentiated from those seen after splenectomy, which may have a similar pattern. The

LATE HEMATOLOGIC COMPLICATIONS AFTER TREATMENT OF HODGKIN'S DISEASE

Table 4-4. Autoimmune Hemolytic Anemia (AIHA)

Reference (Year)	No. Pts./ Series	Tx HD	Active HD at Time of AIHA	Months from Dx HD to Dx AIHA	Coombs'/ Overt Hemolysis	Tx AIHA	Result
Brown et al.[204] (1949)	1/	A	yes	*0	1/2	SP	PR(+)
Wasserman et al.[223] (1955)	8/104	S-B	(?)	20	1/2	S-B	PR
		A(spleen)	no	*-5	(?)/2	A	NR(+)
		A	no	*-2	0/2	SP-A	R(+)
		?	yes	*0	0/2	none	R(spont)
		A-B	yes	*0	0/2	A-B	NR(+)
		A-B	no	*-12	1/2	A-S	PR
		S-B	(?)	48	0/2	S-B	R(+)
		(?)	(?)	8	(?)/2	S	R(+)
Kyle et al.[213] (1959)	†7/	(?)	no	*-2	(?)/2	(?)	(?)
		(?)	yes	*0	1/2	(?)	(?)
		(?)	yes	2	0/2	(?)	(?)
		(?)	yes	*0	0/2	(?)	(?)
		(?)	yes	*0	1/2	(?)	(?)
		(?)	yes	*0	1/2	(?)	(?)
		(?)	no	*-216	1/2	(?)	(?)
Videbaek[222] (1962)	2/	S-B	yes	*0	1/2	S-B	PR(+)
		A-B	(?)	60	1/2	(?)	(?)
Payet et al.[218] (1964)	1/	(?)	no	48	(?)	(?)	(?)
Dacie[209] (1967)	1/	S	yes	*0	1/2	SP-P	(+)
Eisner et al.[210] (1967)	†6/219 (+4 additional)	A	yes	38	1/2	O	P
		S-B-A	yes	0.5	1/2	S	R(+)
		(?)	yes	132	1/2	A	R(+)
		A	yes	94	1/2	A-S	R
		(?)	yes	*0	1/2	S-SP	R(+)
		(?)	yes	10	1/2	A-S	P(+)
		(?)	yes	5	1/2	O	P(+)
		(?)	yes	13	1/2	S-A	P(+)
		(?)	yes	41	1/?	(?)	(?)
		(?)	yes	84	1/?	S	(+)
Miller[217] (1967)	†5/109						
Pirofsky[219] (1968)‡	†3/-	(?)	yes	*0	(?)	(?)	(?)
		(?)	yes	*0	(?)	(?)	(?)
		(?)	yes	*0	(?)	(?)	(?)
	†10/-	(?)	(?)	(3-132) range	(?)	(?)	(?)
Osta et al.[282] (1970)	1	A	yes	*4	1/2	S	R(+)
Garratty et al.[225] (1972)	1/-	A	(?)	17	1/(?)	(?)	(?)
Jones[212] (1973)	2/-	A(splenic)	yes	20	1/2	S-B	R(+)
		SP	yes	20	1/2	S-B	R
Garratty et al.[211] (1974)	3/-	A	yes	168	1/2	S	PR
		S	no	10	1/2	S	PR(+)
		SP	no	*-12	1/2	S	(?)
Stojcevski[220] (1974)	†6/-	S-B	yes	9	1/2	S-B	R
		(?)	(?)	(?)	1/2	(?)	(?)
		(?)	(?)	(?)	1/2	(?)	(?)
		(?)	(?)	(?)	1/2	(?)	(?)
		S-B	yes	*0	1/2	S-B	NR(+)
		(?)	(?)	(?)	0/2	(?)	(?)

Table 4-4. Autoimmune Hemolytic Anemia (AIHA) Continued

Reference (Year)	No. Pts./ Series	Tx HD	Active HD at Time of AIHA	Months from Dx HD to Dx AIHA	Coombs'/ Overt Hemolysis	Tx AIHA	Result
Chu et al.[208] (1976)	1	(?)	yes	*0	1/2	S	PR
May et al.[216] (1976)	1	C	yes	*0	1/2	S	PR
Rosenthal[389] (1978)	1	A	yes	*0	1/2	S-SP	PR
Kedar et al.[201] (1979)	1	C	yes	*0	1/2	CM	R
Levine et al.[214] (1980)	7/71	B	yes	*0	1/	B	R
		B	yes	46	1/2	S-B	R
		B	yes	*0	1/2	B	R
		B	yes	32	1/	B	R
		B	yes	30	1/	B	NR(+)
		B	yes	*0	1/	B	R
		B	yes	30	1/2	B	R
Bjorkholm et al.[203] (1982)	(4)1/-	SP	no	*−108	0→1/2	S-SP	R
Weitberg et al.[224] (1984)	1/-	B	yes	96	1/2	B	(?)
Kempin (1989)	(3)1/-	C	no	24	1/2	S	R
			yes	32	(?)	S-SP-B	R

*initial presentation/antedated diagnosis
†complete information not available on these patients
‡13 cases out of a series of 234 cases of autoimmune hemolytic anemia
R = remission (AIHA)
P = partial remission (AIHA)
NR = non-responding AIHA
(+) = death
S = steroids
SP = splenectomy
(?) = information unavailable
A = radiotherapy
B = chemotherapy
C = combined modality
(1) = direct Coombs' positive
(2) = overt hemolytic anemia
(3) = two episodes
(4) = chronic relapsing AIHA: primary splenic presentation of HD

white-blood-cell count may be increased. The platelet count is generally normal. Serologically, a direct and indirect antiglobulin test (Coombs' test) is positive with the antibody functioning as a panagglutinin. Occasionally, only an antibody directed against complement is responsible for a positive test, with an apparent absence of immunoglobulin on the surface. Approximately 10% of immunohemolytic anemias have a negative antiglobulin test, which is related most often to potent antibodies with low membrane density. A serum haptoglobin was subnormal in 4 of 8 patients with overt hemolysis in one series.[210] The lactic acid dehydrogenase level is always elevated. An increased lysozyme may be present if increased monocyte-macrophage activity is partially responsible for the destruction.

The appearance of an immunohemolytic anemia in a previously treated patient does not necessarily represent definitive evidence for relapse (Fig. 4-2), although at least 50% of late onset immunohemolytic anemias are associated with recurrent disease (Table 4-4). The immunohemolytic anemia may be isolated or be associated with another immunocytopenia (Fig. 4–2). If anemia appears, a vigorous work-up for recurrent disease, including a splenectomy if no obvious disease is found, is necessary. The latter can in fact be helpful in improving red-cell survival in spite of the absence of disease.

Treatment of immunohemolytic anemia does not differ from that in other lymphoproliferative diseases. Treatment of the underlying disease is the most effective therapy for the complication. Frequently, however, no recurrent disease is found. A corticosteroid is administered (i.e., prednisone 1 mg/kg/PO/daily) until a maximum response is obtained. This is generally observed after several weeks. Folic acid (1 mg/PO/daily) is also administered. If patients are kept in bed during this period of time, only rarely are blood transfusions necessary, even at low levels of hemoglobin. If a satisfactory result is not achieved and a splenectomy has not been performed, this should be done. Occasionally, splenic irradiation may be useful. The absence of Howell-Jolly bodies on a blood smear from a splenectomized patient suggests the presence of accessory splenic tissue, and a search for this should be undertaken since its removal may be necessary. Cytotoxic therapy may be considered if corticosteroids or splenectomy are unsuccessful. Either single alkylating agent therapy, or azathioprine may be tried first. If unsuccessful, an empiric trial of MOPP or another antiHodgkin's disease regimen can be used because the majority of late AIHAs are seen with recurrent disease. High-dose gammaglobulin has been successfully employed in certain cases of AIHA and may be tried.[227] Recently, danazol has been shown to be effective in treating AIHA, and this agent may be employed.[228] Lastly, a trial of radiation therapy (irradiation of abdominal Hodgkin's disease, total nodal irradiation) may be attempted if all else fails.

Immune-mediated thrombocytopenia may antedate the diagnosis, occur simultaneously at presentation, or occur late in the course of the Hodgkin's disease as a harbinger of relapse or in the apparently cured patient (Figs. 4–2 and 4–3).[229–242] In Table 4–5, 35 cases have been collected from the literature, of which seven (20%) significantly antedated or occurred at the time of diagnosis. Sensitization of platelets by platelet-specific immunoglobulin or the deposition on the platelet surface of immune complexes and their subsequent removal by the monocyte-macrophage system[243] represent the pathogenic mechanisms of decreased platelet survival. The subclass IgG_1 is found in highest concentration in the idiopathic variety, followed by IgG_2, IgG_3, and IgG_4.[244] Platelet associated immunoglobulin (PAIg) has been reported in several series of patients with Hodgkin's disease who developed immune thrombocytopenia;[230,234,245] its disappearance was documented when the patient achieved remission of the Hodgkin's disease.[245] Serum antibodies against platelets have also been described in this setting.[201,235,236,240,245] Although biochemical determinations of the antibody, by gel chromatography and splenic lymphocyte cultures with harvesting of the antibody,[246] suggest that the immunoglobulin is directed against a specific membrane antigen, this has not been identified. The observation that serum or platelet eluates from a significant number of patients with ITP binds to normal platelets but not to those from patients with Glanzmann's thrombasthenia[242,247] suggests that the antibody may have specificity for the platelet glycoprotein IIb-IIIa complex, which is absent or present in decreased amounts on the platelet membrane in this disorder.[248] One patient in this series was diagnosed as having Hodgkin's disease and an ITP-like syndrome (platelet count 10,000 × 10^6/liter, increased marrow megakaryocytes, increased amounts of platelet-associated IgG). An autoantibody was detected; it was directed against the glycoprotein IIb-IIIa complex. This ITP was noted in the setting of recurrent Hodgkin's disease. It is not known whether a common antigenic determinant, such as glycoprotein IIb or glycoprotein IIIa, is shared by the platelet/megakaryocyte and Hodgkin's cell, or if the appearance of the antibody is a reflection of disordered immunoregulation.

Immune thrombocytopenia presents most commonly with the appearance of purpura, particularly petechiae on the torso and extremities. Hematuria, gastrointestinal bleeding, and epistaxis may also occur. If present concurrently with the diagnosis of Hodgkin's

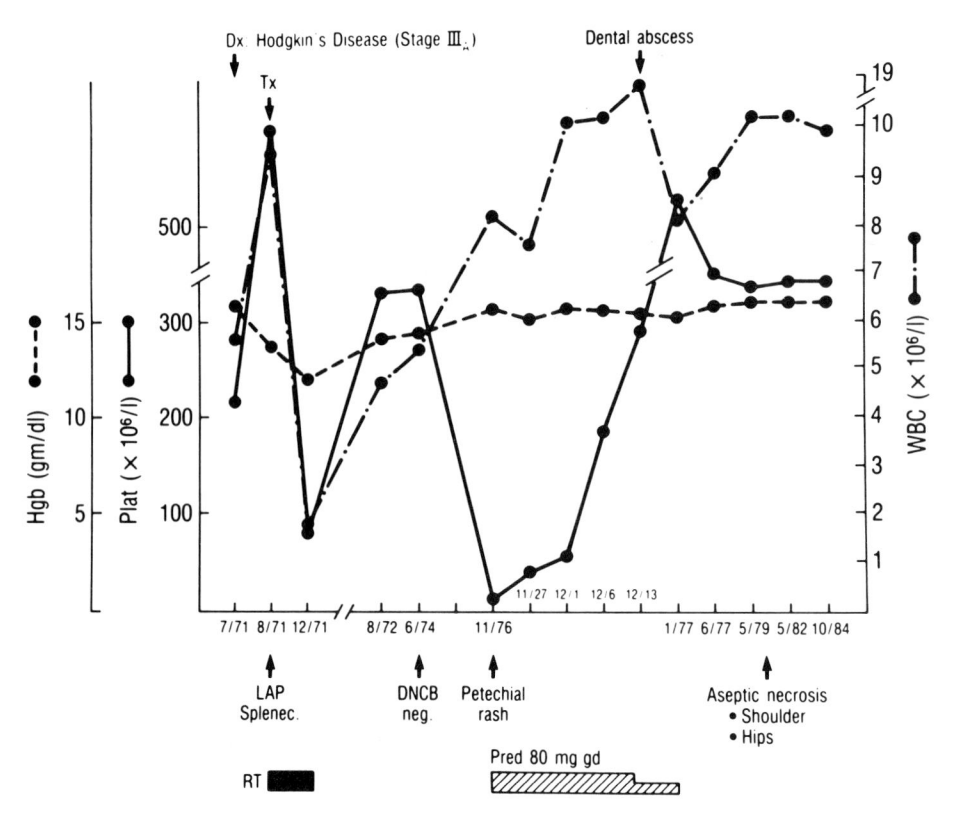

Fig. 4–3. Male patient, age 49, with idiopathic thrombocytopenic purpura (ITP) in setting of Hodgkin's disease.

disease, symptoms related to Hodgkin's disease are observed as well. Symptoms of anemia, such as pallor and fatigue, are also present if bleeding is significant. Splenomegaly is generally absent in the idiopathic thrombocytopenic syndrome. When present, it is difficult (in the absence of platelet antibody tests) to attribute the thrombocytopenia to an immune cause, rather than hypersplenism (secondary thrombocytopenic purpura).[250] Laboratory evaluation reveals a decreased platelet count and a normal red- and white-blood-cell count. Occasionally a Coombs' test will be positive if combined AIHA and ITP are present. AIHA was concommittantly present in two patients in a series (Table 4–5), and one patient serially developed ITP, followed by AIHA, and subsequently ITP at relapse (Fig. 4–2). No evidence of early myeloid forms or leukoerythroblastic blood smear was noted. Laboratory evaluation of the thrombocytopenic patient is outlined in Table 4–6. Measurements of serum antiplatelet antibodies and PAIg are the best methods used to detect the platelet-immunized state.[251] Its presence, if active disease and thrombocytopenia were present, might conceivably function as a tumor marker and its disappearance as a measure of the remission state.[230] One must distinguish this immune-mediated thrombocytopenia from the thrombocytopenia associated with treatment and the rare complication of thrombotic thrombocytopenic purpura.[252,253]

Once the diagnosis of immune thrombocytopenia is made, the patient begins corticosteroids (i.e., prednisone, 1 mg/kg/PO/ daily). A diagnostic work-up for recurrent disease is undertaken if the patient is thought to be in remission. Prednisone is continued until a maximum response is achieved and, as is the case with immunohemolytic anemia, this may take several weeks. The steroid dose is then tapered slowly, and if recurrent Hodgkin's disease is not documented, it may be discontinued with the patient in apparent remission. Splenectomy may be necessary if it

Table 4–5. Immune Thrombocytopenia (ITP) in Patients Treated for Hodgkin's Disease

Reference (Year)	No. Pts./ Series	Tx HD	Active HD	Months from Dx HD to Dx ITP	Tx/ITP	Result
Doan et al.[250] (1960)	4/-	—	—	—	—	—
Eisner et al.[210] (1967)	(*)1/-	—	yes	†0	—	—
Rudders et al.[239] (1972)	3/134	(1) A (2) A (3) B	yes no yes	48 24 †0	S/SP S/SP S/I/SP	R (+) P
Hamilton et al.[233] (1973)	1/-	A	yes	35	S/I/SP	R
Jones[212] (1973)	2/-	(1) SP (2) (?)	no no	(1) 37 (2) 132	S/I S/SP	R R
Khilanani et al.[236] (1973)	1/-		yes	†0	S/I/SP	R
Rudders[238] (1974)	(*)1/-	C	yes			
Antonio et al.[229] (1976)	1/-	A	no	32	S	R
Fink et al.[232] (1976)	3/-	(1) A (2) A (3) A	no; yes no yes	(1)† – 4/24 (2) 6 (3) 48	S/SP/S/I/B S/I/SP	R R P
Julia et al.[235] (1976)	1/-	A	no		S	R
Weitzman et al.[241] (1977)	1/-	C	yes	180	S/B	(+)
Cohen[231] (1978)	6/-	(1) A (2) C (3) C (4) C (5) C (6) A	(1) no (2) no (3) no (4) no (5) no (6) no	(1) 96 (2) 144 (3) 120 (4) 313 (5) 18 (6) 36	(1) S (2) S (3) S/I (4) S (5) S/I (6) S/I/S	P R R R R R
Kedar et al.[201] (1979)	2/-	(1) C (2) C	 no	52 81	S S	P R
Hassidim et al.[234] (1979)	1/-	B	yes	20	S/I/SP	P
Waddell et al.[240] (1979)	2/-	(1) SP (2) C	yes no	†0 6	S/B S	R (+)
Kirsher et al.[237] (1980)	2/-	(1) A (2) A	(1) no (1) no	(1) 36 (1) 41	(1) S (1) S	R R
Berkman et al.[230] (1983)	1/-	SP/B	yes	†0	B	R
Kempin (1989)	2/-	(1) C/SP-B (2) A-SP	no/yes no	(1)† – 11/73 (2) 64	 S	R/R R

*AIHA (in addition to ITP)
†Initial presentation/antedated diagnosis of Hodgkin's disease
R = remission ITP
P = partial remission ITP
(+) = death
S = steroids
SP = splenectomy
I = immunosuppressive
A = radiotherapy
B = chemotherapy
C = combined modality
S = splenectomy
(?) = Information not given

Table 4–6. Laboratory Evaluation of Suspected Immune Thrombocytopenia In Patients with Hodgkin's Disease

Complete blood count, reticulocyte count, and platelet count
Bone marrow aspirate and biopsy
Cytogenetics
Coombs' test
Antinuclear antibody
Sedimentation rate
Complete coagulation profile
Platelet survival study
Platelet autoantibody tests
　PAIg *indirect*
　　• clot retraction
　　• platelet migration inhibition
　　• platelet agglutination
　　• platelet lysis
　　• serotonin release
　　• platelet factor 3 availability
　PAIg *direct*
　　• direct binding
　　• two stage assays
　　• platelet lysates

has not already been performed and if steroid therapy cannot be stopped, if there are complications with its usage, or if there is a question of recurrent disease. Alternatives to splenectomy include splenic irradiation and immunosuppressive therapy. The latter will be in the form of chemotherapy if recurrent disease is documented. Bleomycin has been successfully employed in a patient with Hodgkin's disease in "remission," who subsequently developed ITP.[254] Danazol and vincristine may also be tried if steroids are ineffective. Gammaglobulin therapy may be employed as well.[255]

Autoimmune neutropenia is a rarely described disorder of Hodgkin's disease, with only three documented cases in the world's literature. Two cases occurred in the setting of active Hodgkin's disease, the first at diagnosis,[256] and the second at relapse.[224] Splenectomy transiently improved the neutrophil count, as did corticosteroids. MOPP therapy was associated with longer lasting control. In 1987, an asplenic patient developed immune neutropenia while in remission;[257] this occurred four years after mantle-radiation therapy for Stage IIA nodular sclerosing disease. The neutrophil count spontaneously was corrected. The presence of neutropenia unrelated to treatment should lead to a search for recurrent disease. Treatment should then be directed towards Hodgkin's disease, if it is present. If the patient is in remission, no treatment is indicated unless there are recurrent infections.

SECONDARY HEMATOPOIETIC MALIGNANCY

MYELODYSPLASIA AND LEUKEMIA

In addition to a decreased hematopoietic mass and abnormalities of immunoregulation, more profound changes may occur in bone-marrow tissue, resulting in myelodysplastic states and leukemia. These changes are the most serious long-term effects of antineoplastic therapy and are being increasingly observed after therapy for Hodgkin's disease.[145,149,150,258–292] Myelodysplastic states may result in mild pancytopenia, with no bone marrow abnormalities, only subtle changes, or in progressively abnormal bone-marrow maturation with an increase in apparently malignant myeloid and erythroid precursors.[293–295] Myelodysplastic syndromes with apparently normal bone-marrow morphology are probably common and consist of abnormalities in maturation representing intrinsic cellular defects as well as a decrease in normal stem cell mass. These latter states can be investigated by cytogenetics and by in vitro marrow culture techniques.[296–297] Cytogenetic abnormalities, such as increased breaks, aberrant response to CSFs, and in vitro growth inhibitors, are the earliest recognizable abnormalities. Such abnormalities may be seen in a small number of cells within an ostensibly normal stem-cell population or may be present in all hematopoietic cells. It is not known if the former states represent reversible changes with the possibility of gradual disappearance of the abnormal clone, or if the latter states represent premalignant hematopoiesis. A multistep pathogenesis of the myelodysplastic syndrome has been postulated based on studies combining cytogenetics and G6PD heterozygote analysis.[298] The incidence of mild dysmyelopoiesis in Hodgkin's disease patients is not known. Recent studies of Hodgkin's disease patients with more advanced dysmyelopoiesis ("preleukemia")[283,284] suggest a frequency of 2.5%. No calculation of cumulative risk for this complication was performed. All patients within this group (10 of 391) had previously been treated with chemotherapy and seven of those ten received radiotherapy as well.

Clinically, no symptoms related to mild dysmyelopoietic states are present, although a blunted response to hematopoietic stress during periods of infection or bleeding may signal the appearance of the syndrome. As more severe changes progressively occur, various degrees of pancytopenia may be present[291,294] with symptoms, most often related to progressive anemia (RA = refractory anemia). Thus, fatigue, shortness of breath, and tachycardia are not uncommon accompaniments of these disorders. Abnormalities in thrombopoiesis may be present with purpura, bleeding gums, epistaxis, and hematuria representing troublesome problems. Infections generally herald the next stages of dysmyelopoiesis with increased blast forms (RAEB = refractory anemia with excess blasts), and frank leukemia.

Laboratory evaluation of dysmyelopoiesis demonstrates either pancytopenia or a combination of cytopenias.[294,299,300] Abnormalities of red cell morphology on blood smears (anisopoikilocytosis, tear-drop forms, macrocytosis, schistocytes) are common (Fig. 4–4a). In 1987, the extent of increase in the mean corpuscular volume during chemotherapy was shown to be of prognostic significance for the development of secondary leukemia,[301] suggesting an early injury to erythroid precursors. Nucleated red blood cell forms, occasionally megaloblastoid, are observed, and the reticulocyte count is either decreased or inappropriately low for the degree of anemia. Neutrophils are increased, normal, or decreased, and Pelger-Huet forms are not uncommon. More immature white blood cell forms are occasionally seen, including a rare myeloblast. Auer rods are rarely noted. Monocytosis is occasionally observed. Platelets are commonly decreased with occasional large, bizarre forms noted (Fig. 4–4a). Examination of the bone marrow discloses a hypercellular to normocellular specimen. Megakaryocytes may be normal, increased, or decreased. There is a shift to more immature myelopoiesis with myeloblasts representing less than 5% of the nucleated cells. Erythropoiesis is mildly to frankly megaloblastic with binucleate and four-leaf-clover forms occasionally noted. Large nuclear remnants are seen in more mature red cell forms. Ringed sideroblasts are commonly seen.[47,150,277,283,295,302] Electron microscopy of myeloid, erythroid, and megakaryocytic precursors may show significant abnormalities.[303] Abnormalities that may distinguish primary from secondary dysmyelopoietic states are more of a quantitative than qualitative nature and include hypocellularity, increased fibrosis, ringed sideroblasts, and difficulty in aspiration of the marrow.[293]

Serum B12, folate, iron stores, and leukocyte alkaline phosphatase are generally normal. About 20% of cases may demonstrate an increased serum and urine muramidase.[304] An elevated fetal hemoglobin (HbF) level may be observed.[305] Lactic dehydrogenase is often increased, representing ineffective erythropoiesis. Total bilirubin is generally normal, as are haptoglobins. In vitro marrow-culture techniques reveal decreased colony formation, impaired responsiveness to CSFs, and lack of inhibition of colony growth by prostaglandin and interferon. Erythropoietin and CSF levels (serum and urine) are generally increased, a reflection of the poor responsiveness of the marrow to normal control mechanisms.

Cytogenetic abnormalities are common, particularly involvement of chromosomes 5, 7, and 17.[306-309] In one series of patients with "unexplained" cytopenias of an idiopathic nature, 77% of patients with cytogenetic abnormalities underwent an evolution into acute leukemia.[307] Karyotypic evolution and the presence of complex cytogenetic abnormalities[307,310] in the dysmyelopoietic syndrome are indications of a leukemic evolution, especially in an alkylating agent-treated patient (seven of eight patients in Anderson's series).[299,311] Two patients with Hodgkin's disease are described in this series, both received chemotherapy and one received radiation therapy—both developed acute leukemia. The survival from the diagnosis of dysmyelopoiesis was 8 and 34 months respectively. The cytogenetic abnormalities were complex (46XY,-2,-5,-7,+(1;17)(q24;p13)+mar1+mar2+r;46XX,del(7)(q11),

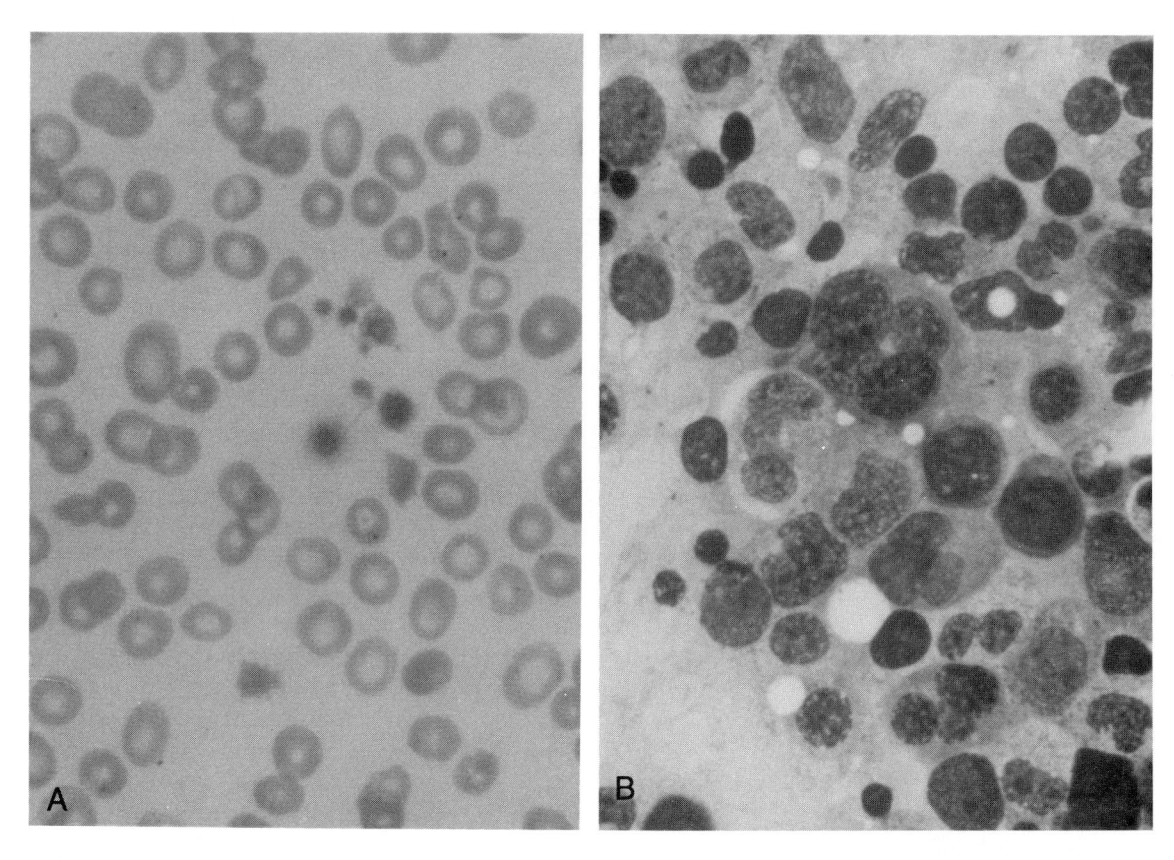

Fig. 4-4. (A) Blood smear demonstrates severe neutropenia, anisopoikilocytosis, schistocytes, Howell-Jolly bodies, and large platelet forms. (B) Bone-marrow smear demonstrates dyserythropoiesis with megaloblastic, multinucleate red-cell precursors, several degranulated myelocytes, and metamyelocytes.

t(9;?)(p22;?). The latter patient had no response to chemotherapy (details not given); the former was untreated. Survival from the diagnosis of leukemia was 3 and 7 months respectively. The presence of cytogenetic abnormalities in the idiopathic variety of dysmyelopoiesis has prognostic significance with respect to survival.[312] In one series, ten patients with Hodgkin's disease developed severe dysmyelopoietic syndrome; 50% of these patients were later diagnosed with acute leukemia. All of these patients had characteristic cytogenetic abnormalities.[313] Of the five patients who did not develop leukemia, at least two died of severe cytopenia.

The treatment of the myelodysplastic syndrome, in the absence of increased blast forms, poses difficult problems for the clinician because of one's hesitancy to use an aggressive antileukemia approach or even modest cytotoxic therapy if there is no clearcut evidence of neoplasia. Although the evolution of this syndrome into acute leukemia is relatively frequent, the time until, as well as the degree of, cytopenia is variable, and a period of observation is reasonable. Once blood supportive therapy beomes necessary, a trial of pyridoxine (150 mg/day/3 months), androgens, (oxymethalone 300 mg/day/3 months), or corticosteroids (prednisone 60 mg/day/3 to 4 weeks),[314] alone or in combination as "marrow-failure cocktails," may be used.[294] Although their efficacy is doubtful, some patients have appeared to respond with decreased blood-support needs.[294,315] Whether or not these apparent improvements are a part of the natural history of this disorder is unknown. The use of biologic response modifiers, such as retinoic acid[316] and endotoxin,[317] are approaches that were tried in the early 1980s, with some modest success in the syndrome of refractory anemia with excess blasts. Although spontaneous remissions and stabilization with no blood replace-

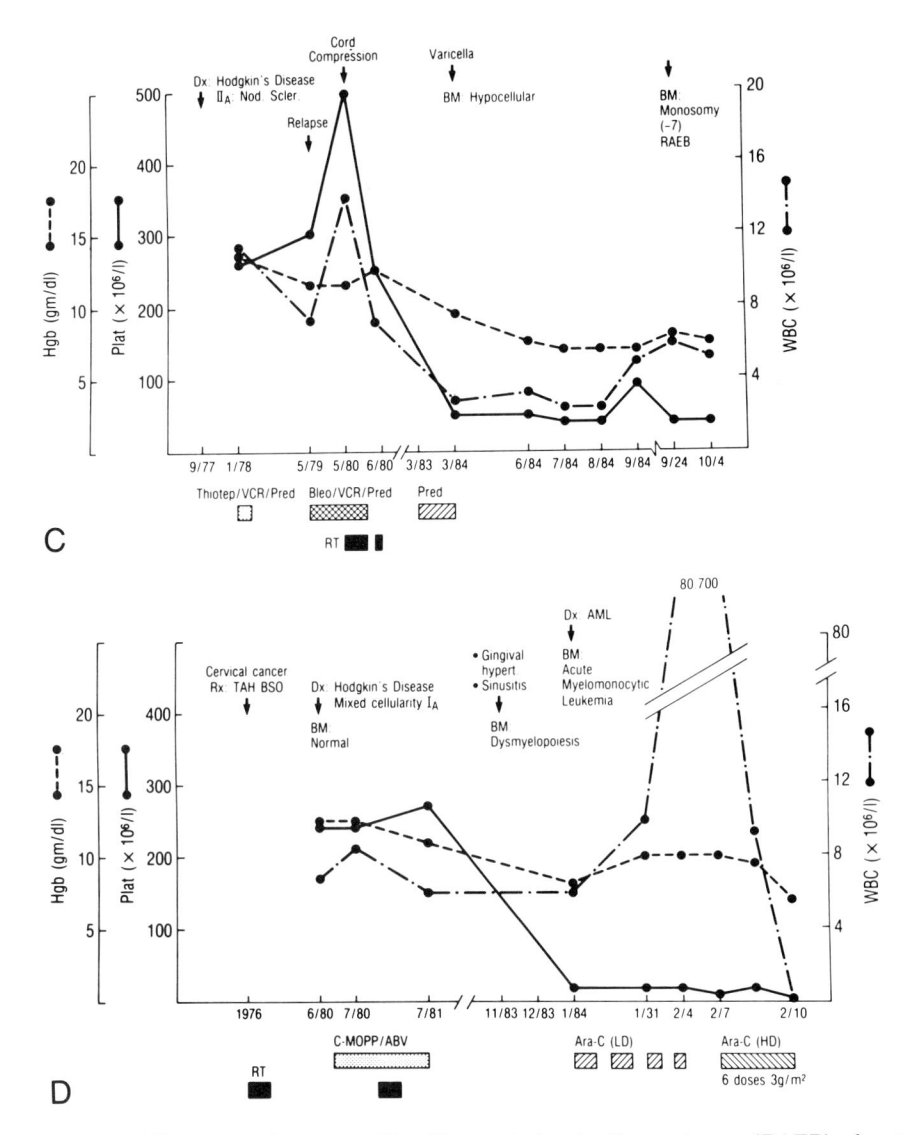

Fig. 4-4 Continued. (C) Male patient, age 49, with myelodysplastic syndrome (RAEB) after treatment of Hodgkin's disease. (D) Female patient, age 43, with acute myelogenous leukemia after treatment of Hodgkin's disease.

ment requirements may occur, the persistence of thrombocytopenia with bleeding and increased red-cell transfusions generally leads one to a more aggressive treatment approach. Low-dose cytosine arabinoside[318] and granulopoietic growth factors (GM-CSF, G-CSF) are presently being employed.[398] New differentiating agents such as HMBA may be useful in future trials.[319]

An absolute increase in marrow-blast forms (greater than 5%) with pancytopenia signals the presence of a refractory anemia with excess blasts (RAEB).[283,284,293] The time frame of this evaluation is noted in Figure 4-4C. Pancytopenia is somewhat more pronounced than in the refractory anemia syndrome and blasts are frequently seen on blood smears. Often, a higher proportion of blasts is seen in the peripheral blood than one might expect from examining the bone marrow.[293] Anemia is present in almost all patients, and thrombocytopenia is common. Neutropenia may be present and many neutrophils appear to be degranulated. The leukocyte alkaline phosphatase (LAP) score may be low, and myeloperoxidase is occasionally lacking. A mon-

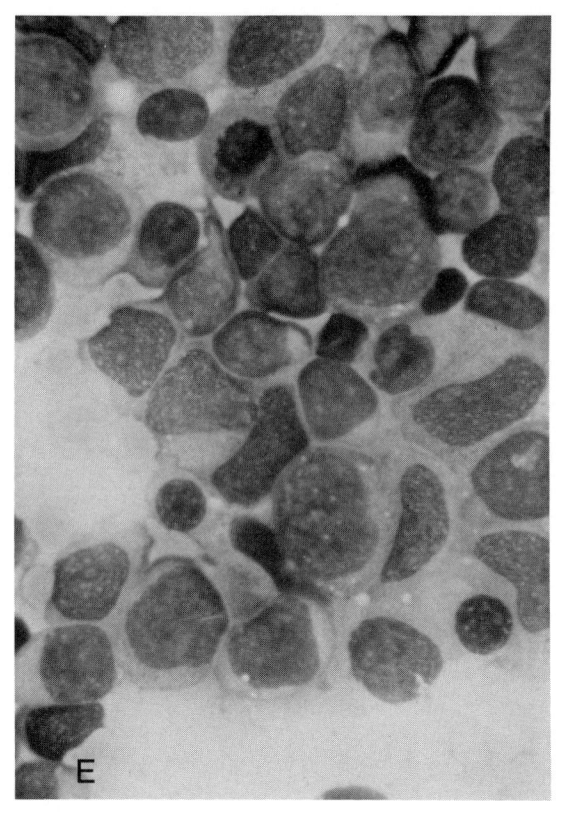

Fig. 4–4 Continued. (E) Hypercellular bone marrow almost totally replaced with myeloblasts and monoblasts.

ocytosis may be present and if pronounced (greater than $1 \times 10^9/l$) it defines the syndrome of chronic myelomonocytic leukemia.[293] Examination of the bone marrow demonstrates an obvious increase in blast forms with the presence of Auer rods occasionally noted. Myelopoiesis is abnormal with degranulated myeloid precursors.[320] Erythropoiesis is megaloblastic, and it is occasionally difficult to determine if blasts are of myeloid or erythroid derivation. If the latter predominates, then the syndrome is equivalent to that of erythroleukemia. Electron microscopy of erythroid precursors and megakaryocytes demonstrates a variety of abnormalities.[321,322]

Although not all patients with RAEB progress to frank myeloblastic leukemia, the syndrome must be considered preleukemic. In several series of patients, most of whom developed idiopathic rather than therapy-related RAEB, between 28 and 64% developed acute leukemia.[323–325] Important prognostic variables in the idiopathic groups include in vitro growth pattern, in vivo diffusion chamber growth, cytogenetic abnormalities, myeloid versus erythroid dysplasia, and the presence of ringed sideroblasts.[295] The presence of abnormal growth in in vitro systems, ringed sideroblasts with predominantly erythroid dysplasia, and myeloid dysplasia, are correlated with the development of acute leukemia.[326] Similar abnormalities have been described in patients with leukemia who are in apparent remission and may represent the earliest defects in leukemic hematopoiesis.[388] It is obvious that as the blast percentage in the marrow increases, the clinical manifestations will be similar to those of acute leukemia. In general, anemia dominates the clinical picture.

Bleeding manifestations are more common than in refractory anemia and occasionally represent a major problem. As the blast count increases with subsequent inhibited myelopoiesis, sensitivity to infections, particularly cellulitis and pneumonias, becomes a problem (RAEBIT = refractory anemia with excess blasts in transformation). This syndrome occurred in 6 of 391 patients following treatment for Hodgkin's disease.[283] An evolution from refractory anemia was observed in three of six, and three of six developed acute leukemia. Spontaneous remission and/or stabilization of disease is less likely to occur in this syndrome, and a significant proportion of patients will die of cardiovascular and infectious complications without developing acute leukemia.

Treatment of RAEB is similar to that of refractory anemia, except aggressive therapy is often necessary because of the more profound marrow failure associated with RAEB. Pyridoxine, androgens,[323] and prednisone are administered, often with no therapeutic results. As noted above, retinoic acid may be tried.[316] Because of the aggressive nature of this disease, cytotoxic approaches are often undertaken. Standard antileukemia therapy using cytosine arabinoside[323] and combinations of cytosine arabinoside, anthracyclines, and thioguanine are responsible for a small percentage of remissions. High morbidity and mortality, however, are often the cost of this treatment. Armitage et al.[105] reported on 13 patients with RAEB, of whom one was treated with radiation and chemotherapy for Hodgkin's disease. This patient had both ringed sideroblasts and Auer rods in the bone marrow and a blast count of 21%. Treatment with a combination of doxorubicin, cytosine arabinoside and thioguanine did not result in remission, and the patient survived for only 1 month after therapy. Of the entire group of 13 patients, three achieved remission, with survival of 1 to 37+ months. The successful induction regimens employed were DP (daunorubicin, prednisone), TADPO (thioguanine, ara-C, daunorubicin, prednisone, vincristine), and AT (ara-C, thioguanine). Cytosine arabinoside, either using standard dose[323,325] or a high dose[327] (as in secondary leukemias) may be tried. More recently, low dose continuous infusion cytosine arabinoside has been used successfully in this syndrome and is probably the drug schedule of choice.[318,328] The exact mode of its activity when given in low dose is unclear. Both cytotoxic and cell differentiation[318] properties may play a role. GM-CSF and G-CSF as well as differentiating agents such a HMBA are also being used in this disorder.[319,398] In young patients who develop RAEB, an aggressive treatment approach is certainly warranted, allogeneic bone-marrow transplantation being the treatment of choice.[330] Although only a minority of patients will have a compatible HLA match for marrow transplantation, with newer techniques of marrow preparation, such as lectin separation to prevent graft versus host disease, it is not inconceivable that donors with minor mismatches will be available more readily.

Once the blast count in the bone marrow is greater than 30%, acute leukemia is considered established and the clinical picture of severe marrow failure with anemia, infection, and bleeding results (Fig. 4–4d, 4–4e). Reports of patients who developed acute leukemia after treatment of Hodgkin's disease are summarized in Table 4–7. The cumulative risk and actual/expected (relative) risk of developing secondary leukemia (S-ANLL) after treatment of Hodgkin's disease can be determined when large series of patients have been studied long enough to establish incidence rates to compare with a control population. Table 4–8 outlines the risk data of the largest series of patients. Stanford University Medical Center analyzed the survival of 690 patients with Hodgkin's disease beginning 1 year after the initial diagnosis.[275] The actuarial risks of developing acute leukemia at 5 and 7 years were 1.5 and 2% respectively. These figures are in agreement with those reported from the Southeastern Cancer Study Group[263] and the Task Force for Malignant Lymphoma (Bologna).[262] Reports from Boston and Europe have appeared showing cumulative risks of 5.5% at 6 years,[331,332] 9.9% at 9 years,[283,284] and 9.1% at 12 years in certain treatment modality categories.[258] The National Cancer Institute recently updated the survival and relapse data on 192 patients treated between 1964 and 1975.[333] Leukemia-related complications (ANLL, MDS, AA) developed in 12 patients. The cumulative risk at 5 and 10 years was 3% and 10% respectively. The highest risk of development (peak incidence) occurred at 6 years ("critical window" is 2 to 12 years). Indirectly, the most important factor in explaining the increased incidence of this complication is the improvement in survival of patients whose lives have been prolonged sufficiently, so that the number of patients at risk has increased dramatically over the last two decades. This improvement in survival is a result of increasingly more aggressive therapeutic approaches, with respect to radiation therapy, chemotherapy, and their combined usage (combined modality treatment). During the era of minimal therapy for Hodgkin's disease, eight cases of S-ANLL out of 4591 patients were reported, an incidence of 0.18%.[271] This figure was obtained by reviewing a large series of patients with Hodgkin's disease between 1938 and 1970. Borum reviewed the incidence of acute leukemia in Hodgkin's disease, accumulating 16 cases prior to 1969, with the remaining 161 cases since 1970.[268] In 1974, Sahakian et al.[286] reviewed the world's literature, documenting 22 cases since the initial report by Craver in 1936.[335] Between 1977 and 1987, 10 studies with a total of 6256 cases of Hodgkin's disease[258,260,262,275,331,336-339] reported 104 S-ANLL's with an incidence of 1.6%, a nearly eightfold increase when compared to earlier studies.

A number of factors have been directly implicated in this increase, including radiation therapy, chemotherapy, and their combined

Table 4-7. Leukemias After Treatment of Hodgkin's Disease

Reference (Year)	No. Pts./ Series	Tx HD	Age	Type Leuk.	Months From Dx HD to MDS	Months From MDS to Leuk	Active HD	Months to Dx ANLL	Tx Leuk	Response	Survival (Mos.)
Lacher et al.[278] (1963)	1/-	CM	23	AUL	*	*	*	30	*	NR	.1
Berg[145]† (1967)	0/1,129	*	*	*	*	*	*	*	*	*	*
Newman et al.[281] (1970)	4/-	CM RT	26–65	ANLL	59 (mean)	7 (mean)	1/4	19–228	*	NR	.1
Osta et al.[282] (1970)	1/-	CM	59	ANLL	*	*	+	9	NO	*	.1
Steinberg et al.[288] (1970)	2/-	CM	30–26	ANLL/M-6	*	*	*	108–180	*	*	1–2
Chan et al.[274] (1972)	3/-	CM RT	28–58	ANLL/AUL	*	*	*	60–144	*	*	5.5
Weiden et al.[291] (1973)	3/-	CM RT	16–51	ANLL/AUL	18–84	3–11	1/3	22–95	2/3	NR	.5–1
Sahakian et al.[286] (1974)	3/-	CM CTH	30–49	ANLL	74–94	2–10	3/3	10–96	2/3	NR	1–6
Canellos et al.[272] (1975)	2/452	CM	*	*	*	*	*	*	*	*	*
Cadman et al.[271] (1977)	4/-	CM RT	27–48	ANLL	97	10	0/4	43–107	3/4	NP	1–12
Brody et al.[269] (1977)	3/-	*	22–48	ANLL	*	*	*	8–100	*	*	*
Coleman et al.[275] (1977)	9/680	CM	12–56	ANLL/RAEB	18–84	0–10	3/9	19–91	1/9	CR	1+–6
Neufeld et al.[339] (1978)	2/232	CM	51–57	ANLL	*	*	*	37–48	*	*	*
Toland et al.[290] (1978)	21/659	CM CTH	*	ANLL	*	*	*	*	*	*	*
Coltman et al.[336] (1982)											
Auclerc et al.[260] (1979)	21/2000	CM CTH	5–73 (mean = 37)	ANLL/ALL	*	*	6/21	24–128 (mean = 90)	*	5/24 CR	.25–15
Casciato et al.[273] (1979)	4/-	CM CTH	22–57	ANLL/AUL	26–36	26–36	1/4	35–99	2/4	NR	1–3
Foucar et al.[277] (1979)	2/-	CM	19–31	ANLL	*	*	1/2	35–123	2/2	1/2PR	1–22

Study	Cases	Modality	Age	Type							
Baccarini et al.262 (1980)	7/613	CM CTH	26–63	ANLL/M-6	2–76	3–25	1/7	12–83	6/7	NR	1–12
Valagussa et al.331 (1980)	9/764	CM CTH	*	ANLL	*	*	0/9	20–127	9/9	*	1 (median)
Boivin et al.264,265 (1981, 1984)	21/–	CM CTH RT	10–67	ANLL/AUL	*	*	*	22–150	*	*	*
Glicksman et al.338 (1982)	10/178	CM CTH	*	ANLL	*	*	*	*	*	*	*
Aisenberg258 (1983)	8/408	CM CTH	21–51	ANLL	*	*	1/8	42–132	*	*	*
Bartolucci et al.263 (1983)	3/–	CTH	38–73	ANLL	*	*	*	49–77	*	*	*
Tester et al.395**	9/473	CM CTH	19–35	ANLL/CML	*	*	3/9	36–139	3/9	*	5 (median)
Austin-Seymour et al.261 (1984)	2/52	*	60–75	ANLL	*	*	*	*	*	*	*
Pedersen-Bjergaard et al.284 (1984)	7/	CM CTH RT	22–73	ANLL	38–105	5–8	4/7	14–120	3/7	2/7CR	3–14+
Schomberg et al.287 (1984)	2/169	CTH CM	28–37	ANLL	*	*	*	32–60	2/2	2/2NR	.25–1
Tabilio et al.289 (1984)	1	CM	50	AMEGL	*	*	*	48	1/1	1/1NR	.5
Doreen et al.337 (1986)	6	CM CTH	32–70	ANLL/MPD	*	*	2/6	24–108	4/6	*	*
Blayney et al.333 (1987)	12/192	CM CTH	*	*	*	*	*	*	*	*	*

*Details not given
**Does not include 5 cases of refractory cytopenias
†1948–1962 (Memorial Hospital)
CM = Combined modality
CTH = Chemotherapy
RT = Radiotherapy
ANLL = Acute nonlymphocytic leukemia
AUL = Acute undifferentiated leukemia
M-6 = Erythroleukemia
RAEB = Refractory anemia with excess blasts
AMEGL = Acute megakaryoblastic leukemia
MPD = Myeloproliferative disease
MDS = Myelodysplastic syndrome
NR = No response
PR = Partial response
CR = Complete response

Table 4–8. Risk of Developing Leukemia After Treatment of Hodgkin's Disease

Reference	Number of Patients	Cumulative Risk (%) (Years)						Relative Risk
		5	6	7	9	10	12	
Coleman et al.[275] (1977)	690	1.5±0.6		2.0±0.6				
RXT only	320	0.0		0.0				
CHT + RXT	330	2.9±1.2		3.9±1.2				
CHT only	30	0.0		0.0				
Neufeld et al.[339] (1978)	232							40
CHT + RXT	174							
Toland et al.[290] (1978)	643							302
NR + SC	134							—
NR + IC	115							257
SR + NC	106							—
SR + SC	357							—
SR + IC	162							253
IR + NC	99							—
IR + SC	209							816
IR + IC	43							1049
Baccarani et al.[262] (1980)	613							
RXT only	117		0.0					
CHT + RXT	344		2.04					
CHT only	152		2.0					
Valagussa et al.[331] (1980)	764					2.4		
RXT only	236	0.0				0.0		
CHT + RXT	492	1.4				3.5		
CHT only	36	5.5						
Boivin§ et al.[264] (1981)	1,553							
No intensive therapy								7.7
Intensive IR, no IC								15
IC, no IR								40
IC, IR								290
Coltman et al.[336] (1982)	659							
RXT only	95	0	0	0				
CHT + RXT	283	3.4	4.1	6.4				
CHT only	102	6.2	6.2	6.2				
Salvage CHT	179	3.2	6.0	7.7				
Age <20	127	2.4	2.4	2.4				
Age 20–29	237	1.7	1.7	1.7				
Age 30–39	139	3.0	3.0	4.8				
Age ≥40	153	7.8	3.8	20.7				
Glicksman et al.[338] (1982)	798							
RXT only	133							
CHT + RXT	429							
CHT only	369							
Age <40	499						2.9(±2.0)†	122
Age 40–59	216						11.8(±5.8)	214
Age 60+	82						6.4(±4.8)	75
Symptoms A	196						2.0(±1.5)	117
Symptoms B	600						7.2(±3.2)	139
Stage III	285						4.6(±4.0)	79
Stage IV	511						6.3(±2.7)	162

Table 4–8. Risk of Developing Leukemia After Treatment of Hodgkin's Disease (continued)

Reference	Number of Patients	Cumulative Risk (%) (Years)						Relative Risk
		5	6	7	9	10	12	
Induction								
MOPP/MVPP	292	9.9(±4.3)						255
BOPP/COPP, CVPP	260	9.9(±9.0)						82
Post-Induction								
Unmaintained	198						0	0
Velban	217						1.0(±1.0)	45
Velban + Induct	139						1.1(±1.1)	82
CLB±OP	155						14.9(±5.7)	463
Radiotherapy								
No RXT	369						7.5(±3.9)	147
IF	180						2.7(±2.7)	130
EF	67						4.2(±4.1)	183
TNI	133						0	0
Pedersen-Bjergaard et al.[283] (1982)	391	3.9(±1.3)			9.9±2.9			
RXT only	79	0						0
CHT + RXT								1.4
CHT only								1
Age <40					8.6±5.6			0.3
Age >40					39.5±10.1			
Age 40–59								2.2
Age >59								3.2
Stage IA								0.6
Stage IB								0
Stage IIA								1.1
Stage IIB								0
Stage IIIA								1
Stage IIIB								0.9
Stage IVA								0
Stage IVB								2.3
Aisenberg[258] (1983)	408						4.9	
RXT only	188						0	
MOPP + RXT	220						9.1	
Stage I, II, III	188						2.6	
Stage IV	24						37.2	
Age <40	173						5.4	
Age >40	47						33.1	
N Relapse	138						2.8	
Relapse	82						18.0	
Bartolucci et al.[263] (1983)	209							185
CHT only	209							185
POST-IND CHT	88	8.1±5.51†						338.5
Age <30	93							0
Age 30–49	64	2.6±2.60						213.6
Age 50–79	52	16.7±9.89						249.9
Symptoms A	37							0
Symptoms B	172	6.3±3.20						255.1
Stage 2	6							0
Stage 3	102	7.9±4.65						269.5
Stage 4	101	2.2±2.2						98.0

Table 4–8. Risk of Developing Leukemia After Treatment of Hodgkin's Disease (continued)

Reference	Number of Patients	Cumulative Risk (%) (Years)						Relative Risk
		5	6	7	9	10	12	
Boivin et al.[265] (1984)	2591							
IC								136
IC + IR								125
IC ± XRT								140
No IC								3
No IC + IR								7
No IC + XRT								2
Drugs utilized								
NM, Proc, VCR								90
NM, Proc, VLB								100
NM, Proc, VCR, VLB								160
Tester et al.[395] (1984)	473							
RXT						0		0
RXT + CHT						6		1.6
CHT						2		0.5
RXT + CHT (salvage)						9		3.5
<30						1.4		1.2
30–39						4.1		1.0
40–49						0		0
≥50						0		0

*Actuarial risk
†Life Table Estimate (4.34 years mean follow up)
§IC = 3 or more drugs, cyclical; no IC = All other chemotherapy or none
CHT = Chemotherapy
RXT = Radiotherapy
No RXT = No radiotherapy
SC = Some chemotherapy
IC = Intensive chemotherapy
SR = Some radiotherapy
IR = Intensive radiotherapy
NC = No chemotherapy
NM = Nitrogen mustard
Proc = Procarbazine
VCR = Vincristine
VLB = Velban
CLB = Chlorambucil
POST-IND CHT = Post-induction chemotherapy
OP = Vincristine and prednisone

usage. The actuarial risks for combined modality in the Stanford series were 2.9% ± 1.2% and 3.9% ± 1.2% at 5 and 7 years respectively, compared to a figure of 0% with either modality alone.[275] Although no leukemias were seen in the radiation-only group, at least five well documented case reports in which radiotherapy was the only treatment modality used have been reported.[279,291,341] A 1984 update of a collaborative study of 460 stage I and II Hodgkin's disease patients, which used involved-field (IF) and extended-field (EF) radiation as initial therapy, reported 5 of 220 and 1 of 240 leukemias in the IF and EF groups respectively.[342] All cases, however, occurred in patients receiving salvage chemotherapy after documentation of disease progression (6 of 167 patients). It would appear that the relative risk of developing S-ANLL after radiation therapy alone is no different from the rest of the population.[279,338,341] The small number of case reports after radiation therapy alone, although heartening, may reflect a time lag in leukemogenesis using this modality of treatment, and 20-year follow-up studies will be needed to conclude that radiation treatment alone does not result in an increase in incidence when compared to those that are naturally occurring.

Chemotherapy and combined modality approaches appear to be the major risk factors for leukemia. A number of studies have addressed the relative risk of various treatment modalities (Table 4–8). In one study, intensive chemotherapy, with or without radiation therapy, carried an estimated relative risk of 136.[265] A similar RR for intensive chemotherapy, with or without intensive radiation therapy (125 and 140 respectively), was observed. Intensive radiotherapy, without intensive chemotherapy, carried a relative risk of seven and when only modest chemotherapy or modest radiotherapy was used this decreased to three and two, respectively. The experience of the Cancer and Leukemia Group B is similar,[338] with a relative risk of 147 for chemotherapy alone, 130 for chemotherapy and involved-field irradiation, and 183 for chemotherapy and extended-field radiation. The Southwest Oncology Group reported a significantly higher relative risk for various treatment modalities ranging from 257 to 1049 for chemotherapy, with or without intensive radiotherapy, and 302 for all treatments combined.[290] Intensive radiotherapy, modest chemotherapy, or modest radiotherapy and modest chemotherapy combined carried no increased risk of leukemia. This observation is similar to that of the Boston Study, which found no leukemia in patients treated with radiation therapy alone or in patients treated with six cycles of MOPP and extended-field irradiation.[258] A 1985 report, however, found S-ANLL in a patient treated with three cycles of MOPP and IF radiation; this casts some doubt on the concept that modest combined modality treatment may be free of leukemia risk.[343]

The NCI reported that of 12 leukemia-related complications, 11 had received combined modality and only one patient developed this complication after MOPP alone.[333] In 1986, members of this group recommended the use of radiation as an adjuvant only for patients at high risk after MOPP therapy.[267] The contribution of individual agents to the relative risk calculation has been addressed by several authors. The use of nitrogen mustard, procarbazine, and vincristine carried a relative risk of 90, with the addition of vinblastine increasing this to 150.[264] In one study non-nitrosurea combinations were found to have a significantly higher risk,[338] an unusual observation, considering the known leukemogenic properties of this class of compounds. Another important factor in increasing the risk of leukemia includes relapse after initial therapy, which necessitates salvage therapies.[258] A group of patients in one study demonstrated a cumulative risk of 18% at 12 years. Thus far, using ABVD as front-line therapy has not been associated with an increase in leukemia,[332] suggesting that its use in salvage programs is almost imperative for those trying to decrease this complication. Leukemia has been associated with ABVD combined with radiotherapy, demonstrating the leukemogenic effect of this modality.[292,346]

Maintenance therapy is also likely to increase the leukemia risk,[338] as is advanced age,[258,261,263,283,338] particularly in the 40 to 75 age group. The importance of the age factor is emphasized by a 33.1% incidence at 12 year follow-up for this age group, versus a 5.4% incidence for younger patients.[258] This age dependence was not observed in a recent NCI update.[395] Advanced stage at diagnosis is also associated with a significantly increased risk (37.2% for stage IV patients at 12 years versus 2.6% in stages I, II, III).[258,337] Limiting the degree of combined-modality therapy according to prognostic factors may ultimately result in less leukemia.[343,347,396] Unfortunately, this may occur at the cost of decreased survival from Hodgkin's disease.

Almost all leukemias seen are acute non-lymphocytic, with myeloblastic leukemia predominating. Reports of monocytic leukemia,[348] erythroleukemia,[349] promyelocytic leukemia,[260] acute lymphoblastic leukemia,[260,264] chronic lymphocytic leukemia,[350,351] chronic myelogenous leukemia,[352,395] and lymphosarcoma-cell leukemia[353] have also appeared. The frequency of the more common leukemias is shown in Table 4–9. Using electron microscopic analysis and monoclonal antibodies, several cases of megakaryoblastic leukemia with myelofibrosis were reported in 1984.[289]

The time until onset of acute leukemia after

Table 4–9. Type of Acute Leukemia in 301 Reported Patients with Hodgkin's Disease*

Myeloblastic	135	(45)
Promyelocytic	4	(1)
Myelomonocytic	54	(18)
Monocytic	24	(8)
Erythroleukemia	26	(9)
Nonlymphocytic	25	(8)
Lymphoblastic	20	(7)
Undifferentiated	9	(3)
Other (lymphosarcoma cell leukemia, etc.)	4	(1)
Total	301	(100)

*From: Grunwald HW, Rosner F: Acute myeloid leukemia following treatment of Hodgkin's disease. A review. Cancer 50:676–683, 1982.

Table 4–10. Cytogenetic Abnormalities Noted in Hodgkin's Disease Patients Developing Dysmyelopoietic Syndromes and Secondary Leukemia[306–313,340,354,390,391]

47,XY,+8
46,XX,−7,−16,−21,+der t(2:7)(cen:cen),del(2)(q33),del(11)(q22),+11p+,14p+,+t(21;21;21;16)(21q22;21q11,q22;21q11q22;16p13)
45,XX,−7,inv(1)(p36q13)/46,XX,−7,+8,inv(1)
45,XY,−7
44,XY,−7,−16,17p+,20q−/43,XY,−5,−7,−12,−16,4p+,17p+,20q−,+mar1/43;XYq+
45XY,−5,−7,del(3)(p13),+der(5)t(5;17)q11^2;q11)
45XY,−7,del(5)(q13?)/t(12?:17?)(q13?:p12?)
45,XY,−7,del(3)(p13?),del(8)(q22),del(16)(p12)
44,XY,−2,−3,−6,−12,−15,−21,−22,?del(?)(p11),del(11)(?p14),t(14;?)(q32;?),t(17;?)(p13;?),del(22)(?q11),+5mar/43,same,−7
44,XY,−5,−6,−7,−8,−17,+t(17;?),+2mar
45,XX,−7
46,XX,−7,+mar
48,XX,+2,+8
45,XX,−5,−7,−10,+2mar
46,XY,−7,+t(1q7p)/46XY,−5,+8,−22,del(7)(q22),+t(21q22q)
45,XY,9q−,12p−

treatment varies considerably from series to series, ranging from 3 to greater than 10 years (Table 4–7). This variation is a reflection of differences in treatment modalities, with respect to the use of radiation and chemotherapy, stage of disease, necessity for salvage therapy, and age. Approximately 75% of patients with acute leukemia seen after treatment for Hodgkin's disease present with a myelodysplastic syndrome and 25% have a de novo presentation.[283] This myelodysplastic state may last for a variable period, but as noted above, most patients with the more severe syndromes (RAEB) will develop acute leukemia.[283]

Once leukemia is present, the diagnosis is generally not a problem. All changes on the blood smear noted during the myelodysplastic syndrome will be more pronounced. The white-blood-cell count may be elevated, normal, or decreased, with a variable number of blast forms, either myeloblasts or monoblasts noted. Auer rods may be seen[281,282] and early myeloid forms are common. The blood smear will show significant red-cell abnormalities, with schistocytes and nucleated red-blood cells. Platelets are generally decreased. The bone-marrow examination will demonstrate a greater than 30% infiltration by blast forms, with a concomitant decrease in normal myeloid, erythroid, and megakaryocytic precursors (Fig. 4–4e). Numerous cytogenetic abnormalities have been described in these S-ANLLs (Table 4–10),[313,354,355] particularly abnormalities of chromosome numbers 5 and 7.

Deciding when to treat a patient with secondary leukemia with specific chemotherapy depends on the rapidity of leukemic progression, age, and activity of Hodgkin's disease. Recent observations of the relationship of treatment outcome to karyotypic analysis[284] may establish guidelines for undertaking therapy. Because age is such an important determinant of survival in acute leukemia, the younger age of the Hodgkin's disease population should, theoretically, result in more satisfactory remission rates than in secondary leukemias seen after treatment of solid tumors. Because treatment regimens differ, reported results of antileukemia chemotherapy in both situations are variable, and it is difficult to determine the actual remission induction rate for leukemia seen after treatment of any specific primary cancer. In a 1984 study of eight patients with S-ANLL (primary tumor not specified) who received daunorubicin, cytosine arabinoside, and thioguanine (DAT), five patients (62%) achieved a complete remission, but these were of short duration (median: 2.8 months; range: 1.5 to 3.9 months).[357] Of the greater than 300 reported cases of secondary leukemias in patients initially treated for Hodgkin's disease,[149] enough details are available in only 36 cases to determine responses to therapy. Table 4–11 outlines the results compiled from the literature of antileukemia therapy in patients previously treated for Hodgkin's disease. Analysis is complicated because of the different treatment programs used, variable ages of patients, and the lack of knowledge with respect to aggressiveness of support facilities. In 1977, Cadman et al.[271] recorded, in a series of 109 cases of secondary leukemia in Hodgkin's disease, 77 patients who had been treated with antileukemia therapy (details of therapy not given). A complete remission was documented in five cases (6.5%). Pedersen-Bjergaard et al.[284] described seven patients with Hodgkin's disease (ages 22–73), one of whom received radiation therapy alone and developed S-ANLL. Three of these patients received daunomycin and cytosine arabinoside (doses not given), and two achieved complete remissions lasting 3 and 9 months. One of these two had a normal karyotype and one had a $-5, -7, -10, +2$ minimal angle resolution (mar) karyotype. Schomberg et al.[287] described two patients who developed ANLL after treatment for Hodgkin's disease (one receiving TNI plus chemotherapy; the other chemotherapy alone). Both failed to achieve remission (induction regimen not described) and died early in induction. Càsciato et al.[273] compiled a total of 33 cases in the literature, of which only one patient was alive at the time of their review. The median survival range was 1 to 12 months. All cases were reported prior to 1976, and many had actually occurred several years before anthracyclines were commonly used as part of antileukemia chemotherapy. Foucar et al.[277] reported on two patients treated with combined modality; one achieved a partial remission and survived for 22 months after the diagnosis of leukemia, and one died after 1 month. Both received daunorubicin and cytosine arabinoside. Coleman et al.[275] reported on one patient who achieved a complete remission with DAT. Three others were treated (details not given) without effect. Valagussa et al.[331] were unsuccessful in inducing any remissions with DAT in eight patients. Androgens and corticosteroids were successful in inducing a remission in one of nine patients. Anderson et al.[299] were unsuccessful in inducing a remission in one patient treated with an anthracycline and cytosine arabinoside. Rowley et al.[354] reported on nine patients with secondary ANLL, of whom six were treated with either Ara-C/TG, DAT, doxorubicin/Ara-C/TG, or hydroxyurea. No responses were noted and survival was short from the diagnosis of leukemia, with a median survival of 4 months (range: 0 to 12 months). One patient had a persistent dysmyelopoietic syndrome until death. Bloomfield et al.[357] reported on 12 patients with Hodgkin's disease who developed S-ANLL. They were treated with an anthracycline and cytosine arabinoside. The response rate and survival could not be determined from this report (part of a series of 49 S-ANLL cases). Of 22 patients with prior hematologic malignancy, however, 32% achieved a remission.

In older patients over age 50, the decision to treat is based on the inability of transfusional therapy and antibiotics to permit a reasonably satisfactory lifestyle. Because patients are sensitive to the effects of cytosine arabinoside, a 14-day course of low-dose (20 mg/m^2/IV) continuous infusion is justifiable as an initial approach.[328] If a partial response is obtained, a second course may be given to achieve a complete remission. The role of maintenance therapy is unclear in this situation. If low-dose Ara-C is ineffective, a standard induction therapy should be used. This may consist of daunomycin, cytosine arabinoside, and thioguanine. High-dose cytosine arabinoside has been used successfully in patients with secondary leukemia.[327] Palliative control of elevated white-blood-cell counts can often be achieved with the use of hydroxyurea.

The goal of treatment of secondary leukemia in a young patient otherwise cured of Hodgkin's disease should be eradication, and an aggressive approach is justified. With complete remission rates (using chemotherapy) ranging from 0 to 25% and survival rarely lasting 1 year in the series cited, every effort should be made, particularly in patients less than 50 years of age, to take advantage of bone-marrow transplantation. If a syngeneic or allogeneic bone-marrow donor is available,

Table 4-11. Treatment Results of Secondary Leukemias in Hodgkin's Disease

Reference (Year)	Tx HD	Months to Dx Sec. Leuk.	Tx Sec. Leuk.	Result	Survival (Mos.)
Newman et al.[281] (1970)	CM	228	6-MP	PR	3
Weiden et al.[291] (1973)	RT	43	BMT*	NR	17 days
	RT	22	Oxymethalone	NR	1
Sahakian et al.[286] (1974)	CM	96	Ara-C/TG	NR	6
	CM	84	Ara-C/TG	NR	6
Cadman et al.[271] (1977)	CM	107	P	NR	3
	RT	83	Ara-C/TG/CTX (VCR/P/MTX)(D)	NR	6
Larsen et al.[279] (1977)	RT	23	D/Ara-C/VCR/TG/ MTX/CTX		2
	CM	100			6
	CM	79			6
Coleman et al.[275] (1977)‡	CM	36	DAT	CR	1
Foucar et al.[277] (1979)	CM	123	D/Ara-C	NR	1
	CM	35	D/Ara-C	PR	22
Valagussa et al.[331] (1980)	CM	30–127	DAT	NR	?
	CM		DAT	NR	?
	CM		DAT	NR	?
	CM		DAT	NR	?
	CM		DAT	NR	?
	CM		DAT	NR	?
	CM		DAT	NR	?
	CM		DAT	NR	?
	CTH	20	And/C	CR	?
Anderson et al.[299] (1981)	CTH	50	none	—	3
	CM	56	A/Ara-C	NR	7

Study						
Armitage et al.[105] (1981)†	CM	?	AD/Ara-C/TG	NR	1	
Pedersen-Bjergaard[283] (1982)	CM		D/Ara-C	NR	?	
	CM		D/Ara-C	CR	?	
	CM	18–111				
	CM					
	CM					
	CM					
	RT	14	D/Ara-C	CR	?	
Schomberg et al.[287] (1984)	CTH	60	DAT	NR	8 days	
	CM	32	•HU/L	NR	6 weeks	
			•Cranial RT			
			•VCR/D/Ara-C/P			
Tabilio et al.[289] (1984)	CM	52	LD Ara-C	NR	2 weeks	
Kempin (1989)	CM	42	LD Ara-C→HD Ara-C	NR	1	

A = Anthracycline
C = Corticosteroid
D = Daunorubicin
L = Leukeran
P = Prednisone
AD = Adriamycin
HU = Hydroxyurea
LD = Low-dose
TG = Thioguanine
6-MP = 6-Mercaptopurine
And = Androgen
Ara-C = Cytosine arabinoside
BMT = Bone marrow transplantation
CTX = Cytoxan
DAT = Daunorubicin, Ara-C, thioguanine
MTX = Methotrexate
VCR = Vincristine
CM = Combined modality
RT = Radiotherapy
CTH = Chemotherapy
*no leukemia at autopsy
†RAEB
‡details of therapy available on only one of nine cases reported

Table 4–12. Non-Hodgkin's Lymphoma (NHL) After Treatment of Hodgkin's Disease

Reference (Year)	No. Pts/Series	Tx HD	Months from Dx HD to Dx NHL (m)	Histol.	Tx NHL	Results	Survival (Mos.)
Burns et al.[353] (1971)	1/-	C	43	LSL	SA	D	*
Toland et al.[290] (1978)	1/643	C	*	DPDL	*	*	*
D'Agostino[373] (1979)	1/-	A	65	N-DHL	B	*	*
Krikorian et al.[377] (1979)	5/579	C	44–124	DHL, DUL	CHOP/BACOP	1/5 PR	*
Spaulding et al.[381] (1979)	1/-	B	48	DHL	*	*	*
Andrieu et al.[367] (1980)	1/-	C	90	Burkitt's	*	*	*
Kim et al.[376] (1980)	3/-	A,B	36–72	DPDL, NHL, NPDL	MOPP, CVP BCVPP	2/3 CR	23+–65+
Valagussa et al.[331] (1980)	1/764	C	16	DHL	*	*	*
Lowenthal et al.[379] (1981)	1/-	C	89	DHL (T)	CHOP	D	*
Bergsagel et al.[369] (1982)	4/780	A	*	DUL	*	*	*
Aisenberg[258] (1983)	1/408	C	72	DHL	*	*	*
Henry-Amar et al.[365] (1983)	3/334	C	120–180	Burkitt's	*	2/3 AL	*
Armitage et al.[368] (1983)	5/242	A,B,C	12–54	DHL, LL, IMMUNO	CHOP, COPP, BMT	2/5 AL(CR)	1–11+
Austin-Seymour[261] (1984)	1/52	*	*	*	*	*	*
Caya et al.[385] (1984)	1/-	A	12	MF	VLB, ST, PUVA, CCNU, BLEO	D	60
Boivin et al.[265] (1984)	1/2591	C	27	*	*	*	*
Hutchinson[342] (1984)	4/460	A	*	*	*	*	*

Tester et al.[395] (1984)	4/473	A,B,C	11–141	DHL, DUL PLASMA	*	*	0–31 (D)
Jacquillat et al.[375] (1984)	4/-	B,C	24–48	DHL,LL	VLB, CYT, BLEO, PROC, RUFO, TT	2/4CR	*
Schomberg et al.[287] (1984)	1/169	A	42	DHL	COPA/CHOPP	*	*
Rotenberg et al.[380] (1984)	1/-	A	96	DML	MOPP/RT	PR	*
Gowitt et al.[374] (1985)	3/-	B,C	84–192	L-TC	ABVD, RT, BCVPP	*	*
List et al.[378] (1986)	2/-	A	108–144	DUL, IMMUNO	COMLA, PROMACE, MOPP	2/2D	2–5
Dorreen et al.[337] (1986)	6/529	A,B	24–180	MF, Burkitt's, IMMUNO, LP	MOPP	2/6AL	*

AL - Alive D - Dead
*Details not given
A - Radiotherapy
B -Chemotherapy
C - Combined modality
MF - Mycosis fungoides
L-TC - T-Cell lymphoma
LP - Immunocytoma
LSL - Lymphosarcoma cell leukemia
DPDL - Diffuse poorly differentiated lymphoma
DHL - Diffuse histiocytic lymphoma
DUL - Diffuse undifferentiated lymphoma
NPDL - Nodular poorly differentiated lymphoma
LL - Lymphoblastic lymphoma
IMMUNO - Immunoblastic sarcoma
RUFO - Rufomycin
SA - Single agent
PR - Partial response
CR - Complete response
DML - Diffuse mixed lymphoma
PLASMA - Plasmacytoma

bone marrow-transplantation after high-dose chemotherapy and radiation offers the best opportunity for long-term survival.[358] Although the achievement of a complete remission prior to bone-marrow transplantation is recommended in de novo acute leukemia, it is not certain that this is necessary in the dysmyelopoietic states or secondary leukemias. Bone-marrow transplantation between unmatched individuals is not yet available for routine use. If a bone-marrow donor is not available, standard chemotherapy induction regimens can be used and more aggressive approaches using high-dose cytosine arabinoside in combination are justified. Palliative approaches in this young population as initial therapy are not justified because of the high mortality associated with this complication. Although it is premature to recommend that all patients being treated for Hodgkin's disease have their own bone marrow cryopreserved prior to therapy, patients in high-risk groups should be considered for this (age greater than 40, stage IV-nonmarrow involved relapse cases).

OTHER SECONDARY HEMATOPOIETIC TUMORS

It has been recognized for a number of years that patients receiving immunosuppressive therapy for a variety of non-neoplastic diseases are at risk of developing non-Hodgkin's lymphomas. This was initially observed in patients receiving renal allografts in whom azathioprine and prednisone were administered to prevent graft rejection.[359] The predominant lymphoma was diffuse histiocytic lymphoma, with central nervous system involvement the most common sign at initial presentation. Similar reports have appeared in patients receiving cardiac allografts treated with cyclosporine[360] and in patients in whom T-cell depletion is used to prevent graft versus host disease after bone marrow transplantation.[361] Ebstein-Barr virus (EBV) was implicated in this latter report based on the finding of EBV genomic material incorporated within the lymphoma cells. In a large series of renal transplant patients,[359] the median time until the appearance of these secondary tumors was 14 months, a considerably shorter time than is observed for the appearance of secondary leukemias. Patients who suffer from congenital deficiencies of cellular and humoral immunity also appear to be at increased risk of developing non-Hodgkin's lymphomas.[167] In 1984, it was observed that an increasing number of lymphomas, particularly Burkitt's lymphoma, were occurring in patients with acquired immunodeficiency syndrome (AIDS).[362] Hodgkin's disease has now been reported in association with this syndrome.[363] It is clear from these observations, therefore, that any patient receiving immunosuppressive therapy or in whom an immunosuppressed state is present, either congenitally or through acquisition, is at risk of developing these tumors.

Lymphomas and other solid tumors are being recognized with increasing frequency in patients with Hodgkin's disease treated with intensive therapy.[285,364,365] The initial observation of the appearance of a non-Hodgkin's lymphoma in patients with Hodgkin's disease was reported in 1977[366] and since then a total of 52 patients (Table 4–12) have been reported in the world's literature.[261,264,265,271,287,337,353,366-369,371-381] Almost all of these cases have occurred in patients receiving combined-modality therapy (radiation and chemotherapy) or chemotherapy alone. Although animal models have demonstrated the occurrence of lymphoma after radiation therapy (see above), this has only been observed in several case reports of secondary lymphomas in Hodgkin's disease.[287,376] The etiology of lymphomas observed after treatment of Hodgkin's disease is not known, although several explanations are possible. The appearance of non-Hodgkin's lymphomas in patients with Hodgkin's disease may represent a spectrum of the natural history of the disease and whatever is responsible for the appearance of Hodgkin's disease is likewise responsible for the lymphoma. The profound immunosuppression of Hodgkin's disease, both de novo and treatment related, may allow oncogenic viruses to proliferate and produce lymphomas. List et al. have demonstrated Epstein-Barr viral DNA in the genome of two B-cell lymphomas seen after treatment of Hodgkin's disease.[378] Chronic immunostimulation as a result of the presence of either "Hodgkin's disease antigens" or altered-self antigens may permit a lymphoid clone to undergo autonomous proliferation. The therapy itself may induce the lymphomas. Support for the latter explanation derives from the atomic bomb experience,[382] and animal experiments,[116,118,164,165] where radiation alone appears to have been responsible for the development of lymphomas.

Almost all non-Hodgkin's lymphomas reported in patients treated for Hodgkin's disease are diffuse large-cell lymphomas. Both B- and T-cell phenotypes have been reported.[371,374,379] Nodular lymphomas, multiple myeloma,[394] lymphoblastic lymphomas,[375] Kaposi's sarcoma[269,383,384] and mycosis fungoides[337,385] have been reported in association with this tumor. Almost all reported cases of mycosis fungoides have antedated or occurred simultaneously with the diagnosis of Hodgkin's disease. The risk of development of a non-Hodgkin's lymphoma has been estimated by studies at Stanford University as 0.3%, 0.6%, and 4.4% at 5, 7, and 10.3 years after the diagnosis of Hodgkin's disease.[377] Risk estimates for patients receiving combined-modality treatment were higher, with a maximum of 15.2% at 10.3 years. The risk of developing lymphoma appears to be higher than that for acute leukemia previously reported from this group.[275] The Southwest Oncology Group reported one non-Hodgkin's lymphoma among 643 patients with all stages of Hodgkin's disease.[290] Schomberg et al.[287] recently reported one case of non-Hodgkin's lymphoma (diffuse histiocytic lymphoma, DHL) from a group of 169 patients. This patient received only radiation therapy. The recent update of the Collaborative Study which used IF and EF radiotherapy for Hodgkin's disease,[342] reported four cases (4 of 460 patients) of non-Hodgkin's lymphoma (type and prior therapy not specified). Therefore, this complication, in most series, occurs less frequently than acute leukemia, and its association with one form of therapy is less clear.

The clinical presentation of these lymphomas does not appreciably differ from that of other non-Hodgkin's lymphomas; however, extranodal sites may be more frequent. Although secondary leukemias appear to go through a prodromal phase, with diverse abnormalities of the blood smear and blood count noted before symptoms appear, the "hidden anatomy" of lymph nodes only permits a diagnosis when the disease is obvious. Clonal evolution is almost certainly occurring in lymph nodes and would only be found if serial gene rearrangement studies were done.[386] The time until development of secondary lymphoma appears to be similar to that seen for secondary acute leukemias, with a range of 24 to 89 months after the diagnosis of Hodgkin's disease. In a patient with Hodgkin's disease who is in apparent remission for several years and then develops an enlarged lymph node—particularly in a previously adequately irradiated area—the possibility of a second lymphoma should be considered, and rebiopsy is mandatory. Likewise, the onset of abdominal complaints several years after an initially localized supradiaphragmatic Hodgkin's disease presentation suggests the possible development of an intra-abdominal lymphoma.

In those cases that are reported, patients' response to treatment for non-Hodgkin's lymphoma appears similar to the results of treatment for ANLL. Phenotypic analysis has demonstrated that a number of these patients have a poor prognosis (lymphoblastic, T cell, immunoblastic) and it is not surprising that their response has been less than optimal with standard chemotherapy approaches. The response to treatment of the intermediate-grade lymphomas, particularly the B-cell large-cell lymphomas, is similar to the treatment of de novo large-cell lymphomas. MOPP,[376] BCVPP,[376] CVP,[376] CHOP,[187] and a combination of vincristine, prednisone, cytoxan, L-asparaginase, and daunorubicin[375] have all been used successfully to achieve remissions in the more favorable phenotypes; several of these remissions have been long lasting. Therefore, if possible, such patients should be aggressively treated in hopes of eradicating this second malignancy.

REFERENCES

1. Koller, P.C., and Doak, S.M.A. Serial transplantation of haematopoietic tissue in irradiated hosts. *In*

Cellular Basis and Aetiology of Late Somatic Effects of Ionizing Radiation, edited by R.V.C. Harris. New York, Academic Press 1963, pp. 59–64.
2. Siminovitch, L., Till, J.E., McCulloch, E.A. Decline in colony-forming ability of marrow cells subjected to serial transportation into irradiated mice. J. Cell. Physiol. 64:23–32, 1962.
3. Vos, O., and Dolmans, M.J.A.S. Self-renewal of colony forming units (CFU) in serial bone marrow transplantation experiments. Cell Tissue Kinet. 5:371–385, 1972.
4. Micklem, H.S., Ogden, D.A., and Payne, A.C. Aging, hemopoietic stem cells, and immunity. In Haematopoietic Stem Cells. Ciba Found. Symp. 13:285–301, 1973.
5. Mauch, P., Botnick, L.E., Hannon, E.C. et al. Decline in bone marrow proliferative capacity as a function of age. Blood 60:245–252, 1982.
6. Ogden, D.A., and Micklem, H.S. The fate of serially transplanted bone marrow cell populations from young and old donors. Transplantation 22:287–293, 1976.
7. Hodgson, G.S., and Bradley, T.R. Properties of haematopoietic stem cells surviving 5-fluorouracil treatment: evidence for a pre-CFU-S cell. Nature 281:381–382, 1979.
8. Magli, M.C., Iscove, N.N., and Odartchenko, N. Transient nature of early haematopoietic spleen colonies. Nature 295:527–529, 1982.
9. Metcalf, D., Johnson, G.R., and Nicola, N.A. Separation and commitment of hemopoietic stem and progenitor cells. In "Hemopoietic Stem Cells," Alfred Benzon Symposium 18, edited by Killman, S.A., Cronkite, E.P., and Muller-Berat, C.N. Copenhagen Munksgaard, 1983, p 65.
10. Reincke. U., Hannon, E.C., Rosenblatt, M., and Hellman, S. Proliferative capacity of murine hematopoietic stem cells in vitro. Science 215:1619–1622, 1982.
11. Dicke, K.A., Van Noord, M.J., Maat, B. et al. Identification of cells in primate bone marrow resembling the hemopoietic stem cell in the mouse. Blood 42:195–208, 1973.
12. Dexter, T.M., Allen, T.D., and Lajtha, L.G. Conditions controlling the proliferation of haemopoietic stem cells in vitro. J. Cell. Physiol. 91:335–344, 1977.
13. Hocking, W.G., and Gold, D.W. Long term human bone marrow cultures. Blood 56:118–124, 1980.
14. Ihle, J.N., Keller, J., Greenberger, J.S., et al. Phenotypic characteristics of cell lines requiring interleukin 3 for growth. J. Immunol. 129:1377–1383, 1982.
15. Golde, D.W., Finley, T.N., and Cline, M.J. Production of colony-stimulating factor by human macrophages. Lancet 2:1397–1399, 1972.
16. Okabe, T., Fryisawa, M., Igudo, H. et al. Establishment of a human colony-stimulating factory producing cell line from an undifferentiated large cell carcinoma of the lung. Cancer 54:1024–1029, 1984.
17. Takeda, A., Suzumori, K., Sugimoto, Y., et al. Clear cell carcinoma of the ovary with colony-stimulating-factor production. Occurrence of marked granulocytosis in a patient and nude mice. Cancer 54:1019–1023, 1984.
18. Troxell, M.L., Mills, G.M., and Allen, R.C.: The hypereosinophilic syndrome in acute lymphocytic leukemia. Cancer 54:1058–1061, 1984.
19. Golde, D.W., Bersch, N., Quan, S.G., and Lusis, A.J. Production of erythroid potentiating activity by a human T-lymphoblast cell line. Proc. Natl. Acad. Sci. USA 77:593–596, 1980.
20. Fauser, A.A., Messner, H.A., Lusis, A.J., and Golde, D.W. Stimulatory activity for human pluripotent hemopoietic progeniters produced by a human T-lymphocyte cell line. Stem Cells 1:78–80, 1981.
21. Gillis, S., and Watson, J. Biochemical and biological characterization of lymphocyte regulatory molecules V. Identification of an interleukin 2-producing human leukemia T cell line. J. Exp. Med. 152:1709–1719, 1980.
22. Kalyanaram, V.S., Sarngadharan, M.G., Robert-Guroff, M., et al. A new subtype of human T-cell leukemia virus (HTLV-II) associated with a T-cell variant of hairy cell leukemia. Science 218:571–573, 1982.
23. Lusis, A.J., Quon, D.H., and Golde, D.W. Purification and characterization of a human T-lymphocyte derived granulocyte macrophage colony-stimulating factor. Blood 57:13–21, 1981.
24. Weisbart, R.H., Billing, R., and Golde, D.W. Neutrophil migration inhibition activity produced by a unique T lymphoblast cell line. J. Lab. Clin. Med. 93:622–626, 1979.
25. Gordon, M.Y., Kearney, L., and Hibbin, J.A. Effects of human marrow stromal cells on proliferation by human granulocytic (GM-CFC), erythroid (BFU-E), and mixed (Mixed-CFC) colony forming cells. Br. J. Haematol. 53:317–325, 1983.
26. Greenberg, B.R., Wilson, F.D., and Woo, L. Granulopoietic effects of human bone marrow fibroblastic cells and abnormalities in the "Granulopoietic Microenvironment." Blood 58:557–564, 1981.
27. Quesenberry, P.J., and Gimbrone, M.A. Jr. Vascular endothelium as a regulator of granulopoiesis: Production of colony-stimulating activity by cultured human endothelial cells. Blood 56:1060–1067, 1980.
28. Wolf, N.S. The haemopoietic microenvironment. Clin. Haematol. 8:469–500, 1979.
29. Ascensao, J.L., Vercellotti, G.M., Jacob, H.S., and Zanjani, E.D. Role of endothelial cells in human hematopoiesis: modulation of mixed colony growth in vitro. Blood 63:553–558, 1984.
30. Bergby, G., McCall, E., Jetmalani, S., et al. A monokine (MRA) regulates production of CSA by fibroblasts, endothelial cells, and T-lymphocytes. Blood (abstr), 60-94a(suppl), 1982.
31. Reincke, U., Hsieh, P., Mauch, P. et al Cell types associated with fibronectin in long-term mouse bone marrow cultures. J. Histochem. Cytochem. 30:235–244, 1982.
32. Balducci, L., Little, D.D., Glover, N.G., et al. Gran-

ulocyte reserve in cancer and malnutrition. Ann. Int. Med. 98:610–611, 1983.
33. Jacobson, W., Sidman, R.L., and Diamond, L.K. The effect of testosterone on the uptake of tritiated thymidine by the bone marrow of children. Ann. NY Acad. Sci. 149:389–405, 1968.
34. Golde, D.W., Bersch, N., Chapra, I.J., and Cline, M.J. Thyroid hormones stimulate erythropoiesis in vitro. Br. J. Haematol. 37:173–177, 1977.
35. Hollander, C.S., Thompson, R.H., Barrett, P.V.D., and Berlin, N.L. Repair of the anemia and hyperlipedemia of the hypothyroid dog. Endocrinology, 81:1007–1017, 1967.
36. Waldmann, T.A., Weissman, S., and Levin, E.H. Effect of thyroid administration on erythropoiesis in the dog. J. Lab. Clin. Med. 59:926–931, 1962.
37. Peschle, C., Zanjani, E.D., Gidari, A.S., et al. Mechanism of thyroxine action on erythropoiesis. Endocrinology 89:609–612, 1971.
38. Fuhr, J.E., and Dunn, C.D.R. Thyroid hormones and protein synthesis in fetal mouse liver erythroid cells. Exp. Hemat. 78:490–494, 1979.
39. Jones, P.A.E., Miller, F.M., Worwod, M., and Jacobs, A. Ferritinaemia in leukaemia and Hodgkin's disease. Br. J. Cancer 27:212–217, 1973.
40. Najean, Y., Dresch, C., and Ardaillon, N.: Trouble de l'utilization du fer hemoglobinique au cours des maladies de Hodgkin's evolutines. Nouv. Rev. Fr. Hematol. 7:739–747, 1967.
41. Al-Ismail, S., Cavill, I., Evans, I.H., et al. Erythropoiesis and iron metabolism in Hodgkin's disease. Br. J. Cancer 40:365–370, 1979.
42. Beamish, M.R., Ashley, Jones P., Trevett, D., et al. Iron metabolism in Hodgkin's disease. Br. J. Cancer 26:444–452, 1972.
43. Kampschmidt, R.F. Leukocyte endogenous mediator. J. Reticuloendothelial Soc. 23:287–297, 1978.
44. VanSnick, J.L., Masson, P.L., and Heremans, J.F. The involvement of lactoferrin in the hyposideremia of acute inflammation. J. Exp. Med. 140:1068–1084, 1974
45. Bowman, W.D. Abnormal ("ringed") sideroblasts in various hematologic and non-hematologic disorders. Blood 18:662–671, 1961.
46. Hines, J.D., and Grasso, J.A. The sideroblastic anemias. Semin. Hematol. 7:86–106, 1970.
47. Khaleeli, M., Keane, W.M., and Lee, G.R. Sideroblastic anemia in multiple myeloma: a preleukemic change. Blood 41:17–25, 1973.
48. Brownstein, M.H., and Scherl, B.A. Hodgkin's disease with erythrocytosis. Arch. Int. Med. 117:689–691, 1966.
49. Levinson, B., Walter, B.A., Wintrobe, M.M., and Cartwright, G.E. A clinical study of Hodgkin's disease. Arch. Int. Med. 99:519–535, 1957.
50. Lipson, R.L., Bayrd, E.D., and Watkins, C.H. The postsplenectomy blood picture. Am. J. Clin. Pathol. 32:526–532, 1959.
51. Hirsh, J., and Dacie, J.W. Splenectomy, thrombocytosis, and thromboembolism. Br. J. Haematol. 12:44–53, 1966.
52. Hoagland, H.C. Hematologic complications of cancer chemotherapy. Semin. Oncol. 9:95–102, 1982.
53. Laszlo, J., and Kremer, W.B. Hematologic effects of chemotherapeutic drugs and radiation. In Cancer Medicine, edited by Holland, J.F., and Frei, E III. Philadelphia, Lea & Febiger, 1973, pp. 1099–1115.
54. Lohrmann, A.P., and Schreml, W. Cytotoxic drugs and the granulopoietic system. Recent Results Cancer Res. 81:15–154, 1982.
55. Botnick, L.E., Hannon, E.C., Vigneulle, R., and Hellman, S. Differential effects of cytotoxic agents on hematopoietic progenitors. Cancer Res. 41:2338–2342, 1981.
56. Osband, M., Cohen, H., Cassady, J.R., and Jaffe, N. Severe and protracted bone marrow dysfunction following long-term therapy with methyl-CCNU (abstr). Proc. Am. Soc. Clin. Oncol. 18:303, 1977.
57. Botnick, L.E., Hannon, E.C., and Hellman, S. Limited proliferation of stem cells surviving alkylating agents. Nature 262:68–70, 1976.
58. Botnick, L E., Hannon, E.C., and Hellman, S. Multisystem stem cell failure after apparent recovery from alkylating agents. Cancer Res. 38:1942–1947, 1978.
59. Hellman, S., Botnick, L.E., Hannon, E.C., et al. Proliferative capacity of murine hematopoietic stem cells. Proc. Natl. Acad. Sci. USA 75:490–494, 1978.
60. Schofield, R. The relationship between the spleen colony-forming cell and the hematopoietic stem cell. A hypothesis. Blood Cells 4:7–25, 1978.
61. Botnick, L.E., Hannon, E.C., and Hellman, S. Late effects of cytotoxic agents on the normal tissues of mice. Front. Radiat. Ther. Onc. 13:36–47, 1979.
62. Morley, A., Trainor, K., and Blake, J. A primary stem cell lesion in experimental chronic hypoplastic marrow failure. Blood 45:681–688, 1975.
63. Rudd, P., Fries, J.F., and Epstein, W.V. Irreversible bone marrow failure with chlorambucil. J. Rheumatol. 2:421–429, 1975.
64. Hellman, S., Botnick, L.E. Stem cell depletion: an explanation of the late effects of cytotoxins. Int. J. Radiat. Oncol. Biol. Phys. 2:181–184, 1977.
65. Trainor, K.J., Seshadri, R.S., and Morley, A.A. Residual marrow injury following cytotoxic drugs. Leuk. Res. 3:205–210, 1979.
66. Boggs, D.R., Athens, J.W., Cartwright, G.E., and Wintrobe, M.M. The different effects of vinblastine sulfate and nitrogen-mustard upon neutrophil kinetics in the dog. Proc. Soc. Exp. Biol. Med. 121:1085–1090, 1966.
67. Host, H. Comparative effects of cyclophosphamide, nitrogen mustard, and total body irradiation on survival and on white blood cells in rats. Radiat. Res. 27:638–651, 1966.
68. Host, H. Regeneration of bone marrow cells in rats following cyclophosphamide or total body irradiation. Acta. Radiol. Ther. Phys. Biol. 4:337–352, 1966.
69. Fink, M.E., and Calabresi, P. The granulocyte response to an endotoxin (Pyrexal) as a measure of functional marrow reserve in cancer chemotherapy. Ann. Intern. Med. 57:732–742, 1962.
70. Baisogolov, G.D., and Isaev, I.G. Bone marrow he-

matopoiesis in the irradiated area with combined chemo and radiation therapy. Radiobiol. Radiother. (Berlin) 22:44–48, 1981.
71. Rubin, P., Scarantino, C.W. The bone marrow organ: the critical structure in radiation-drug interaction. Int. J. Radiat. Oncol. Biol. Phys. 4:3–21, 1978.
72. Hellman, S., and Hannon. E. Effects of adriamycin on the radiation response of murine hematopoietic stem cells. Radiat. Res. 67:162–167, 1976.
73. Till, J.E., and McCulloch, E.A. A direct measurement of the radiation sensitivity of normal mouse bone marrow cells. Radiat. Res. 14:213, 1961.
74. Rubin, P., Landman, S., Mayer, E., et al. Bone marrow regeneration and extension after extended field irradiation in Hodgkin's disease. Cancer 32:699–711, 1973.
75. Knospe, W.A., Blom, J., and Crosby, W.H. Regeneration of locally irradiated bone marrow—I Dose dependent long term changes in the rat, with particular emphasis upon vascular and stromal reaction. Blood 28:398–415, 1966.
76. Nelson, D.F., Chaffy, J.T., and Hellman, S. Late effects of x-irradiation on the ability of mouse bone marrow to support hematopoiesis. Int. J. Rad. Onc. Biol. Phys. 2:39–45, 1977.
77. Knospe, W.H., and Crosby, W.H. Aplastic anaemia: A disorder of the bone marrow sinusoidal microcirculation rather than stem-cell failure. Lancet 1:20–22, 1971.
78. Greenberger, J.S., Klassen, V., Kase, K., et al. Effects of low dose rate irradiation on plateau phase bone marrow stromal cells in vitro: Demonstration of a new form of non-lethal physiologic damage to support of hematopoietic stem cells. Int. J. Rad. Oncol. Biol. Phys. 10:1027–1037, 1984.
79. Sykes, M.P., Chu, F.C.H., Savel, H., et al. The effects of varying dosages of irradiation upon sternal marrow regeneration. Radiology 83:1084–1088, 1964.
80. Sykes, M.P., Sanel, H., Chu, F.C.H., et al. Long-term effects of therapeutic irradiation upon bone marrow. Cancer 17:1144–1148, 1964.
81. Goswitz, F.A., Andrews, G.A., and Kniseley, R.M. Effects of local irradiation (Co 60 Teletherapy) on the peripheral blood and bone marrow. Blood 21:605–619, 1963.
82. Slanina, J., Musshoff, K., Rahner, T., and Stiasny, R. Long-term side effects in irradiated patients with Hodgkin's disease. Int. J. Rad. Oncol. Biol. Phys. 2:1–19, 1977.
83. Atkinson, H.R. Bone marrow distribution as a factor in estimating radiation to the blood-forming organs.—A survey of present knowledge. J. Coll. Radiol. Aust. 6:149–154, 1962.
84. Parker, R.G., and Berry, H.C. Late effects of therapeutic irradiation on the skeleton and bone marrow. Cancer 37:1162–1171, 1976.
85. Parmentier C., Morardet, N., and Tubiana, M. Late effects on human bone marrow after extended field radiotherapy. Int. J. Radiat. Oncol. Biol. Phys. 9:1303–1311, 1983.

86. Sacks, E.L., Goris, M.L., Glatstein, E., et al. Bone marrow regeneration following large field radiation: Influence of volume, age, dose, and time. Cancer 42:1057–1065, 1978.
87. Tubiana, M., Frindel, E., Croizal, H., and Parmentier, C. Effects of radiations on bone marrow. Pathol. Biol. 27:326–334, 1979.
88. Vogel, J.M., Kimball, H.R., Foley, H.T., et al. Effect of extensive radiotherapy on the marrow granulocyte reserves of patients with Hodgkin's disease. Cancer 21:798–804, 1968.
89. Knospe, W.H., Rayudu, V.M.S., Cardello, M., et al. Bone marrow scanning with ^{52}Iron (^{52}Fe). Cancer 37:1432–1442, 1976.
90. Kun, L.E., and Johnson, R.E. Hematologic and immunologic status in Hodgkin's disease five years after radical radiotherapy. Cancer 36:1912–1916, 1975.
91. Hellman, S., and Fink, M.E. Granulocyte reserve following radiation therapy as studied by the response to a bacterial endotoxin. Blood 25:310–324, 1965.
92. Sherins, R.J., and DeVita, V.T. Jr. Effect of drug treatment for lymphoma on male reproductive capacity: Studies of men in remission after therapy. Ann. Intern. Med. 79:216–220, 1973.
93. Steinglass, P., Gordon, A.S., and Charipper, H.A. Effect of castration and sex hormones on the blood of the rat. Proc. Soc. Exp. Biol. Med. 48:167–177, 1941.
94. Chapman, R.M., Sutcliffe, S.B., and Malpas, J.S. Cytotoxic-induced ovarian failure in women with Hodgkin's disease. I. Hormone Function. JAMA 242:1877–1881, 1979.
95. Schilsky, R.L., Sherins, R.J., Hubbard, S.M., et al. Long-term follow-up of ovarian function in women treated with MOPP chemotherapy for Hodgkin's disease. Am. J. Med 71:552–556, 1981.
96. Sobrinko, L., Levine, R., and DeConti, R. Amenorrhea in patients with Hodgkin's disease treated with antineoplastic agents. Am. J. Obstet. Gynecol. 109:135–139, 1971.
97. Warne, G.L., Fairley, K.F., Hobbs, J.B., and Martin, F.I.R. Cyclophosphamide-induced ovarian failure. N. Eng. J. Med. 289:1159–1162, 1973.
98. Fuks, Z., Glatstein, E., Marsa, G.W., et al. Long-term effects of external radiation on the pituitary and thyroid glands. Cancer 37:1152–1161, 1976.
99. Tudhope, G.R., and Wilson, G.M. Anaemia in hypothyroidism. Q. J. Med. 29:513–537, 1960.
100. Wardrop, C., and Hutchison, H.E. Red-cell shape in hypothyroidism. Lancet i:1243, 1969.
101. Simone, J.V., Abildgaard, C.F., and Schulman, I. Blood coagulation in thyroid dysfunction. N. Eng. J. Med. 273:1057–1061, 1965.
102. Metcalf, D. Regulation of self-replication in normal and leukemic stem cells, in Normal and Neoplastic Hematopoiesis, edited by Golde, D., and Marks, P. New York, Alan R. Liss, 1983, pp. 141–156.
103. Sacks, L. Control of normal cell differentiation and phenotype reversion of malignancy in myeloid leukemia. Nature 274:535–539, 1978.

104. Koeffler, H.P. Induction of differentiation of human acute myelogenous leukemia cells: therapeutic implications. Blood 62:709–721, 1983.
105. Armitage, J.O., Dick, F.R., Needleman, S.W., and Burns, C.P. Effect of chemotherapy for the dysmyelopoietic syndrome. Cancer Treat. Rev. 65:601–605, 1981.
106. Arthur, D.C., and Bloomfield, C.D. Partial deletion of the long arm of chromosome 16 and bone marrow eosinophilia in acute nonlymphocytic leukemia: A new association. Blood 61:994–998, 1983.
107. Harris, R.E., Seo, I.S., Provisor, D., et al. Acute myeloblastic leukemia two years after diagnosis of non-Hodgkin lymphoma. Med. Pediatr. Oncol. 7:303–308, 1979.
108. Burny, A., Bex, F., Chantrenne, H., et al. Bovine leukemia virus involvement in enzootic bovine leukosis. Adv. Cancer. Res. 28:251–311, 1978.
109. Gallo, R.C., Gallagher, R.E., Wong-Staal, F., et al. Isolation and tissue distribution of type-C virus and viral components from a gibbon ape (Hylobates lar) with lymphocytic leukemia. Virology 84:359–373, 1978.
110. Gardner, M.B., Henderson, B.E., Estes, J.D., et al. The epidemiology and virology of C-type virus-associated hematological cancers and related diseases in wild mice. Cancer Res. 36:574–580, 1976.
111. Kawakami, T.G., Theilen, G.H., Dungworth, D.L., et al. "C" type viral particles in plasma of cats with feline leukemia. Science 158:1049–1050, 1967.
112. Baltimore, D. RNA-dependent DNA polymerase in virions of RNA tumour viruses. Nature 226:1209–1121, 1970.
113. Hayward, W.S., Neel, B.G., and Astrin, S.M. Activation of a cellular onc gene by promoter insertion in ALV-induced lymphoid leukosis. Nature 290:475–480, 1981.
114. DeKlein, A., VanKessel, A.G., Grosveld, G., et al. A cellular oncogene is translocated to the Philadelphia chromosome in chronic myelocytic leukemia. Nature 300:765–767, 1982.
115. Ribacchi, R., and Giraldo, C. Leukemia virus release in chemically or physically-induced lymphomas in BALB/c mice. Natl. Cancer Inst. Monogr. 22:701–711, 1966.
116. Conklin, J.W., Upton, A.C., Christenberry, K.W., and McDonald, T.P. Comparative late somatic effects of some radiomimetic agents and x-rays. Radiat. Res. 19:156–168, 1963.
117. Kaplan, H.S. Leukemia and lymphoma in experimental and domestic animals. Ser. Haematol. 7:94–163, 1974.
118. Loutit, J., and Carr, T. Lymphoid tumours and leukaemia induced in mice by bone-seeking radionuclides. Int. J. Radiat. Biol. 33:245–263, 1978.
119. Kaplan, H.S., Carnes, W.H., Brown, M.B., and Hirsch, B.B. Indirect induction of lymphomas in irradiated mice. I. Tumor incidence and morphology in mice bearing nonirradiated thymic grafts. Cancer Res. 16:422–425, 1956.
120. Decleve, A., Niwa, O., Gelmann, E., and Kaplan, H.S. Radiation activation of endogenous leukemia viruses in cell culture: Acute x-ray irradiation. In Biology of Radiation Carcinogenesis, edited by Yukas, J.M., Tennant, R.W., and Regan, J.D. New York, Raven Press, 1976, pp. 217–225.
121. MacMahon, B. Prenatal x-ray exposure and childhood cancer. J. Natl. Cancer Inst. 28:1173–1191, 1962.
122. March, H.C. Leukemia in radiologists ten years later. Am. J. Med. Sci. 242:137, 1961.
123. Moloney, W.C. Leukemia and exposure to x-ray: A report of six cases. Blood 14:1137–1142, 1959.
124. Murray, R., Heckel, P., and Hempelmann, L.H. Leukemia in children exposed to ionizing radiation. N. Eng. J. Med. 261:585–589, 1959.
125. VanSwaay, H. Aplastic anemia and myeloid leukaemia after irradiation of the vertebral column. Lancet 2:225–227, 1955.
126. Finch, S.C. The study of atomic bomb survivors in Japan. Am. J. Med. 66:899, 1979.
127. Kamada, N., and Uchino, H. Preleukemic states in atomic bomb survivors in Japan. Blood Cells 2:57–65, 1976.
128. Toolis, F., Potter, B., Allan, N.C., and Langlands, A.O. Radiation-induced leukemias in ankylosing spondylitis. Cancer 48:1582–1585, 1981.
129. Alderson, M.R., and Jackson, S.M. Long term follow-up of patients with menorrhagia treated by irradiation. Br. J. Radiol. 44:295–298, 1971.
130. Berk, P.D., Goldberg, J.D., Silverstein, M.N., et al. Increased incidence of acute leukemia in polycythemia vera associated with chlorambucil therapy. N. Eng. J. Med. 304:441–447, 1981.
131. McEndy, D.P., Boon, M.C., and Furth, J. Induction of leukemia in mice by methylcholanthrene and x-rays. J. Natl. Cancer. Inst. 3:227–247, 1942.
132. Dexter, T.M., Schofield, R., Lajtha, L.G., and Moore, M. Studies on the mechanism of chemical leukaemogenesis. Br. J. Cancer. 30:325–331, 1974.
133. Fraumeni, J.F., and Miller, R.W. Drug-induced cancer. J. Natl. Cancer Inst. 48:1267–1270, 1972.
134. Schmahl, D., and Habs, M. Experimental carcinogenesis of antitumor drugs. Cancer Treat. Rev. 5:175–184, 1978.
135. Aksoy, M., Erdem, S., and Dincol, G. Leukemia in shoe-workers exposed chronically to benzene. Blood 44:837, 1974.
136. Cohen, H.J., and Huang, A.T.F. A marker chromosome abnormality: Occurrence in chloramphenicol-associated acute leukemia. Arch. Int. Med. 132:440–433, 1973.
137. Jensen, M.K., and Roll, K. Phenylbutazone and leukaemia. Acta. Med. Scand. 178:505–513, 1965.
138. Gavwerky, C.E., and Golde, D.W. Lithium enhances growth of human leukemia cells in vitro. Br. J. Haematol. 51:431–438, 1982.
139. Cameron, S. Chlorambucil and leukemia (letter). N. Eng. J. Med. 296:1065, 1977.
140. O'Gara, R.W., Adamson, R.H., Kelly, M.G., and Dalgaard, D.W. Neoplasms of the hematopoietic system in nonhuman primates: Report of one spontaneous tumor and two leukemias induced by procarbazine. J. Natl. Cancer Inst. 46:1121–1130, 1971.
141. Rosner, F., and Grunwald, H.W. Cytotoxic drugs and leukemogenesis. Clin. Haematol. 9:663–681, 1980.
142. Walpole, A.L. Carcinogenic action of alkylating agents. Ann. NY Acad. Sci. 68:750–761, 1958.

143. Weisburger, J.H., Griswald, D.P., Prejean, J.D., et al. The carcinogenic properties of some of the principal drugs used in clinical cancer chemotherapy. Recent Results Cancer Res. 52:1–17, 1975.
144. Kelly, M.G., O'Gara, R.W., Yancey, S.T., and Botkin, C. Induction of tumors in rats with procarbazine hydrochloride. J. Natl. Cancer Inst. 40:1027–1051, 1968.
145. Berg, J.W. The incidence of multiple primary cancers. Development of further cancer in patients with lymphomas, leukemias, and myeloma. J. Natl. Cancer Inst. 38:741–752, 1967.
146. Karchmer, R.K., Amare, M., Larsen, W.E. et al. Alkylating agents as leukemogens in multiple myeloma. Cancer 33:1103–1107, 1974.
147. Kyle R.A., Pierre, R.V., Bayrd, E.D. Multiple myeloma and acute leukemia associated with alkylating agents. Arch. Intern. Med. 135:185–192, 1975.
148. Rosner, F., and Grunwald, H. Multiple myeloma and Waldenstrom's macroglobulinemia terminating in acute leukemia. A review with emphasis on karyotypic and ultrastructural abnormalities. NY State J. Med. 80:558–570, 1980.
149. Grunwald, H.W., and Rosner, F. Acute myeloid leukemia following treatment of Hodgkin's disease. Cancer 50:676–683, 1982.
150. Rosner, F., and Grunwald, H. Hodgkin's disease and acute leukemia. Am. J. Med. 58:339–353, 1975.
151. Collins, A.J., Bloomfield, C.D., Peterson, R.A., and McKenna, R.W. Acute nonlymphocytic leukemia in patients with nodular lymphoma. Cancer 40:1748–1754, 1977.
152. O'Donnell, J.F., Bereton, H.D., Greco, F.A., et al. Acute non-lymphocytic leukemia and acute myeloproliferative syndrome following radiation therapy for non-Hodgkin's lymphoma and chronic lymphocytic leukemia: clinical studies. Cancer 44:1930, 1979.
153. Zarrabi, M.H., Rosner, F., and Bennett, J.M. Non-Hodgkin's lymphoma and acute myeloblastic leukemia. A report of 12 cases and review of the literature. Cancer 44:1070–1080, 1979.
154. Zarrabi, M.H., Rosner, F., and Bennett, J.M. Acute leukemia and non-Hodgkin's lymphoma. N. Eng. J. Med. 298:280, 1978.
155. Catovsky, D., and Galton, D.A.G. Myelomonocytic leukemia supervening on chronic lymphocytic leukaemia. Lancet 1:478–479, 1971.
156. Kempin, S., Lee, B.J. III, Thaler, H.T., et al. Combination chemotherapy of advanced chronic lymphocytic leukemia: The M-2 protocol (Vincristine, BCNU, Cyclophosphamide, Melphalan, and Prednisone). Blood 60:1110–1121, 1982.
157. Grunwald, H., and Rosner, F. Acute leukemia and immunosuppressive drug use. A review of patients undergoing immunosuppressive therapy for non-neoplastic diseases. Arch. Int. Med. 139:461–466, 1979.
158. Kempin, S., Sundaresan, N., Shapiro, W.B., and Arlin, Z. Acute nonlymphocytic leukemia following treatment of malignant glioma. J. Neurosurg. 60:1287–1290, 1984.
159. Muller, W., and Brandis, M. Acute leukemia after cytotoxic treatment for nonmalignant diseases in childhood. A case report and review of the literature. Eur. J. Pediatr. 136:105–108, 1981.
160. Rosner, F., Carey, R.W., and Zarrabi, M.H. Breast cancer and acute leukemia: Report of 24 cases and review of the literature. Am. J. Hematol. 4:151, 1978.
161. Zarrabi, M.H., and Rosner, F. Acute myeloblastic leukemia following treatment for non-hematopoietic cancers: Report of 19 cases and review of the literature. Am. J. Hematol. 7:357–367, 1979.
162. Lilly, F., Duran-Reynals, M.L., and Rowe, W.P. Correlation of early murine leukemia virus titer and H-2 type with spontaneous leukemia in mice of the BALB/c × AKR Gross: A genetic analysis. J. Exp. Med. 141:882–889, 1975.
163. Mayer, A., and Dorsch-Hasler, K. Endogenous MuLV infection does not contribute to onset of radiation or carcinogen-induced murine thymoma. Nature 295:253–255, 1982.
164. Kaplan, H.S. Influence of age on susceptibility of mice to the development of lymphoid tumors after irradiation. J. Natl. Cancer Inst. 9:55, 1948.
165. Kaplan, H.S. Influence of thymectomy, splenectomy, and gonadectomy on incidence of radiation-induced lymphoid tumors in strain C57 black mice. J. Natl. Cancer Inst. 11:83–90, 1950.
166. Law, L.W. Effect of gonadectomy and adrenalectomy on the appearance and incidence of spontaneous lymphoid leukemia in C58 mice. J. Natl. Cancer Inst. 8:157–159, 1947.
167. Waldman, T.A., Strober, W., and Blaese, R.M. Immunodeficiency disease and malignancy. Various immunologic deficiencies of man and the role of immune processes in the control of malignant disease. Ann. Int. Med. 77:605–628, 1972.
168. Bjorkholm, M., Holm, G., Defaire, U., and Mellstadt, H. Immunological defects in healthy twin siblings of patients with Hodgkin's disease. Scand. J. Haematol. 19:396–400, 1977.
169. Clapp, N.K., and Yumas, J.M. Suggested correlation between radiation-induced immunosuppression and radiogenic leukemia in mice. J. Natl. Cancer Inst. 51:1211–1215, 1973.
170. Honto, D.W., Frizzera, G., Gail-Peczalska, K.J., et al. Epstein-Barr virus-Induced B-cell lymphoma after renal transplantation: acylovir therapy and transition from polyclonal to monoclonal B-cell proliferation. N. Eng. J. Med. 306:913–918, 1982.
171. Schneck, S.A., and Penn, I. De novo brain tumors in renal-transplant recipients. Lancet 1:983–986, 1971.
172. Tchermia, G., Mielot, F., Subtil, E., and Parmentier, C. Acute myeloblastic leukemia after immunodepressive therapy for primary nonmalignant disease. Blood Cells 2:67–80, 1976.
173. Till, M., Rapson, N., and Smith, P.G. Family studies in acute leukaemia in childhood: A possible association with autoimmune disease. Br. J. Cancer 40:62–71, 1979.
174. Ten-Bensel, R.W., Stadlan, I.M., and Krivit, W. The

development of malignancy in the course of the Aldrich syndrome. J. Pediatr. *68*:761–767, 1968.
175. Aisenberg, A.C. Manifestations of immunologic unresponsiveness in Hodgkin's disease. Cancer Res. *26*:1152–1160, 1966.
176. Aisenberg, A.C. Studies on delayed hypersensitivity in Hodgkin's disease. J. Clin. Invest. *41*:1964–1970, 1962.
177. Pick, A.I., Duer, D., Kessler, H., et al. Delayed hypersensitivity and lymphocyte transformation in patients with Hodgkin's disease and granulomas. Cancer *41*:2192–2196, 1978.
178. Aisenberg, A.C., and Leskowitz, S. Antibody formation in Hodgkin's disease. N. Eng. J. Med. *93*:1269–1272, 1963.
179. Mendins, J.R., Dehortius, R.J., Messner, R.P., et al. Family distribution of lymphocytoxins in Hodgkin's disease. Ann. Int. Med. *84*:151–156, 1976.
180. Reed, D.M. On the pathological changes in Hodgkin's disease with special reference to its relation to tuberculosis. Johns Hopkin's Hospital Rev. *10*:133–196, 1902.
181. Winkelstein, A., Mikulla, J.M., Sartiano, G.P., and Ellis, L.D. Cellular immunity in Hodgkin's disease: Comparison of cutaneous reactivity and lymphoproliferative responses to phytohemagglutinin. Cancer *34*:549–553, 1974.
182. Young, R.C., Carder, M.P., Haynes, H.A., and DeVita, V.T. Delayed hypersensitivity in Hodgkin's disease. Am. J. Med. *52*:63–72, 1972.
183. Romagnani, S., Maggi, E., Bragotti, R., et al. Altered proportion of Tμ- and Tγ-cell subpopulations in patients with Hodgkin's disease. Scand. J. Immunol. *7*:511–514, 1970.
184. Case, D.C., Hansen, J.A., Corrales,E., et al. Depressed in vitro lymphocyte responses to PHA in patients with Hodgkin's disease in continuous long remissions. Blood *49*:771–778, 1977.
185. Miller, D.G. Patterns of immunological deficiency in lymphomas and leukemias. Ann. Int. Med. *57*:703–716, 1962.
186. Dinsmore, R.E., Straus, D.J., Pollack, M.S., et al. Fatal graft-versus host disease following blood transfusion in Hodgkin's disease documented by HLA typing. Blood *55*:831–834, 1980.
187. Joachim, H.L., Cooper, M.C., Hellman, G.C. Lymphomas in men at high risk for acquired immunodeficiency syndrome (AIDS). Cancer *56*:2831–2842, 1985.
188. Huber, C., Michlmayr, G., Falkensamer, M., et al. Increased proliferation of T-lymphocytes in the blood of patients with Hodgkin's disease. Clin. Exp. Immunol. *21*:47–53, 1975.
189. Longmire, R.L., McMillan, R., Yelenosky, R., et al. In vitro splenic IgG synthesis in Hodgkin's disease. N. Eng. J. Med. *289*:763–767, 1973.
190. Cohen, S., Fisher, B., Yoshida, T., and Bettigole, R.E. Serum migration-inhibitory activity in patients with lymphoproliferative diseases. N. Eng. J. Med. *290*:882–886, 1974.
191. Kass, L., and Votow, M.L. Eosinophilia and plasmacytosis of the bone marrow in Hodgkin's disease. Am. J. Clin. Pathol. *64*:248–250, 1975.
192. deMulder, P.H.M., dePauw, B.E., Van deVen, E.C., et al. Monocyte-mediated antibody-dependent cellular cytotoxicity in malignant lymphoma and solid tumors. Cancer *53*:2444–2449, 1984.
193. Bukowski, R.M., Naguchi, S., Hewlett, J.S., and Deodhar, S. Lymphocyte subpopulations in Hodgkin's disease. Am. J. Clin. Path. *65*:31–39, 1976.
194. Knowles, D.M. III, Hapler, J.P., and Jakobiec, F.A. T-lymphocyte subpopulations in B-cell-derived non-Hodgkin's lymphomas and Hodgkin's disease. Cancer *54*:644–651, 1984.
195. Aisenberg, A.C., and Wilkes, B.M. Lymph node T-cells in Hodgkin's disease: Analysis of suspensions with monoclonal antibody and rosetting techniques. Blood *59*:522–527, 1982.
196. Martin, J.M.E., and Warnke, R.A.: A quantitative comparison of T-cell subsets in Hodgkin's disease and reactive hyperplasia. Frozen section immunohistochemistry. Cancer *53*:2450–2455, 1984.
197. Amlot, P.L., Prissell, B., Staney, J.M., et al. Correlation between immune complexes and prognostic factors in Hodgkin's disease. Clin. Exp. Immunol. *31*:166–175, 1978.
198. Dunbar, J.A. Injury to large lymphoid cells in Hodgkin's disease. Lancet *1*:222–223, 1975.
199. DeSousa, M., Yang, M., Lopes-Corrales, E., et al. Ecotaxis: The principle and its application to the study of Hodgkin's disease. Clin. Exp. Immunol. *27*:143–149, 1977.
200. Hansen, N.E., and Karle, H. Elevated plasma lysozyme in Hodgkin's disease: An indicator of increased macrophage activity? Scand. J. Haematol. *22*:173–178, 1979.
201. Kedar, A., Khan, A.B., Mattern, J.Q.A. II., et al. Autoimmune disorders complicating adolescent Hodgkin's disease. Cancer *44*:112–116, 1979.
202. Lanier, R.L., and Amare, M. Autoimmune cytopenias in Hodgkin's disease. Rocky Mountain Med. J. *76*:165–168, 1979.
203. Bjorkholm, M., Holm, G., and Merk, K. Cyclic autoimmune hemolytic anemia as a presenting manifestation of splenic Hodgkin's disease. Cancer *49*:1702–1704, 1982.
204. Brown, R.J.K., and Meynell, M.J. Haemolytic anaemia associated with Hodgkin's disease. Lancet *2*:835–836, 1949.
205. Carpentieri, U., Daeschner, C.W., and Haggard, M.E. Immunohemolytic anemia and Hodgkin disease (letter). Pediatrics *70*:320–321, 1982.
206. Case Records of the Massachusetts General Hospital, Case 24-1978. N. Eng. J. Med. *298*:1407–1412, 1978.
207. Cazenave, J.P., Gagnon, J.A.E., Girouard, E., and Bastarache, A. Autoimmune hemolytic anemia terminating seven years later in Hodgkin's disease. Can. Med. Assoc. J. *109*:748–752, 1973.
208. Chu, J.Y., McElfresh, A.E., and Waeltermann, B.S. Autoimmune hemolytic anemia as a presenting manifestation of Hodgkin disease. J. Pediatr. *89*:429–430, 1976.

209. Dacie, K.V. The Hemolytic Anemias, Part 3, Second Edition. New York, Grune and Stratton, 1967, pp. 719–754.
210. Eisner, E., Ley, A.B., and Mayer, K. Coombs' positive hemolytic anemia in Hodgkin's disease. Ann. Intern. Med. 66:258–273, 1967.
211. Garratty, G., Petz, L.D., Wallerstein, R.O., and Fudenberg, H.H. Autoimmune hemolytic anemia in Hodgkin's disease associated with anti-I^T. Transfusion 14:226–231, 1974.
212. Jones, SE. Autoimmune disorders and malignant lymphoma. Cancer 31:1092–1098, 1973.
213. Kyle, R.A., Kiely, J.M., and Stickney, J.M. Acquired hemolytic anemia in chronic lymphocytic leukemia and the lymphomas. Survival and response to therapy in twenty seven cases. Arch. Int. Med. 104:61–67, 1959.
214. Levine, A.M., Thornton, P., Forman, S.J., et al. Positive Coomb's test in Hodgkin's disease: significance and implications. Blood 55:607–611, 1980.
215. Matthias, J. Haemolytic anemia in leukaemia and lymphoma: incidence, prognostic significance, and effect of treatment. Tenth Congress of the International Society of Haematology, Stockholm, 1964. (Abst: 52).
216. May, R.B., and Bryan, J.H. Autoimmune hemolytic anemia and Hodgkin's disease. J. Pediatr. 89:428–429, 1976.
217. Miller, D.G. The association of immune disease and malignant lymphoma. Ann Intern. Med. 66:507–521, 1967.
218. Payet, M., Sankale, M., Linhard, J., et al. Ictere hemolytique premonitoire d'une maladie de Hodgkin chez un africain. Presse. Med. 72:1665, 1964.
219. Pirofsky, B. Autoimmune hemolytic anemia and neoplasia of the reticuloendothelium with a hypothesis concerning etiologic relationships. Ann. Int. Med. 68:109–121, 1968.
220. Stojcevski, R. Haemolytic anaemia in malignant lymphoreticuloendothelial diseases. Haematologia 8:507–516, 1974.
221. Trinick, R.H. Lymphocytes and intravascular haemolysis: Lancet i:225, 1949.
222. Videbaek, A. "Auto-immune" haemolytic anaemia in some malignant systemic diseases. Acta. Med. Scand. 171:463–476, 1962.
223. Wasserman, L.R., Stats, D., Schwartz, L., and Fudenberg, H. Symptomatic and hemopathic hemolytic anemia. Am. J. Med. 18:961–989, 1955.
224. Weitberg, A.B., and Harmon, D.C. Autoimmune neutropenia, hemolytic anemia, and reticulocytopenia in Hodgkin's disease. Ann. Int. Med. 100:702–703, 1984.
225. Garratty, G., Haffleigh, B., Dalziel, J., and Petz, L.D. An IgG anti-I^T detected in a caucasian American. Transfusion 12:325–329, 1972.
226. Lewis, F.B., Schwartz, R.S., and Dameshek, W. X-irradiation and alkylating agents as possible "trigger" mechanisms in the autoimmune complications of malignant lymphoproliferative disease. Clin. Exp. Immunol. 1:3–11, 1966.
227. Leickly, F.E., and Buckley, R.H. Successful treatment of autoimmune hemolytic anemia in common variable immunodeficiency with high-dose intravenous gamma globulin. Am. J. Med. 82:159–162, 1987.
228. Ahn, Y.S., Harrington, W.J., Mylvaganam, R., et al. Danazol therapy for autoimmune hemolytic anemia. Ann. Int. Med. 102:298–301, 1985.
229. Antonio, J., and Sherwood, P.M. Idiopathic thrombocytopenic purpura in Hodgkin's disease after splenectomy. Am. J. Hemat. 1:115–120, 1976.
230. Berkman, A.W., Woog, J.J., Kickler, T.S., and Ettinger, D.S. Serial determinations of antiplatelet antibodies in a patient with Hodgkin's disease and autoimmune thrombocytopenia. Cancer 51:2057–2060, 1983.
231. Cohen, J.R. Idiopathic thrombocytopenic purpura in Hodgkin's disease. A rare occurrence of no prognostic significance. Cancer 41:743–746, 1978.
232. Fink, K., and Al-Mondhiry, H. Idiopathic purpura in lymphoma. Cancer 37:1999–2004, 1976.
233. Hamilton, P.J., and Dawson, A.A. Thrombocytopenic purpura as the sole manifestation of a recurrence of Hodgkin's disease. J. Clin. Pathol. 26:70–72, 1973.
234. Hassidim, K., McMillan, R., Conjalka, M.S., and Morrison, J. Immune thrombocytopenic purpura in Hodgkin's disease. Am. J. Hematol. 6:149–153, 1979.
235. Julia, A., and Miller, S.P. Idiopathic thrombocytopenic purpura in Hodgkin's disease after splenectomy. Am. J. Hematol. 1:115–120, 1976.
236. Khilanani, P., and Al-Sarraf, M. The association of autoimmune thrombocytopenia and Hodgkin's disease. Oncology 28:238–245, 1973.
237. Kirshner, J.J., Zamkoff, K.W., and Gottlieb, A.J. Idiopathic thrombocytopenic purpura and Hodgkin's disease: report of two cases and a review of the literature. Am. J. Med. Sci. 280:21–28, 1980.
238. Rudders R.A. Autoimmune thrombocytopenic purpura in Hodgkin's disease. N. Eng. J. Med. 290:49–50, 1974.
239. Rudders, R.A., Aisenberg, A.C., and Schiller, A.L. Hodgkin's disease presenting as "idiopathic" thrombocytopenic purpura. Cancer 30:220–230, 1979.
240. Waddell, C.C., and Cimo, P.L. Idiopathic thrombocytopenic purpura occurring in Hodgkin's disease after splenectomy: report of two cases and review of the literature. Am. J. Hemat. 7:381–387, 1979.
241. Weitzman, S., Dvilansky, A., and Yanai, I. Thrombocytopenic purpura as the sole manifestation of recurrence in Hodgkin's disease. Acta. Haemat. 58:129–133, 1977.
242. Woods, V.L. Jr, Oh, E.H., Mason, D., and McMillan, R.: Autoantibodies against the platelet glycoprotein IIb/IIIa complex in patients with chronic ITP. Blood 63:368–375, 1984.
243. Shulman, N.R. Weinrach, R.S., Libre, E.P., and Andreus, H.L. The role of the reticuloendothelial system in the pathogenesis of idiopathic thrombocy-

topenic purpura. Trans. Assoc. Am. Physicians 78:374–390, 1965.
244. Rosse, W.F., Adams, J.P., and Yount, W.J. Subclass of IgG antibodies in immune thrombocytopenic purpura (ITP). Br. J. Haematol. 46:109–114, 1980.
245. Kaden, B.R., Rosse, W.F., and Hauch, T.W. Immune thrombocytopenic purpura in lymphoproliferative disorders. Blood 53:545–551, 1979.
246. McMillan, R., Longmire, R.L., Yelenosky, R., et al. Immunoglobulin synthesis in vitro by splenic tissue in idiopathic thrombocytopenic purpura. N. Eng. J. Med. 286:681–684, 1972.
247. VanLeeuwen, E.F., VanderVen, J. ThM, Engelfriet, C.P., and Yon dem Borne, A.E.G.K. Specificity of autoantibodies in autoimmune thrombocytopenia. Blood 59:23–26, 1982.
248. Nurden, A.T., and Caen, J.P. Different glycoprotein abnormalities in thromboasthenic and Bernard-Soulier platelets. Semin. Hematol. 16:234–250, 1979.
249. Metcalf, D. Regulator-induced suppression of myelomonocytic leukemic cells: clonal analysis of early cellular events. Int. J. Cancer 30:203–210, 1982.
250. Doan, C.A., Bouroncle, B.A., and Wiseman, B.K. Idiopathic and secondary thrombocytopenic purpura. Clinical study and evaluation of 381 cases over a period of 28 years. Ann. Int. Med. 53:861–876, 1960.
251. Hymes, K., Shulman, S., and Karpatkin, S. A solid-phase radioimmunoassay for bound anti-platelet antibody. J. Lab. Clin. Med. 94:639–648, 1979.
252. Crain, S.M., and Choudhury, A.M. Thrombotic thrombocytopenic purpura in a splenectomized patient with Hodgkin's disease. Am. J. Med. Sci. 280:35–40, 1980.
253. Dumoulin-Lagrange, M., Tulliez, H., Diebold, J., et al. Purpura thrombotique thrombocytopenique (PTT) associe a une maladie de Hodgkin (MdH). Nouv. Rev. Fr. Hematol. 25:275–276, 1983.
254. Phillips, E.A., Kempin, S., Reich, L., and Clarkson, B. Bleomycin for the treatment of immune cytopenia. N. Eng. J. Med. 302:1031, 1980.
255. Bussel, J.B., and Hilgartner, M.W. The use and mechanism of action of intravenous immunoglobulin in the treatment of immune haematologic disease. Br. J. Haematol. 56:1–7, 1984.
256. Hunter, J.D., Logue, G.L., and Joyner, J.T. Autoimmune neutropenia in Hodgkin's disease. Arch. Intern. Med. 142:386–388, 1982.
257. Heyman, M.R., and Walsh, T.J. Autoimmune neutropenia and Hodgkin's disease. Cancer 59:1903–1905, 1987.
258. Aisenberg, A.C. Acute nonlymphocytic leukemia after treatment for Hodgkin's disease. Am. J. Med. 75:449–454, 1983.
259. Arseneau, J.C., Canellos, G.P., Johnson, R.E., and DeVita, V.T. Risk of new cancers in patients with Hodgkin's disease. Cancer 40:1912–1916, 1977.
260. Auclerc, G., Jacquillat, C., Auclerc, M.F., et al. Post-therapeutic acute leukemia. Cancer 44:2017–2025, 1979.
261. Austin-Seymour, M.M., Hoppe, R.T., Cox, R.S., et al. Hodgkin's disease in patients over sixty years old. Ann. Int. Med. 100:13–18, 1984.
262. Baccarani, M., Bosi, A., and Papa, G. Second malignancy in patients treated for Hodgkin's disease. Cancer 46:1735–1740, 1980.
263. Bartolucci, A.A., Liu, C., Durant, J.R., and Gams, R.A. Acute myelogenous leukemia as a second malignant neoplasm following the successful treatment of advanced Hodgkin's disease. Cancer 52:2209–2213, 1983.
264. Boivin, J.F., and Hutchinson, G.B. Leukemia and other cancers after radiotherapy and chemotherapy for Hodgkin's disease. J. Natl. Cancer Inst. 67:751–760, 1981.
265. Boivin, J.F., Hutchinson, G.B., Lyden, M., et al. Second primary cancers following treatment of Hodgkin's disease. J. Natl. Cancer Inst. 72:233–241, 1984.
266. Bolla, M., Sotto, J.J., Barjhoux, R., et al. Complications nongonadiques de l'association chimioradiotherapie dans la maladie de Hodgkin: A propos d'une serie de quatre-vinqt-trois observations. Sem. Hop. Paris 58:204–208, 1982.
267. Bookman, M.A., and Longo, D.L. Concomitant illness in patients treated for Hodgkin's disease. Cancer Treat. Rev. 13:77–111, 1986.
268. Borum, K. Increasing frequency of acute myeloid leukemia complicating Hodgkin's disease: A review. Cancer 46:1247–1252, 1980.
269. Brody, R.S., Schottenfeld, D., and Reid, A. Multiple primary cancer risk after therapy for Hodgkin's disease. Cancer 40:1917–1926, 1977.
270. Brody, R.S., and Schottenfeld, D. Multiple primary cancers in Hodgkin's disease. Semin. Oncol. 7:187–201, 1980.
271. Cadman, E.C., Capizzi, R.L., and Bertino, J.R. Acute nonlymphocytic leukemia. A delayed complication of Hodgkin's disease therapy: Analysis of 109 cases. Cancer 40:1280–1296, 1977.
272. Canellos, G.P., DeVita, V.T., Arseneau, J.C., et al. Second malignancies complicating Hodgkin's disease in remission. Lancet i:947–949, 1975.
273. Casciato, D., and Scott, J.L. Acute leukemia following prolonged cytotoxic agent therapy. Medicine 58:32–47, 1979.
274. Chan, B.W.B., and McBride, J.A. Hodgkin's disease and leukemia. Can. Med. Assoc. J. 106:558–561, 1972.
275. Coleman, C.N., Williams, C.J., Flint, A., et al. Hematologic neoplasia in patients treated for Hodgkin's disease. N. Eng. J. Med. 297:1249–1252, 1977.
276. Doby, H., Genot, J.Y. Imbert, M., et al. Myelodysplasia and leukemia related to chemotherapy and/or radiotherapy—a hematological study of 13 cases. Value of macrocytosis as an early sign of bone marrow injury. Clin. Lab. Haematol. 2:111–119, 1980.
277. Foucar, K., McKenna, R.W., Bloomfield, C.D., et al. Therapy related leukemia. A panmyelosis. Cancer 43:1285–1296, 1979.
278. Lacher, M.J., and Sussman, L.N. Leukemia and Hodgkin's disease. Ann. Int. Med. 59:369–378, 1963.

279. Larsen, J., and Brincker, H. The incidence and characteristics of acute myeloid leukaemia arising in Hodgkin's disease. Scand. J. Haematol. 18:197–206, 1977.
280. Nelson, D.F., Cooper, S., Weston, M.G., and Rubin, P. Second malignant neoplasms in patients treated for Hodgkin's disease with radiotherapy or radiotherapy and chemotherapy. Cancer 48:2386–2393, 1981.
281. Newman, D.R., Moldanado, J.E., Harrison, E.G. Jr., et al. Myelomonocytic leukemia in Hodgkin's disease. Cancer 25:128–134, 1970.
282. Osta, A., Wells, M., Viamonte, M., and Harkness, D. Hodgkin's disease terminating in acute leukemia. Cancer 26:795–799, 1970.
283. Pedersen-Bjergaard, J., and Larsen, S.O. Incidence of acute nonlymphocytic leukemia, preleukemia, and acute myeloproliferative syndrome up to 10 years after treatment of Hodgkin's disease. N. Eng. J. Med. 307:965–971, 1982.
284. Pedersen-Bjergaard, J., Philip, P., Pedersen, N.T., et al. Acute nonlymphocytic leukemia, preleukemia, and acute myeloproliferative syndrome secondary to treatment of other malignant diseases. Cancer 54:452–462, 1984.
285. Razis, D.V., Diamond, H.D., and Craver, L.F. Hodgkin's disease associated with other malignant tumors and certain non-neoplastic diseases. Am. J. Med. Sci. 238:327–335, 1959.
286. Sahakian, G.J., Al-Mondhiry, H., Lacher, M.J., and Connolly, C.E. Acute leukemia in Hodgkin's disease. Cancer 33:1369–1375, 1974.
287. Schomberg, P.J., Evans, R.G., Banks, P.M., et al. Second malignant lesions after therapy for Hodgkin's disease. Mayo Clin. Proc. 59:493–497, 1984.
288. Steinberg, A.H., Geary, G.G., and Crosby, W.H. Acute granulocytic leukemia complicating Hodgkin's disease. Arch. Int. Med. 125:496–498, 1970.
289. Tabilio, A., Herrera, A, D'Agay, M.F. et al. Therapy-related leukemia associated with myelofibrosis. Blast cell characterization in six cases. Cancer 54:1382–1391, 1984.
290. Toland, D.M., Coltman, C.A., Jr., and Moon, T.E. Second malignancies complicating Hodgkin's disease: The Southwest Oncology Group experience. Cancer Clin. Trials 1:27–33, 1978.
291. Weiden, P.L., Lerner, K.G., Gerdes, A., et al. Pancytopenia and leukemia in Hodgkin's disease: Report of three cases. Blood 42:571–577, 1973.
292. Yahalom, J., Voss, R., Leizerowitz, R., et al. Secondary leukemia following treatment of Hodgkin's disease: Ultrastructural and cytogenetic data in two cases with a review of the literature. Am. J. Clin. Pathol. 80:231–236, 1983.
293. Bennett, J.M., Catovsky, D., Daniel, M.T., et al. Proposals for the classification of the myelodysplastic syndromes. Br. J. Haematol. 51:189–199, 1982.
294. Linman, J.W., and Bagby, G.C. Jr: The preleukemic syndrome: clinical and laboratory features, natural course, and management. Blood Cells 2:11–31, 1976.
295. Rosenthal, D.S., Moloney, W.C. Refractory dysmyelopoietic anemia and acute leukemia. Blood 63:314–318, 1984.
296. Dicke, K.A., Spitzer, G., and Verma, D.S. The value of in vitro culture in diagnosis and prognosis in preleukemia and oligoblastic leukemia. In Preleukemia, edited by Schmalze, F.S., and Hellneyel, K.P. Berlin, Springer-Verlag, 1977, pp. 118–122.
297. Senn, J.S., and Pinkerton, P.H. Defective in vitro colony formation by human bone marrow preceding overt leukaemia. Br. J. Haematol. 23:277–281, 1972.
298. Raskind, W.H., Tarumali, N., Jacobon, R., et al. Evidence for a multistep pathogenesis of a myelodysplastic syndrome. Blood 6:1318–1323, 1984.
299. Anderson, R.L., Bagby, G.C. Jr., Richert-Boe, K., et al. Therapy-related preleukemic syndrome. Cancer 47:1867–1871, 1981.
300. Bernard, J. Les aplasies pre-leucemiques. Nouv. Rev. Fr. Hematol. 9:41–48, 1969.
301. DeGramont, A., Louvet, C., Krulik, M., et al. Erythrocyte mean corpuscular volume during cytoxic therapy as a predictive parameter of secondary leukemia in Hodgkin's disease. Cancer 59:301–304, 1987.
302. Kitahara, M., Cosgriff, T.M., and Eyre, H. Sideroblastic anemia as a preleukemic event in patients treated for Hodgkin's disease. Ann. Int. Med. 92:625–627, 1980.
303. Breton-Gorius, J. Abnormalities of granulocytes and megakaryocytes in preleukemic syndromes. In Preleukemia, edited by Schmalze, F., and Hellriegel, K.P. Berlin, Springer-Verlag, 1977, pp. 24–53.
304. Youman, J.D. III, Saarin, M.I., and Linman, J.W. Diagnostic value of muramidase (lysozyme) in acute leukemia and preleukemia. Mayo Clin. Proc. 45:219–228, 1970.
305. Newman, D.R., Pierre, R.V., and Linman, J.W. Studies on the diagnostic significance of hemoglobin F levels. Mayo Clin. Proc. 48:199–202, 1973.
306. Nowell, P.C. Cytogenetics of preleukemia. Cancer Genet. Cytogenet. 5:265–278, 1982.
307. Nowell, P.C., and Finan, J. Chromosome studies in preleukemic states: IV. Myeloproliferative versus cytopenic disorders. Cancer 42:2254–2261, 1978.
308. Sokal, G., Michaux, J.L., Vanden Berghe, H., et al. A new hematologic syndrome with a distinct karyotype: The 5q-chromosome. Blood 46:519–533, 1975.
309. Streuli, R.A., Testa, J.R., Vardiman, J.W., et al. Dysmyelopoietic syndrome: sequential clinical and cytogenetic studies. Blood 55:636–644, 1980.
310. Degnan, T., Weiselberg, L., Schulman, P., and Budman, D. Dysmyelopoietic syndrome. Current concepts. Am. J. Med. 76:122–128, 1984.
311. Anderson, R.L., and Bagby, G.C. Jr. The prognostic value of chromosome studies in patients with preleukemic syndrome (hemopoietic dysplasia). Leuk. Res. 6:175–181, 1982.
312. Pierre, R.V. Cytogenetic studies in preleukemia: studies before and after transition to acute leukemia in 17 subjects. Blood Cells 1:163–170, 1975.
313. Rowley, J.D., Golomb, H.M., and Vardiman, J. Non

random chromosomal abnormalities in acute non-lymphocytic leukemia in patients treated for Hodgkin's disease and non-Hodgkin's lymphomas. Blood 50:759–770, 1977.
314. Bagby, G.C. Jr., Gabourel, J.D., and Linman, J.W. Glucocorticoid therapy in the preleukemic syndrome (hemopoietic dysplasia): identification of responsive patients using in vitro techniques. Ann. Int. Med. 92:55–58, 1980.
315. Hoagland, H.C., and Linman, J.W. Pyridoxine-responsive anemia: A preleukemic manifestation? Minn. Med. 55:891, 1972.
316. Gold, E.J., Mertelsmann, R.H., Itri, L.M., et al. Phase I clinical trial of 13-cis-retinoic acid in myelodysplastic syndromes. Cancer Treat. Rep. 67:981–986, 1983.
317. Metcalf, D. Clonal extinction of myelomonocytic leukemic cells by serum from mice injected with endotoxin. Int. J. Cancer 25:233–255, 1980.
318. Wisch, J.S., Griffin, J.D., and Kufe, D.W. Response of preleukemic syndromes to continuous infusion of low-dose cytarabine. N. Eng. J. Med. 309:1599–1602, 1983.
319. Reuben, R.C. Studies on the mechanism of action of hexamethylene bisacetamide, a potent inducer of erythroleukemic differentiation. Biochim. Biophys. Acta. 588:310–321, 1979.
320. Breton-Gorius, J., Coquin, Y., Vilde, J.L., and Dreyfus, B. Cytochemical and ultrastructural studies of aberrant granules in the neutrophils of two patients with myeloperoxidase deficiency during a preleukemic state. Blood Cells 2:187–209, 1976.
321. Maldonado, J.E., Maigne, J., and Lecog, D. Comparative electron-microscopic study of erythrocyte line in refractory anemia (preleukemia) and myelomonocytic leukemia. Blood Cells 2:167–185, 1976.
322. Maldonado, J.E., and Pintado, T. Ultrastructure of the megakaryocytes in refractory anemia and myelomonocytic leukemia. In Platelets: Production, Function, Transfusion, and Storage, edited by Baldini, M.G., and Ebbe, S. New York, Grune and Stratton, 1974, pp. 104–114.
323. Cooperative Group for the Study of Aplastic and Refractory Anemias. Refractory anemia with excess of blast cells: prognostic factors and effect of treatment with androgens or cytosine arabinoside. Results of a prospective trial in 58 patients. Cancer 44:1976–1982, 1979.
324. Dreyfus, B. Preleukemic states. Definition and classification. Refractory anemia with excess of myeloblasts in the bone marrow. Blood Cells 2:33–55, 1976.
325. Najean, Y., and Pecking, A. Refractory anemia with excess of blast cells: prognostic factors and effects of treatment with androgens or cytosine arabinoside. Cancer 44:1976–1982, 1979.
326. Francis, G.E., Miller, E.J., Wonke, B., et al. Use of bone marrow culture in prediction of acute leukaemic transformation in preleukemia. Lancet 1:1409–1412, 1983.
327. Preisler, H.D., Early, A.P., Raza, A., et al. Therapy of secondary acute nonlymphocytic leukemia with cytarabine. N. Eng. J. Med. 308:21–23, 1983.
328. Mufti, G.J., Oscier, D.G., Hemlin, J.J., and Bell, A.J. Low doses of cytarabine in the treatment of myelodysplastic syndrome and acute myeloid leukemia. N. Eng. J. Med. 309:1653–1654, 1983.
329. Castaigne, S., Daniel, M.T., Tully, H., et al. Does treatment with Ara-C in low dosage cause differentiation of leukemic cells? Blood 62:85–86, 1983.
330. Appelbaum, F.R., Storb, R., Raberg, R.E., et al. Allogenic marrow transplantation in the treatment of preleukemia. Ann. Int. Med. 100:689–693, 1984.
331. Valagussa, P., Santoro, A., Kenda, R., et al. Second malignancies in Hodgkin's disease: A complication of certain forms of treatment. Br. Med. J. 280:216–219, 1980.
332. Valagussa, P., Santoro, A., Fossati-Bellani, F., et al. Absence of treatment-induced second neoplasms after ABVD in Hodgkin's disease. Blood 59:488–494, 1982.
333. Blayney, D.W., Longo, D.L., Young, R.C., et al. Decreasing risk of leukemia with prolonged follow-up after chemotherapy and radiotherapy for Hodgkin's disease. N. Eng. J. Med. 316:710–714, 1987.
334. Bennett, N.B., Ogston, C.M., and McAndrew, G.M. The thyroid and fibrinolysis. Br. Med. J. IV:147–148, 1967.
335. Craver, L.F. Clinical manifestations and treatment of leukemia. Am. J. Cancer. 26:124–136, 1936.
336. Coltman, C.A. Jr, and Dixon, D.O. Second malignancies complicating Hodgkin's disease: A Southwest Oncology Group 10-year follow-up. Cancer Treat. Rep. 66:1023–1033, 1982.
337. Dorreen, M.S., Gregory, W.M., Wrigley, P.F.M., et al. Secondary primary malignant neoplasms in patients treated for Hodgkin's disease at St. Bartholomew's Hospital. Hematolog. Oncol. 4:149–161, 1986.
338. Glicksman, A., Pajak, T.F., Gottlieb, A., et al. Second malignant neoplasms in patients successfully treated for Hodgkin's disease: A Cancer and Leukemia Group B study. Cancer Treat. Rep. 66:1035–1044, 1982.
339. Neufeld, H., Weinerman, B.H., and Kemei, S. Secondary malignant neoplasms in patients with Hodgkin's disease. JAMA 239:2470–2471, 1978.
340. Berger, R., Bernheim, A., Wehs, H.J., et al. Cytogenetic studies on acute monocytic leukemia. Leukemia Res. 4:119–127, 1980.
341. DeGramont, H., Louvet, C., Krulik, M., et al. Preleukemic changes in cases of nonlymphocytic leukemia secondary to cytotoxic therapy. Analysis of 105 cases. Cancer 58:630–634, 1986.
342. Hutchinson, G.B. (A Collaborative Study). Radiotherapy of Stage I and II Hodgkin's disease. Cancer 54:1928–1942, 1984.
343. Zittoun, R., Andebert A., Hoerni, R., et al. Extended versus involved fields irradiation combined with MOPP chemotherapy in early clinical stages of Hodgkin's disease. J. Clin. Oncol. 3:207–214, 1985.
344. Dukes, P.P., and Goldwasser, E. Inhibition of eryth-

ropoiesis by estrogens. Endocrinology 69:21–29, 1961.
345. Jepson, J., and Lowenstein, L. Inhibition of the stem-cell action of erythropoietin by oestradial. Proc. Soc. Exp. Biol. Med. 123:457–460, 1966.
346. Papa, G., Mauro, F.R., Anselmo, A.P., et al. Acute leukemia in patients treated for Hodgkin's disease. Br. J. Haematol. 58:43–52, 1984.
347. Coltman, C.A. Jr, Montague, E., and Moon, T.E. Chemotherapy and total nodal radiotherapy in pathological stage IIB, IIIA and IIIB Hodgkin's disease. In Adjuvant Therapy of Cancer, edited by Salmon, S.E., and Jones, S.E. Amsterdam, Elsevier/North Holland, 1977, pp. 529–536.
348. Gulati, S., Mertelsmann, R., Gee, T., et al. Analysis of multiple cell markers in acute leukemia complicating Hodgkin's disease. Cancer 46:725–729, 1980.
349. Durant, J.R., and Tassoni, E.M Coexistent Di-Guglielmo's leukemia and Hodgkin's disease: A case report with cytogenetic studies. Am. J. Med. 254:824, 1967.
350. Bezwoda, W.R., Bernstein, R., Pinto, M., and Mendelow, B. B-cell chronic lymphatic leukemia in Hodgkin's disease. A report of two patients with unusual chromosome features. Cancer 59:761–766, 1987.
351. Han, T. Chronic lymphocytic leukemia in Hodgkin's disease. Cancer 28:300–305, 1971.
352. Ezdinli, E.Z., Sokal, J.E., Aungst, C.W., et al. Myeloid leukemia in Hodgkin's disease: chromosomal abnormalities. Ann. Int. Med. 71:1097–1104, 1969.
353. Burns, C.P., Stjernholm, R.L., Kellermeyer, R.W., et al. Hodgkin's disease terminating in acute lymphosarcoma cell leukemia: A metabolic study. Cancer 27:806–811, 1971.
354. Rowley, J.D., Golomb, H.M., Vardiman, J.W., et al. Nonrandom chromosome abnormalities in acute leukemia and dysmyelopoietic syndromes in patients with previously treated malignant disease. Blood 58:759–767, 1981.
355. Sandberg, A.A., Abe, S., Kowalczyk, J.R., et al. Chromosomes and causations of human cancer and leukemia. I. Cytogenetics of leukemias complicating other diseases. Cancer Genet. Cytogenet. 7:95–136, 1982.
356. Schwartz, R.S., Mackintosh, F.R., Halpern, J., et al. Multivariate analysis of factors associated with outcome of treatment for adults with acute myelogenous leukemia. Cancer 54:1672–1681, 1984.
357. Bloomfield, C.D., Preisler, H., Cuttner, J., et al. Treatment-induced acute non-lymphocytic leukemia (T− ANLL): Response to cytarabine-anthracycline therapy. Blood 60:152a, 1982.
358. DeWitte T., Blacklock, H.A., Prentice, H.G., et al. Allogeneic bone marrow transplantation in a patient with acute myeloid leukemia secondary to Hodgkin's disease. Cancer 53:1507–1508, 1984.
359. Penn, I., and Starzl, T.E. A summary of the status of the novo cancer in transplant recipients. Transplant Proc. 4:719–732, 1972.
360. Cleary, M.L., Warnke, R., and Sklar, J. Monoclonality of lymphoproliferative lesions in cardiac-transplant recipients. Clonal analysis based on immunoglobulin-gene rearrangements. N. Eng. J. Med. 310:477–482, 1984.
361. Shearer, W.T., Ritz, J., Finegold, M.J., et al. Epstein-Barr virus-associated B-cell proliferation of diverse clonal origins after bone marrow transplantation in a 12-year-old patient with severe combined immunodeficiency. N. Eng. J. Med. 312:1151–1159, 1985.
362. Ziegler, J.L., Beckstead, J.A., Volderding, P.A., et al. Non-Hodgkin's lymphoma in 90 homosexual men. Relation to generalized lymphadenopathy and the acquired immunodeficiency syndrome. N. Eng. J. Med. 311:565–570, 1984.
363. Robert, N.J., and Schneiderman, H. Hodgkin's disease and the acquired immunodeficiency syndrome. Ann. Int. Med. 101:142–143, 1984.
364. Arseneau, J.C., Sponzo, R.W., Levin, D.L., et al. Nonlymphomatous malignant tumors complicating Hodgkin's disease. Possible association with intensive therapy. N. Eng. J. Med. 287:1119–1122, 1972.
365. Henry-Amar, M. Second cancers after radiotherapy and chemotherapy for early stages of Hodgkin's disease. J. Natl. Cancer Inst. 71:911–916, 1983.
366. Kim, H., Hendrickson, M.R., and Dorfman, R.F. Composite lymphoma. Cancer 40:959–976, 1977.
367. Andrieu, J.M., Casassus P., Bayle-Weisgerber, C., et al. Lymphome de type Burkitt survenant apres une maladie de Hodgkin. Nouv. Presse Med. 19:1175, 1980.
368. Armitage, J.O., Dick, F.R., Goeken, V.A., et al. Second lymphoid malignant neoplasms occurring in patients treated for Hodgkin's Disease. Arch. Intern. Med. 143:445–450, 1983.
369. Bergsagel D.E., Alison, M.A., Brown, T.C., et al. Results of treating Hodgkin's disease without policy of laparotomy staging. Cancer Treat. Rep. 66:717–731, 1982.
370. Mirand, E.A., and Gordon, A.S. Mechanism of estrogen action in erythropoiesis. Endocrinology 78:325–332, 1966.
371. Boucheix, C., Zittorin, R., Reynes, M., et al. Atypical T-cell leukemia terminating Hodgkin's disease. Cancer 44:1403–1407, 1979.
372. Cardinali, G., and Eusebi, V. Hodgkin's disease and nodular lymphoma. Haematologica (Pavia) 60:236–240, 1975.
373. D'Agostino, R.S. Non-Hodgkin's lymphoma after radiotherapy for Hodgkin's disease. N. Eng. J. Med. 301:1289, 1979.
374. Gowitt, G.T., Chan, W.C., Brynes, R.K., and Hoffner, L.T. T-cell lymphoma following Hodgkin's disease. Cancer 56:1191–1196, 1985.
375. Jacquillat, C., Khayat, D., Desprez-curely, J.P., et al. Non-Hodgkin's lymphoma occurring after Hodgkin's disease. Cancer 53:459–462, 1984.
376. Kim, H.D., Bedetti, C.D., and Boggs, D.R. The development of non-Hodgkin's lymphoma following therapy for Hodgkin's disease. Cancer 46:2596–2602, 1980.
377. Krikorian, J.G., Burke, J.S., Rosenberg, S.A., and Kaplan, H.S. Occurrence of non-Hodgkin's lym-

phoma after therapy for Hodgkin's disease. N. Eng. J. Med. 300:452–458, 1979.
378. List, A.F., Greer, J.P., Cousar, J.B., et al. Non-Hodgkin's lymphoma after treatment of Hodgkin's disease: Association with Epstein-Barr virus. Ann. Int. Med. 105:668–673, 1986.
379. Lowenthal, R.M., Harlow, R.W.H., Mead, A.E., et al. T-cell non-Hodgkin's lymphoma after radiotherapy and chemotherapy for Hodgkin's disease. Cancer 48:1586–1589, 1981.
380. Rotenberg, Z., Weinberger, I., Fuchs, Y., et al. Elevation of serum lactic dehydrogenase levels as an early marker of occult malignant lymphoma. Cancer 54:1379–1381, 1984.
381. Spaulding, M.B., Mogavero, H., and Montes, M. Non-Hodgkin' lymphoma after chemotherapy for Hodgkin's disease. N. Eng. J. Med. 301:384–385, 1979.
382. Nishiyama, H., Anderson, R.E., Ishimuru, T., et al. The incidence of malignant lymphomas and multiple myeloma in Hiroshima and Nagasaki atomic bomb survivors, 1945–1965. Cancer 32:1201–1309, 1973.
383. Jacquillat, C., Auclerc, G., Weill, M., et al. Acute leukemia, Kaposi's sarcoma, epitheliomas, complicating 30 observations of Hodgkin's disease. Proc. Am. Assoc. Cancer Res. 17:247, 1976.
384. Moertel, C.G., and Hagedorn, A.B. Leukemia or lymphoma and coexistant primary malignant lesions: A review of the literature and a study of 120 cases. Blood 12:788–802, 1957.
385. Caya, J.G., Choi, M., Tieu, T.M., et al. Hodgkin's disease followed by mycosis fungoides in the same patient. Case report and literature review. Cancer 53:463–467, 1984.
386. Arnold, A., Cossman, J., Bakhski, A., et al. Immunoglobulin-gene rearrangements as unique clonal markers in human lymphoid neoplasms. N. Eng. J. Med. 309:1593–1599, 1983.
387. Orr, P.R. Haemorrhage in myxoedema coma. Lancet ii:1012–1015, 1962.
388. Peschle, C., Konwalinka, G., Geissler, D., et al. Studies of myelopoiesis in vitro on blood and bone marrow cells of patients with acute leukemia in long-term remission. Leuk. Res. 7:397–406, 1983.
389. Rosenthal, D. Presentation of case. N. Eng. J. Med. 298:1407–1412, 1978.
390. Rowley, J.D. Identification of a translocation with quinacrine fluorescence in a patient with acute leukemia. Ann. Genet. 16:109–112, 1973.
391. Rowley, J.D., Golomb, H.M., Vardiman, J., et al. Further evidence for a non-random chromosomal abnormality in acute promyelocytic leukemia. Int. J. Cancer 20:869–872, 1977.
392. Rowley, J.D. Chromosome abnormalities in acute leukemia. Ann. Rev. Genet. 14:17–39, 1980.
393. Rowley, J.D., and Testa, J.R. Chromosome abnormalities in malignant hematologic diseases. Adv. Cancer Res. 36:103–148, 1982.
394. Sacks, P.V., Tavassoli, M., and Eastlund, D.T. Simultaneous occurrence of myeloma and Hodgkin's disease. Acta. Haematol. 55:118–122, 1976.
395. Tester W.J., Kinsella, T.J., Waller, B., et al. Second malignant neoplasms complicating Hodgkin's disease: the National Cancer Institute experience. J. Clin. Oncol. 2:762–769, 1984.
396. Tubiana, M., Henry-Amer, M., and Hayat, M. Long term results of the EORTC randomized study of irradiation and vinblastine in clinical stages I and II of Hodgkin's disease. Eur. J. Cancer. Clin. Oncol. 15:645–657, 1979.
397. Vilpo, J.A., and Nordman, E.M. Haematologic evaluation after radiation therapy in Hodgkin's disease. Acta. Radiol. Oncol. Radiat. Phys. Biol. 17:209–217, 1978.
398. Vadhan-Raj, S., Keating, M., Le Maistre, A., et al. Effects of recombinant human granulocyte macrophage colony stimulating factor in patients with myelodysplastic syndromes. N. Eng. J. Med. 317:1545–1552, 1987.

CHAPTER 5

Immunocompetence in Patients with Hodgkin's Disease

MAGNUS BJÖRKHOLM
GÖRAN HOLM
HÅKAN MELLSTEDT

The outcome of patients with Hodgkin's disease has improved greatly since the introduction of modern staging procedures and treatment. Most patients under the age of 50 recover and will eventually be considered cured. The prolonged relapse-free survival time, however, has uncovered certain late therapy-related complications. A broad spectrum of acute and late unwanted effects related to radiotherapy (RT) and cytotoxic drug therapy (CT) and surgical or other staging procedures have to be considered complications of Hodgkin's disease survival. Long-term survivors may also have certain constitutional features, which are uninfluenced by the tumor and its treatment. Such patient characteristics may predispose them for tumor development and influence the course of disease. Certain constitutional features of Hodgkin's patients may accordingly be manifested before any form of diagnostic or therapeutic intervention or they may develop in "cured" patients without any relation to therapy. Consequently, these effects cannot be fully isolated as long as we need the presently used diagnostic and therapeutic modalities in the clinical evaluation and treatment of Hodgkin's disease. Among other factors, the premorbid immunocompetence of the patient may be important in this context. Some effects of radiotherapy, cytotoxic drug therapy, and splenectomy may persist for a long time and hamper identification of the inherent characteristics of Hodgkin's patients.

UNTREATED HODGKIN'S DISEASE PATIENTS

The immunodeficiency state associated with Hodgkin's disease was first reported by Reed.[1] Parker et al.[2] and Steiner[3] were the first to postulate that the susceptibility to tuberculosis in Hodgkin's patients might reflect an immunologic derangement. Since then, numerous studies have confirmed the depression of delayed skin hypersensitivity, not only to tuberculin, but also to other recall antigens and neoantigens such as dinitrochlorobenzene (DNCB) in a high proportion of untreated patients.[4] The proportion of anergic patients is higher in advanced disease.[5,6] A strong correlation exists between the delayed skin hypersensitivity to purified protein derivative (PPD) and the in vitro lymphocyte stimulation induced by the same antigen.[6-8]

BLOOD LYMPHOCYTE SUBPOPULATIONS

The relationship between lymphocytopenia and Hodgkin's disease was first recognized by Bunting in 1914[9] and was confirmed by Uddströmer[10] and Sears.[11] Westling[12] observed lymphocyte counts below $0.8 \times 10^9/L$ in 17% of the patients in a retrospective study. In confirmation of these results, lymphocyte counts below $1.0 \times 10^9/L$ have been noted in 17 to 19% of untreated patients by several groups.[13-16] The corresponding figure for age-matched healthy controls is 5%.[17] Moreover, the mean total number of lymphocytes is lower in patients than in age-matched healthy controls (Tables 5–1 and 5–2).[16]

Most studies have reported slightly reduced or normal relative counts of circulating T lymphocytes, as revealed by rosetting of sheep red blood cells (SRBC; E+ cells) or by anti-T-cell sera.[6,7,18-29] Because patients are often lymphocytopenic, it appears that an absolute T-lymphocytopenia is common in untreated Hodgkin's patients.

Bobrove et al.,[20] however, found about 60% of T cells in both patients and controls using an anti-T-cell serum while the percentage of E+ cells was reduced in the patients. Later Fuks et al.[22,30] showed that the E-rosetting capacity was normalized after incubation for 18 to 24 hours in fetal-calf serum, but not in adult-human or bovine serum. Renewed exposure of Hodgkin's disease lymphocytes to 20% of Hodgkin's disease serum again suppressed their rosette formation. These data, however, remain controversial.[31]

The lymphocytopenia is mainly attributed to lack of T cells carrying receptors for the Fc fragment of IgM (Tμ cells) while IgG Fc receptor-carrying T cells (Tγ cells) are present in normal or raised numbers leading to a low Tμ/Tγ ratio.[26,32,33] In addition, blood T lymphocytes defined by the OKT4 monoclonal antibody ("inducer/helper") are low (Table 5–2).[25,27,34] A slight reduction of OKT8+ cells is also noted.

We may therefore conclude that untreated Hodgkin's patients exhibit lymphocytopenia, which is mainly ascribed to a reduction of OKT4+ T-cells and to the partly overlapping Tμ cell population.

BLOOD LYMPHOCYTE FUNCTIONS

Blood lymphocytes of untreated Hodgkin's patients are poorly activated by mitogens and antigens, which preferentially stimulate T cells.[7,21,24,35-42] They are also poor responders in the allogeneic mixed lymphocyte reaction (MLR).[43-47] Furthermore, the proliferative response of T lymphocytes cultured with autologous non-T lymphocytes (autologous MLR) is usually impaired or absent.[47-49] Lymphocyte-mediated cytotoxicity induced by lectins or by IgG antibodies to target-cell antigens is subnormal.[8,50] Also, the spontaneous lymphocyte-mediated killing of tissue-culture cells as determined by the ^{51}Cr release assay or by the single-cell cytotoxicity assay (NK cell-like activity) is commonly impaired, particularly in patients with advanced disease[8,51-55] (unpublished findings). Cytotoxicity was poorly augmented by interferon-α.

LYMPHOCYTES ACTIVATED IN VIVO

Freshly isolated blood lymphocytes contain a few cells that synthesize DNA in tissue culture without stimulants. The DNA synthesis of such cells declines rapidly with time. These characteristics indicate that the cells have become activated in vivo. Increased numbers of spontaneously activated blood lymphocytes, as denoted by autoradiography or total DNA synthesis, is a common finding in untreated Hodgkin's patients (Table 5–3).[4,29,56-61] The majority of the in vivo activated lymphocytes are large cells of low-specific gravity with basophilic cytoplasm and often prominent nucleoli.[7,57,61,62] Cells with similar characteristics may also be present in patients with non-Hodgkin's lymphoma or solid cancers[63-65] or with nonmalignant conditions, including infections, autoimmune diseases, and postvaccination states.[66-68]

The surface characteristics of in vivo activated blood lymphocytes in Hodgkin's disease have been studied by rosetting techniques in combination with autoradiography.

Table 5-1. Blood Lymphocyte Counts in Relation to Clinical Stage, Histopathology, and Symptoms in Untreated Patients with Hodgkin's Disease (Mean ± SD)

	Clinical Stage				Histopathology‡				Symptoms		Controls§
	I (n=32)	II (n=32)	III (n=39)	IV (n=24)	LP (n=21)	NS (n=49)	MC (n=43)	LD (n=11)	A (n=72)	B (n=55)	(n=167)
Total lymphocyte counts (log No/mm³)	3.12±0.20	3.13±0.26	3.00±0.38	3.06±0.22*	3.09±0.32	3.07±0.33	3.07±0.26	3.04±0.15	3.13±0.21	3.01±0.35†	3.22±0.20
Total E⁺ cell counts (log No/mm³)	2.83±0.30	2.92±0.31	2.86±0.29	2.84±0.19	2.90±0.26	2.85±0.34	2.85±0.25	2.82±0.15	2.89±0.27	2.83±0.30	3.04±0.21

*p <0.05 (Student's t-test; refers to comparison between stage I/II and III/IV patients).
†p <0.05 (Student's t-test; refers to comparison between patients without (A) and with constitutional symptoms (B)).
‡LP = Lymphocyte predominance; NS = Nodular sclerosis; MC = Mixed cellularity; LD = Lymphocyte depletion (3 patients were histologically unclassified).
§All patient values differ significantly from control values.

Table 5-2. Blood Lymphocyte Subpopulations in Untreated Patients with Hodgkin's Disease

Lymphocyte Subpopulations	Percentage (mean ± SD)		Total number/mm³ (log-value ± SD)	
	Patients (n = 60)	Controls (n = 50)	Patients (n = 60)	Controls (n = 50)
Total lymphocyte counts	—	—	3.10 ± 0.23	3.20 ± 0.20‡
E-binding	68.1 ± 11.2	69.4 ± 6.5	2.97 ± 0.25	3.07 ± 0.18*
Fc-binding	16.8 ± 7.1	10.9 ± 5.6†	2.30 ± 0.23	2.28 ± 0.30
OKT3+	63.6 ± 11.9	68.2 ± 8.7*	2.90 ± 0.26	3.05 ± 0.24‡
OKT4+	42.3 ± 12.3	49.0 ± 11.7†	2.71 ± 0.29	2.88 ± 0.28†
OKT8+	24.0 ± 10.0	23.9 ± 8.3	2.44 ± 0.30	2.56 ± 0.27†
OKT4+/OKT8+ ratio	2.18 ± 1.45	2.38 ± 1.25		

*p <0.05 (Student's t-test)
†p <0.01
‡p <0.001

Cells carrying receptors for SRBC or C3b, or cells that lack such receptors have been identified.[62,69,70] The high spontaneous activity in the non-T-cell population may be inhibited by T cells that are present in the same high-density fraction.[71]

CLINICAL CORRELATIONS OF BLOOD LYMPHOCYTE COUNTS AND FUNCTIONS

Although lymphocytopenia is present in all clinical stages, it tends to be more pronounced in patients with advanced disease (Table 5–1).[7,12,16,21,24,72,73] Patients with B symptoms usually have lower lymphocyte counts than asymptomatic cases (Table 5–1),[15,16,29,73] which may account for the lower rate of stage III/IV disease in the latter.[16] Severe lymphocytopenia has been reported in patients with lymphocyte deplete histopathology.[74] Most studies, however, have been unable to confirm an association between histopathology and blood lymphocyte counts (Table 5–1).[16,24,38,73] Age and sex do not influence lymphocyte counts either.[16,24,72,73]

Lymphocyte DNA synthesis induced by concanavalin A (ConA), and to a lesser extent by pokeweed mitogen (PWM) and PPD, declines with age in untreated Hodgkin's disease (Fig. 5–1). In general, the mitogen and antigen response in vitro is lower in patients with B symptoms and advanced disease. Most blood lymphocyte functions do not correlate with the histopathologic picture.[6,16,38,72]

A high spontaneous lymphocyte DNA synthesis is closely related to advanced disease and B symptoms in Hodgkin's disease (Table 5–3),[24,29,61,75] as well as in patients with nonHodgkin's lymphoma.[65] The spontaneous blood lymphocyte DNA synthesis increases with spleen weight in patients with uninvolved spleens.[76]

ANTIBODY-MEDIATED IMMUNITY

It is generally agreed that B-lymphocyte functions are well preserved in untreated Hodgkin's disease, except in patients with generalized disease. Thus, blood B lymphocytes defined as cells carrying surface membrane-bound immunoglobulins are normal or slightly depressed, though individual variation is often greater than in healthy controls.[7,23,24,72] However, immunoglobulin synthesis by blood lymphocytes after activation with PWM or *Staphylococcus aureus* in vitro was significantly reduced in untreated Hodgkin's patients.[77]

A study with direct implications on B-cell functions in Hodgkin's disease was recently published by Souhami et al.[78] They investigated the specific antibody response in cultures of mononuclear cells stimulated with varicella-zoster antigens. In contrast to splenic cell cultures, blood cells from untreated patients did not produce antibodies. The defect was shown to be attributable to the blood B cells; the authors suggested that an abnormality in B-cell circulation, with localization of antibody-producing B cells in spleen and lymph nodes, is a feature of untreated and treated Hodgkin's disease.

Table 5–3. Schematic Presentation of Spontaneous Blood Lymphocyte DNA Synthesis in Hodgkin's Patients in Relation to Clinical Variables and Disease Status*

| | Untreated Patients | | | | | | | | Complete Remission Patients | | | Patients in Relapse | Elderly Healthy Controls† |
| | Stage | | Systemic Symptoms | | Histopathology | | | | Years After End of Therapy | | | | |
	I–II	III–IV	Absent	Present	LP	NS	MC	LD	1–3	4–9	>10		
All	↑	↑↑↑	↑	↑↑↑	↑	↑↑	↑↑	↑↑↑	↑	↑	↑	↑↑	(↑)

*The arrows denote the degree of increment in comparison to age-matched healthy controls
†In comparison to healthy individuals below the age of 50

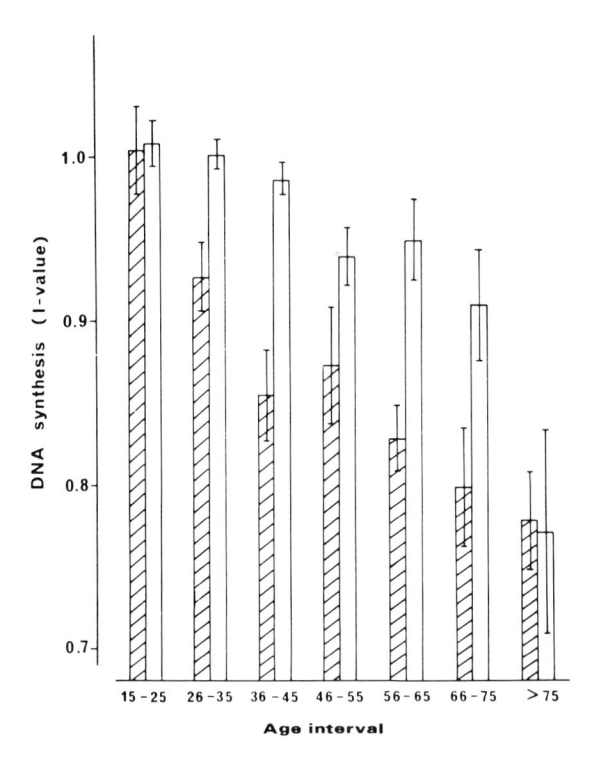

Fig. 5-1. Age dependency of blood lymphocyte DNA synthesis induced by 20 μg/ml of Con A in patients (▨; n = 127) and controls (☐; n = 167). (From: Björkholm, M., Wedelin, C., Holm, G. et al. Immune status of untreated patients with Hodgkin's disease and prognosis. Cancer Treat. Rep. 66:705, 1982.)

The literature on specific antibody production in cases of untreated Hodgkin's disease is abundant.[4,72,79] The secondary-antibody response is essentially normal, with the possible exception of severely ill patients. Furthermore, the primary antibody response is normal or only moderately suppressed.[72,79] Thus, the antibody titers after vaccination with *Haemophilus influenzae* type B are normal.[80] Also the IgG and IgM antibody response to flagellin from *Salmonella adelaide* was normal in untreated patients (unpublished results).

Serum immunoglobulin concentrations are usually normal in untreated patients, but low or high levels have been reported (Table 5–4).[72,81,82] Thus, in a recent published series of 182 untreated patients, 13 patients had subnormal IgG (three with only low IgG), 26 patients had a low IgA (15 with only low IgA) and 19 had a low IgM (8 with only low IgM).[16]

IgG and IgA concentrations were higher in patients with B symptoms (Table 5–4). Low IgG and IgM were seen in patients with large tumor-involved spleens.[16] Serum IgD concentrations were increased in 50 to 65% of Hodgkin's patients.[83,84] Serum IgE tended to increase, particularly in patients with advanced disease or with impaired delayed skin hypersensitivity to recall antigens.[81,85]

SOME CONFOUNDING FACTORS IN STUDIES OF LONG-TERM SURVIVORS

Since certain blood lymphocyte functions are strongly associated with age in untreated Hodgkin's disease (Fig. 5–1), knowledge of normal immunologic aging is highly relevant in studies of long-term survivors. The immune system undergoes significant changes during the life cycle of an individual, and the age-related regressive changes of the thymus are well known.[86,87] Waning of delayed hypersensitivity to recall antigens and to neoantigens such as DNCB has also been noted in the aging man.[88,89] While there is no age-dependent reduction of blood-lymphocyte counts, T-lymphocyte counts seem to diminish with increasing age.[17,89–92] Blood-lymphocyte blastogenesis and DNA synthesis induced by T-cell mitogens decline in adults over 30 years and are severely impaired in healthy persons over 70 years (Fig. 5–1).[17,88,89,93–95] In contrast, the spontaneous DNA synthesis is slightly increased in older persons (Table 5–3).[17]

T lymphocytes from aged individuals have low activity of 5-nucleotidases and cyclic adenosine monophosphates (cAMP) activity, together with a high level of cyclic guanosine monophosphate activity (cGMP).[96,97] In addition, T lymphocytes from the elderly become more sensitive to prostaglandin E_2 (PGE_2) and irradiation, but more resistant to inhibition by hydrocortisone and histamine.[98–100] A decreased production of interleukin-2 and diminished sensitivity to the same mediator may partly explain the impaired blastogenesis of lymphocytes from the elderly.[101]

Table 5–4. Immunoglobulin Levels in Untreated Patients with Hodgkin's Disease in Relation to Stage, Histopathology and Symptoms (g/L; Mean ± SD)

Immunoglobulin Class	Clinical Stage				Histopathology*				Symptoms		Reference Values
	I (n=44)	II (n=43)	III (n=53)	IV (n=42)	LP (n=25)	NS (n=67)	MC (n=66)	LD (n=17)	A (n=103)	B (n=79)	
IgG	12.3±3.3	12.7±3.1	13.1±5.2	12.6±5.0	11.6±3.8	13.9±4.1‡	12.0±4.4	12.6±4.8	12.0±3.5	13.6±5.0†	7.0–15.0
IgA	1.8±0.9	1.7±0.9	1.9±1.4	2.2±2.0	1.6±1.0	1.9±1.1	1.9±1.5	2.6±2.4	1.7±1.0	2.2±1.7†	0.8–3.8
IgM	1.1±0.8	1.0±0.6	0.9±0.6	1.0±1.0	1.2±1.1	1.0±0.6	0.9±0.6	1.1±0.7	1.0±0.7	1.0±0.8	0.4–2.0

*7 patients were histologically unclassified

†$p < 0.05$ (significance level refers to patients without symptoms (A) compared to patients with symptoms (B); Student's t-test)

‡$p < 0.05$ (significance level refers to LP patients compared to NS patients)

Antibody production against T-dependent antigens decreases to a greater degree and at an earlier age than the response to T-independent antigens, suggesting a decrease of T-helper cell activity.[95] The increased frequency of autoantibodies may be secondary to a T-suppressor-cell defect rather than a specific B-cell defect.[102-105] These observations suggest that the primary age-related effect on the immune system is a decrease in T-cell functional capacity, resulting in impaired immune regulation.

The normal decline in T-cell functions with age, which may be partly related to the patient's genetic background,[4,95,106] could have important bearings on the effects of anticancer therapy on immunity. Thus, the effects of cytotoxic drug therapy and radiotherapy or those initiated by the tumor itself may particularly depress the immune system in certain individuals, eventually leading to long-lasting or irreversible damage. Such unpredictable effects may severely hamper the interpretation of studies comparing two different patient populations. This is the situation when a group of patients studied before treatment is compared to a group of long-term survivors. A preferable approach is to monitor the same group of patients given a uniform treatment. Even in this situation, however, the effects of "normal aging" on immunity add to disease-associated and therapy-related effects.

Finally, there seems to be a general association between cell-mediated immunodeficiency and a poor prognosis in cancer patients.[107-111] This is most probably explained by the deterioration of immune defense in advanced stages of cancer.[112-115] Thus, patients who are available for immunologic studies a long time following termination of therapy form a select group; they have a favorable prognosis, possibly the result of specific characteristics in regard to immunity before and after treatment.

EFFECTS OF IRRADIATION ON THE IMMUNE SYSTEM

Effects of radiation, whether direct or indirect, are random. The major biologic consequences of therapeutic radiation are those concerned with reproductive integrity. Inhibition or delay of DNA synthesis is generally acknowledged as representative of critical consequences of radiation injury to all dividing cells, including lymphocytes. This, however, has not been proven. Other effects, like interruption of the normal metabolic pathways and injury to the plasma membrane (edema), are also likely to contribute to the detrimental effects of radiation.[116,117] Many factors influence the biologic consequences of radiation, for instance the effects of whole body radiation are qualitatively and quantitatively different from those caused by localized or regional radiation. Furthermore, radiation does not only kill lymphocytes, but may also affect the homing potential of lymphoid cells.[118]

Therapeutic irradiation induces lymphocytopenia and a profound depression of immune functions, which manifest soon after the initiation of treatment.[119-123] Among blood cells, the lymphocyte shows a most exquisite radiosensitivity, and blood lymphocytopenia can be induced by extracorporeal irradiation of peripheral blood.[121,124-127] Bone-marrow stem cells, which are the precursors of all lymphoid cells, are also highly radiosensitive.[127] We do not know to what degree irradiation damage of lymphocytes in blood/lymphatic vessels, lymphoid tissues, or bone marrow contributes to therapy-induced lymphocytopenia.[128,129] In general, the degree of lymphopenia depends on target volume, exposure dose, and underlying structures in the irradiated field. Moreover, factors such as age, clinical stage, and type of malignancy may influence the radiation-induced lymphocyte deficiency.[120] Most lymphocytes killed by ionizing radiation die a reproductive death (i.e., they lose the capacity for sustained proliferation and die during attempted mitotic division). There are, however, highly radiosensitive cells that succumb during interphase.

The significant radiosensitivity of lymphocytes is illustrated by the induction of lymphopenia in animals after whole-body exposure to as little as 2.5 Gy.[119,130] Interphase death may explain the decrease in number of recirculating lymphocytes within one hour after exposure to a LD50 of X-ray radiation.

Subpopulations of T- and B-lymphocytes appear to have different degrees of radiosensitivity. In mice, B cells seem to be more radiosensitive and recover faster than T cells. Most lymphocytes surviving interphase death are T cells. The radiosensitivity of lymphocytes decreases with differentiation from precursor to effector cells. Like activated cytotoxic T-cells, however, primed T-helper cells include radiosensitive subpopulations.[130] Differences in radiosensitivity also exist among human blood T-lymphocyte subpopulations. Tγ lymphocytes are more radiosensitive than Tμ cells.[131,132] However, subsets with a varying degree of radiosensitivity have also been described in the OKT4+ and OKT8+ cell populations.[133]

The immunosuppressive effects of irradiation are well documented but refer primarily to animal research. The rate at which a particular dose is given and the time intervals between doses seems to be of greater importance than the total dose. Upon stimulation by an antigen or mitogen, T and B cells acquire some degree of radioresistance, presumably as a result of activation of repair mechanisms preventing interphase death. Such repair accounts for tolerance to irradiation and eventual resistance, particularly in tumor cells.[130–132] Tγ-cell induced suppression of phytohaemagglutinin (PHA)-induced mitotic response of other T-lymphocyte subsets was abolished by pretreatment with 1.0 Gy.[132] Furthermore, significant differences have been observed in terms of radiosensitivity in and between antigen-induced and mitogen-induced T-cell helpers.[134,135] Irradiation (4.5 Gy) induced a severe depression of the in vitro mitotic response to T- and B-cell antigens. The recovery was found to be subnormal, even at 8 weeks after irradiation, with a clear tendency towards a faster restitution of the B-cell response.[136]

Many early studies in animals have demonstrated the suppressive effect of irradiation on the humoral antibody response.[118] Because it is generally considered that macrophage functions (including antigen presentation) are relatively resistant to irradiation, as is antibody production, it appears that radiotherapy-induced inhibition of the antibody response mainly depends on the radiosensitivity of unstimulated lymphocytes. The primary antigen response is depressed when the antigen is injected shortly before or immediately after irradiation. The inductive phase of the antibody response, rather than the productive phase, seems to be more vulnerable to radiation. In general, the secondary antibody response appears to be more radioresistant than the primary response.[118,130]

THYMUS IRRADIATION

The role of thymus irradiation in immunosuppression has been studied by comparing the effects on lymphocyte counts and subpopulations as well as functions in patients receiving radiotherapy including or excluding the thymus. Although no studies using monoclonal antibodies in the identification of lymphocyte subsets have been published, most studies support the concept that irradiation of the thymus seems to have little influence on the acute and late effects of lymphocyte counts and functions.[120,137–140] We cannot, however, rule out the possibility that adult involution of the thymus due to irradiation has detrimental effects on the human immune system. This is because radiotherapy induces a severe and longstanding depression of lymphocyte counts and functions, which may mask the subtle effects of "thymectomy"; these effects may not manifest until long after treatment. Surgical thymectomy may also induce a higher degree of T-cell impairment than "medical thymectomy" induced by irradiation.[141] Hence, the thymic milieu necessary for T-lymphocyte maturation does not appear to be particularly damaged by irradiation to the thymus; this, however, sharply contrasts the results of animal experiments.[122,142]

LYMPHOCYTE SUBPOPULATIONS

Most modern plans of Hodgkin's disease treatment have followed standardized protocols for radiotherapy. Usually, a fractionated total dose of 40 Gy is distributed either as total-nodal irradiation or as mantle or inverted Y-field treatment.[72] Most patients monitored by immunologic tests have been treated according to these principles. Limited information is available, however, to evaluate the immunosuppressive effects in relation to localization and extension of the radiation fields.

The acute effects of radiotherapy on blood lymphocytes have been amply documented. Shortly after completion of radiotherapy, lymphocytes, including T and B cells, are severely depleted.[143–146] Following mantle and para-aortic irradiation there is an acute and significant diminution of OKT4+ cells, while the fraction of OKT8+ cells remains constant.[147]

Blood lymphocyte counts, including T cells, tend to increase following treatment. During the first year, however, there seems to be little or no recovery[26,143–145,147] and T lymphocytopenia is frequently encountered 1 to 10 years following termination of radiotherapy (Table 5–5).[75,143,144,148–158] No consistent correlation between the degree of T lymphocytopenia and the treatment technique or the time interval from completion of treatment has been reported.[143,144,151,159] Interestingly, Steele and Han[154] observed suppressed total T-lymphocyte counts in a group of Hodgkin's patients examined 2 years or more after therapy, while patients with nonHodgkin's lymphoma did not have significantly lower numbers of T cells.

In nine patients tested 10 to 28 years following termination of radiotherapy, the total number of blood lymphocytes was significantly lower than that of an age-matched control group.[159] In this study, a group of patients with seminoma testis, who had received comparable doses of irradiation 10 to 12 years before testing, had normal lymphocyte counts. In many patients with good prognoses, however, lymphocyte counts exceeding pretreatment levels are reached 5 to 10 years or more following curative radiotherapy (Fig. 5–2).

Efforts have recently been made to answer the question of whether there is a varying degree of radiosensitivity within the T-cell population in Hodgkin's disease patients. In 56 patients, the large majority of who received radiotherapy, relative and absolute values of $T\mu$ cells were significantly decreased in comparison with normal controls and untreated patients.[155] In contrast, the percentages of $T\gamma$ cells were increased in treated patients, while the absolute numbers of $T\gamma$ cells were essentially unchanged. In spite of a continuous but slow rise, blood $T\mu$ cell counts remained low in many patients in complete remission for at least 5 years.[155,156] Recently, Herrmann et al.[158] observed a significant decrease of OKT4+ cells 19 to 28 months after radiotherapy or radiotherapy and cytotoxic drug therapy. OKT8+ and Leu7+ (marker for NK cells) cell counts were normal. OKT3+ and OKT4+ lymphocytes, but not OKT8+ cells, also remained low in patients in long-term remission (5 years or more) (Table 5–5).[157] It must be stressed that phenotyping of T cells as $T\mu$ and $T\gamma$ cells or as OKT4+ and OKT8+ cells does not strictly delineate T-helper or T-suppressor activities.[160–162] Nevertheless, the reduction of OKT4+ cells and $T\mu$ cells in the blood of patients with active or treated Hodgkin's disease is well documented and may have bearing on the immunosuppression seen before and after therapy. A few of the studies cited above have included only a minor fraction of patients

Table 5–5. Blood Lymphocyte Subpopulations in Patients with Hodgkin's Disease in Unmaintained Remission 5 to 22 (Mean = 11) Years Following Therapy

Lymphocyte Subpopulations	Percentage (mean ± SD)		Total Number/mm³ (log-value ± SD)	
	Patients (n = 21)	Controls (n = 50)	Patients (n = 21)	Controls (n = 50)
Total lymphocyte counts	—	—	3.23 ± 0.17	3.20 ± 0.20
E-binding	63.8 ± 7.9	69.4 ± 6.5†	3.03 ± 0.17	3.07 ± 0.18
OKT3+	61.8 ± 13.4	68.2 ± 8.7*	3.00 ± 0.25	3.05 ± 0.24
OKT4+	38.9 ± 13.8	49.0 ± 11.7†	2.79 ± 0.29	2.88 ± 0.28
OKT8+	27.0 ± 10.1	23.9 ± 8.3	2.65 ± 0.28	2.56 ± 0.27
OKT4+/OKT8+ ratio	1.76 ± 1.13	2.38 ± 1.25	—	—

*p <0.05 (Student's t-test)
†p <0.01

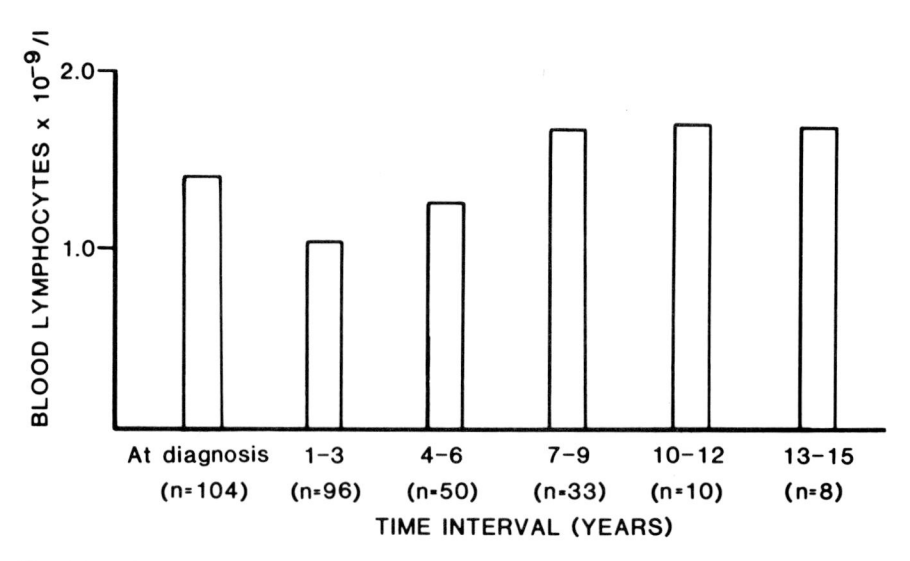

Fig. 5–2. Total lymphocyte counts (mean) in HD patients before and repeatedly after curative (in the majority of patients) radiotherapy.

given cytotoxic drug therapy. Furthermore, a varying proportion of patients have been splenectomized. In many publications, however, it has been impossible to identify patients who were splenectomized and/or given cytotoxic drug therapy. The influence of splenectomy is discussed separately in this chapter.

The immediate absolute B lymphocytopenia following radiotherapy seems to normalize within the first 1 or 2 years after therapy.[26,147,151,158,163] After this time, relative B-cell counts are frequently increased; increased absolute B-cell numbers appear to be common in disease-free survivors of Hodgkin's.[26,143,151,153,154,157,164] However, patients who undergo continuous cytotoxic drug therapy for more than 10 years have essentially normal total B-lymphocyte counts.[152,159]

T-CELL FUNCTIONS

Most functional studies of blood lymphocytes in Hodgkin's disease patients following radiotherapy, with or without cytotoxic drug therapy, involve patients not examined prior to therapy. Fuks et al.[143] observed little or no recovery of phytohemagglutinin (PHA), ConA, and tetanus-toxoid stimulation in a large group of patients tested 1 to 10 years after completion of treatment (the large majority had received radiotherapy). In contrast, the response of the allogeneic MLR, which was significantly impaired during the first 2 years after treatment, was normalized in patients in continuous complete remission for more than 5 years. Impairment of mitogen stimulation of blood lymphocytes in long-term survivors in continuous complete remission and in those who have been off treatment for at least 5 years has been confirmed repeatedly.[152–154,157,159,165] In one study, four out of nine Hodgkin's patients in complete and unmaintained remission for more than 10 years after termination of radiotherapy displayed severe blood T-lymphocyte defects.[159] A few early reports, however, described normal or close to normal PHA stimulation in remission patients.[37,166,167]

Few studies have included patients who were tested both before and after treatment. The immediate effect of radiotherapy on Hodgkin's patients is a profound reduction of the in vitro stimulation of blood lymphocytes by mitogens, antigens, and allogeneic cells.[151,168,169] In a prospective study, 19 patients were retested 15 to 18 months after termination of TNI. ConA- and PPD-induced lymphocyte DNA synthesis remained low and largely unchanged in comparison to the pretreatment levels.[151] These results were confirmed in a large series of patients retested

2 to 56 months following termination of radiotherapy. The responses to ConA and PPD, but not to PWM, were significantly reduced shortly after total-nodal irradiation. The mitogen response did not increase with time after treatment, as it did with PPD stimulation.[144]

Eleven patients followed for 8 to 11 years following termination of therapy (8 of 11 received total-nodal irradiation) showed a decreased lymphocyte response to PWM, but only slightly reduced activation by ConA and PPD (Fig. 5–3). This patient group, however, had displayed only subtle, if any, lymphocyte abnormalities before therapy.

The deficient autologous MLR in some untreated patients persists in a large proportion of patients following termination of radiotherapy. Although there was a tendency to improve after therapy, low activity was found in patients free of disease up to 15 years after treatment.[48] No consistent inhibition by suppressor cells or serum factors was observed. The authors concluded that the impairment of autologous MLR, at least in some patients, is the result of a reduction or dysfunction of responder T cells and not the result of a defect of autologous stimulator cells. Similar results were reported by Begemann et al.[47] These authors, however, observed that the autologous MLR of lymphocytes from healthy persons was inhibited by the addition of Hodgkin's disease serum. Sera from patients in long-term remission were as inhibitory as sera from patients with active disease.

To summarize, T-cell functional impairment persists in most Hodgkin's patients, during long-term remission following radiotherapy.

NONLYMPHOID TUMORS

Lymphocytopenia is observed in cancer patients after radiotherapy with 5 to 10 Gy to the pelvic area (cervical, ovarian, endometrial cancer),[137] to the spine (medulloblastoma),[127] or to iliac and paraortic lymph nodes (seminoma testis).[129] In patients receiving radiotherapy after mastectomy and patients given it to head and neck tumors, a moderate lymphopenia is usually observed after 20 Gy.[107,137,139,170] In a prospective study of 39 patients with various malignancies, the fall in lymphocyte count was exponential through-

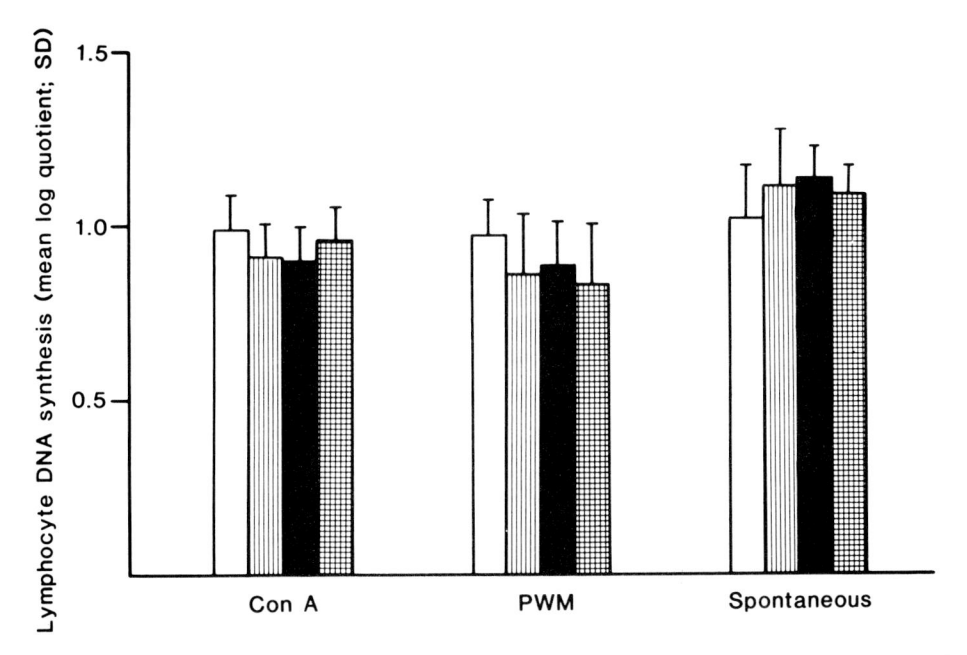

Fig. 5–3. Blood lymphocyte DNA synthesis (spontaneous- and Con A- [20 μg/ml] and PMW- [1 μg/ml] induced) in 11 patients at diagnosis (▦), 1 to 3 years (■), and 8 to 11 years (▦) following curative TNI and controls (□). The spontaneous DNA synthesis remained high and that induced by PWM decreased (p < 0.05; Wilcoxon test) as compared to controls. For explanation of log quotient see Wendelin, C. et al.[17]

out the period of irradiation.[171] Lymphocytopenia did not depend on the site of irradiation and occurred even if the bone marrow and thymus were not irradiated. The effect was related to volume of tissue treated.

Recovery from lymphocytopenia is variable, but the nadir is often reached at completion of irradiation or shortly thereafter.[127,137] The lymphocyte numbers started to increase within three months following termination of therapy.[172] Lymphocytopenia may persist for 2 to 8 years in patients with mammary carcinoma after local radiotherapy[173,174] and in patients with various malignancies treated by regional irradiation.[140,159,175] Lymphocyte counts were reported to be restored 9 to 12 years following radiotherapy for endometrial carcinoma.[176]

Radiotherapy-induced lymphocytopenia involves both T and B cells. Blood B lymphocytes and other non-T cells are drastically reduced by radiotherapy. B-lymphocyte counts, however, recover rapidly and are often normal after ½ to 3 years.[175-178] In contrast, blood T cells are repopulated at a slow rate and low counts are frequently encountered even 5 years or more after irradiation.[120,129,140,159,176] In 1982, Petrini et al.[179] reported that the Tγ cell population was more extensively depleted than other T-cell subsets immediately following radiotherapy for mammary carcinoma. However, the proportions of T-cell subsets determined by monoclonal antibodies were not changed. Approximately one year later, Tγ cells and Leu2+ cells had increased, while Tμ and Leu3+ cells did not recover, leading to decreased ratios between Tμ and Tγ cells or Leu2+ and Leu3+ cells.[179,181]

A large number of studies of patients with various cancers have reported a reduction of blood lymphocyte stimulation by mitogens, antigens, and allogeneic lymphocytes during or shortly after radiotherapy.[107,109,170,182-184]

Lymphocyte stimulation started to recover 6 to 8 weeks after completion of treatment.[107,109] The PHA stimulation did not improve in patients with poor clinical effects of treatment. Patients in long-standing (1 to 12 years) radiotherapy-induced remission usually displayed normal PHA-induced lymphocyte transformation.[182,184,185] Patients with cured laryngopharyngeal cancer, however, had subnormal in vitro lymphocyte reactivity to PHA 4 to 15 years following radiotherapy, which is in contrast to the normal response found in patients treated by surgery.[138]

Radiotherapy-induced suppression of mitogen-induced stimulation has not been confirmed consistently. In a rather large series of patients with primary carcinoma of the breast, PHA-induced lymphocyte incorporation of C-thymidine-14 increased approximately one year after treatment and was significantly higher than the pretreatment response after 2 years.[174] However, PPD-induced lymphocyte stimulation was reduced one month after completion of radiotherapy, but reached pretreatment levels within half a year.

The abrogation of lymphocyte reactivity in vitro following lymphoid irradiation has also been verified in patients with rheumatoid arthritis and pelvospondylitis.[183,186,187] The mitogen responses recovered within one year, while the restitution of antigen stimulation was slower.[187]

In summary, untreated patients with solid cancer show impaired in vitro blastogenesis of blood lymphocytes induced by mitogens, antigens, and allogeneic lymphocytes, which is usually stage dependent.[109,115] Irradiation further depresses blood lymphocyte stimulation, which is gradually restored to pretreatment or higher levels in the majority of "cured" patients within 5 years. The initial decrease of lymphocyte stimulation by PHA and ConA following radiotherapy was prevented by the addition of indomethacin to the cultures.[188] Furthermore, mitogen-treated lymphocytes from recently irradiated patients were found to be more sensitive to the inhibition by PGE_2 than normal lymphocytes. The induction of PGE_2 production by radiotherapy-treated monocytes-macrophages may contribute to the radiotherapy-induced lymphocyte defect.

NONHODGKIN'S LYMPHOMA

Blood lymphocytes from untreated nonleukemic patients with nonHodgkin's lymphoma are poorly stimulated to DNA synthesis by PHA, PWM, and ConA.[23,65,189-193] PPD stimulation is also low.[65] The proliferative response to allogeneic lymphocytes, however, seems to be normal or only moderately depressed.[192,194] In contrast, the autologous MLR was lower in nonHodgkin's lymphoma patients with an active disease than in patients with an inactive disease.[194] In general, mitogen, antigen, and allogeneic lymphocyte stimulation was more depressed in patients in advanced clinical stages.[65,190] A severe lymphocyte deficiency was also seen in patients with diffuse lymphoma.[190,192] However, no difference in mitogen- and antigen-induced lymphocyte DNA synthesis was observed histopathologically between patients with a low- and high-grade malignancy.[65,193]

Information concerning blood lymphocyte counts and functions in patients with nonHodgkin's lymphoma following radiotherapy as the single mode of treatment is sparse. The general effects, however, seem to be similar to those described in radiotherapy treated cancer. Thus, total lymphocyte and T-cell counts were reduced in irradiated patients with a diffuse histiocytic (large cell) lymphoma and a high-grade malignant lymphoma, according to Kiel.[65,192,193] As in other cancer patients given radiotherapy, lymphocytopenia was mainly the result of a reduction of OKT4+ cells. The latter study included 28 patients retested in early unmaintained complete remission (7 months after cessation of therapy) and eight who were studied after a long-term complete remission (2 or more years). Total lymphocytes and T cells increased, especially in patients in long-term complete remission. Pretreatment levels were not reached however.[195,196]

Patients with nonHodgkin's lymphoma who achieve a complete remission following radiotherapy and/or cytotoxic drug therapy seem to recover their mitogen-induced proliferative responses.[191,195-197] In the study by Lindemalm et al.,[195] patients in their first complete remission with normal mitogen-induced lymphocyte stimulation remained disease-free while patients who relapsed during the observation period had lymphocytopenia and reduced lymphocyte responses to mitogens and antigens. These observations may suggest that the deficient lymphocyte stimulation in nonHodgkin's lymphoma is an effect of the tumor and related to the tumor burden. This conclusion is supported in a study by Yonkonsky et al.[198] They treated patients with nonHodgkin's lymphoma who had failed to respond to cytotoxic therapy with low-dose fractionated total-body irradiation. The mitogen-induced lymphocyte proliferation was restored in patients who entered clinical remission following radiotherapy, whereas it remained unchanged in nonresponders with progressive diseases.

Generally, therapeutic radiotherapy in cancer patients induces an acute reduction of T and B cells, which is gradually normalized. Major differences exist, however, between the recovery rates of subpopulations. Blood non-T lymphocytes and T cells phenotypically defined as "suppressor" cells recover more rapidly than "helper" T cells. This pattern can also be seen in nonmalignant conditions following radiotherapy. While T lymphocytopenia is commonly present after 5 years, normal lymphocyte counts are frequently observed 10 years after radiotherapy. Radiotherapy also leads to functional impairment of blood lymphocytes. After the initial depression, there is a recovery phase of varying length depending on the function. The degree of suppression and its quality and duration are probably influenced by many factors, such as radiation dose, mode of application and field localization, extension, and various undefined disease-related factors. Analysis of such multivariant factors has not routinely been performed.

An important question concerns the possible differences between Hodgkin's disease, nonHodgkin's lymphoma, and other cancers with regard to restitution of the immune apparatus after radiotherapy. Because of the complex interaction among multiple relevant factors, no definite answer can be given. Available data, however, seem to support a more complete restoration of immune functions in patients with nonlymphoid cancers and nonHodgkin's lymphoma than in Hodgkin's cases. In support of this tentative interpretation are the authors' results regarding Hodgkin's and nonHodgkin's lymphoma. Patients with nonHodgkin's lymphoma regained normal lymphocyte capacity shortly after achieving a continuous complete remission. A full normalization in Hodgkin's cases was only encountered in patients studied after many years in complete remission and with normal or only moderately impaired pretreatment lymphocyte characteristics.

In 1982, Rotstein et al.[199] studied untreated Hodgkin's disease and patients with non-Hodgkin's lymphoma with regard to the responsiveness of blood lymphocytes to PHA and ConA following exposure to varying doses of ionizing radiation in vitro. They observed that lymphocytes from 19 of 20 nonHodgkin's lymphoma patients exhibited the same pattern of radiosensitivity as those of healthy donors (i.e., one cell population was relatively radiosensitive and one was relatively radioresistant). The latter subpopulation was not detected in patients with Hodgkin's disease.

IMMUNOSUPPRESSIVE EFFECTS OF CHEMOTHERAPEUTIC AGENTS

The immunosuppressive effects of antineoplastic drugs have been the subject of numerous studies.[200] The most commonly used combination chemotherapy for Hodgkin's disease is the MOPP regimen and variants thereof.[201] Among these drugs, cyclophosphamide and glucocorticosteroids have been extensively studied. Alkylating agents have multiple effects on the cell. Interaction with DNA by cross linking of nucleotides is the most important biologic effect. Alkylation leads to latent DNA damage, which manifests and kills the cell when it enters DNA synthesis. Metabolic transformation of cyclophosphamide is required for immunosuppressive activity. Cyclophosphamide-treated lymphocytes are killed when stimulated to proliferation. It, therefore, has its main effect on the proliferative phase of the immune response. Repair mechanisms may eliminate the DNA damage by cyclophosphamide.

Cyclophosphamide suppresses cell-mediated and humoral-immune responses, particularly if given during the first week after immunization when there is rapid proliferation of specifically activated lymphocytes.[202]

Cyclophosphamide metabolites seem to have profound effects on the in vitro responsiveness of human lymphocytes to PHA, ConA, and PWM.[203] High concentrations caused suppression, while low doses augmented stimulation. It is suggested that cyclophosphamide acts on regulatory T-cell subpopulations.[202] As judged from studies of the PWM-induced plaque-forming cell response against SRBC, human B cells appeared to be most sensitive to cyclophosphamide, followed by the suppressor T cells, with relative resistance of the helper T cells.[204]

Blood B cells may also become selectively suppressed in patients with non-neoplastic immune-mediated diseases during treatment with a chronic low-dose (2 mg/kg/day) cyclophosphamide.[205] The PWM-induced immunoglobulin secretion was drastically reduced, while T-cell functions, measured by blastogenic responses to PHA, ConA, and PWM, were not suppressed. The patients had lymphocytopenia without selective depletion of B- or T-cell subsets. Moreover, low or intermediate doses of cyclophosphamide (100 to 600 mg/m^2) administered intravenously temporarily reduced circulating B lymphocytes and produced transient depression of OKT8, MI, and Ia positive cells in patients with malignant melanoma.[206] With higher doses, all T cells were affected.

Glucocorticosteroids have pronounced effects on inflammatory reactions in man. Man, however, belongs to the corticosteroid-resistant species and the effects on immunity are less pronounced.[207] The administration of single injections of 40 to 60 mg prednisone results in blood lymphocytopenia and monocytopenia after 4 to 6 hours, which is caused by a redistribution of cells into other lymphoid compartments. Recirculating T lymphocytes, particularly Tγ cells are selectively depleted.[207] Glucocorticoids suppress T-cell stimulation by mitogens, antigens, and allogeneic cells in vitro. Thymocyte mitogenesis seems to be more corticosteroid-sensitive than mitogenesis of blood lymphocytes.[208] Activated human T cells may be killed by moderate concentrations of glucocorticoids.[207] In contrast to cyclophosphamide, glucocorticosteroids reduce the OKT4+/OKT8+ lymphocyte ratio by selectively depleting OKT4+ cells.[206] Cutaneous delayed hypersensitivity is suppressed by inhibition of recruitment of monocytes-macrophages and by inhibition of lymphokine effects on the macrophages. Glucocorticoid effects on immunoglobulin synthesis and complement metabolism are less clinically significant.

It may be concluded that cyclophosphamide affects humoral and cellular immune functions.[209] Low doses may augment immunologic responses, probably by inhibition of suppressor cells. Glucocorticoids have major anti-inflammatory effects and suppress T-cell functions to some extent, while their effect on antibody production is weak.

LYMPHOCYTE SUBPOPULATIONS

Lymphocytopenia following cytotoxic drug therapy for Hodgkin's disease has been widely recognized. In a study of patients with stage IIIB Hodgkin's disease (five were splenectomized and two were previously given radiotherapy), a sharp fall of blood T and B cells was noted after one week.[210] There was no selective depression of T-lymphocyte subpopulations. The pretreatment levels were reached within 6 weeks. In only one study of previously untreated patients with advanced Hodgkin's was no reduction of blood T cells noted shortly after MOPP cytotoxic drug therapy.[211]

A moderate to severe T-cell depletion was observed in stage III and IV patients during and 2 to 12 months after cytotoxic drug therapy.[75,163] This has been confirmed in a prospective study by van Rijswik et al.[212] who monitored 20 previously untreated patients with stage III and IV Hodgkin's disease before modified MOPP cytotoxic drug therapy, after three courses, and within 3 months after the sixth course. There was no change in B cells and non-T non-B cells. T lymphocytopenia was also observed 2 years or more after cytotoxic drug therapy.[213] In another prospective study, 11 stage III/IV patients, tested before treatment and on average 1.5 years (3 to 36 months) after termination of cytotoxic drug therapy, T-lymphocyte counts were lower following therapy than before therapy.[144]

Lymphocyte counts were not restored in nonsplenectomized Hodgkin's patients 5 years after MOPP.[214] Moreover, T lymphocytes remained low in 28 long-term survivors (median disease-free interval after the completion of all therapy was 6.5 years).[215] There was no tendency towards normalization of the T-cell percentage with increasing disease-free survival. B-cell numbers were normal.

T lymphocytopenia in cytotoxic drug therapy-treated long-term survivors seems to primarily be the result of a reduction of Tμ and/or OKT4+ cells (Table 5–5).[34,156,157]

In summary, aggressive combination cytotoxic drug therapy induces an acute reduction of T and B lymphocytes in Hodgkin's patients. T lymphocytopenia, however, can be detected in a large proportion of cured patients 1 to 12 years after cessation of cytotoxic drug therapy. A reduction of Tμ and OKT4+ cells is seen in long-term survivors with Hodgkin's after such therapy.

LYMPHOCYTE FUNCTIONS

In a prospective study, lymphocyte-DNA synthesis induced by mitogens, antigens, and allogeneic lymphocytes declined during or immediately after six courses of MOPP.[212] PHA-induced proliferation was partially restituted during complete remission, though the pretreatment levels were not reached 1 to 2 years after cytotoxic drug therapy. Moreover, functional blood lymphocyte defects may persist many years after therapy.[213,215] Thus, lymphocyte proliferation induced by PHA, ConA, antigens, and allogeneic cells assessed in 28 long-term survivors with Hodgkin's disease remained subnormal during continuous complete remission 1 to 13 years after treatment with MOPP. The mitogen-induced DNA synthesis, however, was still lower in another group of patients who had received MOPP plus radiotherapy.[215] These authors also studied 16 patients with advanced diffuse-histiocytic lymphoma in complete remission after treatment with comparable cytotoxic drug therapy. Interestingly, the mitogen response in this patient group was identical to that of the control group. Thus, the lymphocyte defect seen in Hodgkin's patients during unmaintained complete remission does not appear to be a consequence of combination cytotoxic drug therapy. This conclusion is further corroborated by a prospective study in which 11 Hodgkin's patients were treated for ConA, PWM, and

PPD-induced DNA synthesis before and up to 3 years following termination of modified MOPP therapy.[144] The lymphocyte response remained on the low pretreatment level and no restitution with time was observed. Moreover, blood lymphocytes from cured Hodgkin's patients exhibited a higher sensitivity to ConA-activated suppressor cells from normal donors than did cells from healthy controls and long-term survivors with diffuse histiocytic lymphoma.[216] The increased suppressor sensitivity did not tend to normalize when the free interval increased from 1.5 to 12 years.

It may be concluded that persistent abnormalities of T-cell functions can be detected in long-term survivors of Hodgkin's disease following curative cytotoxic drug therapy.

DISEASES OTHER THAN LYMPHOMA

Despite the improved clinical effects of combination cytotoxic drug therapy in recent years, only select patient groups are available for studies of immune functions in disease-free survivors. This may have important implications with regard to the findings and their interpretation.

Treatment of rheumatoid arthritis with continuous low-dose oral cyclophosphamide induced a reduction of lymphocyte counts, which was reversible after drug withdrawal.[217] In patients with various solid tumors, Harris et al.[112] observed that the degree of absolute cell-number reduction and rate of recovery were similar for T and B lymphocytes after a short intensive course of cytotoxic drug therapy. Following termination of therapy, children with leukemia had blood T and B lymphocytopenia. B lymphocytes increased during the following 3 months, while T cells were essentially unchanged up to 4 months. Thereafter, T cells rose gradually to normal levels within one year.[112] Adjuvant chemotherapy given to breast-cancer patients as 12 cycles of chlorambucil/cyclophosphamide, methothrexate, and 5-fluorouracil caused a progressive lymphocytopenia.[218,219] Also here, the restitution of non-T cells was faster than for T cells. After two courses of cytotoxic drug therapy the Leu3+/Leu2+ ratio was reduced and remained so throughout the period of study.[181]

The severe depression of humoral and cell-mediated immune functions following short intensive multiple-drug cytotoxic therapy courses in cancer patients is well documented.[112,220] The long-term situation is less clear, but the general impression is that an almost complete restoration of immune function will occur following cessation of successful cytotoxic drug therapy protocols.[112,221]

DELAYED HYPERSENSITIVITY IN HODGKIN'S DISEASE

A partial restitution of delayed skin reactivity takes place in patients cured after radiotherapy and cytotoxic drug therapy.[143,148] Many patients, however, remain anergic (to neoantigens in particular) a long time following termination of therapy.[5,144,145,211–213,222] The persistent skin anergy in many patients is partly related to the aggressiveness of treatment.

HUMORAL IMMUNITY IN HODGKIN'S DISEASE

Only limited information is available regarding the influence of treatment on humoral immunity in Hodgkin's disease. The antibody response after vaccination with *Haemophilus influenzae* type B was reduced in patients who had received radiotherapy and cytotoxic drug therapy, whereas the titers were unaffected by radiotherapy and only slightly reduced by cytotoxic drug therapy alone.[80] In contrast, Sybesma et al.[223] found no correlation between mode of treatment and antibody response to influenza A (Hongkong) virus. The antibody titers after immunization of untreated Hodgkin's patients with pneumococcal polysaccharide vaccine were normal.[224,225] Radiotherapy and cytotoxic drug therapy, however, suppressed a subsequent antibody response. Suppression was most pronounced following total-nodal irradiation plus cytotoxic drug therapy.[224,226] The antibody response recovered with time after therapy and became normal in several patients after 3 years.[227] Furthermore, splenectomized and nonsplenectomized patients did not differ in preimmunization antibody titers or antibody responses to pneumococcal polysaccharides. The mechanisms for the suppression of humoral immunity are not known.

Following curative radiotherapy and cytotoxic drug therapy, serum IgG, IgA, and IgE concentrations are slightly decreased.[81,82,144] The reduction of serum IgM in complete remission patients may be more pronounced. Splenectomy may partly contribute to the decline in serum IgM concentrations.[80–82,144] IgD concentrations decreased in patients who achieved complete remission but not in nonresponders. Splenectomized patients displayed higher IgD concentrations than nonsplenectomized patients.[81,83,84]

In summary, treated and possibly cured patients with Hodgkin's disease often have reduced serum IgM levels and a poor antibody response after immunization with microbial antigens.

INFLAMMATORY REACTIONS IN HODGKIN'S DISEASE

COMPLEMENT

Individual complement factors and CH_{50} are usually normal or elevated.[79] High concentrations of the total hemolytic complement, C3 and C4, appear to be associated with widespread disease and B symptoms.[228] Complement activity is usually normalized in complete remission,[80,229,230] however, one study explained that patients given the most aggressive therapy had higher concentration of complement factors than those treated less vigorously.[80] Moreover, persistently raised serum complement levels were observed in stage IV patients in complete remission,[230] which may indicate the presence of residual disease.

PHAGOCYTIC CELLS

Blood polymorphonuclear leukocytes and monocytes are normal or increased in Hodgkin's patients.[16,72] Monocyte production in the bone marrow of untreated patients is raised; it returns to normal during long-term complete remission.[231] The phagocytic activity of polymorphonuclear leukocytes and monocytes appears to be normal or increased,[232–235] though decreased activity has also been reported.[236] Nitroblue-tetrazolium reduction by phagocytic cells in untreated Hodgkin's disease patients may be normal or high.[232,235,237]

Cytotoxic drug therapy appears to depress neutrophil migration. Chemotactic, candidacidal, and bactericidal activities were frequently inhibited in patients before and after cytotoxic drug therapy.[234,235,238,239] These functions were normal in long-term survivors.

Monocyte-macrophage cytotoxicity in untreated Hodgkin's disease may be low,[51] normal,[240] or increased.[241,242] The discrepancy between these results may be attributed, in part, to the differences in the effector cell populations employed. No statement regarding this monocyte function in patients following therapy can be made.

LYMPHOCYTES ACTIVATED IN VIVO FOLLOWING CURATIVE TREATMENT IN HODGKIN'S DISEASE

Most studies have shown that the increased in vivo activation of lymphocytes in untreated Hodgkin's patients tends to normalize following successful treatment.[58,150,151,159,168] In one study, however, the spontaneous DNA synthesis rose in patients responding to cytotoxic drug therapy, whereas it decreased in nonresponders.[212] Moreover, the "spontaneous" lymphocyte activity did not normalize completely in disease-free long-term survivors after therapy (Table 5–3, Fig. 5–3).[144] One tentative explanation is a residual undetected tumor in some long-term clinical disease-free survivors.[243] This is further supported by the observation that activated lymphocytes are increased in numbers during relapse (Table 5–3).[58,244] Other explanations, however, are offered in the following section (Fig. 5–4).

EFFECTS OF SPLENECTOMY

The indications for splenectomy in patients with malignant lymphoma have generally

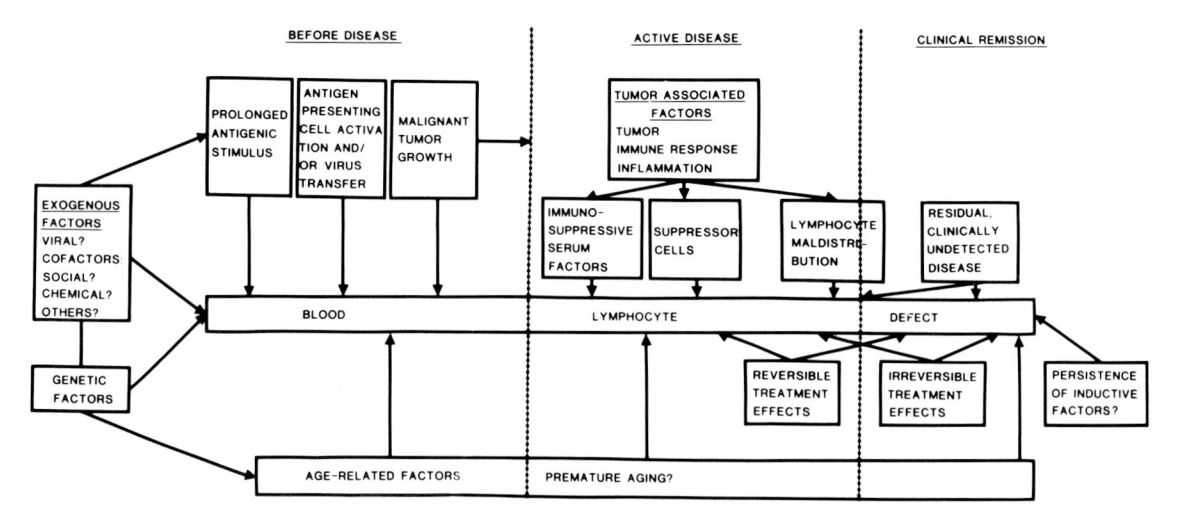

Fig. 5–4. Schematic and tentative model for lymphocyte deficiency and etiology in Hodgkin's disease.

included the presence of painful bulky splenomegaly or unequivocal evidence of hypersplenism. Furthermore, exploratory laparotomy with splenectomy was introduced in Hodgkin's disease as a diagnostic measure to assess the extent of abdominal disease.[245] The approach has led to an improved clinical and immunologic understanding of Hodgkin's disease. Splenectomy, however, may be associated with acute and late surgical complications and an increased risk of septicemia as a result of encapsulated bacteria, which are predominantly pneumococci.[246–248] Functional hyposplenism can also be induced by irradiation to the spleen, which hampers evaluation of the long-term immunologic effects of splenectomy.[249] With splenectomy, 20 to 25% of the phagocytic cell mass of the body is removed, leading to a diminished capacity for clearing circulating bacteria.[250] In addition, splenectomy following traumatic rupture, in connection with gastrointestinal surgery and for nonmalignant hematologic conditions, leads to a depression of the plasma IgM concentration.[251–254]

Removal of the spleen may result in persistent blood-cell abnormalities. Neutrophilia, lymphocytosis, eosinophilia, and thrombocytosis are regular findings after splenectomy, but cell counts tend to return to normal over weeks to months if other hematologic disorders are not present.[255]

The following characteristics of blood lymphocytes have been described in patients investigated 3 to 5 years following splenectomy: (1) Elevated numbers of T and B lymphocytes;[254,256] (2) A relative increase of EA-rosette-forming cells[256] and Tγ cells;[254] and (3) Normal or enhanced mitogen-induced DNA synthesis.[256,257]

HODGKIN'S DISEASE

The results of early studies have suggested that splenectomized Hodgkin's patients, even if previously treated with cytotoxic drug therapy, experience less hematologic depression (also with respect to lymphocyte counts) than nonsplenectomized patients undergoing radiotherapy.[258,259] Cytotoxic drug therapy used in the management of lymphoma may be better tolerated after splenectomy for anemia, leukopenia, or thrombocytopenia.[260–262] However, nontherapeutic splenectomy as part of the staging procedure did not improve the possibility of administering planned amounts of drugs during initial combination cytotoxic drug therapy in patients with Hodgkin's or nonHodgkin's lymphoma.[212,263]

Lymphocyte Subpopulations

Blood lymphocyte counts usually increase shortly after splenectomy, but before radiotherapy and cytotoxic drug therapy.[146,168,232,264–266] The effects on lymphocyte subpopulations, however, may be complex and related to a variety of clinical factors.

Thus, Diehl et al.[266] observed increased B cells, but no change in T-cell counts following staging splenectomy in 22 patients with favorable prognoses (i.e., without splenic tumor involvement). In contrast, patients with tumor-involved spleens showed only moderate lymphocytosis and no change of B cells. The long-term effects of splenectomy in Hodgkin's patients treated by radiotherapy, cytotoxic drug therapy or both, include increased T and B lymphocyte counts.[267] Among patients given total-nodal irradiation, early splenectomy prevented or mitigated the therapy-induced decline in lymphocyte counts 3 years after termination of therapy.[144,146,264,268] Prior splenectomy appeared to ameliorate the persisting T lymphocytopenia following radiotherapy in long-term survivors of Hodgkin's disease.[144,154,268]

To summarize, early removal of the spleen causes a relative increase in lymphocyte counts (both T and non-T cells), which can also be observed in patients in long-term remission. This effect seems to be partly related to splenic weight and tumor involvement. One possible mechanism may be the inhibition of a continuous elimination of lymphocytes by the spleen.[244] Alternatively, splenectomy may alter the distribution of lymphocytes, which is discussed in the next section.

Lymphocyte Functions

The PWM- and PHA-induced lymphocyte DNA synthesis essentially remained at the pretreatment level in patients tested 7 to 10 days after splenectomy.[264,265] The PHA response, however, increased significantly in stage III and IV patients who had spleen weights ranging from 140 to 543 g in one of these studies.[265] No consistent influence on the in vitro lymphocyte activation by mitogens, antigens, and allogeneic lymphocytes was observed in patients studied before and 5 to 30 days after splenectomy.[42,168] In a similar study of 22 patients, the spontaneous lymphocyte-DNA synthesis increased, while the response to PHA and ConA decreased 4 to 63 days after splenectomy in patients without splenic tumor involvement.[266] In contrast, these lymphocyte functions remained unchanged after splenectomy in patients with splenic tumor involvement.

The responding capacity of lymphocytes in MLR after completion of six courses of cytotoxic drug therapy was lower in splenectomized than in nonsplenectomized patients.[212] No long-term effects of splenectomy on spontaneous, mitogen or antigen-induced lymphocyte-DNA synthesis and leukocyte migration inhibition have been observed.[144,154,214,268] In one study, however, splenectomized patients showed a decreased mitogen response of blood lymphocytes after radiotherapy, cytotoxic drug therapy, or combined-modality treatment.[267] The state of delayed hypersensitivity is not influenced by splenectomy.[168,269]

Serum Immunoglobulins

No immediate reduction of serum IgM was observed after splenectomy.[168,265] A progressive fall in serum IgM after radiotherapy and cytotoxic drug therapy observed in long-term survivors was slightly potentiated by prior splenectomy.[144,214,267,268] A gradual and unexplained fall in IgM has also been reported in women with advanced breast cancer who were treated with multiple-drug cytotoxic drug therapy[110,218] and in patients with nonHodgkin's lymphoma.[270] Also, the IgA concentration declined irrespective of splenectomy.[144,146,212]

In summary, splenectomy seems to protect patients from therapy-induced lymphocytopenia and it contributes to the delayed reduction of serum IgM. No major changes in delayed skin hypersensitivity or T-cell functions in vitro can be ascribed to splenectomy. The asplenic state, reduced IgM levels, and possibly impaired B-cell responses contribute to the persistent life-long threat of overwhelming postsplenectomy infections in splenectomized patients with Hodgkin's disease.

EFFECTS OF IMMUNOPOTENTIATING THERAPY IN UNTREATED AND TREATED PATIENTS WITH HODGKIN'S DISEASE

The T-cell defect is a hallmark of Hodgkin's disease that has attracted the interest of immunologists and clinicians. If the anergy is closely linked to the disease process, improvement of immune reactivity might have important bearings on patient outcome. Clinicians have, therefore, attempted to confer immunity to anergic patients by treatment with nonspecific immunopotentiating measures. Although active immunization with BCG may induce tuberculin sensitivity in anergic Hodgkin's patients,[271] spontaneous fluctuations of immune status secondary to changes in disease activity, treatment effects, and boost effects of repeated skin testing may confound such findings.[4,72,272]

Transplantation of fetal thymic tissue resulted in a rise of total lymphocyte counts, normalization of tuberculin-skin sensitivity, and increased PHA reactivity in five previously treated Hodgkin's patients with advanced disease.[273] The prompt restoration of immune functions was associated with incomplete regression of lymphadenopathy and organomegaly. We, however, were unable to identify immunologic improvement in a patient with progressive Hodgkin's disease after fetal thymus transplantation. Apart from a transient fall in high body temperature, there was no clinical improvement (unpublished findings). Improvement of T-cell functions and delayed skin hypersensitivity has been reported in previously untreated and treated Hodgkin's patients following the administration of thymic extracts.[274,275,72]

The antihelminthic drug levamisole and a number of other chemical and biologic agents have been used as immunomodulators in Hodgkin's disease. So far, however, the information is limited,[276-281] though available data may indicate that thymus transplantation and administration of thymic extracts or levamisole have nonspecific immunopotentiating effects, both in untreated and treated Hodgkin's patients. No influence of such treatment on the long-term clinical course has been described.

IMMUNE FUNCTIONS OF HODGKIN'S DISEASE PATIENTS IN REMISSION FOLLOWING SUCCESSFUL TREATMENT

Untreated Hodgkin's patients display a widespread immunodeficiency, which mainly affects T-cell functions. A similar, but less pronounced, immunodeficiency is usually encountered in untreated patients with nonHodgkin's lymphoma or other solid cancers. Treatment with radiotherapy and cytotoxic drug therapy have twofold effects on the immune status of patients. Firstly, by curing the patients, tumor and tumor-associated immunosuppressive factors may be removed, which tends to normalize the immune capacity of the patients. This effect is, however, counteracted by the immunosuppressive action of the treatment itself. This is particularly important after radiotherapy, which may cause long-lasting immunosuppression. The immune status of "cured" tumor patients is therefore a net effect of these various factors. Bearing this in mind, the following general conclusions may be drawn regarding the immune status of long-term survivors with Hodgkin's disease:

1. Blood T cells are low, which is mainly because of a lack of $T\mu$ and/or OKT4+ cells.
2. Blood lymphocytes are poorly stimulated to blastogenesis and DNA synthesis by mitogens and allogeneic as well as autologous lymphocytes. In contrast, antigen-induced lymphocyte stimulation may recover, though at a slower rate than in other patient categories receiving the same type of treatment.
3. The high "spontaneous" blood lymphocyte-DNA synthesis in untreated patients decreases following therapy. Completely normal activity is not reached in all patients.
4. Serum factors that inhibit lymphocyte stimulation gradually disappear, with the possible exception of lymphocytotoxic serum activity, which is encountered in complete remission patients.[282]
5. A substantial proportion of cured Hodgkin's patients eventually regain the ability to express delayed hypersensitivity to recall antigens and to a lesser degree to neoantigens.
6. Immunoglobulin concentrations, particularly IgM levels, are reduced.
7. Primary, and to a lesser extent secondary, antibody responses are depressed,

but a slow restoration with time is observed.
8. Splenectomy appears to mitigate the therapy-induced reduction of blood T cells and may also potentiate the decline in serum IgM concentration.

The existence of a persistent T-cell defect in cured Hodgkin's patients is further corroborated by the fact that patients treated by surgery alone also display these abnormalities.[159] Furthermore, a high spontaneous and a decreased mitogen-induced blood lymphocyte-DNA synthesis before institution of therapy is associated with a poor prognosis in Hodgkin's disease.[6,24,29,59] Thus, long-term survivors who are available for follow-up studies may belong to a patient population with relatively well preserved lymphocyte capacity.

IMPLICATIONS AND CONSEQUENCES OF IMMUNE DEFICIT IN DISEASE-FREE HODGKIN'S PATIENTS

PRE- AND POST-TREATMENT IMMUNE STATUS IN RELATION TO PROGNOSIS

Notwithstanding the partial lack of knowledge concerning the mechanisms of immunoincompetence on Hodgkin's disease and the relationship between immunologic impairment and the disease process, efforts have been made to correlate the immune status of Hodgkin's patients with prognosis. Despite the vast literature on Hodgkin's disease, a rather limited number of studies using modern principles for staging and therapy have focused on whether some components of the pretreatment immune status of Hodgkin's patients might be useful predictors of prognosis. Still fewer studies are available concerning the post-treatment immune status of Hodgkin's patients in relation to prognosis. In short, pretreatment responses to DNCB and recall antigens seem to have no[6,40,283] or only limited prognostic impact.[72,284] Lymphocytopenia has been thought to be associated with a poor prognosis,[13,285] but subsequent studies of large patient series have been unable to confirm this claim.[6,29,73] This seems to also be true for total and relative numbers of T cells.[6] An increased spontaneous blood lymphocyte DNA synthesis and a decreased mitogen-induced blood lymphocyte-DNA synthesis before treatment have been shown to be associated with a dismal prognosis.[6,24,29,59] Similar findings have been achieved by other authors,[26,286] while others have been unable to verify such an association.[40] The plausible reasons for this discrepancy are discussed in detail.[6,29]

Many Hodgkin's disease patients in clinical remission have decreased lymphocyte responses to stimulation with mitogens and allogeneic and autologous lymphocytes. Thus, it seems highly improbable to achieve any prognostic information by repeating these tests.[72,144] De Sousa et al.,[287] however, reported a persistently low PHA response after treatment in eight children who had subsequent relapses. The same reasoning is also true for lymphocyte counts and subpopulations. Since some patients in remission revert to anergy during subsequent relapses, the delayed skin hypersensitivity seems to correlate directly with disease activity and indirectly with prognosis.[4,72,288] The clinical usefulness of repeated skin tests, however, is limited.[72,212] In parallel, the spontaneous lymphocyte DNA synthesis and the presence of various serum factors are closely correlated to disease activity. Thus, these tests may be useful in defining complete remission.[144,289] Unfortunately, data are too sparse to base any meaningful opinion concerning the ability of these tests to estimate future patient outcome.

IMMUNODEFICIENCY AND INCREASED RISK OF SECOND MALIGNANCIES

The epidemiologic and clinical aspects of second neoplasms in Hodgkin's patients are discussed extensively in this book, while only restricted aspects are examined in this chapter. There can be little doubt that the present epidemic of acute nonlymphocytic leukemia in treated Hodgkin's patients is mainly caused by MOPP and similar drug combinations. Radiotherapy may potentiate the leukemogenic effect of combination chemotherapy, however, only a moderately increased risk of secondary leukemia has been observed following radiotherapy as single treatment.[290]

The incidence of post-treatment leukemia appears to be higher in heavily treated patients and in patients above the age of 40 and/or with stage IV disease. Since many patients with these characteristics at presentation will relapse and eventually die from progressive Hodgkin's disease,[291,292] the incidence of secondary leukemias is likely to increase with the increasing cure rate. Elderly patients with advanced disease also have a vast impairment in T-cell immunity.[6,29] Thus, the question to be addressed is whether immunologic impairment is in some way related to the increased risk of secondary leukemias. An increased incidence of leukemia and lymphoma has been noted in patients with depressed immune function, in both naturally occurring immunodeficiency diseases like Bruton's sex-linked agammaglobulinemia, congenital hypogammaglobulinemia, ataxia telangiectasia, and Wiskott-Aldrich syndrome and, more recently, in transplant recipients given immunosuppressive therapy.[293,294] Furthermore, several reports of multiple cases of hematologic malignancies in families with an increased frequency of immunologic abnormalities have been published. These, however, mostly involve lymphoma or chronic lymphocytic leukemia.[295,296] The hematologic neoplasms induced by cytotoxic drug therapy probably arise in a complex interplay with several other factors, including genetic predisposition, impaired immune-host defense mechanisms, activation of oncogenic viruses, and a lack of factors regulating cell growth. It is rather well established that patients with a previous malignancy run an increased risk to develop another primary neoplasm regardless of the type of treatment given.[297,298] It should also be considered that an increased incidence of acute nonlymphocytic leukemia has been observed in patients given cytotoxic drug therapy for cancers other than Hodgkin's disease (i.e., nonHodgkin's lymphoma, multiple myeloma, and ovarian carcinoma;[299] conditions that are not known to be associated with persistent T-cell defects). Furthermore, in a series of 182 untreated patients, 11 patients (6%) reported a previous malignancy that was confirmed by medical records.[16] The expected number of primary malignancies was calculated to be 13.8. This further supports aggressive cytotoxic drug therapy as the probable cause of the increase in secondary leukemias in treated Hodgkin's patients. Thus, available data may not be interpreted as evidence for an association between defect cell-mediated immunity and an increased risk of secondary leukemia.

Another, and in many aspects more important, issue is whether treatment and its detrimental immunologic effects may enhance a conceivable constitutional risk to develop Hodgkin's disease. In other words, are Hodgkin's patients more prone to develop de novo Hodgkin's disease than the normal population? This might be anticipated if there is a constitutional/genetic basis for the evolution of Hodgkin's disease. To fully resolve this issue, not only Hodgkin's disease specific markers in general,[300] but also clonal markers will be needed. In the future, molecular genetic analyses will be demanded to differentiate between relapsing and de novo Hodgkin's disease. What we call late relapses are relatively rare 5 years or more following successful treatment. However, limited numbers of patients have survived 15 years or more following the introduction of modern radiotherapy and chemotherapy. Consequently, it remains to be seen whether this patient category will retain its low probability of "relapse."

POST-TREATMENT IMMUNODEFICIENCY AND SUSCEPTIBILITY TO INFECTION

Historically, tuberculosis was the first infection to be associated with Hodgkin's disease.[10] In fact, Carl Sternberg[301] stated that Hodgkin's disease was a variant of tuberculosis in his paper "Über eine eigenartige unter dem Bilde der Pseudolekämie verlaufende Tuberkulose des Lymfatischen Apparate." Since then, other organisms, which also depend in large part on an intact cell-mediated immune capability for control, have been frequently encountered in patients with Hodgkin's disease. They include varicella-zoster virus,[302] various fungi,[303] toxoplasmosis,[304] listeriosis,[305] pneumocystosis,[306] and other unusual infections. Paradoxically, the large majority of serious infections during the course of Hodgkin's disease are caused by other organisms, particularly common bacterial pathogens. Because of the acute myelosuppressive effect of both radiotherapy and cytotoxic drug therapy, this seems a logical finding.[303,307] In addition, an increased incidence of bacterial infections is observed later in the course of disease in patients who are "cured" of the disease. Among identifiable factors predisposing patients to infection are high age, advanced disease, and prior extensive radiotherapy and cytotoxic drug therapy.[303,308] *Streptococcus pneumoniae* is the most common organism causing serious infection. The pattern of infections resembles that associated with primary immunoglobulin deficiencies and B-cell neoplasms in which humoral immunity is often impaired.[309] The effects of radiotherapy and/or cytotoxic drug therapy on humoral-immune responses are most likely the major cause of this impairment.

Removal of the spleen predisposes patients to developing septicemia, which is caused predominantly by pneumococci, although other pathogens such as *Haemophilus influenzae*, *Escherichia coli*, and *Staphylococcus aureus* may be isolated. Prior radiotherapy and/or cytotoxic drug therapy increase the risk of developing overwhelming sepsis.[247,310-312] The increased susceptibility is believed to be chiefly related to the loss of mechanical filtration, but decreased serum IgM, properdin, and opsonin concentrations may have contributory effects.[252] In 1981, however, it was stated that deficiencies of complements and antibodies are not sufficient to account for the infection seen in splenectomized individuals.[313] Increased opsonization was required for the clearance of sensitized erythrocytes in splenectomized persons to compensate for the reduced phagocytic capacity of remaining macrophages. Thus, the increased requirement for type-specific antibodies for intravascular clearance in combination with the inability to produce antibodies may be major causative factors in postsplenectomy septicemia. The loss of the filter function of the spleen may in fact be less important than previously anticipated. It is important to bear in mind that irradiation to the spleen causes a splenic functional impairment.[249,314,315] This may, in part, explain the increased frequency of infections caused by encapsulated bacteria in nonsplenectomized patients who have received irradiation to the splenic area.[248,303,316]

MECHANISMS OF THE PERSISTENT T-CELL DEFECT IN HODGKIN'S DISEASE

A number of mechanisms have been proposed to explain the various defects in blood lymphocytes of Hodgkin's patients:

1. Intrinsic T-cell defects.[4,7,32,35,42,144,317-319]
2. Suppressive effects of monocytes and/or T lymphocytes.[317,320-329]
3. Lack of responder or regulator blood T cells caused by destruction, decreased production, and/or maldistribution among lymphoid compartments.[4,76,244,282,330-332]
4. Defect binding of lectins to lymphocytes,[333,334] although this is not generally agreed on.[289,335]
5. A poor survival of cultured Hodgkin's disease lymphocytes has been suggested,[35] which has not however been confirmed.[8,289]
6. Hodgkin's disease sera from patients with active disease inhibit lymphocyte activation by mitogens, antigens, and allogeneic cells. Only a few inhibitory factors have been suggested, such as glucolipids and ferritin.[336,337] In most studies, however, the suppressive components were not isolated.[8,22,30,32,230,282,338-345] A reduction of thymic-hormone activity may also contribute to the lymphocyte deficiency.[32]

A detailed discussion of the previously listed mechanisms and their relative contribution to the immunodeficiencies manifested in Hodgkin's disease are far from the topic of this chapter. Many complex factors, intrinsic T-cell defects included, are likely to contribute to the state of impaired immunity observed in untreated Hodgkin's disease. If a broad battery of tests for T-cell functional activity and serum effects are applied, almost every untreated Hodgkin's patient will exhibit one or more defect. It should be noted that some of the listed mechanisms may not explain the immunodeficiency of disease-free survivors with Hodgkin's disease. Thus, most lymphocyte inhibitory serum factors are only associated with active disease and do not explain the lymphocyte abnormalities in remission patients.[8,289]

LYMPHOCYTE MALDISTRIBUTION AS A TENTATIVE MECHANISTIC MODEL OF IMMUNODEFICIENCY IN UNTREATED AND TREATED HODGKIN'S DISEASE PATIENTS

Among the various mechanisms that have been proposed to explain the defect observed in blood lymphocytes of Hodgkin's patients, only a restricted number may also account for persistent T lymphocytopenia and the depressed response to stimulation by mitogens, allogeneic, and autologous lymphocytes. One attractive possibility that explains the major features of the immunodeficiency during the course of the disease is the lack of responder or regulator blood T cells caused by destruction and/or decreased production or caused by maldistribution among lymphoid compartments.[4,330] The spleen, as the largest single lymphoid organ of the human body, has a central place in the study of neoplastic lymphoreticular diseases. The spleen is a reservoir of recirculating T lymphocytes in normal individuals.[346] As a result, much interest has been focused on the role of the spleen in relation to immunologic impairment in Hodgkin's disease. Tumor-associated factors may elicit both humoral and cell-mediated responses in the spleen to some still unidentified antigen(s).[347,348] A number of studies have shown an increased number of T lymphocytes in the spleens of Hodgkin's patients, particularly in tumor-involved spleens.[25,330,349-353] In addition, increased mitogen responsiveness of splenic lymphocytes has been observed.[46,330,354,355] Since blood lymphocytes constitute only a small fraction of the entire lymphoreticular system, the blood lymphocyte defect may mirror a lymphocyte sequestration in the spleen and lymph nodes. In a group of untreated Hodgkin's patients, a strong inverse correlation existed between spleen weight and lymphocyte DNA synthesis induced by PWM, ConA, and PPD in patients with splenic tumor involvement.[76] In patients with uninvolved spleens, the spontaneous blood lymphocyte DNA synthesis increased with spleen weight.[76] Spontaneously proliferating lymphocytes seem to have a rapid turnover and home towards the spleen.[60] More data are now available concerning human lymphocyte traffic with the success of ^{111}In labeling and tracing and imaging of lymphocytes in man.[332] Recent studies from the same group have shown an increased sequestration of labeled blood lymphocytes of the diseased lymph nodes, suggesting lymphocyte trapping. This sequestration is sufficient to deplete the rest of the lymphoid system of recirculating cells and thus accounts for the immune deficit elsewhere. The increased migration and trapping of T cells in affected tissues suggests that this could be mediated by tumor-associated antigens.[356] It should be observed that, by this rather crude approach, no evidence of spleen sequestration was noted. In a study of children with Hodgkin's disease, Gupta and Tan[357] observed increased relative numbers of Tμ cells immediately following splenectomy. However, pre- and postsplenectomy results of phenotyping blood lymphocytes of adult patients did not show any increase in T cells or redistribution of T-cell subsets identified by monoclonal antibodies.[25,34]

A new approach to studying the possible elimination of lymphocytes by the spleen was presented in 1983; simultaneous evaluation of arterial and venous splenic blood lymphocytes was obtained during diagnostic or therapeutic splenectomy.[244] The percentage of E+ cells in splenic venous blood was lower than that of arterial blood, although no significant differences were found in total lymphocyte or E+ cell counts. The spontaneous lymphocyte-DNA synthesis was lower in venous than in arterial splenic lymphocytes in both untreated and treated patients. Four patients showed a decreased mitogen-induced lymphocyte-DNA synthesis in splenic venous blood, while the reverse was observed in another two. The mechanism for the elimination of mitogen-responsive lymphocytes in the spleen or elsewhere may be provided by the presence of opsonizing serum factors. Sera from 30% of untreated Hodgkin's patients showed lymphocytotoxic activity in the presence of complement against a panel of lymphocytes from 23 healthy normal donors.[282] These patients had lower total lymphocyte- and T-cell counts and a decreased response to mitogens as compared to the remainder. Furthermore, their spontaneous lymphocyte activity was increased. Lymphocytotoxic activity dominated among patients with B symptoms and advanced disease and was often found in patients with large tumor-involved spleens.

IMMUNOLOGIC STUDIES IN FAMILY MEMBERS OF PATIENTS WITH HODGKIN'S DISEASE

The T lymphocytopenia and impairment of T-cell functions in long-term survivors have suggested a persistent T-cell defect in Hodgkin's patients; genetic and/or environmental factors may play a role in initiation and maintenance of the immunodeficiency.[4,151,159,358] Inherent in this hypothesis is the fact that the persistent immunodeficiency is in part unrelated to therapy. Such a hypothesis requires discussion of the following crucial questions:
1. Is the immunodefect in "cured" Hodgkin's disease patients acquired? If so, is it secondary to the tumor- or disease-associated factors that may promote and perpetuate a state of immunologic imbalance in predisposed individuals?
2. Is the immunodeficiency an inherited (genetic?) characteristic of Hodgkin's disease patients? If so, it might be detected in relatives. Moreover, it may predispose one to developing the disease and may modulate its course. An inherited immunodeficiency may also be latent and precipitated by the disease or other factors. Early immunologic aging may contribute.

These questions prompted us to closely evaluate the immunology of healthy relatives of Hodgkin's patients. In an early study, the immunocompetence was investigated in six healthy twins whose monozygotic and dizygotic same-sexed twin partners had died from progressive Hodgkin's disease (on average 7.8 years before the test). Lymphocyte DNA synthesis induced by ConA was significantly reduced in all twins compared to age-matched healthy controls.[358] A less pronounced depression in the lymphocyte response to PWM and PHA was also observed. PPD-induced lymphocyte DNA synthesis was low in three twins who were skin anergic to the same antigen. T and B lymphocyte counts were normal.

We have studied another series of ten twin pairs. The index twin was alive 5 years or more after diagnosis in six pairs. The twin patients displayed the ordinary facets of cured Hodgkins patients—T lymphocytopenia, low OKT4+/OKT8+ ratios, and depressed responses to mitogens. Three out of ten healthy twin brothers/sisters also showed decreased responses to mitogens and antigens and one had an OKT4+/OKT8+ ratio of 0.3. Furthermore, five healthy twins had an increased spontaneous lymphocyte-DNA synthesis, which was also observed in three of the six surviving twins. Lymphocyte impairment was equally common in monozygotic and dizygotic twins (unpublished findings). Thus, the qualitative and quantitative T-cell impairment in this twin series was somewhat lower in comparison to the previous one; this can partly be explained by their lower mean age and the fact that the majority of index twins were long-term survivors.[6,17]

Lymphocyte activation by ConA was also suppressed in approximately 40% of the healthy close relatives to patients with a poor lymphocyte response to ConA.[359] The same frequencies of lymphocyte defects were noted in consanguineous first-degree relatives and spouses. In contrast, the mitogen response was normal in all relatives of patients with normal lymphocyte ConA stimulation. In relatives of ConA hyporesponsive patients, there was a small but statistically significant depression of PWM and PPD stimulation. Ricci and Romagnani[26] found a reduced mitogen-induced DNA synthesis in some of the 74 relatives of the 22 Hodgkin's patients. Dworsky et al.[360] studied immune functions in healthy members of families with multiple lymphoreticular neoplasms and compared them with those of healthy members of families with multiple cancers and families with no history of malignancies. Members of the lymphoma families were frequently skin anergic to *Candida* antigens and showed impaired lymphocyte ConA responses. T-lymphocyte defects were also revealed in a family where three sisters in a sibship of five girls developed Hodgkin's disease over a period of 6 years.[361]

An increased frequency of lymphocyte-reactive immunoglobulins (lymphocytotoxins) have been found in consanguineous and nonconsanguineous relatives of Hodgkin's patients.[362] Lymphocytotoxic activity may be associated with reduced T-cell counts, increased spontaneous blood lymphocyte DNA synthesis and decreased mitogen-induced blood lymphocyte-DNA synthesis in untreated Hodgkin's patients and in healthy family members.[282] In a more recent family study, abnormalities in T-cell function were verified in healthy members in nine of 20 Hodgkin's families. Only one of these 15 individuals was not blood related to the index patient (unpublished findings).

In summary, otherwise healthy persons with a first-degree relative with Hodgkin's disease display a significantly increased frequency of T-cell impairment. These findings have led us to hypothesize that a state of T-cell impairment existed in certain patients prior to the evolution of Hodgkin's disease.

IMMUNOLOGIC IMPAIRMENT AND THE PATHOGENESIS OF HODGKIN'S DISEASE

If one accepts the possible existence of a constitutional T-cell impairment in many Hodgkin's patients and a fraction of their family members, the question to be raised is whether such a defect is related to the pathogenesis of the disease. The weight of evidence suggests that close relatives of patients with Hodgkin's disease have a significantly increased risk of developing Hodgkin's disease compared to those in the general population,[363-366] which seems to contrast the evidence associated with nonHodgkin's lymphoma.[363,365] The risk of developing Hodgkin's disease seems to be concentrated among siblings of young adults with the disease, and the risk is higher among siblings of the same sex.[364,367] Strong arguments supporting a linkage between susceptibility to Hodgkin's disease and the HLA locus have also been reported.[368] A recent review of various patient series confirms the generally admitted trend of higher susceptibility borne by HLA-A1.[369] There are also converging arguments in favor of the prevalence of B5 and B18 in Hodgkin's disease.[370,371] The haplotype A1, B8, predominant in long-term survivors, appears to have a protective effect, while other phenotypes have been associated with a dismal prognosis.[372] Furthermore, accumulating data favor a relationship between genetic background and immune functions in man in general[95,373,374] and specifically in Hodgkin's disease.[375] In several multiple cases in Hodgkin's families, an additional association with immunodeficiency states, autoimmune diseases, and cutaneous T-cell lymphomas and other hematologic neoplasms has been observed.[295,376-378] Marshall et al.[379] investigated a familial aggregate (with HLA typing) of seven cases of Hodgkin's disease and over 600 people in the immediate population. They observed an increased frequency of B18 and a definite increase in A28 in the healthy population. Interestingly, in a prospective study of HLA-antigen phenotypes and lymphocyte abnormalities in Hodgkin's disease, HLA-A28 was the only antigen associated with severe T-cell impairment and a poor prognosis.[375] In a family of seven children, three cases of Hodgkin's disease were observed.[370] They all had the same HLA genotype: A26-B18, A1-B5. Marshall et al.[379] presented a hypothesis based on the concept of a "healthy carrier" state for a possible Hodgkin's agent. They postulated that such an agent might be more frequent in populations with a certain genetic constitution. Recent epidemiologic and immunologic data support the concept that Hodgkin's disease may be initiated by an infection (most probably a virus), and the host responsiveness plays a crucial role in the development of the disease.[4,380] The host responsiveness is thought to be mainly governed by immunologic capacity, which is at least in part genetically controlled.

The evidence for a familial T-cell deficiency in Hodgkin's disease is further corroborated by the results of a recent study on familial longevity and prognosis in Hodgkin's disease patients.[381] This study focused on the influence of familial longevity on the prognosis in 98 Hodgkin's patients followed for a long time. The survival of parents and grandparents of patients above 50 years of age who died from progressive Hodgkin's disease was significantly shorter than that of ancestors of survivors in the same age group. Remarkably, the excess death rate among relatives (less than 70 years) of the deceased patients was mainly caused by tuberculosis, which strongly suggests a T-cell defect. Since progressive Hodgkin's disease is almost without exception associated with a profound T-cell deficiency[4,6] and a short life expectancy is seen among normal subjects with T-cell defects,[17,88] it may be assumed that these Hodgkin's disease relatives also had a T-cell deficiency as a manifestation of premature aging. It might be expected that patients who develop aggressive Hodgkin's disease after the age of 50 have an immunodeficiency state prior to the evolution of disease. If this assumption is true, the main issue is to clarify whether such a condition is related to the pathogenesis of the disease or merely mirrors the patient's ability to cope with this disease and (perhaps more importantly) its treatment.

IMMUNODEFICIENCY IN RELATION TO ETIOLOGY, TUMOR, AND TREATMENT—A HYPOTHESIS

Various well established and tentative factors contributing to the state of immune impairment in long-term survivors with Hodgkin's disease are summarized in Figure 5-4. A fraction of patients who develop Hodgkin's disease may have an inherited (genetically determined) disturbance of immunoregulatory mechanisms and/or blood lymphocyte capacity. Such an impairment may be manifested as an absolute or relative immunodeficiency prior to exposure of inductive agents or the evolution of disease. An etiologic (viral?) agent, possibly in combination with cofactor effects, induces a prolonged immunologic stimulus in susceptible individuals. A defective immune defense may result in a persistent liberation of lymphocyte and macrophage activating factors. Immunocompetent blood lymphocytes are attracted and retained at the site of the reaction, further aggravating the state of immune dysfunction. The persistent release of macrophage activating/growth factors and/or direct virus transfer eventually leads to the development of a cytogenetic error within an antigen-presenting cell[382] and subsequently a monoclonal tumor-cell population will emerge. During active tumor progression, disease-associated factors further aggravate the host's immune impairment by the production of immunosuppressive serum factors and activation of suppressor cells. Lymphocyte maldistribution will add to these effects.

Radiotherapy and cytotoxic drug therapy induce a reversible damage of the immune system. The immune apparatus of Hodgkin's patients, however, may be more vulnerable to the effects of therapy, giving cause to an irreversible immune malfunction. In "cured" Hodgkin's patients, the persistent immunodeficiency may be the result of a constitutional impairment[4,383] and the persistence of inductive factors. Furthermore, residual undetected tumors may sustain the immunodeficiency and thus, in particular, prevent the reconstitution of cell-mediated immunity. Finally, the age-related decrease in lymphocyte capacity, possibly accentuated by premature immunologic aging, is superimposed on the immune impairment of cured patients with Hodgkin's disease.

ACKNOWLEDGEMENTS

This work was supported by grants from the Swedish Cancer Society and the Karolinska Institute Foundations. We thank Ricardo Giscombe, Margareta Söderqvist, and Ove Tullgren, M.D. for their skillful technical and statistical assistance, and we thank Katharina

Arvidsson and Ewa Friberg for preparing the manuscript.

REFERENCES

1. Reed, D.M. On the pathological changes in Hodgkin's disease with special reference to its relation to tuberculosis. Johns Hopkins Hosp. Rep. 10:133, 1902.
2. Parker, F. Jr., Jackson, H. Jr., Fitzhugh. G. et al. Studies of diseases of the lymphoid and myeloid tissues IV. Skin reactions to human and avian tuberculin. J. Immunol 22:277, 1932.
3. Steiner, P.E. Etiology of Hodgkin's disease. II. Skin reaction to avian and human tuberculin proteins in Hodgkin's. Arch. Intern. Med. 54:11, 1934.
4. Björkholm, M. Immunodeficiency in Hodgkin's disease and its relation to prognosis. Scand. J. Haematol. (Suppl.) 33:1, 1978.
5. Advani, S.H. et al. Cellular immunity in Hodgkin's disease. Cancer 43:492, 1979.
6. Björkholm, M., et al. Immune status of untreated patients with Hodgkin's disease and prognosis. Cancer Treat. Rep. 66:701, 1982.
7. Holm, G. et al. Lymphocyte abnormalities in untreated patients with Hodgkin's disease. Cancer 37:751, 1976.
8. Holm, G., Björkholm, M., and Mellstedt, H. Lymphocyte abnormalities and serum factors in Hodgkin's disease. In Naturally-Occurring Biological Immunosuppressive Factors and Their Relationship to Disease. Edited by R.H. Neubauer. Boca Raton, CRC Press, 1979, p 3.
9. Bunting, C.H. The blood picture in Hodgkin's disease. Second paper. Johns Hopkins Hospital Bull. 25:173, 1914.
10. Uddströmer, M. On the occurrence of lymphogranulomatosis (Sternberg) in Sweden, 1915–1931 and some considerations as to its relation to tuberculosis. Acta Tuberc. Pneumol. Scand. (Suppl.) 1:1, 1934.
11. Sears, G.W. The blood in Hodgkin's disease with special reference to eosinophilia. Guys Hosp. Rep. 82:40, 1932.
12. Westling, P. Studies of the prognosis in Hodgkin's disease. Acta Radiol. (Suppl.) 145:1, 1965.
13. Swan, H.T. and Knowelden, J. Prognosis in Hodgkin's disease related to the lymphocyte count. Br. J. Haematol. 21:343, 1971.
14. Eltringham, J.R. and Kaplan, H.S. Impaired delayed hyper-sensitivity responses in 154 patients with untreated Hodgkin's disease. Natl. Cancer Inst. Monogr. 36:107, 1973.
15. MacLennan, K.A. et al. The pretreatment peripheral blood lymphocyte count in 1100 patients with Hodgkin's disease: the prognostic significance and the relationship of the presence of systemic symptoms. Clin. Oncol. 7:333, 1981.
16. Wedelin, C., Björkholm, M., Johansson, B. et al. Clinical and laboratory findings in untreated patients with Hodgkin's disease with special reference to age. Med. Oncol. Tumor Pharmacother. 1:33, 1984.
17. Wedelin, C. et al. Blood T-lymphocyte functions in healthy adults in relation to age. Scand. J. Haematol. 28:45, 1982.
18. Aiuti, F., Lacava, V., Fiorilli, M. et al. Lympho-cyte surface markers in lymphoproliferative disorders. Acta. Haematol. 50:275, 1973.
19. Andersen, E. Depletion of thymus dependent lymphocytes in Hodgkin's disease. Scand. J. Haematol. 12:263, 1974.
20. Bobrove, A.M., Fuks, Z., Strober, S. et al. Quantitation of T an B lymphocytes and cellular immune function in Hodgkin's disease. Cancer 36:169, 1975.
21. Case, D.C. Jr. et al.: Comparison of multiple in vivo and in vitro parameters in untreated patients with Hodgkin's disease. Cancer 38:1807, 1976.
22. Fuks, Z., Strober, S., and Kaplan, H.S. Interaction between serum factors and T lymphocytes in Hodgkin's disease. N. Engl. J. Med. 295:1273, 1976.
23. Heier, H.E. et al. Blood B and T lymphocytes and in vitro cellular immune reactivity in untreated human malignant lymphomas and other malignant tumors. Scand. J. Haematol. 18:137, 1977.
24. Björkholm, M. et al. Prognostic factors in Hodgkin's disease. II. The role of the lymphocyte defect. Scand. J. Haematol. 20:306, 1978.
25. Posner, M.R. et al. Lymphoid subpopulations of peripheral blood and spleen in untreated Hodgkin's disease. Cancer 48:1170, 1981.
26. Ricci, M. and Romagnani. S. Immune status in Hodgkin's disease. In The Immune System: Functions and Therapy of Dysfunction. Edited by G. Doria and A. Eshkol. London, Academic Press, 1980.
27. Romagnani, S. et al. Displacement of T lymphocytes with the "helper/inducer" phenotype from peripheral blood to lymphoid organs in untreated patients with Hodgkin's disease. Scand. J. Haematol. 31:305, 1983.
28. Wedelin, C. On the prognosis in Hodgkin's disease. A Clinical and Immunological Study. Academic thesis. Karolinska Institute. Stockholm, 1982.
29. Wedelin, C. et al. Lymphocyte function in untreated Hodgkin's disease. An important predictor of prognosis. Br. J. Cancer 45:70, 1982.
30. Fuks, Z., Strober, S., King, D.P. et al. Reversal of cell surface abnormalities of T-lymphocytes in Hodgkin's disease after in vitro incubation in fetal sera. J. Immunol. 117:1331, 1976.
31. Gupta, S. Immunodeficiencies in Hodgkin's disease. I. T cell-mediated immunity. Clin. Bull. 11:58, 1981.
32. Schulof, R.S. et al. Multivariate analysis of T-cell functional defects and circulating serum factors in Hodgkin's disease. Cancer 48:964, 1981.
33. Smit, J.W., van der Giessen, M., and Halie, M.R. Fc receptors on lymphocytes from normal donors and patients with lympho-proliferative diseases. Acta Haematol. 70:108, 1983.

34. Lauria, F. et al. Increased proportion of suppressor/cytotoxic (OKT8+) cells in patients with Hodgkin's disease in long-lasting remission. Cancer 52:1385, 1983.
35. Hersh, E.M. and Oppenheim, J.J. Impaired in vitro lymphocyte transformation in Hodgkin's disease. N. Engl. J. Med. 273:1006, 1965.
36. Aisenberg, A.C. Quantitative estimation of the reactivity of normal and Hodgkin's disease lymphocytes with thymidine 2-C-14. Nature 205:1233, 1965.
37. Trubowitz, S., Masek, B., and Del Rosario, A. Lymphocyte response to phytohemagglutinin in Hodgkin's disease, lymphatic leukemia and lymphosarcoma. Cancer 19:2019, 1966.
38. Brown, R.S. et al. Hodgkin's disease. Immunologic, clinical and histologic features of 50 untreated patients. Ann. Intern. Med. 67:291, 1967.
39. Holm, G., Perlmann, P., and Johansson, B. Impaired phytohaemagglutinin-induced cytotoxicity in vitro of lymphocytes from patients with Hodgkin's disease or chronic lymphatic leukaemia. Clin. Exp. Immunol. 2:351, 1967.
40. Young, R.C. et al. Immune alterations in Hodgkin's disease. Effect of delayed hypersensitivity and lymphocyte transformation on course and survival. Arch. Intern. Med. 131:446, 1973.
41. Levy, R. and Kaplan, H.S. Impaired lymphocyte function in untreated Hodgkin's disease. N. Engl. J. Med. 290:181, 1974.
42. Romagnani, S. et al. In vitro lymphocyte response to phytomitogens in untreated and treated patients with Hodgkin's disease. Int. Arch. Allergy Appl. Immunol. 51:378, 1976.
43. Lang, J.M. et al. Mixed lymphocyte reaction as assay for immunological competence of lymphocytes from patients with Hodgkin's disease. Lancet 1:1261, 1972.
44. Rühl, H. et al. Mixed lymphocyte culture stimulatory and responding capacity of lymphocytes from patients with lymphoproliferative diseases. Clin. Exp. Immunol. 19:55, 1975.
45. Björkholm, M., Holm, G., Mellstedt, H. et al. Immunological capacity of lymphocytes from untreated patients with Hodgkin's disease evaluated in mixed lymphocyte culture. Clin. Exp. Immunol. 22:373, 1976.
46. Twomey, J.J., Laughter, A.H., Lazar, S. et al. Reactivity of lymphocytes from primary neoplasms of lymphoid tissues. Cancer 38:740, 1976.
47. Begemann, M., Claas, G., and Falke, H. Impaired autologous mixed lymphocyte reactivity in Hodgkin's disease. Klin. Wochenschr. 60:19, 1982.
48. Engleman, E.G. et al. Autologous mixed lymphocyte reaction in patients with Hodgkin's disease. J Clin. Invest. 66:149, 1980.
49. Zamkoff, K.W., Dock, N.L., Kurec, A.S. et al. Diminished autologous mixed lymphocyte reaction in patients with Hodgkin's disease: evidence for non-T cell dysfunction. Am. J. Haematol. 12:237, 1982.
50. Holm, G., Björkholm, M., Mellstedt, H. et al. Cytotoxic activity of lymphocytes from patients with Hodgkin's disease. Clin. Exp. Immunol. 21:376, 1975.
51. Kohl, S., Pickering, L.K., Sullivan, M.P. et al. Impaired monocyte-macrophage cytotoxicity in patients with Hodgkin's disease. Clin. Immunol. Immunopathol. 15:577, 1980.
52. Gupta, S. and Fernandes, G. Spontaneous and antibody-dependent cellular cytotoxicity by lymphocyte subpopulations in peripheral blood and spleen from adult untreated patients with Hodgkin's disease. Clin. Exp. Immunol. 45:205, 1981.
53. Al-Sam, S., Jones, B.D., Payne, S.V., and Wright, D.H.: Natural killer (NK) activity in the spleen of patients with Hodgkin's disease and controls. Br. J. Cancer 46:806, 1982.
54. Ruco, L.P. et al. Natural killer activity in spleens and lymph nodes from patients with Hodgkin's disease. Cancer Res. 42:2063, 1982.
55. Tursz, T., Dokhelar, M.C., Lipinski, M. et al. Low natural killer cell activity in patients with malignant lymphoma. Cancer 50:2333, 1982.
56. Kuper, S.W. and Bignall, J.R. Tritiated-thymidine uptake by tumour cells in blood. Lancet 1:1412, 1964.
57. Crowther, D., Hamilton Fairley, G., and Sewell, R.L. Lymphoid cells in Hodgkin's disease. Nature 215:1086, 1967.
58. Folb, P.I. and Ramot, B. Autoradiography of activated lymphocytes in the blood in Hodgkin's disease. Isr. J. Med. Sci. 9:923, 1973.
59. Björkholm, M., Holm, G., Mellstedt, H. et al. Immunodeficiency and prognosis in Hodgkin's disease. Acta Med. Scand. 198:275, 1975.
60. Schick, P., Trepel, F., and Begemann, H. On the fate of DNA synthesizing lymphoid blood cells in Hodgkin's disease. Scand. J Haematol. 14:17, 1975.
61. DePauw, B.E. et al. Lymphocyte density distribution profile and spontaneous transformation related to the stage of Hodgkin's disease. Br. J. Haematol. 44:359, 1980.
62. Björkholm, M. et al. Spontaneously DNA synthesizing blood and spleen lymphocytes in Hodgkin's disease. Scand. J. Haematol. 26:97, 1981.
63. Huber, C. et al. DNS-synthetisierende Blutlymphocyten bei Karcinompatiente. Med. Klin. 66:1441, 1971.
64. Heier, H.E. and Godal, T. DNA synthesis in unstimulated blood lymphocytes of patients with untreated malignant lymphomas or other malignant tumors. Scand. J. Haematol. 18:149, 1977.
65. Lindemalm, C. et al. Immunodeficiency and prognosis in patients with non-Hodgkin lymphomas. Acta Radiol. 24:159, 1985.
66. Crowther, D., Hamilton Fairley, G., and Sewell, R.L. Lymphoid cellular responses in the blood after immunization in man. J. Exp. Med. 129:849, 1969.
67. Huber, C. et al. Zytologischer Immunglobulinnachweis an DNS-synthetisierenden blutlymphozyten von Patienten mit Virusinfektionen. Acta. Haematol. (Basel) 45:23, 1971.
68. Al-Balaghi, S., Ström H., and Möller, E. Spontaneous DNA synthesis in rheumatoid arthritis: Evidence of enhanced circulating non-T-cell proliferation. Scand. J. Immunol. 17:521, 1983.

69. Huber, C. et al. Increased proliferation of T lymphocytes in the blood of patients with Hodgkin's disease. Clin. Exp. Immunol. 21:47, 1975.
70. DePauw, B., Wagener, T., Wessels, H. et al. Spontaneous DNA synthesis by subpopulations of lymphocytes in Hodgkin's disease. Eur. J. Cancer 16:1329, 1980.
71. DePauw, B. et al. High spontaneous thymidine incorporation into a non-T lymphocyte population in Hodgkin's disease unmasked after cell fractionation. Cancer 45:516, 1980.
72. Kaplan, H.S. Hodgkin's disease. 2nd Ed. Massachusetts, Harvard University Press, 1980.
73. Hancock, B.W., Dunsmore, I.R., and Swan, H.T. Lymphopenia. A bad prognostic factor in Hodgkin's disease. Scand. J. Haematol. 29:193, 1982.
74. Heier, H.E. and Normann, T. Blood lymphocytes in Hodgkin's disease. Lymphocytopenia related to stages and histological groups. Scand. J. Haematol. 13:199, 1974.
75. Michlmayr, G. T-Lymphozyten und ihre Funktion beim M. Hodgkin. Fortschr. Med. 96:1928, 1978.
76. Björkholm, M., et al. Blood lymphocyte functions in relation to splenic weight and tumor involvement in untreated Hodgkin's disease. Scand. J. Haematol. 25:51, 1980.
77. Romagnani, S. et al. Abnormalities of in vitro immunoglobulin synthesis by peripheral blood lymphocytes from untreated patients with Hodgkin's disease. J. Clin. Invest. 71:1375, 1983.
78. Souhami, R.L., Babbage, J., and Sigfusson, A. Defective in vitro antibody production to varicella zoster and other virus antigens in patients with Hodgkin's disease. Clin. Exp. Immunol. 53:297, 1983.
79. Gupta, S. Immunodeficiencies in Hodgkin's disease. II. B cell immunity, complement system and phagocytic cell system. Clin. Bull. 11:110, 1981.
80. Weitzman, S.A. et al. Impaired humoral immunity in treated Hodgkin's disease. N. Engl. J. Med. 297:245, 1977.
81. Amlot, P.L. and Green, L. Serum immunoglobulins G, A, M, D and E concentrations in lymphomas. Cancer 40:371, 1979.
82. Walzer, P.D., Armstrong, D., Weisman, P., et al. Serum immunoglobulin levels in childhood Hodgkin's disease. Cancer 45:2084, 1980.
83. Corte, G. et al. Correlation of serum IgD level with clinical and histologic parameters in Hodgkin's disease. Blood 52:905, 1978.
84. Gobbi, P.G., Merlini, G., Lattanzio, G. et al. Serum IgD in Hodgkin's disease. Haematologia 66:35, 1981.
85. Rubinstein, E., Sokal, J.E., Reisman, R.E. et al. Relationship of serum total IgE and cell-mediated immunity in patients with Hodgkin's disease. Int. Arch. Allergy Immunol. 55:439, 1977.
86. Walford, R.L. The immunologic theory of aging. Baltimore, Williams & Williams, 1969.
87. Makinodan, T. Immunodeficiencies and ageing. In The Immune System: Functions and Therapy of Dysfunction. Edited by G. Doria and A. Eshkol. London, Academic Press, 1980.
88. Roberts-Thomson, T.C., Whittingham, S., Youngchaiyud, U. et al. Ageing, immune response and mortality. Lancet 1:368, 1974.
89. Girard, J.P., Paychére, M., Cuevas, M. et al. Cell mediated immunity in an ageing population. Clin. Exp. Immunol. 27:85, 1977.
90. Diaz-Jouanen, E, Strickland, R.G., and Williams, R.C. Jr. Studies of human lymphocytes in the newborn and the aged. Am. J. Med. 58:620, 1975.
91. Clot, J., Charmansson, E., and Brochier, J. Age-dependent changes of human blood lymphocyte subpopulations. Clin. Exp. Immunol. 32:346, 1978.
92. Cobleigh, M.A., Braun, D.P., and Harris, J.E. Age-dependent changes in human peripheral blood B cells and T-cell subsets: Correlation with mitogen responsiveness. Clin. Immunol. Immunopathol. 15:162, 1980.
93. Weksler, M.E. and Hütteroth, T.H. Impaired lymphocyte function in aged humans. J. Clin. Invest. 53:99, 1974.
94. Fixa, B., Komarkova, O., and Chmelar, V. Ageing and cell-mediated immunity. Gerontologia 21:177, 1975.
95. Greenberg, L.J. Aging and immune function in man: Influence of sex and genetic background. In aging and immunity. Edited by S.K. Singhal, N.R. Sinclair, C.R. Stiller. North Holland, Elsevier Science Publishing Co., 1979.
96. Boss, G.R. et al. Age dependency of lymphocyte ecto-5'-nucleotidase activity. J. Immunol. 125:679, 1980.
97. Tam, C.F. and Walford, R.L. Alterations in cyclic nucleotides and cyclase-specific activities in T lymphocytes of aging normal humans and patients with Down's syndrome. J. Immunol. 125:1665, 1980.
98. Goodwin, J.S. and Messner, R.P. Sensitivity of lymphocytes to prostaglandin E_2. Increase in subjects over age 70. J. Clin. Invest. 64:434, 1979.
99. Goodwin, J.S. Changes in lymphocyte sensitivity to prostaglandin E, histamine, hydrocortisone, and X irradiation with age: Studies in a healthy elderly population. Clin. Immunol. Immunopathol. 25:243, 1982.
100. Delfraissy, J.F. et al. Abolished in vitro antibody response in elderly: Exclusive involvement of prostaglandin-induced T suppressor cells. Clin. Immunol. Immunopathol. 24:377, 1982.
101. Gillis, S., Konak, R., Durante, M. et al. Immunological studies of aging. J. Clin. Invest. 67:937, 1981.
102. Mackay, I.R. Ageing and immunological function in man. Gerontologia 18:285, 1972.
103. Hallgren, H.M., Buckley, C.E., Gilbertsen, V.A. et al. Lymphocyte phytohemagglutinin responsiveness, immunoglobulins and autoantibodies in aging humans. J. Immunol. 3:1101, 1973.
104. Hallgren, H.M. and Yunis, E.S. Suppressor lymphocytes in young and aged humans. J. Immunol 118:2004, 1977.
105. Goodwin, J.S., Searless, R.P., and Tung, K.S.K. Immunological responses of a healthy elderly population. Clin. Exp. Immunol. 48:403, 1982.
106. Benacerraf B. and Germain, R.N. Genetic control of

the immune response. *In* The Immune System: Functions and Therapy of Dysfunction. Edited by G. Doria and A. Eshkol. London, Academic Press, 1980.
107. Slater, J.M., Ngo, E., and Lau, B.H.S. Effect of therapeutic irradiation on the immune responses. Am. J. Roentgenol. *126*:313, 1976.
108. Stefani, S., Kerman, R., and Abbate, J. Immune evaluation of lung cancer patients undergoing radiation therapy. Cancer, *37*:2792, 1976.
109. Rafla, S., Yang, S.J., and Meleka, F. Changes in cell-mediated immunity in patients undergoing radiotherapy. Cancer *41*:1076, 1978.
110. Webster, D.J.T. et al. Effect of treatment on the immunological status of women with advanced breast cancer. Br. J. Cancer *39*:676, 1979.
111. Jenkins, V.K., Dillard, E.A., Olson, M.H. et al. Lymphocyte response and radiation therapy for patients with gynecologic cancer. Gynecol. Oncol. *9*:209, 1980.
112. Harris, J., Sengar, D., Stewart, T. et al. The effect of immunosuppressive chemotherapy on immune function in patients with malignant disease. Cancer *37*:1058, 1976.
113. Wanebo, H.J. Immunologic reactivity in patients with primary operable breast cancer. Cancer *41*:84, 1978.
114. Adler, A., Stein, J., and Ben-Efraim, S. Immunocompetence, immunosuppression, and human breast cancer. II. Further evidence of initial immune impairment by integrated assessment effect of nodal involvement (N) and of primary tumor size (T). Cancer *45*:2061, 1980.
115. Baroni, C.D., Uccini, S., and Ruco, L. Lymphocyte reactivity in malignancies of the lung and of the central and peripheral lymphoid tissues. *In* The Immune System: Functions and Therapy of Dysfunction. Edited by G. Doria and A. Eshkol. London, Academic Press, 1980.
116. McVie, J.G. Immunosuppression. *In* Medical Immunology. Edited by J. Irvine. Edinburgh. Teviot Scientific Publication, 1979.
117. Hellman, S. Principles of radiation therapy. *In* Cancer. Prnciples & Practice of Oncology. Edited by V.T. DeVita, Jr., S. Hellman, S.A. Rosenberg. Philadelphia, J.B. Lippincott, 1982.
118. Anderson, R.E. and Warner, N.L. Ionizing radiation and the immune response. *In* Advances in Immunology. Edited by F.J. Dixon and H.G. Kunkel. New York, Academic Press, 1976.
119. Suter, G.M. Response of hematopoietic systems to X-rays. USAEC Document MDDC-824, 1947.
120. Order, S.E. The effects of therapeutic irradiation on lymphocytes and immunity. Cancer *39*:737, 1977.
121. Hall, E. Radiobiology for the radiologist. 2nd Ed. New York, Harper & Row, 1978.
122. Strober, S. et al. Immunosuppression and tolerance after total lymphoid irradiation (TLI). Transpl. Proc. *12*:477, 1980.
123. Kaplan, H.S.: Selective effects of total lymphoid irradiation (TLI) on the immune response. Transplant. Proc. *13*:425, 1981.
124. Cronkite, E.P. et al. Studies on lymphocytes: 1 Lymphopenia produced by prolonged extracorporeal irradiation of the circulating blood. Blood *20*:203, 1962.
125. Storb, R., Ragde, H., and Thomas, E.D. Extracorporeal irradiation of the blood in baboons. Radiol. Res. *38*:43, 1969.
126. Weeke, E. Extracorporeal irradiation of the blood. Effect of varying transit dose on the degree and the rate of development of lymphopenia. Acta. Med. Scand. *191*:455, 1972.
127. Plowman, P.N. The effects of conventionally fractionated, extended portal radiotherapy on the human peripheral blood count. Int. J. Radiat. Oncol. Biol. Phys. *9*:829, 1983.
128. Rubin, P. et al. Bone marrow regeneration and extension after extended field irradiation in Hodgkin's disease. Cancer *32*:699, 1973.
129. Heier, H.E. The influence of therapeutic irradiation on blood and peripheral lymph lymphocytes. Lymphology *11*:238, 1978.
130. Doria, G., Agarossi, G., and Adorini, L. Selective effects of ionizing radiations on immunoregulatory cells. Immunol. Rev. *65*:23, 1982.
131. Gupta, S. and Good, R.A. Subpopulation of human T lymphocytes. II. Effect of thymopoietin, corticosteroids, and irradiation. Cell. Immunol. *34*:10, 1977.
132. Schwartz, J.L., Darr, J.C., and Gaulden, M.E. Survival and PHA-stimulation of gamma-irradiated human peripheral blood T lymphocyte subpopulations. Mutat. Res. *107*:413, 1983.
133. Thomas, Y. et al. Functional analysis of human T cell subsets defined by monoclonal antibodies. V. suppressor cells within the activated OKT4+ population belong to distinct subset. J. Immunol. *126*:1386, 1982.
134. Agarossi, G., Pozzi, L., Mancini, C. et al. Radiosensitivity of the helper cell function. J. Immunol. *121*:2118, 1978.
135. Lane, H.C., Whalen, G., and Fauci, A.S. Antigen-induced human T cell help. J. Clin. Invest. *72*:636, 1983.
136. Doria, G., DiMichele, A., and Gorini, G. Immune dysfunctions induced by irradiation. *In* The Immune System: Functions and Therapy of Dysfunction. Edited by G. Doria and A. Eshkol. London, Academic Press, 1980.
137. Stratton, J.A. et al. A comparison of the acute effects of radiation therapy, including or excluding the thymus, on the lymphocyte subpopulation of cancer patients. J. Clin. Invest. *56*:88, 1975.
138. Tapley, J.L., Potvin,C., and Chretien, P.B. Prolonged depression of cellular immunity in cured laryngopharyngeal cancer patients treated with radiation therapy. Cancer *35*:638, 1975.
139. Raben, M., Walach, N., Galili, U. et al. The effect of radiation therapy on lymphocyte subpopulations in cancer patients. Cancer *37*:1417, 1976.
140. Hoppe, R.T., Fuks, Z.Y., Strober, S. et al. The long term effects of radiation on T and B lymphocytes in

140. the peripheral blood after regional irradiation. Cancer 40:2071, 1977.
141. Björkholm, M., Holm, G. Johansson, B. et al. T-lymphocyte deficiency following adult thymectomy in man. Scand. J. Haematol. 14:210, 1975.
142. Ernström U., Sandberg, G., and Björkholm, M. Influence of thymectomy, transfer of thymus and bone marrow cells and treatment with thymosin on the depressed splenic release of lymphocytes into the blood after irradiation. Acta. Pathol. Microbiol. Scand. (A) 83:360, 1975.
143. Fuks, Z. et al. Long term effects of radiation on T an B lymphocytes in peripheral blood of patients with Hodgkin's disease. J. Clin. Invest. 58:803, 1976.
144. Björkholm, M. et al. Longitudinal studies of blood lymphocyte capacity in Hodgkin's disease. Cancer 48:2010, 1981.
145. Hancock, B.W. et al. Follow-up studies on the immune status of patents with Hodgkin's disease after splenectomy and treatment, in relapse and remission. Br. J. Cancer 36:347, 1977.
146. Hancock, B.W., Bruce, L., Ward, A.M. et al. The immediate effects of splenectomy, radiotherapy and intensive chemotherapy on the immune status of patients with malignant lymphoma. Clin. Oncol. 3:137, 1977.
147. Posner, M.R. et al. Circulating lymphocyte populations in Hodgkin's disease after mantle and paraaortic irradiation. Blood 61:705, 1983.
148. Kun, L.E. and Johnson, R.E. Hematologic and immunologic status in Hodgkin's disease 5 years after radical radiotherapy. Cancer 36:1912, 1975.
149. Gajl-Peczalska, K.J., Bloomfield, C.D., Sosin, H. et al. B and T lymphocytes in Hodgkin's disease. Clin. Exp. Immunol. 23:47, 1976.
150. King, G.W. et al. Immune function of successfully treated lymphoma patients. J. Clin. Invest. 57:1451, 1976.
151. Björkholm, M., Holm, G., and Mellstedt, H. Persisting lymphocyte deficiencies during remission in Hodgkin's disease. Clin. Exp. Immunol. 28:389, 1977.
152. Case, D.C. et al. Depressed in vitro lymphocyte responses to PHA in patients with Hodgkin's disease in continuous long remissions. Blood 49:771, 1977.
153. Gobbi, M. et al. Immunological study of patients with Hodgkin's disease in long lasting not maintained complete remission. Boll. Ist. Seiroter Milan. 56:144, 1977.
154. Steele, R. and Han, T. Effects of radiochemotherapy and splenectomy on cellular immunity in long-term survivors of Hodgkin's disease and non-Hodgkin's lymphoma. Cancer 42:133, 1978.
155. Romagnani, S. et al. Short and long-term effects of radiation on T-cell subsets in peripheral blood of patients with Hodgkin's disease. Cancer 46:2590, 1980.
156. Karande, A.A., Gulwani, B., Advani, S.H. et al. Subpopulations in human T lymphocytes in patients with Hodgkin' disease before and after treatment. Neoplasma 29:149, 1982.
157. Gattringer, C. and Huber, H. Immunologischer Nachweis und In-vitro-Aktivität von Suppressorzellen. Wiener klin. Wochenschrift 95:138, 1983.
158. Herrman, F. et al. Evaluation of the circulating and splenic lymphocyte subpopulations in patients with non-Hodgkin lymphomas and Hodgkin's disease using monoclonal antibodies. Blut 47:41, 1983.
159. Björkholm, M., Holm, G., and Mellstedt, H. Immunologic profile of patients with cured Hodgkin's disease. Scand. J. Haematol. 18:361, 1977.
160. Moretta, L. et al. Functional analysis of two human T cell subpopulations: Help and suppression of B cell response by T cells bearing receptors for IgM (T_m) or IgG (T_g). J. Exp. Med. 146:184, 1977.
161. Reinherz, E.L. et al. Human T-lymphocyte subpopulations defined by Fc receptors and monoclonal antibodies: A comparison. J. Exp. Med. 151:969, 1980.
162. Reinherz, E.L. et al. Heterogeneity of human T4+ inducer T cells defined by a monoclonal antibody that delineates two functional subpopulations. J. Immunol. 128:463, 1982.
163. Burchardt, K. Immunologische Daten bei der klinischen Einschätzung Morbus Hodgkin. Z. ges. Inn. Med. 36:840, 1981.
164. Engeset, A., Fröland, S.S., Brémer, K. et al. Blood lymphocytes in Hodgkin's disease. Increase of B-lymphocytes following extended field-irradiation. Scand. J. Haematol. 11:195, 1973.
165. Skovmann-Sörensen, O., Schröder, H., Möller-Larsen, A. et al. Cellular and humoral immunity in Hodgkin's disease. I. Patients in continuous long-term remission. Scand. J. Haematol. 27:171, 1981.
166. Hersh, E.M. and Irvin, W.S. Blastogenic responses of lymphocytes from patients with untreated and treated lymphomas. Lymphology 2:150, 1969.
167. Han, T. and Sokal, J.E. Lymphocyte response to phytohemagglutinin in Hodgkin's disease. Am. J. Med 48:728, 1970.
168. van Rijswijk, R.E.N. et al. The influence of splenectomy, radiotherapy and chemotherapy on the immune response in Hodgkin's disease. Neth. J. Med. 19:201, 1976.
169. van Rijswijk, R.E.N., Sybesma, J.P.H., and Kater, L. A prospective study of the changes in immune status following radiotherapy for Hodgkin's disease. Cancer 53:62, 1984.
170. Ideström, K. et al. Changes of the peripheral lymphocyte population following radiation therapy to extended and limited fields. Int. J. Radiat. Oncol. Biol. Phys. 5:1761, 1979.
171. Trask, C.W.L., Llewellyn, I., and Souhami, R.L. The effect of radiotherapy on blood mononuclear cell numbers and phagocytic migration. Clin. Radiol. 31:733, 1980.
172. Stratton, J.A., Fast, P.E., and Weintraub, I. Recovery of lymphocyte function after radiation therapy for cancer in relationship to prognosis. J. Clin. Lab. Immunol. 7:147, 1982.
173. Meyer, K.K. Radiation-induced lymphocyte-immune deficiency. Arch. Surg. 101:114, 1970.
174. Baral, E., Blomgren, H., Petrini, B. et al. Blood lym-

phocytes in breast cancer patients following radiotherapy and surgery. Int. J. Radiat. Oncol. Biol. Phys. 2:289, 1977.
175. Heier, H.E., Christensen, I., Froland, S.S. et al. Early and late effects of irradiation for seminoma testis on the number of blood lymphocytes and their B and T subpopulations. Lymphology 8:69, 1974.
176. Onsrud, M. Whole pelvic irradiation in stage I endometrial carcinoma: Changes in numbers and reactivities of some blood lymphocyte subpopulations. Gynecol Oncol. 13:283, 1982.
177. Campbell, A.C. et al. Characteristics of the lymphopenia induced by radiotherapy. Clin. Exp. Immunol. 23:200, 1976.
178. Petrini, B. et al. Blood lymphocyte subpopulations in breast cancer patients following post-operative adjuvant chemotherapy or radiotherapy. Clin. Exp. Immunol. 38:361, 1979.
179. Petrini, B., Wasserman, J., Glas, U. et al. T lymphocyte subpopulations in blood following radiation therapy for breast cancer. Eur. J. Cancer Clin. Oncol. 18:921, 1982.
180. Petrini, B., Wasserman, J., Blomgren, H. et al. Changes of blood T cell subsets following radiation therapy for breast cancer. Cancer Letters 19:27, 1983.
181. Petrini, B., Wasserman, J., Blomgren, H. et al. The helper/suppressor ratios in chemotherapy and radiotherapy. Clin. Exp. Immunol. 53:255, 1983.
182. Millard, R.E. Effect of previous irradiation on the transformation of blood lymphocytes. J. Clin. Pathol. 18:783, 1965.
183. Chee, C.A., Ilbery, P.L.T., and Rickinson, A.B. Depression of lymphocyte replicating ability in radiotherapy patients. Br. J. Radiol. 47:37, 1974.
184. Twomey, R.L., Catalona, W.J., and Chretien, P.B. Cellular immunity in cured cancer patients. Cancer 33:435, 1974.
185. Haim, N. et al. Immune status in patients cured of breast and gynaecological cancer. Clin. Oncol. 7:141, 1981.
186. Strober, S. et al. The treatment of intractable rheumatoid arthritis with lymphoid irradiation. Int. J. Radiat. Oncol. Biol. Phys. 7:1, 1981.
187. Trentham, D.E. et al. Clinical and immunologic effects of fractionated total lymphoid irradiation in refractory rheumatoid arthritis. N. Engl. J. Med. 305:976, 1981.
188. Maca, R.D. and Panje, W.R. Indomethacin sensitive suppressor cell activity in head and neck cancer patients pre- and post-irradiation therapy. Cancer 50:483, 1982.
189. Lapes, M. et al. Cellular and humoral immunity in non-Hodgkin's lymphoma. Correlation of immunodeficiencies with clinicopathologic factors. Am. J. Clin. Pathol. 67:347, 1977.
190. El-Haddad, S.I. et al. Immune deficiency in Hodgkin's and non-Hodgkin lymphoma. Biomedicine 32:128, 1980.
191. Han, T. and Winnicki, M.S. Indomethacin-mediated enhancement of lymphocyte response to mitogens in treated and untreated Hodgkin's disease and non-Hodgkin's lymphoma. NY State J. Med. 1070, 1980.
192. Anderson, T.C. et al. Immunocompetence and malignant lymphoma: Immunologic status before therapy. Cancer 48:2702, 1981.
193. Lindemalm, C. et al. Blood lymphoyte subpopulations and mitogen responsiveness in relation to prognosis in patients with non-Hodgkin lymphoma. Abstract. ASCO Annual Meeting. Toronto, 1984.
194. Smith, J.B., Knowlton, R.P., and Harris, D.T. Functional aspects of T-cells from patients with non-Hodgkin's lymphoma. Responses to self, TNP-modified self, and alloantigens. Cancer 52:1160, 1983.
195. Lindemalm, C. et al. Longitudinal studies of blood lymphocyte functions in non-Hodgkin lymphomas. Eur. J. Cancer Clin. Oncol. 19:747, 1983.
196. Lindemalm, C. et al. Immunodeficiency and prognosis in patients with non-Hodgkin's lymphomas. Acta. Radiol. (Oncol.) 24:159, 1985.
197. Blomgren, H. et al. Studies on the lymphatic system in long-term survivors treated for Wilms' tumour or non-Hodgkin's lymphoma during childhood. Clin. Oncol. 6:3, 1980.
198. Yonkosky, D.M. et al. Improvement of in vitro mitogen proliferative responses in non-Hodgkin's lymphoma patients exposed to fractionated total body irradiation. Cancer 42:1204, 1978.
199. Rotstein, S. et al. The effect of in vitro irradiation on mitogenic responsiveness of peripheral blood lymphocytes from untreated patients with Hodgkin's disease and non-Hodgkin's lymphoma. Cancer 50:900, 1982.
200. Bach, J.F. The Mode of Action of Immunosuppressive Agents. Edited by A. Neuberger and E.L. Tatum. Amsterdam, North-Holland Publishing Company, 1975.
201. DeVita, V.T., Serpick, A., and Carbone, P.P. Combination chemotherapy in the treatment of advanced Hodgkin's disease. Ann. Intern. Med. 73:881, 1970.
202. Turk, J.L. and Parker, D. Effect of cyclophosphamide on immunological control mechanisms. Immunol. Rev. 65:99, 1982.
203. Sharma, B.S. Effects of cyclophosphamide on in vitro human lymphocyte culture and mitogenic stimulation. Transplantation 35:165, 1983.
204. Stevenson, H.C. and Fauci, A.S. Activation of human B lymphocytes. XII. Differential effects of in vitro cyclophosphamide on human lymphocyte subpopulations involved in B-cell activation. Immunology 39:391, 1980.
205. Cupps, T.R., Edgar, L.C., and Fauci, A.S. Suppression of human B lymphocyte function by cyclophosphamide. J. Immunol. 128:2453, 1982.
206. Bast, R.C., Jr. et al. Contrasting effects of cyclophosphamide and prednisolone on the phenotype of human peripheral blood leukocytes. Clin. Immunol. Immunopathol. 28:101, 1983.
207. Cupps, T.R. and Fauci, A.S. Corticosteroid-medi-

ated immunoregulation in man. Immunol. Rev. 65:133, 1982.
208. Ranelletti, F.O. et al. Modulation of glucocorticoid inhibitory action on human lymphocyte mitogenesis: Dependence on mitogen concentration and T-cell maturity. Cell. Immunol. 76:22, 1983.
209. Ten Berge, R.J.M., van Walbeek, H.K. et Shellekens, P.Th.A. Evaluation of the immunosuppressive effects of cyclophosphamide in patients with multiple sclerosis. Clin. Exp. Immunol. 50:495, 1982.
210. Clay, A., Swain, A., and Trounce, J.R. The effect of quadruple chemotherapy on the peripheral blood lymphocyte populations in Hodgkin's disease. Br. J. Clin. Pharmacol. 4:475, 1977.
211. Alexopoulos, C.G. and Wiltshaw, E. Immunological monitoring during chemotherapy for advanced Hodgkin's disease. Cancer 42:2631, 1978.
212. van Rijswijk, R.E.N., Sybesma, J.P.H.B., and Kater, L. A prospective study of the changes in the immune status before, during, and after multiple-agent chemotherapy for Hodgkin's disease. Cancer 51:637, 1983.
213. Nagel, G.A. et al. Immunprofile bei Patienten mit Morbus Hodgkin in Langzeitremission nach zytostatischer Chemotherapie. Schweiz. Med. Wschr. 109:45, 1979.
214. Hancock, B.W. et al. Immunity in Hodgkin's disease: Status after 5 years' remission. Br. J. Cancer 46:593, 1982.
215. Fisher, R.I. et al. Persistent immunologic abnormalities in long-term survivors of advanced Hodgkin's disease. Ann. Intern. Med. 92:595, 1980.
216. Vanhaelen, C.P.J. and Fisher, R.I. Increased sensitivity of T cells to regulation by normal suppressor cells persists in long-term survivors with Hodgkin's disease. Am. J. Med. 72:385, 1982.
217. Alepa, F.P., Zvaifler, N.J., and Sliwinski, A.J. Immunologic effects of cyclophosphamide treatment in rheumatoid arthritis. Arthritis and Rheum. 13:754, 1970.
218. Strender L-E. et al. Immunologic monitoring in breast cancer patients receiving postoperative adjuvant chemotherapy. Cancer 48:1996, 1981.
219. Strender, L.E. et al. Influence of adjuvant chemotherapy on the blood lymphocyte population in operable breast carcinoma. Acta. Radiol. Oncol. 21:217, 1982.
220. Hersh, E.M. and Oppenheim, J.J. Inhibition of in vitro lymphocyte transformation during chemotherapy in man. Cancer Res. 27:98, 1967.
221. Jones, K.D., Whitehead, R.H., Grimshaw, D. et al. Lymphocyte response to PHA and patient response to chemotherapy in breast cancer. Clin. Oncol. 6:159, 1980.
222. King, G.W., Grozea P.C., Eyre, H.J. et al. Neo-antigen response in patients successfully treated for lymphoma. Ann. Intern. Med. 90:892, 1979.
223. Sybesma, J.P. et al. Antibody response in Hodgkin's disease and other lymphomas related to HL-A antigens, immunoglobulin levels and therapy. Vox Sang. 25:254, 1973.
224. Levine, A.M. et al. Use and efficacy of pneumococcal vaccine in patients with Hodgkin's disease. Blood 54:1171, 1979.
225. Addiego, J.E., Jr. et al. Response to pneumococcal polysaccharide vaccine in patients with untreated Hodgkin's disease. Lancet 2:450, 1980.
226. Siber, G.R. et al. Impaired antibody response to pneumococcal vaccine after treatment for Hodgkin's disease. N. Engl. J. Med. 299:442, 1978.
227. Minor, D.R., Schiffman, G., and McIntosh, L.S. Response of patients with Hodgkin's disease to pneumococcal vaccine. Ann. Intern. Med. 90:887, 1979.
228. Heier, H.E., Carpentier, N.A., Lambert, P.H. et al. Quantitation of serum complement components and plasma C3d in patients with malignant lymphoma: Relation to the stage of the tumor and circulating immune complexes. Int. J. Cancer 21:695, 1978.
229. Rottino, A. and Levy, A.L. Behavior of total serum complement in Hodgkin's disease and other malignant lymphomas. Blood 14:246, 1959.
230. Brandeis, W.E. et al. Circulating immune complexes, complement and complement component levels in childhood Hodgkin's disease. Clin. Exp. Immunol. 39:551, 1980.
231. Meuret, G., Schmitt, E., Tseleni, S. et al. Monocyte production in Hodgkin's disease and non-Hodgkin's lymphoma. Blut 37:193, 1978.
232. Hancock, B.W., Bruce, L., Ward, A.M. et al. Changes in immune status in patients undergoing splenectomy for the staging of Hodgkin's disease. Br. Med. J. 1:313, 1976.
233. Steigbigel, R.T., Lambert, L.H., and Remington, J.S. Polymorphonuclear leukocyte, monocyte, and macrophage bactericidal function in patients with Hodgkin's disease. J. Lab. Clin. Med. 88:54, 1976.
234. Gandossini, M. et al. Neutrophil function during chemotherapy for Hodgkin's disease. Br. J. Cancer 44:863, 1981.
235. Corberand, J. et al. Polymorphonuclear functions in Hodgkin's disease patients at diagnosis, in remission and in relapse. Cancer Res. 42:1595, 1982.
236. Estevez, M.E., Sen, L., Bachmann, A.E. et al. Defective function of peripheral blood monocytes in patients with Hodgkin's and non-Hodgkin's lymphomas. Cancer 46:299, 1980.
237. Hartwich, G. and Eibl, D. Nitroblau-Tetrazolium (NBT)-Test bei Lymphogranulomatose. Med. Klin. 72:1586, 1977.
238. Leb, L. and Merritt, J.A. Decreased monocyte function in patients with Hodgkin's disease. Cancer 41:1794, 1978.
239. Al-Hadithy, H. et al. Neutrophil function in advanced Hodgkin's disease: Effect of therapy. Leuk. Res. 6:261, 1982.
240. Holm, G. et al. Monocyte function in Hodgkin's disease. Clin. Exp. Immunol. 47:162, 1982.
241. Pehamberger, H., Ludwig, H., Pötzi, P. et al. Increased monocyte-mediated antibody-dependent cellular cytotoxicity (ADCC) in Hodgkin's disease. Br. J. Cancer 41:778, 1980.
242. DeMulder, P.H.M. et al. Increased antibody-dependent cytotoxicity mediated by purified mono-

cytes in Hodgkin's disease. Clin. Immunol. Immunopathol. 26:406, 1983.
243. Strum, S.B. and Rappaport, H. The persistence of Hodgkin's disease in long-term survivors. Am. J. Med. 51:222, 1971.
244. Björkholm, M., Holm G., Askergren, J. et al. Lymphocyte counts and functions in arterial and venous splenic blood of patients with Hodgkin's disease. Clin. Exp. Immunol. 52:485, 1983.
245. Glatstein, E., Guernsey, J.M., Rosenberg, S.A. et al. The value of laparatomy and splenectomy in the staging of Hodgkin's disease. Cancer 24:709, 1969.
246. Singer, D.B. Postsplenectomy sepsis. In Perspectives on Pediatric Pathology. H.S. Rosenberg and R.P. Bolands. Chicago, Year Book Medical Publishers, 1973, pp. 185.
247. Askergren, J. and Björkholm, M. Post-splenectomy septicemia in Hodgkin's disease and other disorders. Acta Chir. Scand. 146:569, 1980.
248. Askergren, J. et al. The prognostic effect of early diagnostic splenectomy in Hodgkin's disease: A randomized trial. Br. J. Cancer 42:284, 1980.
249. Coleman, C.N. et al. Functional hyposplenia after splenic irradiation for Hodgkin's disease. Ann. Intern. Med. 96:44, 1982.
250. Schulkind, M.L., Ellis,E.F., and Smith, R.T. Effect of antibody upon clearance of I-125-labelled pneumococci by the spleen and liver. Pediatr. Res. 1:178, 1967.
251. Claret, I., Morales, L., and Montaner, A. Immunological studies in the post splenectomy syndrome. J. Pediatr. Surg. 10:59, 1975.
252. Askergren, J. Splenectomy in Hodgkin's disease. A clinical and immunological study. Academic thesis, Karolinska Institute, Stockholm, 1980.
253. Westerhausen, M. et al. Immunological changes following posttraumatic splenectomy. Blut 43:345, 1981.
254. Graffner, H., Gullstrand, P., and Hallberg, T. Immunocompetence after incidental splenectomy. Scand. J. Haematol. 26:369, 1982.
255. Lipson, R.L., Bayrd, E.D., and Watkins, C.H. The postsplenectomy blood picture. Am. J. Clin. Pathol. 32:526, 1959.
256. Lanng Nielsen, J., Tauris, P., Johnsen, H.E. et al. The cellular immune response after splenectomy in humans. Impaired immunoglobin synthesis in vitro. Scand. J. Haematol. 31:85, 1983.
257. Andersen, V., Cohn, J., and Freiesleben Sörensen, S. Immunologic studies in children before and after splenectomy. Acta. Paediatr. Scand. 65:409, 1976.
258. Di Bella, N.J., Bloom, J., and Slawson, R.G. Splenectomy and hematologic tolerance to irradiation in Hodgkin's disease. Radiology 107:195, 1973.
259. Royster, R.L., Wassum, J.A., and King, E.R. An evaluation of the effects of splenectomy in Hodgkin's disease in patients undergoing extended field or total lymph node irradiation. Am. J. Roentgenol. 120:521, 1974.
260. Lowenbraun, S., Ramsey, H.E., and Serpick, A.A. Splenectomy in Hodgkin's disease for splenomegaly, cytopenias, and introlerance to myelosuppressive chemotherapy. Am. J. Med. 50:49, 1971.
261. Cooper, I.A. et al. The role of splenectomy in the management of advanced Hodgkin's disease. Cancer 34:408, 1974.
262. Adler, S. Stutzman, L., Sokal, J.E. et al. Splenectomy or hematologic depression in lymphocytic lymphoma and leukemia. Cancer 35:521, 1975.
263. Ihde, D.C., DeVita, V.T., Canellos, G.P. et al. Effect of splenectomy on tolerance to combination chemotherapy in patients with lymphoma. Blood 47:211, 1976.
264. Sutherland, R.M., McCredie, J.A., and Inch, W.R. Effect of splenectomy and radiotherapy on lymphocytes in Hodgkin's disease. Clin. Oncol. 1:275, 1975.
265. Wagener, D.J.T., Geestman, E., and Wessels, H.M.C. The influence of splenectomy on the in vitro lymphocyte response to phytohemagglutinin and pokeweed mitogen in Hodgkin's disease. Cancer 36:194, 1975.
266. Diehl, V. et al. Der Einfluss der Splenektomie auf den Immunstatus von Hodgkin-Patienten. Klin. Wochenschr. 56:809, 1978.
267. Schaadt, M. et al. Langzeitauswirkungen der Splenektomie auf den Immunstatus von Hodgkin-Patienten in Abhängigkeit von der Therapieform. Med. Klin. 73:1381, 1978.
268. Björkholm, M., Askergren, J., Holm, G. et al. Long-term influence of splenectomy on immune functions in patients with Hodgkin's disease. Scand. J. Haematol. 24:87, 1980.
269. Rogen-Grgas J. et al. Influence of splenectomy upon immunologic reactivity of patients with Hodgkin's disease. Tumori 67:539, 1981.
270. Opat, P. et al. Humoral and cellular immunity in long-term surviving patients with malignant lymphoma. Neoplasma 27:3, 1980.
271. Sokal, J.E. and Aungst C.W.: Response to BCG vaccination and survival in advanced Hodgkin's disease. Cancer 24:128, 1969.
272. Björkholm, M., Holm, G., and Mellstedt, H. No effect of delayed cutaneous hypersensitivity testing (Multitest) on blood lymphocyte counts and functions. Acta Med. Scand. 214:399, 1983.
273. Marcolongo, R. and Di Paolo, N. Fetal thymic transplant in patients with Hodgkin's disease. Blood 41:625, 1973.
274. Costanzi, J.J. et al. The effect of thymosin on patients with disseminated malignancies. Cancer 40:14, 1977.
275. Martelli, M.F. et al. The in vivo effect of a thymic factor (thymostimulin) on immunologic parameters of patients with untreated Hodgkin's disease. Cancer 50:490, 1982.
276. Levo, Y., Rotter, V., and Ramot, B. Restoration of cellular immune response by levamisole in patients with Hodgkin's disease. Biomedicine 23:198, 1975.
277. Ramot, B., Biniaminov, M., Shoham, C.H. et al. Effect of levamisole on E-rosette-forming cells in vivo and in vitro in Hodgkin's disease N. Engl. J. Med. 294:809, 1976.

278. Berényi, E., Kávai, M., Szabolcsi, M. et al. Levamisole in the treatment of Hodgkin's disease. Acta Med. Acad. Sci. Hung. 36:177, 1979.
279. Rubinstein, A. et al. Possible nonspecific immunopotentiation by 2,4-Dinitrochlorobenzene sensitization in patients with Hodgkin's disease. Oncology 36:23, 1979.
280. Björkholm, M., Holm, G., and Mellstedt, H. Levamisole (LMS) in Hodgkin's disease (HD). Cancer Immunol. Immunother. 8:205, 1980.
281. Lang, J.M. et al. Conversion of skin tests in cancer patients after a short course of treatment with a new immunostimulating compound. Cancer Immunol. Immunother. 8:273, 1980.
282. Björkholm, M. et al. Lymphocytotoxic serum factors and lymphocyte functions in untreated Hodgkin's disease. Cancer 50:2044, 1982.
283. Chang, T.C., Stutzman, L., and Sokal, J.E. Correlation of delayed hypersensitivity responses with chemotherapeutic results in advanced Hodgkin's disease. Cancer 36:950, 1975.
284. De Gast, G.C. and Halie, M.R. Relation of cell-mediated immunity to staging, histology and prognosis in untreated patients with Hodgkin's disease. Neth. J. Med. 19:196, 1976.
285. Aisenberg, A.C. Lymphocytopenia in Hodgkin's disease. Blood 25:1037, 1965.
286. Petrov, M. Degrees of impairment of cell-mediated immune reactivity in Hodgkin's disease. Folia Haematol. 2:201, 1976.
287. DeSousa, M. et al. Immunological parameters of prognosis in childhood Hodgkin's disease (HD). Proc. Am. Soc. Clin. Oncol. 18:333 (abstract), 1977.
288. Aisenberg, A.C. Studies on delayed hypersensitivity in Hodgkin's disease. J. Clin. Invest. 41:1964, 1962.
289. Holm, G. et al. Immunosuppressive serum factors and lymphocyte deficiency in Hodgkin's disease. J. Clin. Lab. Immunol. 1:269, 1979.
290. Aisenberg, A.C. Acute nonlymphocytic leukemia after treatment for Hodgkin's disease. Am. J. Med. 75:449, 1983.
291. Björkholm, M. et al. Prognostic factors in Hodgkin's disease. I. Analysis of histopathology, stage distribution and results of therapy. Scand. J. Haematol. 19:487, 1977.
292. Wedelin, C. et al. Prognostic factors in Hodgkin's disease with special reference to age. Cancer. 53:1202, 1984.
293. Waldmann, T.A., Strober, W., and Blaese, R.M. Immunodeficiency disease and malignancy. Various immunologic deficiencies of man and the role of immune processes in the control of malignant disease. Ann. Intern. Med. 77:605, 1972.
294. Penn, I. Depressed immunity and the development of cancer. Clin. Exp. Immunol. 46:459, 1981.
295. Buehler, S.K. et al. Common variable immunodeficiency, Hodgkin's disease, and other malignancies in a Newfoundland family. Lancet 1:195, 1975.
296. Cohen, H.J. et al. Hairy cell leukemia-associated familial lymphoproliferative disorder. Ann. Intern. Med. 90:174, 1979.
297. Berg, J.W. The incidence of multiple primary cancers. I. Development of further cancers in patients with lymphomas, leukemias and myeloma. J. Natl. Cancer Inst. 38:741, 1967.
298. Bordin, G.M. et al. Multiple primary cancers: relative risk in New Mexico's triethnic population. Cancer 40(suppl 4):1793, 1977.
299. Penn, I. Leukemias and lymphomas associated with the use of cytotoxic and immunosuppressive drugs. In Strategies in Clinical Hematology. Edited by R. Gross and K.P. Hellriegel, 1979.
300. Stein, H. et al. Evidence for the origin of Hodgkin and Sternberg-reed cells from a newly detected small cell population. Haematol. Blood Transfus. 28:407, 1983.
301. Sternberg, C. Über eine eigenartige unter dem Bilde der Pseudolekämie verlaufende Tuberkulose des Lymfatischen Apparate. Zschrift Heilk 19:21, 1898.
302. Goffinet, D.R., Glatstein, E.J., and Merigan, T.C. Herpes zoster-varicella infections and lymphoma. Ann. Intern. Med. 76:235, 1972.
303. Notter, D., Grossman, P., Rosenberg, S.A. et al. Infections in patients with Hodgkin's disease: A clinical study of 300 consecutive adult patients. Rev. Infect. Dis. 2:761, 1980.
304. Vietzke, W.M., Gelderman, A.H., Grimley, P.M. et al. Toxoplasmosis complicating malignancy. Cancer 21:816, 1968.
305. Simpson, J.F., Leddy, J.P., and Hare, J.D. Listeriosis complicating lymphoma. Am. J. Med. 43:39, 1967.
306. Ruskin, J. and Remington, J.S. Pneumocystis carinii infection in the immunosuppressed host. Antimicrob Agents Chemother. 7:70, 1967.
307. Feld, R. and Bodey, G.P. Infections in patients with malignant lymphoma treated with combination chemotherapy. Cancer 39:1018, 1977.
308. Coker, D.D. et al. Infection among 210 patients with surgically staged Hodgkin's disease. Am. J. Med. 75:97, 1983.
309. Twomey, J.J. Infections complicating multiple myeloma and chronic lymphocytic leukemia. Arch. Intern. Med. 132:562, 1973.
310. Robinette, C. and Fraumeni, J.F. Splenectomy and subsequent mortality in veterans of the 1939-45 war. Lancet 2:127, 1977.
311. Gopal, V. and Bisno, A.L. Fulminant pneumococcal infections in "normal" asplenic hosts. Arch. Intern. Med. 137:1526, 1977.
312. Donaldson, S.S., Glatstein, E., and Vosti, K.L. Bacterial infections in pediatric Hodgkin's disease: relationship to radiotherapy, chemotherapy, and splenectomy. Cancer 41:1949, 1978.
313. Hosea, S.W., Brown, E.J., Hamburger, M.I. et al. Opsonic requirements for intravascular clearance after splenectomy. N. Engl. J. Med. 304:245, 1981.
314. Dailey, M.O., Coleman, C.N., and Kaplan, H.S. Radiation-induced splenic atrophy in patients with Hodgkin's disease and non-Hodgkin's lymphomas. N. Engl. J. Med. 302:215, 1980.
315. Dailey, M.O., Coleman, C.N., and Fajardo, L.F.

Splenic injury caused by therapeutic irradiation. Am. J. Surg. Pathol. 5:325, 1981.
316. Shimm, D.S., Linggood, R.M., and Weitzman, S.A. Overwhelming post-splenectomy infection in Hodgkin's disease: pathogenesis and prevention. Clin. Radiol. 34:95, 1983.
317. Han, T. Role of suppressor cells in depression of T lymphocyte proliferative response in untreated and treated Hodgkin's disease. Cancer 45:2102, 1980.
318. Schulof, R.S., Lacher, M.J., and Gupta, S.: Abnormal phytohemagglutinin-induced T-cell proliferative responses in Hodgkin's disease. Blood 57:607, 1981.
319. Fisher, R.I. and Bostick-Bruton, F. Depressed T cell proliferative responses in Hodgkin's disease: role of monocyte-mediated suppression via prostaglandins and hydrogen peroxide. J. Immunol. 29:1770, 1982.
320. Twomey, J.J., Laughter, A.H., Farrow, S. et al. Hodgkin's disease. An immunodepleting and immunosuppressive disorder. J. Clin. Invest. 56:467, 1975.
321. Goodwin, J.S. et al. Prostaglandin-producing suppressor cells in Hodgkin's disease. N. Engl. J. Med. 297:963, 1977.
322. Hillinger, S.M. and Herzig, G.P. Impaired cell-mediated immunity in Hodgkin's disease mediated by suppressor lymphocytes and monocytes. J. Clin. Invest. 61:1620, 1978.
323. Sibbitt W.L., Bankhurst, A.D., and Williams, R.C. Studies of cell subpopulations mediating mitogen hyporesponsiveness in patients with Hodgkin's disease. J. Clin. Invest. 61:55, 1978.
324. Schechter, G.P. and Soehnlen, F. Monocyte-mediated inhibition of lymphocyte blastogenesis in Hodgkin's disease. Blood 52:261, 1978.
325. Amlot, P.L., Chivers, A., Heinzelmann, D. et al. Increased prostaglandin synthesis in Hodgkin's disease: A lymphocyte-monocyte interaction. Adv. Prostaglandin Thromboxane Res. 6:529, 1980.
326. DeShazo, R.D. et al. Evidence for the involvement of monocyte-derived toxic oxygen metabolites in the lymphocyte dysfunction of Hodgkin's disease. Clin. Exp. Immunol. 46:313, 1981.
327. DeShazo, R.D. Indomethacin-responsive mononuclear cell dysfunction in Hodgkin's disease. Clin. Immunol. Immunopathol. 17:66, 1980.
328. Fisher, R.I., Vanhaelen, C., and Bostick, F. Increased sensitivity to normal adherent suppressor cells in untreated advanced Hodgkin's disease. Blood 57:830, 1981.
329. Passwell, J., Levanon, M., Davidsohn, J. et al. Monocyte PGE_2 secretion in Hodgkin's disease and its relation to decreased cellular immunity. Clin. Exp. Immunol. 51:61, 1983.
330. DeSousa, M., Smithyman, A., and Tan, C. Suggested models of ecotaxopathy in lymphoreticular malignancy. Am. J. Pathol. 90:497, 1978.
331. Gupta, S. Subpopulations of human T lymphocytes. XVI. Maldistribution of T cells subsets associated with abnormal locomotion of T cells in untreated adult patients with Hodgkin's disease. Clin. Exp. Immunol. 42:186, 1980.
332. Wagstaff, J. et al. Human lymphocyte traffic assessed by indium-111 oxine labelling: clinical observations. Clin. Exp. Immunol. 43:443, 1981.
333. Amlot, P.L. and Unger, A. Binding of phytohaemagglutinin to serum substances and inhibition of lymphocyte transformation in Hodgkin's disease. Clin. Exp. Immunol. 26:520, 1976.
334. Aisenberg, A.C., Weitzman, S., and Wilkes, B. Lymphocyte receptors or concanavalin A in Hodgkin's disease. Blood 51:439, 1978.
335. Moghe, M.V., Advani, S.H., and Gangal, S.G. Circulating inhibitory factors in Hodgkin's disease: Effect on binding of ^{125}I-PHA to lymphocytes. Indian J. Exp. Biol. 20:517, 1982.
336. Bieber, M.M., Kaplan, H.S., and Strober, S. Polar lipid inhibitor of phytohemagglutinin mitogenesis in the sera of untreated patients with Hodgkin's disease. In Malignant Lymphomas. Etiology, Immunology, Pathology, Treatment. Edited by S.A. Rosenberg and H.S. Kaplan. London, Academic Press, 1982.
337. Ramot, B. A dual mechanism of ERFC blocking in Hodgkin's disease: The possible role of ferritin. In Malignant Lymphomas. Etiology, Immunology, Pathology, Treatment. Edited by S.A. Rosenberg and H.S. Kaplan. London, Academic Press, 1982.
338. Han, T. Effect of sera from patients with Hodgkin's disease on normal lymphocyte response to phytohemagglutinin. Cancer 29:1626, 1972.
339. Moroz, C., Lahat, N., Biniaminov, M. et al. Ferritin on the surface of lymphocytes in Hodgkin's disease patients. A possible blocking substance removed by levamisole. Clin. Exp. Immunol. 29:30, 1977.
340. DelGiacco, G.S. et al. Interference of Levamisole with inhibition of E-Rosette formation by Hodgkin's disease and systemic lupus erythematosus cytotoxic sera. Blood 53:1002, 1979.
341. Ezdinli, E.Z., Simonson, K.L., Simonson, L.G. et al. T and B-RFC inhibiting factor in plasma from patients with active Hodgkin's disease. Cancer 44:106, 1979.
342. Holm, G., Björkholm, M., Mellstedt, H. et al. Suppression of monocyte dependent lymphocyte stimulation by sera from patients with Hodgkin's disease. J. Clin. Lab. Immunol. 7:51, 1982.
343. Moghe, M.V., Advani, S.H., and Gangal, S.G.: Demonstration of inhibitory factors affecting cell-mediated immunity in patients with Hodgkin's disease. Eur. J. Cancer 16:937, 1980.
344. Petrini, M. et al. Serum factors inhibiting some leukocytic functions in Hodgkin's disease. Clin. Immunol. Immunopathol. 23:124, 1982.
345. Sinclair, T. et al. Rosette and blastogenesis inhibition by plasma from Hodgkin's disease and other malignancies. Cancer 51:238, 1983.
346. Ford, W.L. Lymphocyte migration and immune responses. Prog. Allergy 19:1, 1975.
347. Longmire, R.L. et al. In vitro splenic IgG synthesis in Hodgkin's disease. N. Engl. J. Med. 289:763, 1973.
348. McGuire, R.A. et al. Hodgkin's cells and attached

lymphocytes. A possible prognostic indicator in splenic tumor. Cancer 44:183, 1979.
349. Kaur, J., Catovsky, D., Spiers, A.S.D. et al. Increase of T lymphocytes in the spleen in Hodgkin's disease. Lancet 2:800, 1974.
350. Hunter, C.P. et al. Increased T lymphocytes and IgMEA-receptor lymphocytes in Hodgkin's disease spleens. Cell. Immunol. 31:193, 1977.
351. Santoro, A., Caillou, B., and Belpomme, D. T- and B lymphocytes and monocytes in the spleen in Hodgkin's disease: the increase in T lymphocytes in involved spleens. Eur. J. Cancer 13:355, 1977.
352. Pinkus, G.S. et al. Lymphocyte subpopulations of lymph nodes and spleens in Hodgkin's disease. Cancer 42:1270, 1978.
353. Baroni, C.D. et al. Tissue T-lymphocytes in untreated Hodgkin's disease. Morphologic and functional correlations in spleens and lymph nodes. Cancer 50:259, 1982.
354. Tan, C.T.C. et al. In vitro responses of peripheral blood and spleen lymphoid cells to mitogens and antigens in childhood Hodgkin's disease. Cancer Res. 38:886, 1978.
355. Han, T. et al. Splenic T and B lymphocytes and their mitogenic response in untreated Hodgkin's disease. Cancer 45:767, 1980.
356. Crowther, D. and Wagstaff, J. Lymphocyte migration in malignant disease. Clin. Exp. Immunol. 51:413, 1983.
357. Gupta, S. and Tan. C. Subpopulations of human lymphocytes. XIV. Abnormality of T-cell locomotion and of distribution of subpopulations of T and B lymphocytes in peripheral blood and spleen from children with untreated Hodgkin's disease. Clin. Immunol. Immunopathol. 15:133, 1980.
358. Björkholm, M., Holm, G., de Faire, U. et al. Immunological defects in healthy twin siblings to patients with Hodgkin's disease. Scand. J. Haematol. 19:396, 1977.
359. Björkholm, M., Holm, G, and Mellstedt, H. Immunological family studies in Hodgkin's disease. Is the immunodeficiency horizontally transmitted? Scand. J. Haematol. 20:297, 1978.
360. Dworsky, R. et al. Immune function in healthy relatives of patients with malignant disease. J. NCI 60:27, 1978.
361. McBride, A. and Fennelly, J.J. Immunological depletion contributing to familial Hodgkin's disease. Eur. J. Cancer 13:549, 1977.
362. Mendius, J.R. et al. Family distribution of lymphocytotoxins in Hodgkin's disease. Ann. Intern. Med. 84:151, 1976.
363. Razis, D., Diamond, H., and Craver, L. Familial Hodgkin's disease: its significance and implications. Ann. Int. Med. 51:933, 1959.
364. Fraumeni, J.F., Jr. Family studies in Hodgkin's disease. Cancer Res. 34:1164, 1974.

365. Haim, N., Cohen, Y., and Robinson, E. Malignant lymphoma in first-degree blood relatives. Cancer 49:2197, 1982.
366. Kerzin-Storrar, L., Faed, M.J.W., MacGillivray, J.B. et al. Incidence of familial Hodgkin's disease. Br. J. Cancer 47:707, 1983.
367. Grufferman, S.G., Cole, P., Smith, P.G. et al. Hodgkin's disease in sibs. N. Engl. J. Med. 296:248, 1977.
368. Berberich, R.F. et al. Hodgkin's disease susceptibility: Linkage to the HLA locus demonstrated by a new concordance method. Hum. Immunol. 6:207, 1983.
369. Hors, J. and Dausset, J. HLA and susceptibility to Hodgkin's disease. Immunol. Rev. 70:167, 1983.
370. Torres, A. et al. Simultaneous Hodgkin's disease in three siblings with identical HLA-genotype. Cancer 46:838, 1980.
371. Conte, R., Lauria, F., and Zucchelli, P. Short communications. HLA in familial Hodgkin's disease. J. Immunogenet. 10:251, 1983.
372. Osoba, D., et al. The prognostic value of HLA phenotypes in Hodgkin's disease. Cancer 46:1825, 1980.
373. Hallgren, H.M., Kersey, J.H., Dubey, D.P. et al. Lymphocyte subsets and integrated immune function in aging humans. Clin. Immunol. Immunopathol. 10:65, 1978.
374. Björkholm, M., de Faire, U., and Holm, G. Immunologic evaluation of patients with ischaemic heart disease. Genetic determination and relation to disease. Atherosclerosis 36:195, 1980.
375. Björkholm, M. et al. A prospective study of HL-A antigen phenotypes and lymphocyte abnormalities in Hodgkin's disease. Tissue Antigens 6:247, 1975.
376. Fenelly, J.J. and McBride, A. Immunological depletion contributing to familial Hodgkin's disease. Brit. J. Cancer 30:182, 1974.
377. Lynch, H.T. et al. Familial Hodgkin's disease and associated cancer. A clinical-pathological study. Cancer 38:2033, 1976.
378. Greene, M.H. et al. Lymphoma and leukemias in the relatives of patients with mycosis fungoides. Cancer 49:737, 1982.
379. Marshall, W.H. et al. HLA in familial Hodgkin's disease. Results and a new hypothesis. Int. J. Cancer 19:450, 1977.
380. Gutensohn, N. and Cole, P. Epidemiology of Hodgkin's disease. Semin. Oncol. 2:92, 1980.
381. Björkholm, M., Wedelin, C., Holm, G. et al. Familial longevity and prognosis in Hodgkin's disease (HD). Cancer 54:1088, 1984.
382. Fisher, R.I. et al. Neoplastic cells obtained from Hodgkin's disease function as accessory cells for mitogen-induced, human T-cell proliferative responses. J. Immunol. 132:2612, 1984.
383. Fisher, R.I. Implications of persistent T-cell abnormalities for the etiology of Hodgkin's disease. Cancer Treat. Rep. 66:681, 1982.

CHAPTER 6

Infectious Complications of Hodgkin's Disease

DONALD ARMSTRONG
GRACE Y. MINAMOTO

Recent improvements in combination chemotherapy and radiotherapy have significantly improved the long-term prognosis in Hodgkin's disease. The course of the disease, however, is often complicated by infections that can be fatal, especially in patients in the later stages of disease and in those who were considered cured. The infectious complications are generally thought to be secondary to alterations in the immune system by the neoplasm itself and the therapy for the disease.

The immunologic alterations occur in four main categories: T-lymphocytes, B-lymphocytes, splenic dysfunction, and polymorphonuclear leukocytes. Functional and quantitative defects in T lymphocytes occur with the onset of Hodgkin's disease and worsen with later staging at the time of diagnosis and disease progression. These defects are aggravated by treatment, especially radiotherapy, and persist despite remission of the neoplasm; T-lymphocyte function deficits have been shown to persist for as long as 10 to 12 years after successful treatment of Hodgkin's disease, but skin reactivity to recall antigens returns to normal.[1] B-lymphocyte function in untreated Hodgkin's disease, however, is normal. Splenectomy alone does not appear to alter B-lymphocyte function, but in combination with chemotherapy or radiotherapy it decreases B-lymphocyte function, as measured by antibody response to several bacterial antigens.[1] Neutrophil function is altered by adrenocortical steroids,[2] vinca alkaloids,[3] and alkylating agents;[3] the latter two also decrease the neutrophil number. These chemotherapeutic agents can also alter gamma globulin function and may lower total gamma-globulin levels. Table 6–1 lists the organisms showing a particular predilection for patients with Hodgkin's disease with T-cell defects and after splenectomy.

Appropriate therapy for an infection is clearly aided by a specific microbial diagnosis through knowledge of the usual antibiotic susceptibility of that organism. Subsequent sensitivity tests on the isolate may reveal its peculiarities. The lack of a definitive microbial diagnosis should suggest an inadequately drained site of infection or occult infection. Infections in Hodgkin's disease are particularly difficult to evaluate because fever caused by the basic disease is common. Exhaustive attempts to rule out an infectious disease and a response of the fever to therapy directed at

Table 6–1. Microorganisms With a Predilection For Individuals With Hodgkin's Disease

Bacteria	Fungi	Parasites	Virus
Listeria monocytogenes	*Cryptococcus neoformans*	*Pneumocystis carinii*	Herpes simplex
Salmonella spp.	*Histoplasma capsulatum*	*Toxoplasmosis gondii*	Cytomegalovirus
Nocardia asteroides	*Coccidioides immitis*	*Strongyloides stercoralis*	Varicella zoster
Mycobacterium tuberculosis	*Candida albicans*†		Vaccinia
Legionella spp.			
Streptococcus pneumoniae*			
Haemophilus influenzae*			
Neisseria meningitidis			

*Associated with postsplenectomy infections
†Local disease

the Hodgkin's disease are the only means to document that the fever is a consequence of the neoplastic disease. Frequently, the patient appears to tolerate the fever better than would a patient with an infection. The fever of Hodgkin's disease, however, may be accompanied by rigors and an appearance of toxicity, while fever from certain infections such as cryptococcosis may be mild and well tolerated; thus, one can not rely on the fever pattern to make a diagnosis. Infection must always be suspected.

REGIONAL INFECTIONS

INFECTION OF THE CENTRAL NERVOUS SYSTEM

The most common cause of meningitis in patients with Hodgkin's disease at Memorial Sloan-Kettering Cancer Center is *Listeria monocytogenes*, followed by *Cryptococcus neoformans*.[4,5] Meningitis caused by either of these organisms may mimic that of the other. In our experience, cranial nerve palsies are more often associated with cryptococcal than with *Listeria* meningitis. Clinical manifestations of *Listeria* meningitis, however, may be protean and hemiplegia may occur. In overt cases caused by either of these organisms, the patient has signs and symptoms of meningitis;

the more subtle cases may be manifested only by low-grade fever and personality changes.[6] Cryptococcal infection may be unaccompanied by fever, particularly if the patient is being treated with adrenocortical steroids. Thus a personality change alone is sufficient indication for a diagnostic lumbar puncture in a patient with Hodgkin's disease. Lumbar puncture reveals the organism as an encapsulated budding yeast form on india ink preparation (*Cryptococcus*), or as a gram-positive rod on gram stain (*Listeria*) of the cerebrospinal fluid. *Cryptococcus* can be visualized as well on a gram stain as on an india ink smear (Fig. 6–1a and b); using the gram stain, we have seen fewer false positive cerebrospinal fluids. Cellular response of the cerebrospinal fluid in both cryptococcal and *Listeria* infections is primarily mononuclear, but may be polymorphonuclear. The cerebrospinal fluid protein is usually elevated and the glucose content may be diminished.

On gram stain, *Listeria* may be mistaken for gram-positive diplococci or gram-negative rods (Fig. 6–2a and b). A thorough search of the slide for the typical gram-positive rods is necessary. On culture as well as smear, the organism can be confused with diphtheroids. A laboratory report of contamination with diphtheroids in cerebrospinal fluid in an immunosuppressed host should be questioned. If the "diphtheroids" are motile and hemo-

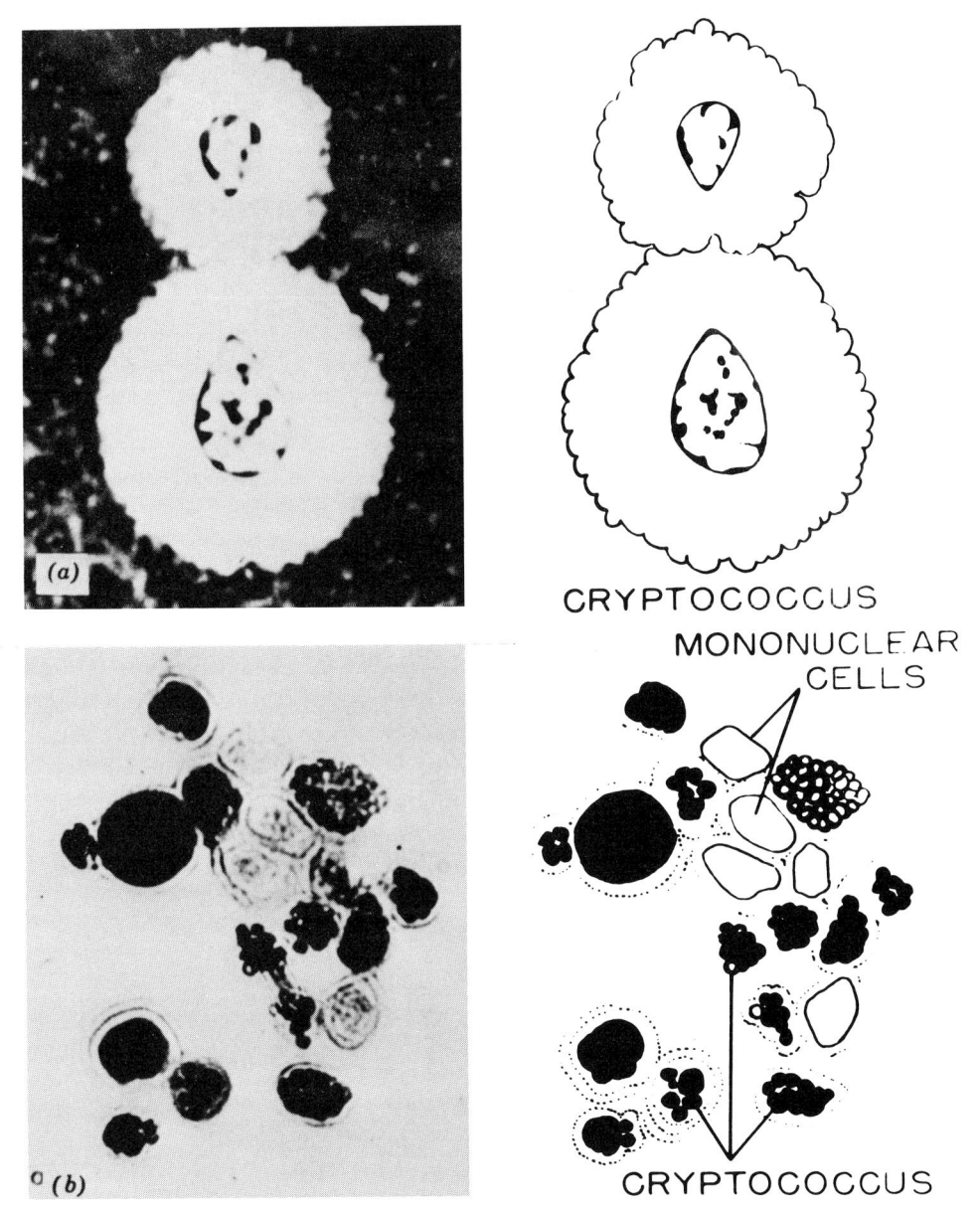

Fig. 6–1. (a) *Cryptococcus neoformans* by the india ink stain. Note two organisms that have just budded. Some of the internal structure can be seen, as well as the large capsule that excludes india ink. (b) *Cryptococcus neoformans* by gram stain. Note the gram-positive internal structures and the large gram-negative capsules. Some of the organisms are budding. Mononuclear cells are interspersed among the cryptococci. (From Armstrong, D., and Chmel, H.: Infectious complications of Hodgkin's disease. *In* Hodgkin's Disease. Edited by M.J. Lacher. New York, John Wiley & Sons, 1976.)

lytic, the organism is *L. monocytogenes*. *Listeria* is frequently isolated from the blood as well as from the cerebrospinal fluid, although infection may be manifested only as a bacteremia without apparent accompanying meningitis.[7] *Listeria* can also cause arthritis, lymphadenitis, and endocarditis. The treatment of choice is intravenous ampicillin 200 mg/kg/day in four to six divided doses or penicillin 300,000 units/kg/day in six divided doses. The infection should be treated for 4 to 6 weeks to avoid relapse. A lower dose of amoxacillin or penicillin (2 to 4 g/day) given orally can be used during the second half of therapy. *Listeria* meningitis has also been treated successfully with trimethoprim-sul-

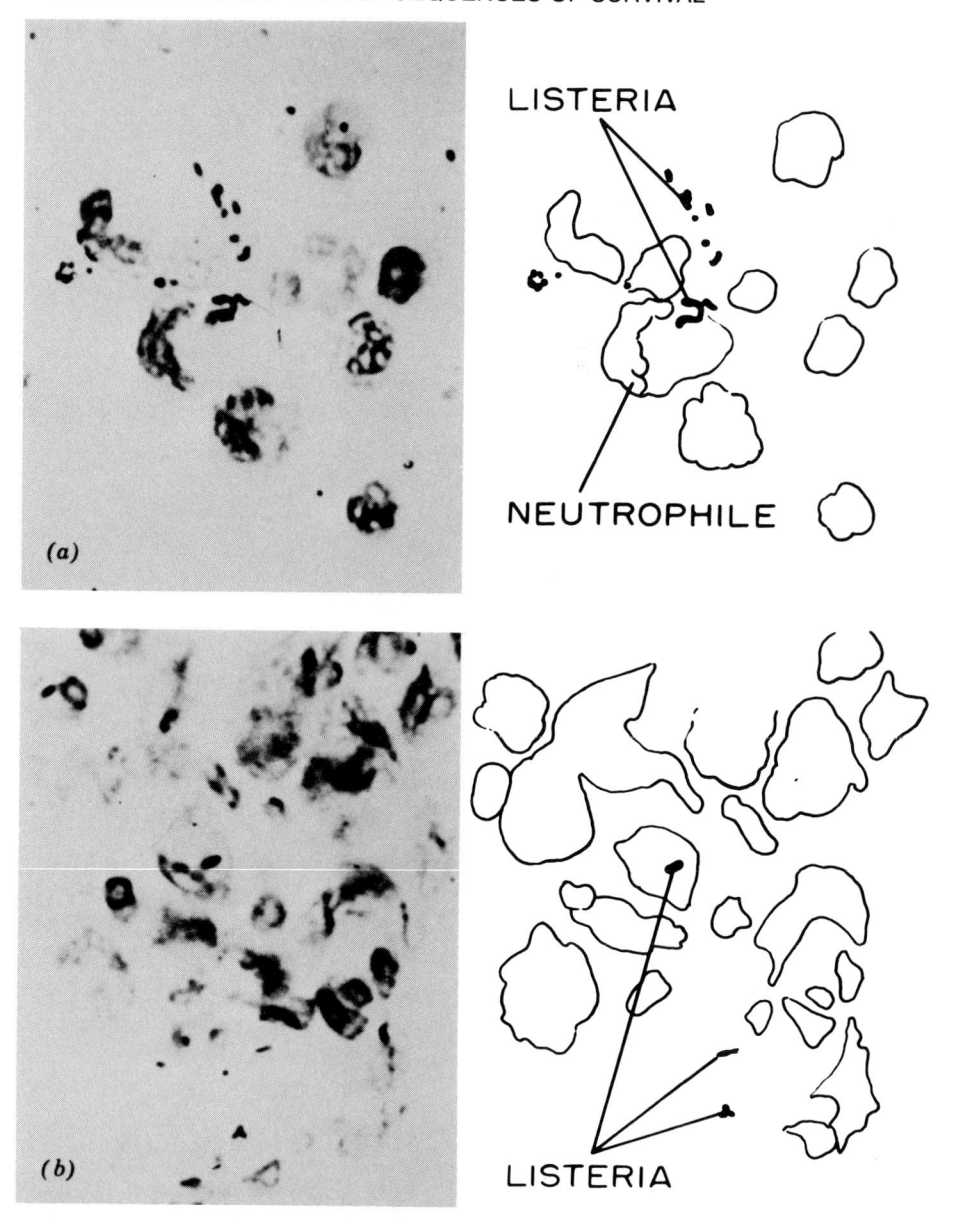

Fig. 6–2. (a) *Listeria monocytogenes*. In this gram stain of cerebrospinal fluid containing *L. monocytogenes*, one organism looks like a gram-negative rod and the other looks like a cluster of three gram-positive cocci, all in the same field. (b) On further searching of the slide, the typical organisms of *L. monocytogenes*, gram-positive diphtheroid rods, are seen. (From Armstrong, D., and Chmel, H.: Infectious complications of Hodgkin's disease. *In* Hodgkin's Disease. Edited by M.J. Lacher. New York, John Wiley & Sons, 1976.)

famethoxazole (Co-Trimoxazole) at a dose of 20 mg/kg of trimethoprim, or with a combination of erythromycin and tetracycline, each at a dose of 2 g/day.[7] The theoretical advantage of this regimen is that protein synthesis of the L forms of the organism is inhibited by these antibiotics.

Cryptococcal meningitis may be difficult to diagnose, because the organism may be difficult to isolate or may grow slowly. We recommend a minimum of 10 ml of cerebrospinal fluid. If the clinical suspicion of *Cryptococcus* is high and the results of the initial lumbar puncture are negative, repeat lumbar punctures with the collection of larger volumes of fluid are mandatory. The diagnosis is aided by the presence of cryptococcal polysaccharide capsular antigens which may be present in the cerebrospinal fluid, blood, or urine in the absence of culturable cryptococcal organisms. Cryptococcosis can also involve the lungs, skin, and bone. Antigens may first be detected in the cerebrospinal fluid at dilutions of 1:128 to 1:512. In every instance in which we have detected antigen in the cerebrospinal fluid, we have been able to isolate the organism. The disappearance of the antigen may be a guide to the success of therapy.

The treatment of choice is a combination of amphotericin B and flucytosine, which is at least as effective as amphotericin B alone and allows for a decrease in amphotericin D dosage.[8] The immediate toxicity of amphotericin B includes reactions of fever, chills, nausea, and vomiting. Rarely, hypotension, cardiac arrhythmias, and bronchial spasm occur during the infusion. Long-term toxicity includes phlebitis at the site of intravenous infusion and renal insufficiency, manifested by rising blood-urea nitrogen and creatinine and falling potassium and magnesium levels. Bone marrow depression, or more rarely hepatotoxicity, may be seen. Flucytosine given alone to patients with normal renal, hematologic, and gastrointestinal function may be associated with nausea, vomiting, and diarrhea, and less often with rash and hepatic and bone marrow dysfunction. In the presence of azotemia or concomitant amphotericin B, leukopenia, thrombocytopenia, and enterocolitis may develop and be fatal.

A test dose of amphotericin B (1 mg) is given in 500 ml of 5% dextrose in water over 4 hours. If there is no reaction, this is followed by a 5-mg dose over 4 to 6 hours. Premedication with diphenhydramine, acetaminophen, or barbiturates may be given to decrease reactions of fever, chills, nausea, and vomiting. Hydrocortisone should be avoided if possible, but rarely, 25 to 50 mg doses may be needed to control severe rigors or high fevers. The dose is then increased by 5 to 10 mg increments every 6 hours until 0.5 to 1.0 mg/kg/dose is reached. The creatinine usually starts to rise at a dose of 1 mg/kg/day. If the patient's clinical response has been favorable after the first one to two weeks, the dose can be doubled and given on alternate days. If not, slowly increasing daily doses should be maintained. For renal insufficiency, the dose of amphotericin B should be decreased by 5- to 10-mg increments, but the drug should be continued. Then renal function usually levels off and starts to normalize. The serum potassium must be closely monitored and supplements given if necessary. Blood levels of antifungal activity against the organism isolated from the patient may be helpful. Fungicidal activity at a 1:2 dilution of serum is usually associated with a favorable therapeutic response. The dose of flucytosine is 25 mg/kg orally every 6 hours. The usual recommended dose of 37.5 mg/kg every 6 hours is seldom tolerated as a result of gastrointestinal toxicity. Blood flucytosine levels should be followed closely and regulated according to renal function. A total of 2.5 to 3.0 g of amphotericin B is usually given, after which cultures should be negative (more prolonged therapy may be necessary to achieve this). At the end of therapy, the antigen titer should be undetectable. In some patients, the titers become stable at levels of 1:8 or 1:16, but do not represent active disease.

Intrathecal amphotericin B in doses of 0.1 to 2 mg/day has been administered in severe cases of cryptococcal meningitis,[9] but controlled studies have not demonstrated an advantage over the intravenous route alone. The intrathecal route can be extremely toxic, resulting in more severe headache and variable radiculopathy (including paresis) in addition to the side effects of intravenous administration. Intrathecal administration is better tolerated if 10 ml of cerebrospinal fluid is drawn into the syringe containing the amphotericin B, allowed to mix, and introduced over 10 minutes.

Intraventricular amphotericin B is the preferable route and has been administered by a catheter attached to a subcutaneous (Omaya) reservoir. This appears to afford higher cerebrospinal fluid levels and better clinical results.[10,11] The reservoir is especially useful in patients who have obstruction and hydrocephalus or who can not tolerate high doses by the intravenous route. The initial dose of 0.05 mg daily is increased by 0.05 mg to 0.10 mg increments until a maintenance dose of 0.5 mg daily is reached. Treatment can be escalated more rapidly with twice daily administration. The drug should be diluted in cerebrospinal fluid and infused slowly. The problem of suprainfection of the reservoir can be diminished with scrupulous care.

Toxoplasma gondii[12,13] and *Nocardia asteroides*[14-16] are two other organisms that must be considered in central nervous system infection in patients with Hodgkin's disease. In infections with the latter organism, a primary pulmonary infection is usually evident. *N. asteroides* may disseminate to the liver, kidneys, heart, bone, and subcutaneous tissues, as well as to the brain. Cerebrospinal fluid findings may suggest a brain abscess, and a significant polymorphonuclear response may be seen without organisms. Brain biopsy may be necessary to make the diagnosis. Any abscess caused by *N. asteroides* should be treated with drainage and a sulfonamide. Sulfadiazine is preferred; initially, 8 g/day should be given, but this can be tapered to 4 g/day after the acute illness is over, or if renal function is not optimal. Adequate hydration is necessary to prevent crystallization of sulfadiazine in the kidneys. The patient should be treated for a minimum of 2 months to avoid recurrence. Co-trimoxazole or cephalosporins such as cefuroxime may be as effective as a sulfonamide alone.

The diagnosis of central nervous system toxoplasmosis is often difficult. In our reviews of toxoplasmosis at Memorial Hospital, Hodgkin's disease was the most frequent underlying neoplasm.[12,13] Toxoplasmosis may also be manifested as myocarditis, pneumonitis, and lymphadenitis, in addition to brain abscess or encephalitis. A serologic diagnosis can be made if there is a fourfold rise in antibody titer; if a single titer is particularly high and the clinical setting sufficiently convincing, empiric therapy should be started. The most commonly available serologic tests are the indirect immunofluorescence test for IgG, which suggests recent infection if the titer is 1:1024 or over, the indirect hemagglutination test, which creates suspicion with a similar titer, and the Sabin-Feldman dye test, which is performed in few laboratories. If IgM antibody titers to toxoplasmosis are increased by the immunofluorescence test ($\geq$ 1:16), this strongly suggests recent infection. The absence of a detectable antibody, however, does not completely rule out toxoplasmosis. In rare instances, in patients with far-advanced Hodgkin's disease, an antibody response is not detectable. Tests to detect circulating antigens[17] could be helpful in such instances. Computed tomographic scan of the brain usually demonstrates one or more ring-enhancing lesions. A positive scan, however, is not diagnostic and if antibody titers are not conclusive, the diagnosis may require brain biopsy with animal inoculation techniques and immunoperoxidase staining for antigen, in addition to routine hematoxylin and eosin and Giemsa stains. It should be stressed that patients with Hodgkin's disease and others with severe mononuclear cell defects may be infected simultaneously or sequentially with two or more organisms, especially facultative or obligate intracellular parasites. Failure to respond or clinical disease that relapses after a specific microbial diagnosis has been made may not represent drug failure, but rather a second infection with another agent. Toxoplasmosis should be treated with a sulfonamide at doses of 4 g/day along with pyrimethamine 25 mg/day after a loading dose of 75 and 50 mg during the first two days of treatment. Patients should be followed for the development of thrombocytopenia. Folinic acid (10 mg/day) should be given to protect against the toxicity of pyrimethamine. Therapy should be continued until 4 to 6 weeks after the resolution of signs and symptoms.

Other central nervous system infections observed in patients with Hodgkin's disease include meningitis caused by *Streptococcus pneumoniae* (Fig. 6-3) or *Haemophilus influenzae* in splenectomized patients, meningitis or brain

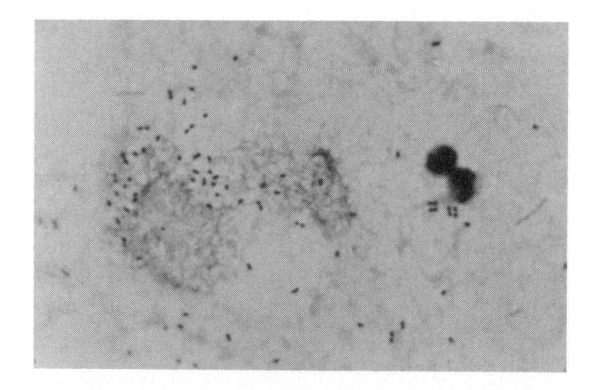

Fig. 6-3. Gram stain of the cerebrospinal fluid of a splenectomized patient with fulminant pneumococcal meningitis and sepsis. The patient had received penicillin prophylaxis prior to the infection.

abscess caused by systemic dissemination of *Strongyloides stercoralis*, subacute measles encephalitis, progressive multifocal leukoencephalopathy, *Salmonella* meningitis, herpes simplex encephalitis, and varicella zoster encephalitis. Meningitis in splenectomized patients may be fulminant and occur despite antibiotic prophylaxis.[18] *Strongyloides stercoralis* may also cause pneumonia or empyema; many patients have a transient pruritic rash, diarrhea, and eosinophilia. The recommended treatment is thiabendazole 25 mg/kg twice daily for 10 to 14 days.[19,20] The optimal duration of therapy is uncertain. Measles encephalitis, which can be preceded by an atypical rash and pneumonia, is characterized by myoclonus, motor and sensory deficits, and lethargy; the diagnosis may be made by brain biopsy, but progressive neurologic deterioration leading to death occurs.[21] Progressive multifocal leukoencephalopathy, caused by papovavirus-JC, has been reported in 18 cases of patients with Hodgkin's disease.[22] Diagnosis is made only by brain biopsy; there is no treatment. *Salmonella* meningitis, usually a disease of children and reported in only 14 adults in the English literature, was observed to be recurrent over 14 weeks in one patient with Hodgkin's disease despite appropriate therapy.[23] Herpes simplex encephalitis occurs only rarely in patients with Hodgkin's disease. Varicella zoster infection of the central nervous system may occur, especially if herpes zoster cranial-nerve involvement is present. The viral infections are discussed in more detail in Chapter 7.

STOMATOPHARYNGITIS

Stomatopharyngitis may be caused by *Streptococcus pyogenes* in people with Hodgkin's disease and in the normal population. Patients with T-lymphocyte defects, especially those on adrenocortical steroids or on broad-spectrum antibiotic therapy, are more inclined to develop local infections with *Candida albicans*. We have seen a number of patients who first developed herpes simplex stomatitis and then became suprainfected by *C. albicans*. Both infections may progress to the upper gastrointestinal tract and in the presence of neutropenia, cause perforation or ulceration with gastrointestinal bleeding. The majority of our patients with severe herpetic involvement of the gastrointestinal tract have had Hodgkin's disease. A potassium hydroxide smear of an oral plaque may show the yeast forms and pseudohyphae of *Candida*. Esophagitis can be diagnosed by barium swallow, but esophagoscopy with biopsy is necessary to determine the etiology.

The treatment of a leukopenic patient with pharyngitis should cover a variety of organisms, including gram-negative enteric organisms and *Pseudomonas aeruginosa*, until the results of cultures are known. A lesion on the roof of the mouth with a black necrotic center may be caused by *P. aeruginosa* or mucormycosis. Scrapings of all lesions should be examined by wet mount for hyphal elements. The rhinocerebral form of mucormycosis, associated with corticosteroid therapy, must be diagnosed and treated promptly if patients are to survive.

PNEUMONIA

Pneumonia in Hodgkin's disease can be caused by the organisms that cause pneumonia in the normal host. As the disease progresses, the patient becomes more immunosuppressed, and if therapy renders the patient leukopenic, gram-negative enteric organisms as well as pneumococci, *Klebsiella pneumoniae*, and staphylococci may cause pneumonia. The first organisms that should be suspected in any patient with Hodgkin's disease and pneumonia are facultative or obligate intracellular parasites. Among the fungi to be expected as causative agents of pneumonia, *Cryptococcus*, *Histoplasma*, and *Coccidioides* must be prominent considerations. *Aspergillus* or *Mucoraceae* may infect patients with advanced disease who have been previously immunosuppressed by chemotherapy.

Infections with higher bacteria like *Nocardia* and tuberculosis can clinically appear similar, causing large areas of infiltration with rapid cavitation. Tuberculosis may appear more like an acute bacterial pneumonia than the usual subacute cavitary disease expected in normal hosts. If the patient has been receiving steroid therapy and has not received prophylactic isoniazid, and if the clinical setting suggests tuberculosis, good sputum specimens should be obtained and the patient treated with isoniazid and rifampin, with the addition of a third antituberculous agent until identification and sensitivities are available. Although the overall prevalence of tuberculosis has decreased significantly over the years, it is still more prevalent in patients with Hodgkin's disease (96 cases of 10,000 versus 3 of 10,000 in normal patients).[24] Multiple sputum specimens may also be necessary to detect *N. asteroides*. The organism grows slowly on culture; it may take 4 to 5 days for colonies to appear. The laboratory should be alerted to the fact that *N. asteroides* is suspected, so that an extensive search for the organism on a gram stain of sputum can be made. A representative gram stain is shown in Figure 6-4. The organisms, particularly in old or poorly stained sputums, may appear to be chains of gram-positive cocci because the gram-positive long branching rod of *N. asteroides* is usually beaded. Rod fragmentation can resemble shorter gram-positive rods or cocci. With the finding of typical organisms on a gram stain, the patient should be treated with a sulfa drug as described earlier and further sputum collected to document the diagnosis by culture. Prompt therapy may be important in preventing the formation of brain abscesses.

Interstitial pneumonias can be caused by the organisms listed in Table 6-2. A specific microbial diagnosis is absolutely essential. Therapy to cover all the infectious and noninfectious causes would be prohibitively toxic. *Pneumocystis carinii*, the most common pathogen causing diffuse infiltrates,[25-28] often occurs during corticosteroid withdrawal. If sputum-specimen examination and cultures are nondiagnostic, bronchoscopy with bronchoalveolar lavage and transbronchial biopsy should be performed. This has a diagnostic yield of approximately 50% in immunosuppressed patients with both localized and diffuse infiltrates.[25,29,30] It has been diagnostic in approximately 95% of cases of pneumonia caused by *P. carinii*. Gallium scans of the lungs are reportedly positive in 93% of patients with *P. carinii* pneumonia and abnormal chest radiograms and in 86% with normal or equivocal chest radiograms.[31] A positive gallium scan, however, is nonspecific in determining the etiology of pneumonia. Open-lung biopsy may be necessary to make a spe-

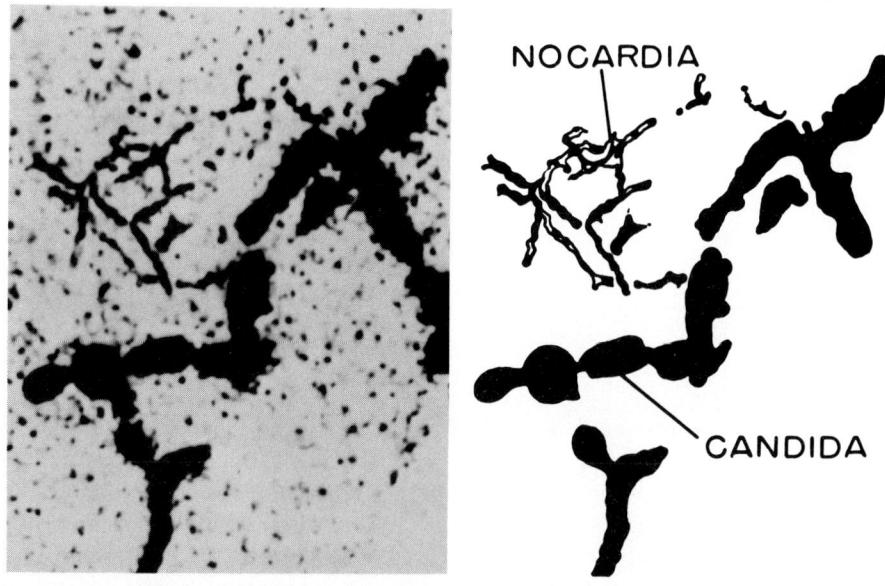

Fig. 6-4. *Nocardia asteroides* and *Candida albicans*. This is the gram stain of a sputum of a patient with Hodgkin's disease IVB, who developed pulmonary cavitary lesions due to *N. asteroides* and, while under therapy for this, became suprainfected with *C. albicans* and subsequently succumbed to the latter infection. The beaded, branching gram-positive rods of *N. asteroides* can be seen in the upper left-hand corner, while the larger yeast forms and pseudohyphae of *C. albicans* can be seen in the lower right-hand corner. (From Armstrong, D., and Chmel, H.: Infectious complications of Hodgkin's disease. *In* Hodgkin's Disease. Edited by M.J. Lacher. New York, John Wiley & Sons, 1976.)

Table 6–2. Causes of Interstitial Pneumonitis in Patients With Hodgkin's Disease

Bacteria	Fungi	Parasites	Viruses
Gram-negative bacilli	*Aspergillus* spp.	*Pneumocystis carinii*	Cytomegalovirus
β-hemolytic streptococci	Mucoraceae	*Toxoplasma gondii*	Herpes simplex
Staphylococcus aureus	*Candida* spp.	*Strongyloides stercoralis*	Measles
Nocardia asteroides	*Cryptococcus neoformans*		Varicella zoster

Neoplastic disease or drugs (e.g., bleomycin), radiation fibrosis, hemorrhage, pulmonary edema, uremia, shock, or oxygen toxicity

cific diagnosis if bronchoscopic studies are not helpful.[32,33] The treatment of choice for *P. carinii* pneumonia is intravenous trimethoprim-sulfamethoxazole (20 mg trimethoprim/kg/day given in 3 to 4 divided doses). If the patient has a sensitivity to sulfa drugs, pentamidine isethionate 4 mg/kg/day is given intravenously or intramuscularly; the former route is preferred to avoid potential bleeding and sterile-abscess formation. Total therapy lasts 2 to 3 weeks. Trimethoprim-sulfamethoxazole may be associated with a rash and leukopenia. Adverse effects of pentamidine include hypoglycemia, renal insufficiency, leukopenia, hypotension, and hypocalcemia; some of these may be lessened considerably by slower infusion.

Therapy for the other infectious causes of interstitial pneumonia is described in Table 6–3.

INTRA-ABDOMINAL INFECTION

Acute abdomens in patients with Hodgkin's disease may be due to the same causes as in the normal population. As with any immunosuppressed host, especially one on corticosteroids, symptoms and signs of an acute abdomen may be minimal. If intra-abdominal infection with bowel flora is diagnosed, drainage (if possible) should be established and treatment initiated with an aminoglycoside and clindamycin to cover aerobic gram-negative flora and penicillin-resistant *Bacteroides fragilis*, respectively. Ampicillin should be used if enterococcal infection is suspected, and a ureidopenicillin or a third-generation cephalosporin if resistant gram-negative enteric infection is suspected. Clostridial sepsis, which usually occurs in the presence of gastrointestinal tumor involvement, can present a striking picture, with alertness despite hypotension, tachycardia out of proportion to fever, and rapid deterioration. Cellulitis may appear in the flanks, axillae, or legs, and become ecchymotic and then crepitant. An aspirate of the area of cellulitis may yield a cherry-red fluid that contains clostridial organisms by gram stain and anaerobic culture. The patient should be treated promptly with 20 million units of penicillin daily and surgical removal of the source of infection, if possible. There is no evidence that clostridial antitoxin is useful in this situation. In our most recent series, only 5 of 11 patients survived clostridial sepsis (Whimbey, E., et al., personal communication). Death usually occurs within the first 24 hours after onset.

Two other organisms that should be considered include *Salmonella*[34] and *Strongyloides*.[19,20] In our review of salmonellosis,[34] 37% of patients had enteritis and 35% were septic. *Salmonella typhimurium* was the most common isolate in both of these presentations. Hyperinfection with *Strongyloides stercoralis* has been reported in patients who have lived in endemic areas. Stool cultures are negative in latent infections, and a duodenal biopsy or string test may be necessary to document the disease. For a patient from an endemic area with a history of strongyloidiasis or unexplained eosinophilia, some clinicians recommend prophylaxis before immunosuppression. The usual clinical manifestation is that of abdominal discomfort, malnourishment, and intractable diarrhea. A high mortality is associated with this infection in the compromised host; therefore, routine stool analysis for ova and parasites should be performed on all patients from en-

Table 6–3. Antimicrobial Agents of Choice for Infections in Hodgkin's Disease*

Infectious Agent	Treatment of Choice — First	Treatment of Choice — Second	Duration
Listeria monocytogenes	Ampicillin 200 mg/kg/day IV in 4–6 divided doses or Penicillin 300,000 units/kg/day IV in 6 divided doses (May administer drug of choice p.o. after 2–3 weeks of IV therapy)	SXT at 20 mg/kg/day IV (of trimethoprim) in 3–4 divided doses plus folinic acid 10 mg/day p.o.	6 weeks
Mycobacterium tuberculosis	INH 300 mg/day p.o. plus RMP 600 mg/day p.o. plus EMB 15 mg/kg/day p.o.	INH 300 mg/day p.o. plus RMP 600 mg/day p.o. × 2 months, then INH 900 mg/day plus RMP 600 mg/day twice weekly	9 months
Nocardia asteroides	Sulfadiazine 90–120 mg/kg/day p.o. in 4–6 divided doses	SXT 10–15 mg (of trimethoprim)/kg/day IV or p.o. in 4 divided doses	2–6 months or longer
Salmonella spp.	Ampicillin 100–200 mg/kg/day IV in 4 divided doses	Chloramphenicol 50 mg/kg/day IV in 4 divided doses or SXT 8–10 mg (of trimethoprim)/kg/day IV in 4 divided doses	2–4 weeks
Cryptococcus neoformans	Amphotericin B: Test dose 1.0 mg IV over 4 hours then increase stepwise q 4 hours to 0.5–1.0 mg/kg/day or twice that dose on alternate days (see text) plus Flucytosine 100 mg/kg/day p.o. in 4 divided doses	Amphotericin B (same dosage as for first choice) **Fluconazole 400 mg/day p.o.	2–3 g total and clinical response
Aspergillus spp.	Amphotericin B (as for C. neoformans)	None	2–3 g total and clinical response
Candida albicans and *tropicalis*	Amphotericin B (as for C. neoformans)	None	2–3 g total and clinical response
Coccidioides immitis	Amphotericin B (as for C. neoformans)	None	2–3 g total and clinical response
Histoplasma capsulatum	Amphotericin B (as for C. neoformans)	None	2–3 g total and clinical response
Pneumocystis carinii	SXT at 20 mg/kg/day (of trimethoprim) IV in 3–4 divided doses plus folinic acid 10 mg/day p.o.	Pentamidine 4 mg of isothionate/kg/day IM or IV	2–3 weeks
Strongyloides stercoralis	Thiabendazole 25 mg/kg p.o. BID × 10–14 days	Mebendazole 100 mg p.o. BID × 3 days	See under drugs of choice
Toxoplasma gondii	Sulfadiazine (as for *Nocardia asteroides*) plus Pyrimethamine 25–75 mg/day p.o. plus folinic acid 10 mg/day p.o.	Trisulfapyrimidines 2–6 g/day p.o. may be substituted for sulfadiazine **Clindamycin 900 mg TID	4–6 weeks after resolution of symptoms

*See chapter 7 for the therapy for viral infections in Hodgkin's disease.
INH: isoniazid; RMP: rifampin; EMB: ethambutol; STM: streptomycin; SXT: trimethoprim-sulfamethoxazole (Co-trimoxazole).
**Experimental

demic areas, and prophylactic therapy with thiabendazole 25 mg twice daily for two days given before the use of immunosuppressive therapy.

may ensue; two weeks of therapy with amphotericin B at 20 to 30 mg daily, decrease in the use of antibiotics, and hydration are curative.

URINARY TRACT INFECTION

The spectrum of urinary tract infections in patients with Hodgkin's disease is similar to that in the general population, except that *Candida* species infections are more common, presumably because these patients are more often hospitalized and receive corticosteroids. If enterococci and *Staphylococcus aureus* are suspected from a gram stain of the urine, oxacillin and high doses of ampicillin should be given (the typical coverage for the more usual gram-negative organisms is inadequate); in the immunosuppressed host, these infections may be life-threatening. *Candida* species can also be visualized well on a gram stain.

The extent of urinary tract infections with *Candida* species is difficult to evaluate, as there may be bladder colonization and candiduria without invasive infection. There is no precise way of establishing invasive renal infection with *Candida*, short of a blood culture or biopsy. We are inclined to treat patients empirically on the basis of clinical suspicion rather than wait for blood cultures to become positive. Results of serologic tests for *Candida* antibody responses, including agglutination and precipitation tests, are often uninterpretable; false negative results can occur because some immunosuppressed hosts can not mount an antibody response, and antibodies may be detectable in the presence of colonization as well as invasive disease. Enzyme immunoassays[35–38] and radioimmunoassays[39,40] are promising for the detection of antigenemia, and gas liquid chromatography has been developed for the quantitation of serum arabinitol[41,42] and mannose[43,44] in candidiasis; however, these assays are not widely available. Candiduria can frequently be attributed to the presence of a urinary catheter and the prolonged use of broad-spectrum antibiotics for bacterial urinary tract infections. Increases in the number of organisms result in clumping of *Candida* in kidney tubules and visible white specks (clumping of organisms) in the urine. Renal insufficiency and oliguria

SKIN INFECTIONS

Skin infections in patients with Hodgkin's disease may be primary or secondary to a systemic infection. Streptococci and staphylococci are among the bacteria causing primary skin infections. Gram-negative organisms (including *Salmonella* species, *Pseudomonas aeruginosa*, *Aeromonas hydrophila*, *Proteus* species, *Klebsiella*, *Enterobacter*, and *Escherichia coli*) in the leukopenic host can cause skin lesions ranging from cellulitis, to a maculopapular rash, to vesicles or bullae, and finally to ecthyma gangrenosum or a red papule, either tender or nontender with a black necrotic center. Various fungi can cause lesions that imitate those caused by bacteria. Maculopapular lesions can be caused by *Candida albicans*, larger indurated papular or ulcerative lesions by *Cryptococcus neoformans*, and skin lesions resembling ecthyma gangrenosum by mucormycosis. Eye involvement with *Candida* species or mucormycosis may be helpful in suggesting the diagnosis; however, similar eye involvement has been seen with *Pseudomonas aeruginosa*. Diffuse macular-papular rashes caused by coccidioidomycosis, histoplasmosis, and toxoplasmosis may be indistinguishable from each other and the rash seen with *Candida* species dissemination. Skin lesions should be aspirated, gram stained, and cultured; potassium-hydroxide wet mount preparation should also be done. If the aspiration fails to reveal the organism, a biopsy should be done for gram stain, culture, and histopathologic examination. Cultural confirmation of the clinical diagnosis becomes mandatory when many different organisms can cause similar skin lesions.

Herpes simplex[45] and herpes zoster are common skin complications in patients with Hodgkin's disease. The lesions are similar. Herpes simplex requires skin precautions during the period of lesion activity. Herpes zoster or chickenpox requires skin and respiratory precautions; either can cause varicella in the susceptible employee who does not have immunity and in the immunosuppressed host who may or may not have had the disease before. The disease is potentially fatal in the latter individual. A review by Guinee et al.[46] showed that most cases of herpes zoster occur during the eight months after starting treatment for Hodgkin's disease. The highest attack rates occurred in patients receiving chemotherapy-radiotherapy-chemotherapy (27.3%), followed by patients on chemotherapy-radiotherapy (19.8%), patients on chemotherapy alone (13.2%), and patients on radiotherapy alone (11.5%). Stage, laparotomy, and histology did not influence the incidence of zoster. This is in contrast to earlier reports that the incidence was greatest in the later stages of the disease.[47-49] Virus cultures of herpes simplex lesions usually become positive within 24 to 48 hours; varicella zoster virus cultures may take 4 days or more. The use of acyclovir topically for local herpes simplex lesions and intravenously for disseminated herpes simplex and varicella zoster disease is recommended.

Rashes caused by viral infections in the immunosuppressed host may be atypical. Measles, although rare since the vaccine became available, may infect the patient with Hodgkin's disease, causing an atypical rash and giant-cell pneumonia. Cytomegalovirus can cause rashes ranging from maculopapular to vesicular. Smallpox vaccine should not be administered to the immunosuppressed host; vaccinia virus may produce local lesions or disseminate, causing a disease similar to smallpox. Persons recently vaccinated should not be exposed to immunosuppressed patients with Hodgkin's diease.

Further details on the virologic complications of Hodgkin's disease are found in chapter 7.

SEPSIS

All the organisms listed in Table 6–1 can cause a clinical picture of sepsis that cannot be differentiated from each other, Hodgkin's disease itself, or the effects of chemotherapy and radiotherapy. The incidence of sepsis and other serious infections is greatest in those patients whose disease is more advanced and who have previously been more aggressively treated (e.g., the risk is higher with total-nodal irradiation plus combination chemotherapy than with total nodal irradiation alone). It is also high in patients who received involved-field radiation, with or without chemotherapy.[50] The decision to treat for possible bacterial sepsis is a matter of clinical judgment. Cultures from all pertinent sources should be obtained in the presence of leukopenia and fever, and empiric broad-spectrum antibiotic therapy begun. Persistent fever, despite such therapy, should signal the possible presence of an invasive infection with *Candida*, *Aspergillus*, *Mucoraceae*, or less commonly occurring fungi or other organisms inadequately covered. The patient should be regularly cultured during fever because it is crucial to make a specific microbial diagnosis. Treatment regimens for organisms showing a predilection for patients with Hodgkin's disease are outlined in Table 6–3.

SPLENECTOMY

The staging splenectomy, when used, has been considered an important risk factor for the development of fulminant infection, especially from organisms such as *Streptococcus pneumoniae* and *Haemophilus influenzae*, even in patients considered to be in remission. In an extensive review of 2795 postsplenectomy patients in 1973,[51] sepsis occurred in 119 patients and 71 patients died as a result of the sepsis; it was concluded that, although an infrequent consequence of splenectomy, such sepsis should be anticipated in all patients, regardless of age or reason for splenectomy. The risk of postsplenectomy infection in Hodgkin's disease at 12 institutions was summarized by Desser and Ultmann in 1972.[52] 1170 splenectomies were performed and 934 of these patients had Hodgkin's disease; 14 episodes of bactermia occurred unrelated to chemotherapy toxicity or to the immediate postoperative period. Six of 14 patients were children; the bacteremia occurred within one year of splenectomy. Gram-positive organisms caused 9 of 14 infections, with pneumococci accounting for seven bacteremic episodes. Gram-negative organisms caused 4 of 14 infections, with *H. influenzae* accounting for two bacteremic episodes. Nine of fourteen bacteremic episodes occurring in Hodgkin's disease were with organisms that usually account for most postsplenectomy infections in patients with other diseases. Other reports have described episodes of fulminant infection in postsplenectomy patients with successfully treated Hodgkin's disease; the distribution of organisms includes pneumococci, other streptococci, *H. influenzae*, meningococci, and gonococci.[53-56] In a 1983 report,[57] *Streptococcus pneumoniae* and *Haemophilus influenzae* were responsible for 46 and 11, respectively, of 145 episodes of postsplenectomy infections in 115 patients. At least 50 of the 115 patients died as a result of the infection. The interval between the splenectomy and the episode of infection ranged from 2 to 119 months, with a median of 21.9 months. The Hodgkin's disease was in complete remission in at least 78 episodes of infection in 48 patients; at least 43 patients were under active treatment for Hodgkin's disease at the time of postsplenectomy infection.

Several reports, however, have suggested that other factors, rather than the splenectomy itself, contribute most to the postsplenectomy infections observed.[50,58,59] In 1983, it was reported[60] that 59 of 210 patients developed serious infection (pneumonia, bacteremia, wound infections, herpes zoster) as long as 5 years after splenectomy. 76% of these infections were associated with other factors, such as disease state, relapse, postoperative state, and the side effects of radiotherapy and chemotherapy (e.g., neutropenia). Among the 47 microbiologically documented infections, a broad spectrum of organisms was observed, with *Streptococcus pneumoniae* in nine episodes and *Haemophilus influenzae* in only two episodes; the overwhelming pneumococcal sepsis syndrome was not observed. Those infections related to splenectomy were generally well tolerated and responsive to therapy.

Based on the available published data, postsplenectomy infection should be anticipated, even in patients in disease remission; however, recent chemotherapy and radiotherapy and the status of the disease are likely to be as important in determining the causative organisms, severity of infection, and empiric treatment. We recommend prophylactic penicillin administration (2 g/day) to Hodgkin's disease patients following splenectomy (see below).

HODGKIN'S DISEASE AND ACQUIRED IMMUNODEFICIENCY SYNDROME (AIDS)

Hodgkin's disease has recently been reported in patients at high risk for acquired immunodeficiency syndrome (AIDS).[61-63] Because Hodgkin's disease is observed in the same age group in which AIDS is usually diagnosed, it is not one of the neoplasms considered in the definition of AIDS. It appears, however, that Hodgkin's disease should be in the differential diagnosis of lymphadenopathy in patients in the risk categories for AIDS. Preliminary findings suggest that the natural history of Hodgkin's disease in such patients may be altered to a more aggressive form and that the prognosis and response to therapy is poorer than in other patients with Hodgkin's disease. The spectrum of infectious complications in these patients broadens to include those seen in patients with AIDS, such as cryptosporidiosis, disseminated cytomegalovirus infection, and disseminated *Mycobacterium avium-intracellulare* infection.

PREVENTION AND TREATMENT OF INFECTION IN HODGKIN'S DISEASE

Improvements in management of the infectious complications of Hodgkin's disease must include measures to treat the immunologic defects caused by the disease and its therapy, because even prompt initiation of antibiotics may fail in treating an infection in an immunologically incompetent host. The neutropenic host is infected by his own flora or environmental flora. There are no convincing controlled studies that suggest that reverse isolation, laminar-flow rooms, and oral nonabsorbable antibiotics to decrease the number of bowel organisms are advantageous.[64,65] Granulocyte transfusions have been used when antibiotics alone are insufficient in the neutropenic patient, but controlled studies have not clearly demonstrated their efficacy.[66-71] The administration of an opsonizing antibody may be necessary for the phagocytosis and killing of the organisms that have a predilection for patients with Hodgkin's disease.[71] It may be necessary to develop globulins that are hyperimmune to these organisms and administer them either prophylactically or therapeutically. (Zoster immunoglobulin is presently recommended within 72 hours of exposure only if there is no history of chickenpox.)

Childhood vaccinations with antigens such as diphtheria, pertussis, and tetanus and the killed polio vaccine are safe and recommended; however, live-virus immunizations such as for mumps, measles, and rubella are to be avoided. Influenzae vaccines are also safe; however, adequate antibody response may require several doses.

Much attention has been focused on the pneumococcal vaccine for the postsplenectomy patient. Although the major effects of Hodgkin's disease are on cellular immunity, the antibody response to vaccination in these patients is not uniform. Antibody responses and prevention of systemic pneumococcal infection appear to be more consistent for hyposplenic patients with sickle cell disease.[72] It has been reported[73] that the vaccine is more likely to provide immunologic response if given prior to splenectomy rather than after splenectomy, radiotherapy, and chemotherapy. The duration of response, however, was variable. Others[74] have reported the development of pneumococcal meningitis in one patient and pneumococcal bacteremia in another, despite vaccination; they also found that postimmunization antibody levels in patients with Hodgkin's disease were significantly lower than those of normal control subjects for 10 of 12 serotypes measured. Antibody response levels tended to continually increase from the time of therapy for Hodgkin's disease. The efficacy of the vaccine is therefore questionable, but administration prior to treatment with radiotherapy and chemotherapy is recommended. Because some patients have had an apparent lowering of their preimmunization antibody levels after immunization, it has been suggested that vaccination not be given less than 10 days prior to chemotherapy or during chemotherapy and radiotherapy.

Penicillin prophylaxis has many advocates,[18,57,75-78] although no controlled studies support this recommendation. Serious and sometimes fatal pneumococcal infections have been reported in patients receiving penicillin prophylaxis and in those in whom the prophylaxis was discontinued.[18,78] It was previously reported[18] that all splenectomized children with Hodgkin's disease at this hospital given prophylactic penicillin have not developed pneumococcal bacteremia. Therefore, administration of prophylactic penicillin in addition to the pneumococcal vaccine is recommended in all splenectomized patients with Hodgkin's disease. The duration of prophylaxis is not established.

Other recommended antimicrobial prophylactic measures in patients with Hodgkin's disease include: oral trimethoprim-sulfamethoxazole for patients on a tapering corticosteroid regimen to prevent *Pneumocystis carinii* pneumonitis;[79] thiabendazole for patients from areas endemic for *Strongyloides* before immunosuppressive therapy; and acyclovir to prevent dissemination of localized herpes zoster infection.

The incidence of infections complicating Hodgkin's disease is high. The diagnosis of infection is often difficult. Because fever associated with the basic neoplastic disease is common, therapy with immunosuppressive agents such as corticosteroids may mask signs and symptoms, and many microorganisms cause infections that are manifested atypically. The basic immunologic defect in Hodgkin's disease is a quantitative and functional defect of T lymphocytes. This makes the host susceptible to a certain group of organisms, for example, obligate or facultative intracellular parasites. Familiarity with the syndromes caused by these microorganisms and their treatment is essential to the management of patients with Hodgkin's disease. Likewise, a knowledge of the syndromes that occur, both infectious and simulating infection, as a result of procedures (e.g., staging with splenectomy) and treatment (e.g., bleomycin-induced interstitial pneumonia) is mandatory. As the neoplastic disease progresses and its treatment intensifies, the patients become more susceptible to a wide variety of organisms, including those which depend on an appropriate neutrophil and antibody response. Every effort should be made to ascertain a specific microbial diagnosis so that prompt specific therapy can be administered. Extraordinary preventive and therapeutic measures must be studied to control infection in these highly susceptible patients.

REFERENCES

1. DeVita Jr., V.T., Jaffe, E.S., and Hellman, S.H. Immunologic abnormalities in patients with lymphoma: Hodgkin's dsease. *In* Cancer: Principles and Practice of Oncology. 2nd Ed. Edited by V.T. DeVita, Jr., S. Hellman, and S.A. Rosenberg. Philadelphia, JB Lippincott Company, 1985, 1656–1657.
2. VonMoeschlin S. et al. Studies on the effects of cortisone and ACTH in phagocytosis of leukocytes and macrophages. Acta Haematol. 9:277, 1953.
3. Hersh, E.M. et al. Host defense mechanisms and their modification by cancer chemotherapy. *In* Methods in Cancer Research. Vol 4. Edited by H. Busch. New York, Academic Press, 1985, 335–451.
4. Chernick, N.L., Armstrong, D., and Posner, J.B. Central nervous system infections in patients with cancer: changing patterns. Cancer 40:268, 1977.
5. Kaplan, M., Rosen, P.P., and Armstrong, D. Cryptococcosis in a cancer hospital: clinical and pathological correlates in forty-six patients. Cancer 39:2265, 1977.
6. Salaki, J.S., Louria, D.B., and Chmel, H. Fungal and yeast infections of the central nervous system: a clinical review. Medicine 63:108, 1984.
7. Louria, D.B. et al. Listeriosis complicating malignant disease: a new association. Ann. Intern. Med. 67:261, 1967.
8. Bennett, J.E. et al. A comparison of amphotericin B alone and combined with flucytosine in the treatment of cryptococcal meningitis. N. Engl. J. Med. 301:126, 1979.
9. Diamond, R.D. and Bennett, J.E. Prognostic factors in cryptococcal meningitis: a study of 111 cases. Ann. Intern. Med. 80:176, 1974.
10. Diamond, R.D. and Bennett, J.E. A subcutaneous reservoir for intrathecal therapy of fungal meningitis. N. Engl. J. Med. 288:186, 1973.
11. Polsky, B. et al. Intraventricular therapy of cryptococcal meningitis via a subcutaneous reservoir. Am. J. Med. 81:24, 1986.
12. Carey, R.M., Kimball, A.C., Armstrong, D. et al. Toxoplasmosis: clinical experiences in a cancer hospital. Am. J. Med. 54:30, 1973.
13. Hakes, T.B. and Armstrong, D. Toxoplasmosis: problems in diagnosis and treatment. Cancer 52:1535, 1983.
14. Young, L.S. et al. Nocardia asteroides infection complicating neoplastic disease. Am. J. Med. 50:269, 1971.
15. Palmer, D.L., Harvey, R.L., and Wheeler, J.K. Diagnostic and therapeutic considerations in Nocardia asteroides infection. Medicine 53:391, 1974.
16. Simpson, G.J. et al. Nocardial infections in the immunocompromised host: a detailed study in a defined population. Rev. Infect. Dis. 3:492, 1981.
17. Araujo, F.G. and Remington, J.S. Antigenemia in recently acquired acute toxoplasmosis. J. Infect. Dis. 141:144, 1981.
18. Chou, M.-Y., Brown, A.E., Blevins, A. et al. Severe pneumococcal infection in patients with neoplastic disease. Cancer 51:1546, 1983.
19. Scowden, E.B., Schaffner, W., and Stone, W.J. Overwhelming strongyloidiasis: an unappreciated opportunistic infection. Medicine 57:527, 1978.
20. Purtilo, D.T., Meyers, W.M., and Connor, D.H. Fatal strongyloidiasis in immunosuppressed patients. Am. J. Med. 56:488, 1974.
21. Wolinsky, J.S., Swoveland, P., Johnson, K.P. et al Subacute measles encephalitis complicating Hodgkin's disease in an adult. Ann. Neurol. 1:452, 1977.
22. Bjerrum, O.W. and Hansen, O.E. Progressive multifocal leucoencephalopathy in Hodgkin's disease. Scand. J. Haematol. 34:442, 1985.
23. Bolivar, R., Bodey, G.P., and Velasquez, W.S. Recurrent salmonella meningitis in a compromised host. Cancer 50:2034, 1982.
24. Kaplan, M.H. et al. Tuberculosis complicating neoplastic disease: a review of 201 cases. Cancer 33:850, 1974.
25. Pennington, J.E. and Feldman, N.T. Pulmonary infiltrates and fever in patients with hematologic malignancy. Am. J. Med. 62:581, 1977.
26. Leight, G.S. and Michaelis, L.L. Open lung biopsy for the diagnosis of acute, diffuse pulmonary infiltrates in the immunosuppressed patient. Chest 73:477, 1978.
27. Stover, D.E. et al. Bronchoalveolar lavage in the diagnosis of diffuse pulmonary infiltrates in the immunosuppressed host. Ann. Intern. Med. 101:1, 1984.
28. Singer, C. et al. Diffuse pulmonary infiltrates in immunosuppressed patients. Am. J. Med. 66:110, 1979.
29. Lauver, G.L., Hasan, F.M., Morgan, R.B., and Campbell, S.C.: The usefulness of fiberoptic bronchoscopy in evaluating new pulmonary lesions in the compromised host. Am. J. Med. 66:580, 1979.
30. Canham, M., Kennedy, T.C., and Merrick, T.A. Unexplained pulmonary infiltrates in the compromised patient. Cancer 53:325, 1983.
31. Barron, T.F. et al. Pneumocystis carinii pneumonia studies by gallium 67 scanning. Radiology 154:791, 1985.
32. Jaffe, J.P. and Maki, D.G. Lung biopsy in immunocompromised patients. Cancer 48:1144, 1981.
33. McCabe, R.E., Brooks, R.G., Mark, J.B.D. et al. Open lung biopsy in patients with acute leukemia. Am. J. Med. 78:609, 1985.
34. Wolfe, M.S., Armstrong, D., Louria, D. et al. Sal-

monellosis in patients with neoplastic disease. Arch. Intern. Med., *128*:456, 1971.
35. Segal, E., Berg, R.A., Pizzo, P.A. et al. Detection of Candida antigen in sera of patients with candidiasis by an enzyme-linked immunosorbent assay-inhibition technique. J. Clin. Microbiol *10*:116, 1979.
36. Harding, S.A., Brody, J.P., and Normansell, D.E. Antigenemia detected by enzyme-linked immunosorbent assay in rabbits with systemic candidiasis. J. Lab. Clin. Med. *95*:959, 1980.
37. Meckstroth, K.L., Reiss, E., Keller, J.W. et al. Detection of antibodies and antigenemia in leukemic patients with candidiasis by enzyme-linked immunosorbent assay. J. Infect. Dis. *144*, 24, 1981.
38. Lew, M.A., Siber, G.R., Donahue, D.M. et al. Enhanced detection with an enzyme-linked immunosorbent assay of Candida mannan in antibody-containing serum after heat extraction. J. Infect. Dis. *145*:45, 1982.
39. Weiner, M.H. and Coats-Stephen, M. Immunodiagnosis of systemic candidiasis: mannan antigenemia detected by radioimmunoassay in experimental and human infections. J. Infect. Dis. *140*:989, 1979.
40. Poor, A.H. and Cutler, J.E. Partially purified antibodies used in a solid-phase radioimmunoassay for detecting candidal antigenemia. J. Clin. Microbiol. *9*:362, 1979.
41. Kiehn, T.E., Bernard, E.M., Gold, J.W.M. et al. Candidiasis: detection by gas-liquid chromatography of D-arabinitol, a fungal metabolite, in human serum. Science *206*:57, 1979.
42. Gold, J.W.M. et al. Serum arabinitol concentrations and arabinitol/creatinine ratios in invasive candidiasis. J. Infect. Dis. *147*:504, 1983.
43. Marier, R.L., Milligan, E., and Fan, Y.-D. Elevated mannose levels detected by gas-liquid chromatography in hydrolysates of serum from rats and humans with candidiasis. J. Clin. Microbiol. *16*:123, 1982.
44. de Repentigny, L., Kuykendall R.J., and Reiss, E. Simultaneous determination of arabinitol and mannose by gas-liquid chromatography in experimental candidiasis. J. Clin. Microbiol. *17*:1166, 1983.
45. Whitley, R.J. et al. Infections caused by herpes simplex virus in the immunocompromised host: natural history and topical acyclovir therapy. J. Inf. Dis. *150*:323, 1984.
46. Guinee, V.F. et al. The incidence of herpes zoster in patients with Hodgkin's disease: an analysis of prognostic factors. Cancer *56*:642, 1985.
47. Schimpff, S. et al. Varicella-zoster infection in patients with cancer. Ann. Intern. Med. *76*:241, 1972.
48. Wilson, J.F., Marsa, G.W., and Johnson, R.E. Herpes zoster in Hodgkin's disease: clinical, histologic, and immunologic correlations. Cancer *29*:461, 1972.
49. Reboul, F., Donaldson, S.S., and Kaplan, H.S. Herpes zoster and varicella infections in children with Hodgkin's disease: an analysis of contributing factors. Cancer *41*:95, 1978.
50. Green, D.M. et al. The incidence of post-splenectomy sepsis and herpes zoster in children and adolescents with Hodgkin's disease. Med. Pediatr. Oncol. *7*:285, 1979.
51. Singer, D.B. Post-splenectomy sepsis. *In* Perspectives in pediatric pathology. Edited by H.S. Rosenberg and R.P. Bolander. Chicago, Year Book Medical Publishers, Vol 1. 1973, 285.
52. Desser, R.K. and Ultmann, J.E. Risk of severe infection in patients with Hodgkin's disease or lymphoma after diagnostic laparotomy and splenectomy. Ann. Intern. Med. *77*:143, 1972.
53. Weitzman, S. and Aisenberg, A.C. Fulminant sepsis after the successful treatment of Hodgkin's disease. Am. J. Med. *62*:47, 1977.
54. Chilcote, R.R. et al. Septicemia and meningitis in children splenectomized for Hodgkin's disease. N. Engl. J. Med. *295*:798, 1976.
55. Curti, A.J., Lin, J.H., and Szabo, K. Overwhelming post-splenectomy infection with Plesiomonas shigelloides in a patient cured of Hodgkin's disease: a case report. Am. J. Clin. Pathol. *83*:522, 1985.
56. Austin, T.W., Sargeant, H.L., and Warwick, O.H. Fulminant gonococcemia after splenectomy. Can. Med. Assoc. J. *123*:195, 1980.
57. Rosner, F. and Zarrabi, M.H. Late infections following splenectomy in Hodgkin's disease. Cancer Invest. *1*:57, 1983.
58. Schimpff, S.C., O'Connell, M.J., Greene, W.H. et al. Infections in 92 splenectomized patients with Hodgkin's disease. Am. J. Med. *59*:695, 1975.
59. Notter, D.T., Grossman, P.L., Rosenberg, S.A. et al. Infections in patients with Hodgkin's disease: a clinical study of 300 consecutive adult patients. Rev. Inf. Dis. *2*:761, 1980.
60. Coker, D.D. et al. Infection among 210 patients with surgically staged Hodgkin's disease. Am. J. Med. *75*:97, 1983.
61. Robert, N.J. and Schneiderman, H. Hodgkin's disease and the acquired immunodeficiency syndrome (Letter to the editor). Ann. Intern. Med. *101*:142, 1984.
62. Schoeppel, S.L. et al. Hodgkin's disease in homosexual men with generalized lymphadenopathy. Ann. Intern. Med. *102*:68, 1985.
63. Ioachim, H.L., Cooper, M.C., and Hellman, G.C. Lymphomas in men at high risk for acquired immune deficiency syndrome (AIDS): a study of 21 cases. Cancer *56*:2831, 1985.
64. Bodey, G.P. Antibiotic prophylaxis in cancer patients: regimens of oral, nonabsorbable antibiotics for prevention of infection during induction of remission. Rev. Infect. Dis. *3*(suppl.):S259, 1981.
65. Pizzo P.A. and Levine, A.S. The utility of protected-environment regimens for the compromised host: a critical assessment. *In* Progress in hematology. Edited by E. Brown. New York, Grune & Stratton, 1977, 311.
66. Clift, R.A. and Buckner, C.D. Granulocyte transfusions. Am. J. Med *76*:631, 1984.
67. Wright, D.G. Leukocyte transfusions: thinking twice. Am. J. Med. *76*:637, 1984.
68. Dutcher, J.P. Granulocyte transfusion therapy. Am. J. Med Sci. *287*:11, 1984.

69. DiNubile, M.J. Therapeutic role of granulocyte transfusions. Rev. Inf. Dis. 7:232, 1985.
70. Winston, D.J., Ho, W.G., and Gale, R.P. Therapeutic granulocyte transfusions for documented infections: a controlled trial in ninety-five infectious granulocytopenic episodes. Ann Intern. Med 97:509, 1982.
71. Keusch, G.T. et al. Role of opsonins in clinical response to granulocyte transfusion in granulocytopenic patients. Am. J. Med. 73:552, 1982.
72. Ammann, A.J. et al. Polyvalent pneumococcal-polysaccharide immunization of patients with sickle-cell anemia and patients with splenectomy. N. Engl. J. Med. 297:897, 1977.
73. Donaldson, S.S. et al. Response to pneumococcal vaccine among children with Hodgkin's disease. Rev. Inf. Dis. 3(Suppl.):S133, 1981.
74. Minor, D.R., Schiffman, G., and McIntosh, L.S. Response of patients with Hodgkin's disease to pneumococcal vaccine. Ann. Intern. Med., 90:887, 1979.
75. Krivit, W. Overwhelming post-splenectomy infection. Am. J. Hematol. 2:193, 1977.
76. Heier, H.E. Splenectomy and serious infection. Scand. J. Haematol. 24:5, 1980.
77. Dickerman, J.D. Splenectomy and sepsis: a warning. Pediatrics 63:938, 1979.
78. Lanzkowsky, P., Shende, A., Karayalcin, G. et al. Staging laparotomy and splenectomy: treatment and complications of Hodgkin's disease in children. Am. J. Hematol. 1:393, 1976.
79. Hughes, W.T. et al. Successful chemoprophylaxis for *Pneumocystis carinii* pneumonitis. N. Engl. J. Med. 297:1419, 1977.

CHAPTER 7

Late Infectious Complications: Viral Infections

BRIAN LEYLAND-JONES
KATHY CLAGETT CARR
PETER O'DWYER

Patients with Hodgkin's lymphoma suffer defects in both humoral and cell-mediated immune systems that make them more prone to a variety of infections. The improved treatment of Hodgkin's disease has led to an increased number of patients surviving with increasingly long survival patterns, and hence an increased likelihood of expression of complications.[25] Infections with Varicella-zoster virus are common in these patients; their incidence in a number of studies is listed in Table 7–1. A review of the effects of treatment intensity and splenectomy on incidence of herpes zoster is presented in Table 7–2.

INCIDENCE AND PREDISPOSING EFFECTS ON INCIDENCE OF HERPES ZOSTER

There have been several excellent studies over many years of the increased incidence of herpes zoster in both Hodgkin's disease and other types of malignancies. In 1924, Pancoast and Pendergrass called attention to the relatively high incidence of herpes zoster in Hodgkin's disease.[3] Schimpff et al., studying 419 patients with cancer over a 2-year period, reported incidences of herpes zoster in 25% of patients with Hodgkin's disease, 8.7% of other lymphoma patients, but in only 1.2% of patients with acute leukemia and 1.8% of patients with solid tumors. The disseminated form of zoster occurred in 31% of cases; localization of zoster was frequently related to a site of prior radiation therapy. Patients with advanced Hodgkin's disease, cutaneous anergy, and recent nodule radiotherapy were inordinately predisposed to zoster. Only 8 of 37 patients had a recurrence.

Goffinet studied 1130 patients with lymphoma seen during a 10-year period.[120] There were 129 cases of varicella-zoster infections (an incidence of 11.4%), including 21 disseminated cases. For Hodgkin's disease itself, the incidence was 15.4%; within the subpopulation that underwent splenectomy, the incidence of herpes-zoster infections was significantly increased, although the survival of this group was apparently unchanged by this infectious complication. Schimpff[40] reviewed the infections that occurred in 92 previously untreated patients with Hodgkin's disease. Herpes zoster developed in 24% of these patients; predisposing factors included gender (female more than male), therapy (radiation plus chemotherapy more than chemotherapy alone), and age (less than 30 years of age more often than 30 to 50 years of age). In this study, splenectomy did not affect either the incidence or severity of infection during a 12+ month period of observation. Mazur and Dolin noted that herpes zoster was largely a source of increased morbidity rather than mortality in a study of 107 hospitalized patients with a variety of illnesses.[118] Predisposing factors for zoster in this study included local irradiation and, occasionally, surgery in subsequently involved areas; more frequently corticosteroid therapy was also associated with disseminated zoster. De Pauw[116] reported an overall incidence of 9.5% herpes zoster in 210 cases of patients with Hodgkin's disease. Patients with the mixed-cellular histologic subtype showed a significantly increased risk ($p < 0.05$) as compared with the total population. Over 90% of the herpes-zoster-varicella infections occurred after termination of treatment. In this study, it was also noted that the combination of chemotherapy with radiotherapy was a predisposing factor.

In another large series, Sokal and Firat conducted a retrospective study of approximately 600 patients with Hodgkin's disease over a 43 year period. 8% were recorded as having had one or more episodes of varicella zoster; the duration of Hodgkin's disease prior to the appearance of zoster lesions ranged from 6 months to 11 years, with a median of 3 years for localized zoster and 4 years for disseminated zoster.[112] In this study, corticosteroid therapy did not appear to be an important predisposing factor. Although localized zoster did not appear to affect survival, patients with disseminated lesions had a median survival of less than one year. In another large study by Guinee,[119] intensity of treatment was a key factor in the incidence of zoster. Thirty-six months after the initiation of treatment in a 717 patient study, patients receiving chemotherapy-radiation-chemotherapy had twice the attack rate (27.3%) of those receiving radiation alone (11.5%). The attack rate in the pediatric age group was significantly greater (26.6%) than in adults (18.7%). The incidence of zoster was not influenced by stage, histology, and laparotomy. Gopal also associated herpes zoster in Hodgkin's disease with more extensive involvement than in the normal population.[121] In 5% of the patients in this study, generalized herpes zoster was seen; this was attributed to the extent of defect of cellular immunity. Monfardini et al.[129] noticed a greater predilection for varicella-zoster infections in the lymphocytic-depleted subtype (26%) and a greater incidence in splenectomized (16%) compared to nonsplenectomized (9%) patients. The incidence of zoster was found to be particularly high in splenectomized patients, both with Hodgkin's (27%) and with nonHodgkin's (15%) lymphomas treated with cyclic-combination chemotherapy. Poussin-Rosillo[125] noted a higher incidence of zoster in a subpopulation of Hodgkin's disease treated with total-nodal irradiation following splenectomy.

One of the larger studies in the pediatric population was conducted by Reboul.[115] The overall frequency of varicella-zoster infections was 34.8%; the occurrence in stage 1 was significantly lower than in other stages. The risk of infection was not significantly increased by previous splenectomy. 56% of patients receiving extensive radiotherapy plus combination chemotherapy developed varicella-zoster infections as compared with 23.8% of patients receiving extensive-field radiotherapy alone. 80% of infections occurred during the first year after completion of treatment. The frequency of disseminated infection was unusually high (27%), but this study did not identify the occurrence of varicella-zoster infection as a poor prognostic sign of either relapse or fatality. Feldman[113] conducted a retrospective study of 1132 children with malignancy and noted that the incidence of zoster infection was highest (22%) in patients with Hodgkin's disease and lowest (0.7%) in patients with acute myelogenous leukemia. Skovby noted a 31% incidence of zoster and a 7% incidence of varicella in a study of 94 children.[14] Although it was again noted that varicella-zoster infection did not impair the overall prognosis, the infection was potentially fatal and de-

Table 7-1. Incidence of Herpes Varicella-Zoster (HV-Z)

Study	Years of Study	Age of Patients (yrs.)	Number of Patients	Episodes of H-VZ Infections	Characteristics of H-VZ Infections	Incidence of H-VZ Infections (%)
Botnick et al.[141]	1969–1975	5–15	50	19	?LHZ—15 DHZ—2 Severe local—2	38.0
Feldman et al.[133]	1969–1972	Children	97	21*	Complications: pneumonitis—1 meningoencephalitis—1 progressive lesions—1	20.6
Reboul et al.[135]	1962–1974	<18	181	69†	LHZ—52 DHZ—14 V—3	34.8‡
Smith et al.[124]	1967–1972	4–20	49	15		30.6
de Pauw et al.[136]	1974–1980	All ages	210	20	LHZ—20 (in all cases limited to skin)	9.5
Goffinet et al.[120]	1959–1969	All ages	592	91	DHZ—13 ?LHZ—78	15.4
Gopal et al.[121]	1976–1978	All ages (50% <30 yrs)	231	32	?mainly LHZ	13.9
Guinee et al.[119]	1978–1981	All ages	717	116	LHZ—84 DHZ—19 unknown—13	16.2§
Mazur & Dolin[138]	1955–1974	All ages	549	26	?LHZ—21 DHZ—5	4.7
Notter et al.[142]	1968–1974	15–65	300	105	LHZ—58 DHZ—47 (Includes V-2; Zoster-1)	35.0
Schimpff et al.[81]	1969–1971	All ages	102	29‖	LHZ—21 DHZ—2 atypical—6	24.5

LATE INFECTIOUS COMPLICATIONS: VIRAL INFECTIONS

Author	Years	Age	Patients	Infection	%
Sokal & Firat[132]	1920–1963	19–72 (1 patient—9 yrs)	600	LHZ—39 DHZ—10 (generalized varicella form eruption without zoster—5)	8.2
Wright & Winer[137]	1954–1958	Average age—30	107	54#	9.3
Ziegler et al.[130]	1967–1971	<15	24	10	16.7
Monfardini et al.[129]	1970–1973	All ages	184	4 Zoster	16.8
Green et al.[131]	1970–1978	<20	72	31 Zoster—Varicella	27.8
Skovby & Sullivan[14]	1970–1978 (some overlap)	Children	94	21** Zoster	38.3
				39†† LHZ—23 DHZ—9 V—7	
Feld & Bodey[127]	1966–1974	Median age—29	144	14 Zoster	9.7
Poussin-Rosillo et al.[125]	1969–1974	13–69	127	53 Zoster	41.7‡‡
Williams et al.[126]	1926–1956	All ages	1992	83 Zoster	4.2
Redón et al.[8]	?	All ages	191	41§§ V—3 Atypical H-Z—2 HZ—36 (DHZ—7)	20.9
Ramot et al.[38]	1969–1976	All ages	108	17‖ Zoster	13.9
Peters et al.[37]	1928–1954	All ages	291	14 Zoster	4.8

*1 patient—2 separate episodes of H-VZ infections: 20 patients.
†6 patients—2 separate episodes of H-VZ infections; 63 patients.
‡36% of LHZ and DHZ occurred in children aged 14–18; 34% in children <13 years.
§26.6% of H-VZ occurred in pediatric population; 18.7% in the adult population.
‖3 patients—2 separate episodes of H-VZ infections; 25 patients.
#49 patients.
**1 patient—2 separate episodes of H-VZ infections.
††3 patients—2 separate episodes of H-VZ infections.
‡‡High incidence of zoster attributed to selection of patients (stage III & IV), amount of radiotherapy used, and the use of chemotherapy.
§§1 patient—2 separate episodes of H-VZ infections.
‖2 patients—2 separate episodes of H-VZ infections.
H-VZ = herpes varicella-zoster; LHZ = localized H-VZ; DHZ = disseminated H-VZ; V = varicella

Table 7-2. Treatment of Hodgkin's Disease Associated With Increased Incidence of H-VZ

Study	Treatment	Number of Patients	Episodes of H-VZ Infections	Incidence of Zoster (%)
Goffinet et al.[120]	Splenectomy	150	33	22.0*
	No splenectomy	442	58	13.1*
	Chemotherapy with MOPP with or without splenectomy	52	15	28.8
	No chemotherapy with or without splenectomy	540	79	14.6
Guinee et al.[119]	Combination chemotherapy-radiotherapy-chemotherapy	185	51	27.3
	Radiotherapy alone	193	22	11.5
	Chemotherapy alone	91	12	13.2
	Chemotherapy then radiotherapy	134	27	19.8
Mazur & Dolin[138]	Splenectomy—19% of all patients with zoster had received a splenectomy			
Schimpff et al.[1]	Radiotherapy	41	13	31.7
	No radiotherapy	37	4	10.8
	Chemotherapy	22	7	31.8
	No chemotherapy	56	10	17.9
	Splenectomy	56	13	23.2
	No splenectomy	46	12	26.1
de Pauw et al.[136]	Radiotherapy alone—15% of all zoster cases had received radiotherapy alone			
	Chemotherapy alone—20% of all zoster cases had received chemotherapy alone			
	Radiotherapy & chemotherapy—65% of all zoster cases had received radiotherapy & chemotherapy			
Feldman et al.[133]	Splenectomy	44	7	15.9†
	No splenectomy	53	14	26.4†
Reboul et al.[133]	Splenectomy	121	46	38.0‡
	No splenectomy	60	16	26.7‡
	Aggressive Treatment—90% of H-VZ cases occurred following aggressive treatment			
Monfardini et al.[129]	Splenectomy	139	26	18.7
	No splenectomy	45	5	11.1
	Combination chemotherapy with or without splenectomy	104	24	23.1
	No chemotherapy with or without splenectomy	80	7	8.8
Green et al.[131]	Initial Treatment:			
	Chemotherapy & radiotherapy	25		46.2
	Radiotherapy alone	50		10.2
	Splenectomy	52		42.8§
	No splenectomy	20		18.3§
Poussin-Rosillo et al.[125]	Splenectomy	71	33	46.5
	No splenectomy	56	20	35.7
Williams et al.[126]	One third of patients developed zoster within 2 months of receiving an alkylating agent on radiotherapy to disease at the same level			
Hoogstratten et al.[2]	Chemotherapy followed by radiotherapy			15.0
	Chemotherapy alone			0
	Total nodal radiotherapy followed by chemotherapy			16.0
	Chemotherapy followed by total nodal radiotherapy			19.0
	Total nodal radiotherapy alone			27.0

*<0.05 but >0.01
†not statistically significant (p >.05)
‡not statistically significant
§difference in incidence possibly due to treatment patient received

served vigorous treatment and support. Finally, Green[131] noted that Hodgkin's disease patients treated initially with irradiation and combination chemotherapy had a significantly greater risk of developing herpes zoster than patients treated initially with only irradiation ($p < 0.05\%$).

In contrast to varicella zoster, herpes simplex is generally observed as a minor infrequent infection in a number of the previous publications.[7,40,123,127] Cytotoxic chemotherapy has been associated with increased oral shedding of herpes-simplex virus (HSV). Rand[17] noted that HSV seropositive outpatients receiving cytotoxic chemotherapy had HSV recovered from throat washings in 7% of patients as compared with only 1.1% in HSV seropositive outpatients not receiving cytotoxic chemotherapy. In the pediatric population, one study revealed that 32.1% of normal children shed herpes-simplex virus at least once during a 6-year study, but herpes labialis was an infrequent physical finding.[16]

Epstein-Barr virus (EBV) has been consistently found to be associated with Hodgkin's disease, both in terms of elevated titer distributions of antibodies against the viral capsid antigen, and in the occurrence of Hodgkin's disease among patients with a history of EBV infectious mononucleosis.[18] Antibody titers to the viral-capsid antigen of EBV were elevated in 39% of Hodgkin's disease patients as compared to only 14% sibling-controls. The incidence of Hodgkin's disease among persons with a history of EBV-infectious mononucleosis is two or three times higher than expected.[18] In the pediatric population, antibodies to EBV-induced early antigens were much more common in Hodgkin's disease (80%) than in controls (9%).[19]

CHARACTERISTICS OF THE INFECTIONS

Arvin evaluated 86 lymphoma patients and noted that they had pre-existing deficiencies in cellular immunity to herpes viruses even before immunouppressive therapy.[31] The duration of suppression appeared to be important in predisposing these patients to reactivation of latent herpes-virus infection.[24,31] In contrast, in 25 patients with acute zoster, uncomplicated recovery from the infection was accompanied by the development of lymphocyte transformation and interferon production to varicella-zoster antigens.

Sokal[112] noted that the distribution of lesions of herpes zoster among Hodgkin's disease patients was not unusual. The thoracic segments were most commonly involved and the sacral segments were least often affected. Furthermore, the course of herpes zoster did not differ from that in the general population; however, morbidity was clearly greater. Generalized eruptions occurred in an unusually high percentage of patients; furthermore, evolution and healing of lesions was unusually slow in many patients.[112] Serious complications were relatively uncommon; however, it should be noted that the more seriously ill patients in this study received large doses of gamma globulin. Scarring and necrosis of the skin were fairly common, and several patients had troublesome postherpetic neuralgia. It has been noted, in the nonmalignant population, that age and trigeminal localization are prognostic factors for duration of postherpetic neuralgia.[15] Unfortunately, Sokal's study was not sufficiently large to make a comparison; indeed, only one patient developed trigeminal-zoster keratitis.

For purposes of comparison, the characteristics of varicella-zoster infections in immunosuppressed patients are well reviewed by Dolin[29] and patients with persistent viral infections are well reviewed by Haywood.[23] In immunosuppressed patients, mortality from visceral infections, especially from herpes-simplex-virus pneumona, is high (above 80%).[27] The clinical manifestations of visceral HSV infection may also involve the esophagus and liver.

TREATMENT

The results of the major randomized trials of antiviral treatment of herpes-viral infections in immunocompromised patients, as of this writing, are summarized in Table 7–3. The phrase "as of this writing" is critical;

Table 7-3. Results of Randomized Trials of Antiviral Treatment of Herpesviral Infections in Immunocompromised Patients (Drug Therapy Compared to Placebo)

Ref.	Treatment	Herpes Infection	Number of Patients (Drug/Placebo)	Viral Clearance	Cessation New Vesicle Formation	Total Pustulation	Total Scabbing	Total Lesion Healing	Defervescence	Acute Pain Response	Post-herpetic Neuralgia	Visceral Complications	Cutaneous Dissemination
Whitley et al.[71]	Ara A	Varicella	19/15	−	+		−	−	+			+	
Whitley et al.[74]		Zoster	47/40	+	+	+(−)				+			
Whitley et al.[75]			63/58	+(−)	+	+	+			+(−)	+	+	+
Whitley[78]		Simplex	39/46	+(−)	+(−)	+(−)	+(−)			+			
Prober et al.[67]	Acyclovir	Varicella	8/12	−			−		+			+	
Balfour et al.[91]		Zoster	52/42	+(1)	+(−)	+(−)	+(−)	−	−	+(−)		+	+
Meyers et al.[70]	Acyclovir (IV)	Simplex	51/46	+			+	+		+			
Chou et al.[57]			5/5	+				+		+			
Whitley et al.[71]	Acyclovir (topical)		33/30	+	−			+*		+*			
Arvin et al.[13]	Human leucemia (IFN)	Varicella	23/21	+	+(−)							+	
Merigan et al.[87]		Zoster	45/45	+†	+†			−		+†	+†	+	+†

*Only patients with extensive lesions derived statistically significant benefit.
†Only seen at high doses of IFN.
Significant improvement seen with drug therapy (+); Some improvement with drug therapy [+(−)]; No difference between placebo and drug (−).
Significant improvement often was seen in a certain population of the patients.

there have been significant advances in antiviral therapy since 1978. The question in the immunocompromised host is no longer whether or not to use antiviral compounds, but rather, which patients should be treated and for how long. The state of the art of treatment is constantly changing. Vidarabine, interferon alpha, and intravenous acyclovir have all demonstrated efficacy in the therapy of herpes zoster in the immunosuppressed host. Studies of oral acyclovir are currently in progress. I will therefore summarize the current recommendations on treatment, recognizing that treatment methods change rapidly.

Three important studies have been done on the treatment of varicella in the immunocompromised host. A study performed by a collaborative antiviral-study group at the National Institute of Allergy and Infectious Diseases randomized vidarabine against placebo within 72 hours of the onset of chickenpox. In the vidarabine group, new lesion formation ceased earlier and defervesced more rapidly than in the placebo group. The incidence of life-threatening complications was significantly lower in the treated arm (5% versus 53%).[77] A similar randomized 20-patient trial evaluated acyclovir.[67] Therapy with acyclovir decreased the development of pneumonitis from 45% to 0%, but had no effect on cutaneous healing or fever. The third study was conducted by Arvin using large doses of interferon early in the disease course.[86] Intramuscular interferon decreased the frequency of visceral complications and prevented progressive disease in children with varicella. Currently, studies are continuing to evaluate recombinant DNA interferons, alone or in combination with antiviral agents, for the management of high-risk varicella patients.[77]

For the treatment of herpes zoster in the immunocompromized patient, Whitley demonstrated that vidarabine was effective in accelerating skin healing, reducing acute pain and post-herpetic neuralgia, and reducing the frequency of complications of acute zoster in immunocompromised patients.[5] Acyclovir is effective in reducing both the progression and complications of acute zoster.[68,69] Acyclovir significantly reduced the frequency of disease progression from 71% to 32% in those with a localized rash and from 22% to 0% in those with a disseminated rash.[68] In this trial, acyclovir did not produce significant differences in the rate of skin healing and pain reduction, perhaps because entry to the trial was not restricted to those beginning treatment within 72 hours of rash onset. Researchers are doing comparative trials of acyclovir and vidarabine.

For the treatment of herpes simplex virus, intravenous acyclovir was quickly shown to be effective in all treatment studies.[47,55,71] In randomized trials, virus shedding was shortened from more than 2 weeks in placebo recipients to 2 to 3 days in the acyclovir recipients. Healing times were also shortened without substantial toxicity. Topical acyclovir has been shown to be virtually equal in efficacy to intravenous acyclovir[71] when only external lesions are evaluated. It should be noted, however, that topical acyclovir does not benefit any infection either originating from, or extending away from, the external cutaneous disease. Oral acyclovir is currently being assessed in randomized trials in marrow-graft recipients. Finally, vidarabine treatment has been shown to be effective for mucocutaneous herpes-simplex virus in immunocompromised patients.[74] The clinical parameters of healing were approximately comparable to those obtained with intravenous acyclovir.

In summary, intravenous acyclovir has been proven to be effective for mucocutaneous herpes-simplex virus infection and is undoubtedly effective for more serious manifestations, such as HSV pneumonia. The efficacy of oral acyclovir in serious HSV infections is currently being assessed. Oral acyclovir, however, is clearly of benefit in mucocutaneous infection and may also be used for HSV esophagitis and gastritis. Because of incomplete absorption, blood levels with oral acyclovir are substantially lower than comparative intravenous treatment, and a higher oral dose is necessary. Finally, topical acyclovir should only be used by those patients with purely external disease and for some patients who cannot accept oral therapy (Meyers[70]). To date, there are no recommended therapies for established cytomegalovirus or Epstein-Barr virus in the immunosuppressed patient.

Table 7-4. Prophylactic Antiviral Therapy With Acyclovir in Immunocompromised Patients

	Acyclovir		Placebo	
	Route of Administration	Number Infected/ Number of Patients	Number Infected/ Number of Patients	References
Herpes Simplex	IV	0/10	7/10	Saral et al.[56]
Herpes Simplex	IV	2/29	15/30	Hann et al.[58]
Herpes Simplex	Oral	1/20	12/20	Anderson et al.[98]
Herpes Simplex	Oral	0/20	13/19	Gluckman et al.[59]
Cytomegalovirus	Oral	0/20	7/19	Gluckman et al.[59]

PROPHYLAXIS

In terms of varicella-zoster prophylaxis, exposure to patients with varicella or zoster should be minimized for all children with lymphoproliferative disorders. Immunoprophylaxis for varicella has been successful, but the unpredictability and low attack rate of zoster makes immunoprophylaxis difficult to implement. Varicella-zoster immunoglobulin should be given to varicella-susceptible persons with a high-risk of severe varicella, ideally within three days of exposure.[93,94] It does not necessarily protect against the virus, but should be expected to modify clinical varicella.

In terms of other agents, transfer factor has been shown to induce at least partial immunity to varicella in children with leukemia; interferon protects simian varicella in monkeys, but its success in man is yet to be demonstrated. Live attenuated varicella vaccine seems now to be the most practical way to prevent severe varicella in high-risk persons, but is still experimental at the present time.

In terms of other therapies, acyclovir (intravenously or oral) and interferon are being tested as prophylaxis in high-risk groups. Proper's study on immunosuppressed children with varicella showed that zoster pneumonitis developed in 45% of placebo-treated patients in comparison with 0% of the acyclovir-treated patients.[67] No evidence of serious acyclovir toxicity was noted. The results of prophylactic antiviral therapy trials with acyclovir are summarized in Table 7-4.

In terms of herpes-simplex virus, Anderson has demonstrated oral-acyclovir prophylaxis in nonHodgkin's lymphoma and acute lymphoblastic leukemia in patients receiving remission-induction chemotherapy. Prophylactic oral acyclovir significantly reduced the incidence of clinical HSV infection from 60% on placebo, to 5% on acyclovir; it also reduced the incidence of viral isolates from 70% on placebo, to 5% on acyclovir.[60] Similarly, Hann has demonstrated the benefit of intravenous acyclovir prophylaxis in 20 patients undergoing allogeneic bone-marrow transplantation and in 39 patients receiving remission-induction chemotherapy for acute leukemia. Acyclovir completely prevented oropharyngeal herpes-simplex-virus infection, compared with a 50% incidence in the placebo arm.[58] Intravenous acyclovir prophylaxis has also been demonstrated in the bone-marrow transplant setting by both Saral[56] and Gluckman.[59]

A randomized placebo-controlled-blind trial of prophylactic interferon alpha has demonstrated protection against herpes labialis in patients undergoing surgical manipulation of the trigeminal root. Therapeutic trials of interferon are underway for herpes-simplex virus infections in immunocompromised patients. At the present time, prophylaxis of herpes-simplex-virus infections continues to be investigational in the immunocompromised host.

The advances in antiviral therapy over the next 5 to 10 years will radically alter both the prophylaxis and treatment recommendations in this chapter.

REFERENCES

1. Schimpff, S.C., O'Connell, M.J., Green, W.H. et al. Infections in 92 splenectomized patients with Hodgkin's disease. Ann. Int. Med. 76:241–254, 1972.
2. Hoogstraten, B., Holland, J.F. Kramer, S. et al.

Combination chemotherapy-radiotherapy for stage III Hodgkin's disease. Arch. Intern. Med. *131*:424–428, 1973.
3. Pancoast, H.K., and Pendergrass, E.P. The occurrence of herpes zoster in Hodgkin's disease. Am. J. Med. Sci. *168*:326–334, 1924.
4. Hope-Simpson, R.E. The nature of herpes zoster: A long-term study and a new hypothesis. Proc. R. Soc. Med. *58*:9–20, 1965.
5. Seiler, H.E. A study of herpes zoster particularly in its relationship to chickenpox. J. Hyg. *47*:253–262, 1949.
6. Rhodes, A.R. Herpes zoster and neoplastic disease. JAMA *236*:2174, 1976.
7. Rosenberg, S.A., Diamond, H.D., Jaslowitz, B. et al. Lymphosarcoma: A review of 1269 cases. Medicine *40*:31, 1961.
8. Redón, J., Montalar, J., Navarro, J.R. et al. Infecciones por herpes virus-varicela en la enfermedad de Hodgkin. Med. Clin. Barcelona. *76*:377–380, 1981.
9. Davis, C.M., VanDersarl, J.V., and Coltman, C.A. Failure of cytarabine in varicella-zoster infections. JAMA *224*:122–123, 1973.
10. Ochocka, M., Chmielewska, D., and Matysiak, M. Isoprinosine in the treatment of herpes virus infections in children with leukaemia and malignant lymphoma. Folia Haematol. (Leipz) *III* (3):343–349, 1984.
11. Geiser, C.F., Bishop, Y., Myers, M. et al. Prophylaxis of varicella in children with neoplastic disease: Comparative results with zoster immune plasma and gamma globulin. Cancer *35*:1027–1030, 1975.
12. Klara, S., Endre, K., Tibor, C. et al. Herpes zoster elofordulása Hodgkin-kóros betefek kozott. Orvosi Hetilap. *124*:1551–1553, 1983.
13. Arvin, A.M., Pollard, R.B., Rasmussen, L.E. et al. Cellular and humoral immunity in the pathogenesis of recurrent herpes viral infections in patients with lymphoma. J. Clin. Invest. *65*:869–878, 1980.
14. Skovby, F. and Sullivan, M.P. Herpes zoster and varicella in children with Hodgkin's disease. Acta Paediatr Scand. *71*:269–273, 1982.
15. de Moragas, J.M. and Kierland, R.R. The outcome of patients with herpes zoster. A.M.A. Arch. Dermatol. *75*:193–196, 1956.
16. Cesario, T.C., Poland, J.D., Wulff, H. et al. Six years experience with herpes simplex virus in a children's home. Am. J. Epidemiol. *90*(8):416–422, 1969.
17. Rand, K.H., Kramer, B., and Johnson, A.C. Cancer chemotherapy associated symptomatic stomatitis—Role of herpes simplex virus (HSV). Cancer *50*:1262–1265, 1982.
18. Evans, A.S. and Gutensohn, N.M. A population-based case-control study of EBV and other viral antibodies among persons with Hodgkin's disease and their siblings. Int. J. Cancer *34*:149–157, 1984.
19. Lange, B., Arbeter, A., Hewetson, J. et al. Longitudinal study of Epstein-Barr virus antibody titer and excretion in pediatric patients with Hodgkin's disease. Int. J. Cancer *22*:521–527, 1978.
20. Cheson, B.D., Samlowski, W.E., Tang, T.T. et al. Value of open-lung biopsy in 87 immunocompromised patients with pulmonary infiltrates. Cancer *55*:453–459, 1985.
21. Collaborative DHPG treatment study group. Treatment of serious cytomegalovirus infections with 9-(1,3-Dihydroxy-2-Propoxymethyl)Guanine in patients with AIDS and other immunodeficiencies. N. Engl. J. Med. *314*(13):801–805, 1986.
22. Bowden, R.A., Sayers, M., Fluornoy, N. et al. Cytomegalovirus immune globulin and seronegative blood products to prevent primary cytomegalovirus infection after marrow transplantation. N. Engl. J. Med. *314*(16):1006–1010.
23. Haywood, A.M. Patterns of persistent viral infections. N. Engl. J. Med. *315*(15):939–948, 1986.
24. Terry, B.A. Hodgkin's disease and non-Hodgkin's lymphomas. Nurs. Clin. North Am. *20*(1):207–217, 1985.
25. Thar, R.L. and Million, R.R. Complications of radiation treatment of Hodgkin's disease. Seminars in Oncology. *7*(2):174–183, 1980.
26. Corey, L. and Spear, P.G. Infections with herpes simplex viruses (Part I). N. Engl. J. Med. *314*(11):686–691, 1986.
27. Corey, L. and Spear, P.G. Infections with herpes simplex viruses (Part II). N. Engl. J. Med. *314*(12):749–757, 1986.
28. Nuss, D.D. Herpes zoster—the best approach. Med. Times *108*:(6):47–52, 1980.
29. Dolin, R., Reichman, R.C., Mazur, M.H. et al. Herpes zoster-varicella infections in immunosuppressed patients. Ann. Intern. Med. *89*:375–388, 1978.
30. Notter, D.T., Grossman, P.L., Rosenberg, S.A. et al. Infections in patients with Hodgkin's disease: A clinical study of 300 consecutive adult patients. Rev. Infect. Dis. *2*:761–800, 1980.
31. Arvin, A.M., Pollard, R.B., Rasmussen, L.E. et al. Cellular and humoral immunity in the pathogenesis of recurrent herpes viral infections in patients with lymphoma. J. Clin. Invest. *65*:869–878, 1980.
32. Hirsch, M.S. and Kaplan, J.C. Antiviral therapy. Sci. Am. *256*:76–85, 1987.
33. Anderson, H., Sutton, R.N.P., and Scarffe, J.H. Cytotoxic chemotherapy and viral infections: the role of acyclovir. J. R. Col. Physicians Lond. *18*(1):51–55, 1984.
34. Brunell, P.A., Ross, A., Miller, L.H. et al. Prevention of varicella by zoster immune globulin. N. Engl. J. Med. *280*(22):1191–1194, 1969.
35. Strander, H., Cantell, K., Carlstrom, G. et al. Clinical and laboratory investigations on man: Systemic administration of potent interferon to man. J. Natl. Cancer Inst. *51*(3):733–742, 1973.
36. Emodi, G., Rufli, T., Just. M. et al. Human interferon therapy for herpes zoster in adults. Scan. J. Infect. Dis. *7*:1–5, 1975.
37. Peters, M.V. and Middlemiss, K.C.H. A study of Hodgkin's disease treated by irradiation. Ontario Inst. Radiother. *79*(1):114–121, 1958.
38. Ramot, B., Modan, M., Berkowitz, M. et al. The relation between therapy and herpes zoster in

Hodgkin's disease. Isr. J. Med. Sci. *14*(10): 1014–1018, 1978.
39. Hoogstraten, B., Holland, J.F., Kramer, S. et al. Combination chemotherapy-radiotherapy for stage III Hodgkin's disease. Arch. Intern. Med. *131*:424–428, 1973.
40. Schimpff, S.C., O'Connell, M.J., Green, W.H. et al. Infections in 92 splenectomized patients with Hodgkin's disease. Am. J. Med. *59*:695–701, 1975.
41. McGregor, R.M. Herpes zoster, chicken-pox and cancer in general practice. Brit. Med. J. *1*:84–87, 1957.
42. Ruckdeschel, J.C., Schimpff, S.C., Smyth, A.C. et al. Herpes zoster and impaired cell-associated immunity to the varicella-zoster virus in patients with Hodgkin's disease. Am. J. Med. *62*:77–85, 1977.
43. Armstrong, R.W., Gurwith, M.J., Waddell, D. et al. Cutaneous interferon production in patients with Hodgkin's disease and other cancers infected with varicella or vaccinia. N. Engl. J. Med. *283*:1182–1187, 1970.
44. Waltuch, G. and Sachs, F. Herpes zoster in a patient with Hodgkin's disease—Treatment with idoxuridine. Arch. Intern. Med. *121*:458–462, 1968.
45. Merselis, Jr. J.G., Kaye, D., and Hook, E.W. Disseminated herpes zoster. Arch. Intern. Med. *113*:679–686, 1964.
46. Shanbrom, E., Miller, S., and Haar, H. Herpes zoster in hematologic neoplasias: Some unusual manifestations. *53*(3):523–533, 1960.
47. Whitley, R.J., Alford, C.A., Hirsch, M.S. et al. and the NIAID Collaborative Antiviral Study Group. Vidarabine versus acyclovir therapy in herpes simplex encephalitis. N. Engl. J. Med. *314*(3):144–149, 1986.
48. Jeffries, D.J. Acyclovir update. Brit. Med. J. *293*:1523, 1986.
49. McKendrick, M.W., McGill, J.I., White, J.E. et al. Oral acyclovir in acute herpes zoster. Brit. Med. J. *293*:1529–1532, 1986.
50. Advances in Therapy Against Herpesvirus Infections in Immunocompromised Hosts. Balfour Jr. HH. (ed.) Proceedings of a Symposium Conducted by the University of Minnesota. University of Minnesota, 1985.
51. McGregor, R.M. Herpes zoster, chicken-pox and cancer in general practice. Brit. Med. J. *1*:84–87, 1957.
52. Lam, M.T., Pazin, G.J., Armstrong, J.A. et al. Hepes simplex infection in acute myelogenous leukemia and other hematologic malignancies: A prospective study. Cancer *48*:2168–2171, 1981.
53. Field, H.J. and Wildy, P. Recurrent herpes simplex: the outlook for systemic antiviral agents. Brit. Med. J. *282*:1821–1822, 1981.
54. Selby, P.J., Powles, R.L., Janeson, B. et al. Parenteral acyclovir therapy for herpesvirus infections in man. Lancet *2*:1267–1270, 1979.
55. Wade, J.C., Newton, B., McLaren, C. et al. Intravenous acyclovir to treat mucocutaneous herpes simplex virus infection after marrow transplantation. Ann. Intern. Med. *96*(3):265–269, 1982.
56. Saral, R., Burns, W.H., Laskin, O.L. et al. Acyclovir prophylaxis of herpes-simplex-virus infections—A randomized, double-blind, controlled trial in bone-marrow-recipients. N. Engl. J. Med. *305*:(2):63–67, 1981.
57. Chou, S. Gallagher, J.G., and Merigan, T.C. Controlled clinical trial of intravenous acyclovir in heart-transplant patients with mucocutaneous herpes simplex infections. Lancet *1*:1392–1394, 1981.
58. Hann, I.M., Prentice, H.G., Blacklock. H.A. et al. Acyclovir prophylaxis against herpes virus infections in severely immunocompromised patients: Randomised double blind trials. Brit. Med. J. *287*:384–388, 1983.
59. Gluckman, E., Lotsberg, J., Devergie, A. et al. Prophylaxis of herpes infections after bone-marrow transplantation by oral acyclovir. Lancet *2*:706–708, 1983.
60. Anderson, H., Scarff, J.H., Sutton, R.N.P. et al. Oral acyclovir prophylaxis against herpes simplex virus in non-Hodgkin's lymphoma and acute lymphoblastic leukaemia patients receiving remission induction chemotherapy. A randomised double blind placebo controlled trial. Brit. J. Cancer *50*:45–49, 1984.
61. Hirsch, M.S. and Schooley, R.T. Treatment of herpesvirus infections (Part I). N. Engl. J. Med. *309*(16):963–970, 1983.
62. Hirsch, M.S. and Schooley, R.T. Treatment of herpesvirus infections (Part II). N. Engl. J. Med. *309*(17):1034–1039, 1983.
63. De Clercq, E., Descamps, J., Verheist, G. et al. Comparative efficacy of antiherpes drugs against different strains of herpes simplex virus. J. Infect. Dis. *141*(5):563–574, 1980.
64. Straus, S.E., Rooney, J.F., Sever, J.L. et al. Herpes simplex virus infection: biology, treatment, and prevention. Ann. Intern. Med. *103*:404–419, 1985.
65. Sutton, R.N.P., Itzhaki, R.F., Christophers, J. et al. Virus infections in immunocompromised patients: Their importance and their management. R. Soc. Med. *78*:100–105, 1985.
66. Peyramond, D., Denoyel, G.A., Philip, T. et al. Les Infections á virus varicelle-zoster chez l'enfant immunodéprimé—Traitment par acyclovir et controles. Arch. Fr. Pediatr. *40*:95–99, 1983.
67. Prober, C.G., Kirk, L.E., and Keeney, R.E. Acyclovir therapy of chickenpox in immunosuppressed children—a collaborative study. J. Pediatr. *101*(4):622–625, 1982.
68. Balfour, Jr. H.H., Bean, B., Laskin, O.L. et al. The Burroughs Wellcome collaborative acyclovir study group. N. Engl. J. Med. *308*(24): 1448–1453, 1983.
69. Balfour, Jr. H.H., McMonigal, K.A., and Bean, B. Acyclovir therapy of varicella-zoster virus infections in immunocompromised patients. J. Antimicrob. Chemother. *12*(Suppl. B):169–179, 1983.
70. Meyers, J.D., Wade, J.C., Mitchell, C.D. et al. Multicenter collaborative trial of intravenous acyclovir for treatment of mucocutaneous herpes simplex virus infection in the immunocompromised host. Am. J. Med.—Acyclovir Symposium *73*(1A):229–235, 1982.

71. Whitley, R.J., Levin, M., Barton, N. et al. Infections caused by herpes simplex virus in the immunocompromised host: Natural history and topical acyclovir therapy. J. Infect. Dis. *150*(3):323–329, 1984.
72. Mitchell, C.D., Bean, B., Gentry, S.R. et al. Acyclovir therapy for mucocutaneous herpes simplex infections in immunocompromised patients. Lancet *1*:1389–1392, 1981.
73. Straus, S.E., Seidlin, M., Takiff, H. et al. Oral acyclovir to suppress recurring herpes simplex virus infections in immunodeficient patients. Ann. Intern. Med. *100*:522–524, 1984.
74. Whitley, R.J., Spruance, S., Hayden, F.G. et al. and the NIAID Collaborative Antiviral Study Group. Vidarabine therapy for mucocutaneous herpes simplex virus infections in the immunocompromised host. J. Infect. Dis. *149*(1):1–8, 1984.
75. Whitley, R.J., Ch'ien, L.T., Dolin, R. et al. and the Collaborative Antiviral Study. Adenine arabinoside therapy of herpes zoster in the immunosuppressed. N. Engl. J. Med. *294*(22):1193–1199, 1976.
76. Grissom, J.A., Durant, J.R., Whitley, R.J. et al. Thymic hyperplasia in a case Hodgkin's disease. South. Med. J. *76*(9):1189–1192, 1983.
77. Whitley, R., Hilty, M., Haynes, R. et al. and the NIAID Collaborative Antiviral Study Group. Vidarabine therapy of varicella in immunosuppressed patients. J. Pediatr. *101*(1):125–131, 1982.
78. Whitley, R.J., Soong, S-J., Dolin, R. and the NIAID Collaborative Antiviral Study Group. Early vidarabine therapy to control the complications of herpes zoster in immunosuppressed patients. N. Engl. J. Med. *307*(16):971–975, 1982.
79. Shepp, D.H., Dandliker, P.S., de Miranda, P. et al. Activity of 9-[2-Hydroxy-1-(hydroxymethyl)ethoxymethyl]guanine in the treatment of cytomegalovirus pneumonia. Ann. Intern. Med. *103*:368–373, 1985.
80. Mavlight, G.M. and Talpaz, M. Cimetidine for herpes zoster. N. Engl. J. Med. (Correspondence) *310*(5):318–319, 1984.
81. Schimpff, S.C., Fortner, C.L., Greene, W.H. et al. Cytosine arabinoside for localized herpes zoster in patients with cancer: Failure in a controlled trial. J. Infect. Dis. *130*(6):673–676, 1974.
82. Luna, M.A. and Lifhtiger, B. Disseminated toxoplasmosis and cytomegalovirus infection complicating Hodgkin's disease. Am. J. Clin. Pathol. *55*:499–505, 1971.
83. Gruson, S., Mouchnino, G., Reinert, P.H. et al. Varicells et zonas chez 83 enfants traités pour une affection maligne. Arch. Fr. Pediatr. *38*:337–343, 1981.
84. Busk, C.M.A., Earl, H.M., Wrigley, P.F.M. et al. Triple drug therapy of herpes zoster infection occurring in patients with reticulo-endothelial neoplasia—a preliminary study. J. Antimicrob. Chemother. *6*:733–736, 1980.
85. Sulliger, J.M., Imbach, P., Barandun, S. et al. Varicella and herpes zoster in immunosuppressed children: Preliminary results of treatment with intravenous immunoglobulin. Helv. Paediat. Acta. *39*:63–70, 1984.
86. Arvin, A.M., Kushner, J.H., Feldman, S. et al. Human leukocyte interferon for the treatment of varicella in children with cancer. N. Engl. J. Med. *306*(13):761–765, 1982.
87. Merigan, T.C., Rand, K.H., Pollard, R.B. et al. Human leukocyte interferon for the treatment of herpes zoster in patients with cancer. N. Engl. J. Med. *298*(18):981–987, 1978.
88. Arvin, A.M., Feldman, S., and Merigan, T.C. Human leukocyte interferon in the treatment of varicella in children with cancer: a preliminary controlled trial. Antimicrob. Agents Chemother. *13*(4):605–607, 1978.
89. Arvin, A.M. Interferon as an antiviral and anti-tumor therapeutic agent. Ophthalmology *87*(12):1236–1238, 1980.
90. Jordan, G.W., Fried, R.P., and Merigan, T.C. Administration of human leukocyte interferon in herpes zoster. I. Safety, circulating antiviral activity, and host responses to infection. J. Infect. Dis. *130*(1):56–62, 1974.
91. Balfour, Jr. H.H., Bean, B., Mitchell, C.D. et al. Acyclovir in immunocompromised patients with cytomegalovirus disease—a controlled trial at one institution. Am. J. Med. *73*(1A):241–248, 1982.
92. Kornhuber, B., Kropp, H., Ribeiro-Ayeh, J. et al. Zur Sicherheit der varizellenprophylaxe mit varizellen-zoster-immunoglobulin. Monatsschr Kinderheilkd. *130*:27–29, 1982.
93. Gershon, A.A., Steinberg, S., and Brunell, P.A. Zoster immune globulin—a further assessment. N. Engl. J. Med. *290*(5):243–245, 1974.
94. Stevens, D.A. and Merigan, T.C. Zoster immune globulin prophylaxis of disseminated zoster in compromised host—a randomized trial. Arch. Intern. Med. *140*:52–54, 1980.
95. Orenstein, W.A., Heymann, D.L., Ellis, R.J. et al. Prophylaxis of varicella in high-risk children: dose-response effect of zoster immune globulin. J. Pediatr. *98*(3):368–373, 1981.
96. Hutter, Jr. J.J., Minnich, L.L., and Ray, C.G. Varicella-zoster antibody titers in children with leukemia and lymphoma—relationship of titer to varicella-zoster infection. Am. J. Dis. Child. *138*:56–59, 1984.
97. Mann, I.M., Prentice, H.G., Blacklock, H.A. et al. Acyclovir prophylaxis against herpes virus infections in severely immunocompromised patients: randomised double blind trial. Brit. Med. J. *287*:384–388, 1983.
98. Anderson, H., Scarffe, J.H., Sutton, R.N.P. et al. Oral acyclovir prophylaxis agaist herpes simplex virus in non-Hodgkin's lymphoma and acute lymphoblastic leukaemia patients receiving remission induction chemotherapy. A randomised double blind, placebo controlled trial. Br. J. Cancer *50*:45–49, 1984.
99. Fauci, A.S., Macher, A.M., Longo, D.J. et al. Acquired immunodeficiency syndrome: Epidemiologic, clinical, immunologic, and therapeutic considerations. Ann. Intern. Med. *100*:92–106, 1984.
100. LaCamera, D.J., Masur, H., and Henderson, D.K.

The acquired immunodeficiency syndrome. Nursing Clinics of North America. 20(1):241–256, 1985.
101. Safai, B., Mike, V., Giraldo, G. et al. Association of Kaposi's sarcoma with second primary malignancies. Cancer 45:1472–1479, 1980.
102. Longo, D.L., Steis, R.G., Lane, H.C. et al. Malignancies in the AIDS patient: natural history, treatment strategies, and preliminary results. Ann. N.Y. Acad. Sci. 437:421–430, 1984.
103. Purtilo, D.T. Immunopathology of infectious mononucleosis and other complications of Epstein-Barr virus infections. Pathol. Annu. 15(Pt. 1):253–299, 1980.
104. Ho, M., Miller, G., Atchison, R.W. et al. Epstein-Barr virus infections and DNA hybridization studies in posttransplantation lymphoma and lymphoproliferative lesions: The role of primary infection. J. Infect. Dis. 152(5):876–886, 1985.
105. Starlz, T.E., Nalesnik, M.A., Porter, K.A. et al. Reversibility of lymphomas and lymphoproliferative lesions developing under cyclosporin-steroid therapy. Lancet 1:583–587, 1984.
106. Flechner, S.N. Cyclosporine: A new and promising immunosuppressive agent. Urol. Clin. North Am. 10(2):263–275, 1983.
107. Lymphoma in organ transplant recipients. (Editorial) Lancet 1:601–603, 1984.
108. Lacher, M.J. Hodgkin's disease and infectious mononucleosis: Is there a causal association. A Cancer Journal for Clinicians 31(6):359–364, 1981.
109. Gallo, R.C. and Gelmann, E.P. In search of a Hodgkin's disease virus. N. Engl. J. Med. 304(3):169–170, 1981.
110. McVay, Jr. J.R. Infection and Hodgkin's disease. Lancet 2:589–590, 1981.
111. Krause, J.R. and Kaplan, S.S. Bone marrow findings in infectious mononucleosis and mononucleosis-like diseases in the older adult. Scand. J. Haematol. 28:15–22, 1982.
112. Sokal, J.E. and Firat, D. Varicella-zoster infection in Hodgkin's disease. Am. J. Med. 39:452–463, 1965.
113. Feldman, S., Hughes, W.T., and Kim, H.Y. Herpes zoster in children with cancer. Am. J. Dis. Child. 126:178–184, 1973.
114. Schimpff, S. Serpick A., Stoler B. et al. Varicella-zoster infection in patients with cancer. Ann. Intern. Med. 76:241–254, 1972.
115. Reboul, F., Donaldson, S.S., and Kaplan, H.S. Herpes zoster and varicella infections in children with Hodgkin's disease. Cancer 41:95–99, 1978.
116. DePauw, B.E., Janssen, J. Th. P., and Haanen, C. Occurrence of herpes zoster varicella infections after completion of treatment of Hodgkin's disease. Neth. J. Med. 26:301–303, 1983.
117. Wright, E.T. and Winer, L.H. Herpes zoster and malignancy. Arch. Dermatol. 84:110–112, 1961.
118. Mazur, M.H. and Dolin, R. Herpes zoster at the NIH: A 20 year experience. Am. J. Med. 65:738–744, 1978.
119. Guinee, V.F., Guido, J.J., Pfalzgraf, K.A. et al. The incidence of herpes zoster in patients with Hodgkin's disease—An analysis of prognostic factors. Cancer 56:642–648, 1985.
120. Goffinet, D.R., Glatstein, E.J., and Merigan, T.C. Herpes zoster-varicella infections and lymphoma. Ann. Intern. Med. 76:235–240, 1972.
121. Gopal, R., Advani, S.H., Dinshaw, K.T. et al. Herpes-zoster in malignancy. Jr. Asso. Phys. Ind. 28:125–132, 1980.
122. Botnick, L.E., Goodman, R., Jaffe, N. et al. Stages I–III Hodgkin's disease in children—results of staging and treatment. Cancer 39:599–603, 1977.
123. Notter, D.T., Grossman, P.L., Rosenberg, S.A. et al. Infections in patients with Hodgkin's disease: A clinical study of 300 consecutive adult patients. Rev. Infect. Dis. 2:761–800, 1980.
124. Smith, K.L., Johnson, D., Hustu, O. et al. Concurrent chemotherapy and radiation therapy in the treatment of childhood and adolescent Hodgkin's disease. Cancer 33:38–46, 1974.
125. Poussin-Rosillo, H., Nisce, L.Z., and Lee, B.J. Complications of total nodal irradiation of Hodgkin's disease stages III and IV. Cancer 42:437–441, 1978.
126. Williams, H.M., Diamond, H.D., and Craver, L.F. The pathogenesis and management of neurological complications in patients with malignant lymphomas and leukemia. Cancer 11:76–82, 1958.
127. Feld, R. and Bodey, G.P. Infections in patients with malignant lymphoma treated with combination chemotherapy. Cancer 39:1018–1025, 1977.
128. Skovby, F. and Sullivan, M.P. Herpes zoster and varicella in children with Hodgkin's disease. Acta. Paediatr, Scand. 71:269–273, 1982.
129. Monfardini, S., Bajetta, E., Arnold, C.A. et al. Herpes zoster-varicella infection in malignant lymphomas. Influence of splenectomy and intensive treatment. Europ. J. Cancer 11:51–57, 1975.
130. Ziegler, J.L., Bluming, A.Z., Fass, L. et al. Chemotherapy of childhood Hodgkin's disease in Uganda. Lancet 2:679–682, 1972.
131. Green, D.M., Stutzman, L., Blumenson, L.E. et al. The incidence of post-splenectomy sepsis and herpes zoster in children and adolescents with Hodgkin's disease. Med. Pediatr. Oncol. 7:285–297, 1979.
132. Sokal, J.E. and Firat, D. Varicella-zoster infection in Hodgkin's disease. Am. J. Med.
133. Feldman, S., Hughes, W.T., and Kim, H.Y. Herpes zoster in children with cancer. Am. J. Dis Child. 126:178–184, 1973.
134. Schimpff, S., Serpick, A., Stoler, B. et al. Varicella-zoster infection in patients with cancer. Ann. Intern. Med. 76:241–254, 1972.
135. Reboul. F., Donaldson, S.S., and Kaplan, H.S. Herpes zoster and varicella infections in children with Hodgkin's disease. Cancer 41:95–99, 1978.
136. De Pauw, B.E., Jannsen, J.T., Vaissier P. et al. Occurrence of herpes zoster varicella infections after completion of treatment for Hodgkin's disease. Neth. J. Med. 26:301–303, 1983.
137. Wright, E.T., Winer, L.H. Herpes Zoster and Malignancy. Arch. Dermatol. 84:242, 1961.
138. Mazur, M.H. and Dolin, R. Herpes zoster at the

NIH: a 20 year experience. Am. J. Med. 65:738–744, 1978.
139. Guinee, V.F., Guido, J.J., Pfalzgraf, K.A. et al. The incidence of herpes zoster in patients with Hodgkin's disease. An analysis of prognostic factors. Cancer 56:642–648, 1985.
140. Goffinet, D.R., Glatstein, E.J., and Merigan, T.C. Herpes zoster-varicella infections and lymphoma. Ann. Intern. Med. 76:235–240, 1972.
141. Botnick, L.E., Goodman, R., Jaffe, N. et al. Stages I–III Hodgkin's disease in children. Cancer 39:599–603, 1977.
142. Notter, D.T., Grossman, P.L., Rosenberg, S.A. et al. Infections in patients with Hodgkin's disease: A clinical study of 300 consecutive adult patients. Rev. Infect. Dis. 2(5):761–800, 1980.

CHAPTER 8

The Skeletal System

JULIUS SMITH
HARRY GRIFFITHS

Long-term survivors of Hodgkin's disease may demonstrate a number of complications that involve the skeleton following either radiation therapy or chemotherapy. These complications include scoliosis and kyphosis, slipped capital femoral epiphysis and avascular necrosis, radiation atrophy and osteitis, localized and generalized osteopenia, as well as the occurrence of postirradiation osteochondromas and osteosarcomas. Following a discussion of the pathophysiology of radiation damage to the skeleton, this chapter addresses each of these issues with a review of the literature as well as comments based on our own personal experience.

PATHOPHYSIOLOGY OF RADIATION DAMAGE TO THE SKELETON

It is apparent that the sensitivity of the skeleton to radiation therapy varies depending on the age of the patient. The most sensitive times appear to be under the age of 2 and at about the age of puberty or menarche.[1,2,3,4] The effects of radiation therapy also depend on the total dose of radiation, the duration of therapy, and the number of fractions given. Radiation therapy damages the chondroblasts and small blood vessels; it affects new bone formation of the periosteum as well as enchondral bone growth, causing irregular production of osteoid bone.[1] In the epiphyseal plate, radiation therapy produces arrest of chondrogenesis: failure of absorption of calcified cartilage and bone occurs in the metaphysis and in the diaphysis, modeling errors occur because of decreased periosteal activity.[3] The threshold for radiation damage to bone varies depending on that part of the skeleton irradiated, but the overall threshold dose seems to be 3000 cGy and bone death occurs beyond 5000 cGy.[4] A dose as low as 1540 cGy, however, has caused a fracture of the femoral neck.[5] Other articles have recorded similar observations.[6,7]

The initial theory as to the actual cause of radiation damage to bone was based on the death of cells. Radiation was thought to either kill individual bone cells or to interfere with their metabolism and nutrition. It now appears, however, that radiation osteonecrosis is a secondary effect mediated by damage to the vascular supply of the skeleton.[8] Following irradiation of bone, the initial effect is an inflammatory response, which occurs within a few days of the radiation. This is followed by bone atrophy caused by a combination of blood supply disturbance, interference with the cellular absorption of ions, and absence of essential nutritive substances.[9] The vascular changes following irradiation are the result of both periarterial fibrosis and direct damage to the arterial wall, mainly caused by damage to the vasa vasorum.[10] If the radiation dose is low, resorption of bone occurs, which is followed by neovascularization in 3 to 6 weeks; ultimately new bone formation occurs at 3 to 6 months.[11] On the other hand, if the radiation dose is higher, bone atrophy occurs and complications will ensue, such as scoliosis, pathologic fracture, osteonecrosis, and the formation of radiation-induced tumors.

RADIATION-INDUCED DAMAGE TO THE SPINE AND SCOLIOSIS

The effects of radiation on the spine are similar to those seen in tubular bones and basically are caused by the arrest of chondrogenesis. If the radiation field includes either the direct beam or scatter to only one half of the spine, then a scoliosis ensues. If the field includes the whole of the spine, however, generalized retardation of growth occurs, and this is best shown by measuring the sitting height of the child.[7] Much of the published literature concerns the late effects of radiation for Wilms tumors. Whitehouse[12] reviews four patients who were irradiated up to 20 years previously. His first patient received 3600 cGy over 13 days in 1935 and developed a scoliosis 10 years later, which progressively worsened. Two of his other patients developed scoliosis with a similar latent period following 6000 cGy over 35 days and 3600 cGy over 19 days respectively. His final patient developed lordosis without scoliosis. Rutherford[3] points out that postirradiation scoliosis recognized by a lateral flexion bend with little rotary component (unlike idiopathic scoliosis, which has a large rotary component). Probert[7] reported on 22 children, under the age of 15, who received spinal irradiation: 16 for lymphoma, two for medulloblastoma, and three for leukemia. By measuring the sitting height of the children they were able to show significant retardation in growth in 16 of them (72%). This would worsen if the radiation was given to children under the age of 6 or at the time of puberty. Two of his patients also developed scoliosis in spite of the fact that the radiation field included the whole spine. These and other authors postulate that this form of scoliosis occurs primarily as a result of reactive fibrosis in the soft tissues secondary to the radiation.[7,13,14] In another article, Rubin[14] describes an early experience at Strong Memorial Hospital. A group of patients received radiation therapy for Wilms tumor, neuroblastoma, and medulloblastoma. All of the children were below 16 months of age, 46% developed scoliosis over 10°, of which four cases progressed. These children had all received between 3000 and 5000 cGy over a 3- to 4-week period. Finally, Thomas[15] describes 25 long-term survivors of Wilms tumor. 54% of his patients developed scoliosis (however, only three were symptomatic) following a dose of over 2500 cGy (median dose = 3490 cGy). Five patients developed osseous hypoplasia of the illum and one patient contracted it on the rib. His findings, however, are somewhat questionable because one of his illustrations of "scoliosis" is actually not true scoliosis but is a positional curve. This would suggest that some of the so-called minor postirradiation scolioses are the result of soft tissue changes and fibrosis rather than the result of actual bony damage.

The major growth centers in the vertebral bodies are at the margins of the end plates (i.e., the ring apophyses, which like all growth centers, contan a zone of provisional calcification that bears the brunt of the radiation damage). Retardation of both chondrogenesis and osteogenesis occurs following a dose of 1000 to 2000 cGy and this results in temporary cessation of bone growth and even premature epiphyseal closure.[3,16] Bone changes in the spine are first seen approximately one year following radiation therapy, although they may occur earlier if the dose is greater than 3000 cGy or if the patient is less than 18 months old.[2,3,15] The outcome of radiation to the spine is mild to severe kyphoscoliosis, which may progress until the adolescent growth spurt occurs. At this point, scoliosis usually ceases to progress, although kyphosis may continue to increase.[3] The severity of a radiation-induced kyphoscoliosis also appears to be age-related, with changes being more pronounced if the child receives radiation prior to 2 years of age.[2]

The earliest radiographic evidence of radiation damage to the spine is subcortical lucent zones (equivalent to growth arrest lines in tubular bones), which can produce the appearance of a bone within a bone.[3,7] The vertebral bodies then develop a bulbous contour with central beaking (at a dose of 2000 cGy or more). Irregularity and scalloping of the end plates finally occurs (at a dose of over 3000 cGy).[3] A narrow interpedicular distance has also been described.[3,15] Radiographically, the hallmark of radiation-induced kyphoscoliosis is the irregularity of the end plates (Fig. 8–1a), which often have a wavy pattern that is reminiscent of that seen in Scheurerman's disease. This is often associated with anterior wedging (Fig. 8–1b). The scoliosis occurs primarily because the vertebral bodies fail to grow on one side; this is usually associated with smaller pedicles and laminae than normal. The kyphosis occurs because of the anterior wedging of the involved vertebral bodies. Associated abnormalities can often be seen, such as hypoplasia of the iliac wing or rib cage (Fig. 8–1).

Case History: Scoliosis

Radiation damage to the spine includes damage to the vertebral end plates and the production of a scoliosis convex away from the irradiated side. Figure 8–1 shows the radiation damage to the spine that occurred in an 18-year-old boy who had received radiation therapy for Hodgkin's disease 7 years earlier.

OTHER EFFECTS OF RADIATION ON THE SKELETON

Apart from scoliosis, kyphosis, and avascular necrosis, both localized and general ef-

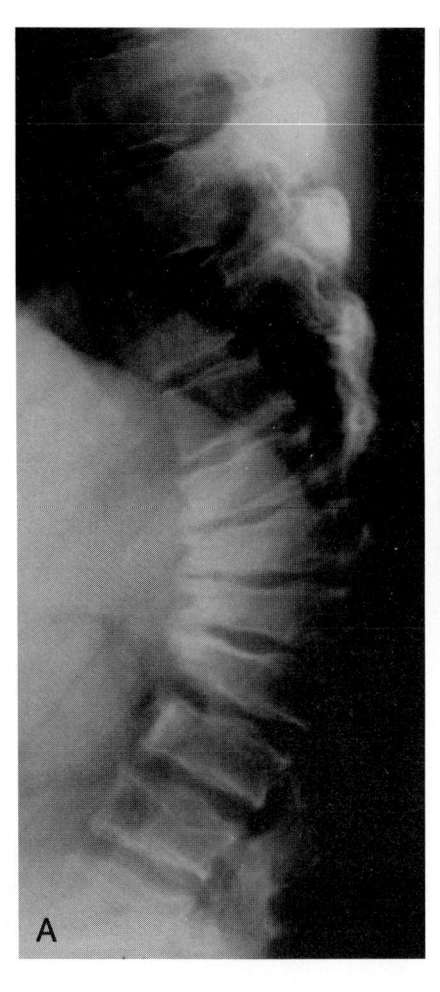

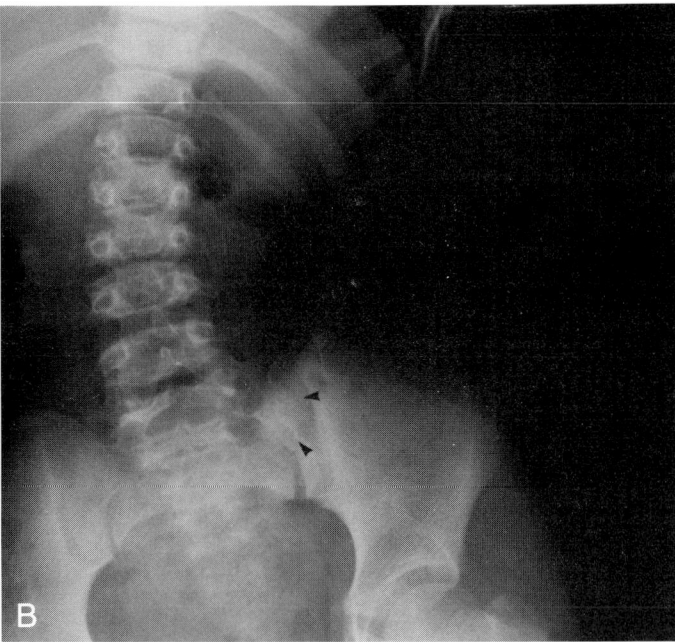

Fig. 8–1. (A) The irregular end plates and wedged vertebral bodies are characteristic of radiation damage to the spine. (B) In the same patient, atrophy of the ribs on the left as well as the scoliosis convex on the right show that the radiation portal was to the left abdomen. Note the osteochondroma on the upper aspect of the left iliac bone (arrows).

fects of irradiation on the skeleton have been described. Although rare, generalized osteoporosis can occur as a result of short-term steroid therapy; osteoporosis also can occur following premature menopause as a result of either radiation to the gonads or chemotherapy itself. Bone atrophy and localized osteoporosis may occur as a direct result of radiation therapy; reactivation of a latent infection has also been described.

GENERALIZED OSTEOPOROSIS

A number of causes may explain early osteoporosis in female patients who have or have had Hodgkin's disease. Steroid therapy is one of the commonest causes of iatrogenic osteoporosis.[17,18] Most patients with Hodgkin's disease, however, only receive relatively low doses of steroids as part of their combined chemotherapy, so generalized osteoporosis is probably rare in this group of patients. Various cytotoxic drugs have been implicated as the cause of unexplained osteoporosis in patients treated with them.[19,20] Premature menopause is becoming a significant factor in long-term survivors of Hodgkin's disease. Since radiation therapy of the ovaries is avoided as often as possible, it appears that combination chemotherapy is now a prime cause of premature menopause and appropriate hormone replacement therapy is now frequently prescribed.

BONE ATROPHY AND OSTEITIS

An effect similar to that seen with radiation to the spine occurs on any growing epiphysis that is irradiated during the treatment of Hodgkin's disease. Atrophy and hypoplasia of the upper ribs and shoulder girdle, lower ribs, and pelvis have all been described.[3,5,8] Because irradiation in Hodgkin's disease is frequently directed to the abdomen, damage to the apophyses of the ribs leads to shortening of the affected rib with premature fusion of its growth plates. Similarly, irradiation to the iliac crest leads to premature fusion and atrophy of that side of the pelvis (Figs. 8–2a and b). Bone atrophy occurs as a result of the arrest of appositional bone growth and cartilage activity, thus producing a complete cessation of bone growth.[3] In young children, acetabular dysplasia and congenital hip dysplasia, coxa valga and vara, as well as leg shortening have all been described as a result of irradation.[2] In older children, hypoplasia of the irradiated bone usually occurs after a dose of at least 2000 cGy.[2] In adults, a greater risk of fractures occurs as a result of radiation, and Dalinka[5] describes a fracture of the femoral neck occurring in a patient 5 months after receiving 1540 cGy. He also describes changes in the sacroiliac joints, including irregularities, sclerosis, widening, and calcification.

Radiation osteitis is a term that applies to the bone changes seen as a result of radiation therapy; it refers to a combination of bone atrophy, secondary osteonecrosis (avascular necrosis), localized osteoporosis, fragmentation, and osteosclerosis. Localized osteoporosis is one of the stages of radiation atrophy and osteitis. Dead bone has the same radiographic appearance as living bone, unless it impacts and collapses when it becomes denser than normal. Localized osteoporosis occurs following irradiation during the healing phase, when a new blood supply grows in and resorption of dead bone occurs.[8,9,10,11,22,23] Localized osteoporosis of the mandible and shoulder girdle is common following the use of high doses of irradiation (i.e., above 5000 cGy) for oropharyngeal carcinoma and breast cancer, but we have not seen localized osteoporosis in patients who have received radiation therapy for Hodgkin's disease.[21,22] Radiation osteitis is more common following high-dose radiation (i.e. over 5000 cGy), and is much less common since supervoltage therapy has become widespread. It was described following axillary radiation for nodal involvement in breast carcinoma.[21,22,23] We have not seen radiation osteitis following irradiation for Hodgkin's disease.

REACTIVATION OF A PREVIOUS INFECTION

Although it is a well known fact that radiation reactivates tuberculosis in the lung, it has rarely been described elsewhere apart from the mandible.[24,25] Recently, however, we have encountered a patient who either developed a new tuberculous infection of the

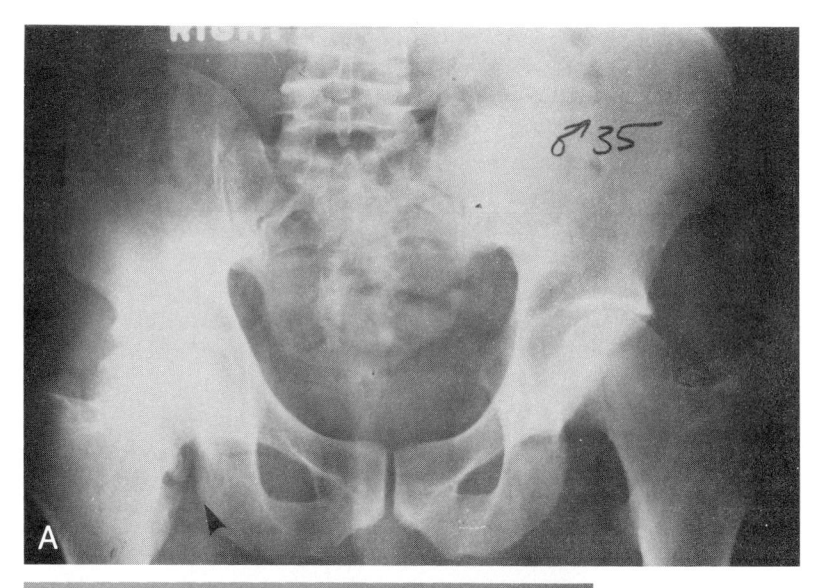

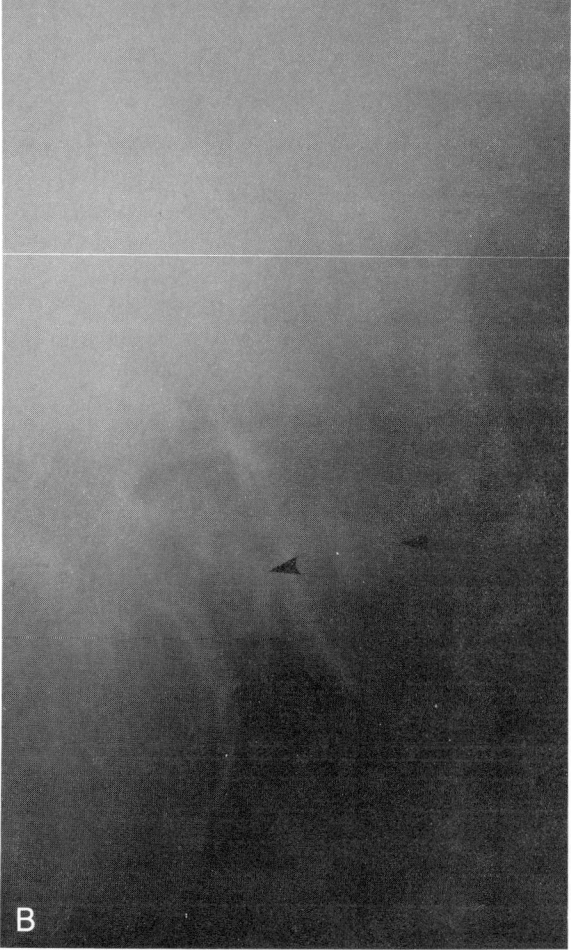

Fig. 8–2. (A) Atrophy of the right half of the pelvis. (B) A ring of osteochondromata surrounds the right femoral neck in the region of the old physeal plate (arrow). (Case courtesy of Dr. Henry Jones, Stanford University.)

spine following irradiation for Hodgkin's disease or reactivated a previous infection (Figs. 8–3a, b, and c).

Case History: Reactive Tuberculous Osteomyelitis in the Spine

Figure 8–3 shows a 40-year-old man who had received a full course of radiotherapy to his para-aortic lymph nodes for Hodgkin's disease four years previously. The disease did not recur, but he recently presented with low-back pain. 400 ml of pus was removed and a percutaneous biopsy was performed; it revealed that *Mycobacterium tuberculosis* was present.

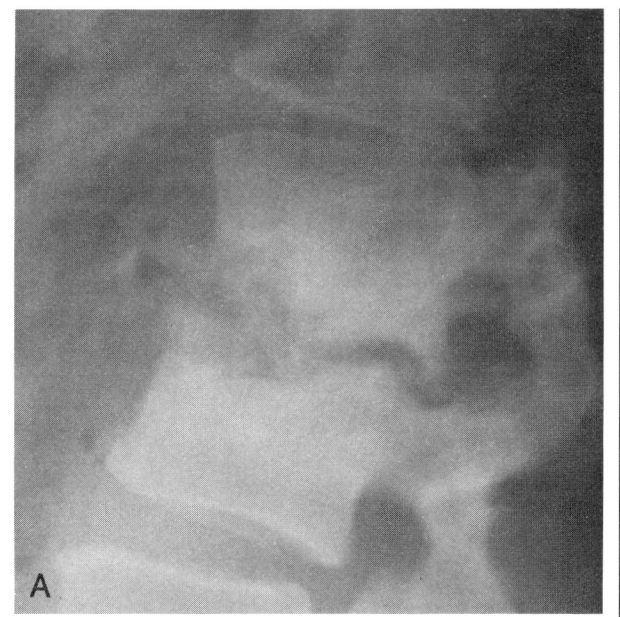

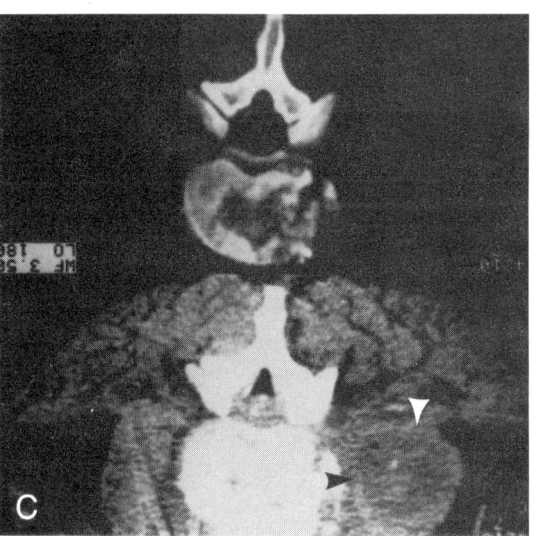

AVASCULAR NECROSIS (OSTEONECROSIS)

Avascular necrosis or osteonecrosis refers to bone death with subsequent fragmentation, usually in a femoral or humeral head. There are many causes of avascular necrosis of the femoral head, including trauma, steroid therapy, caisson disease, and pancreatitis; of the various etiologic factors, either emboli or vascular compromise are the most accepted.[26,27] Since radiation change of bone are thought to be secondary to damage to the microvasculature, causing atrophic changes in the skeleton that weakens the overall structure of the bone, this appears to support mod-

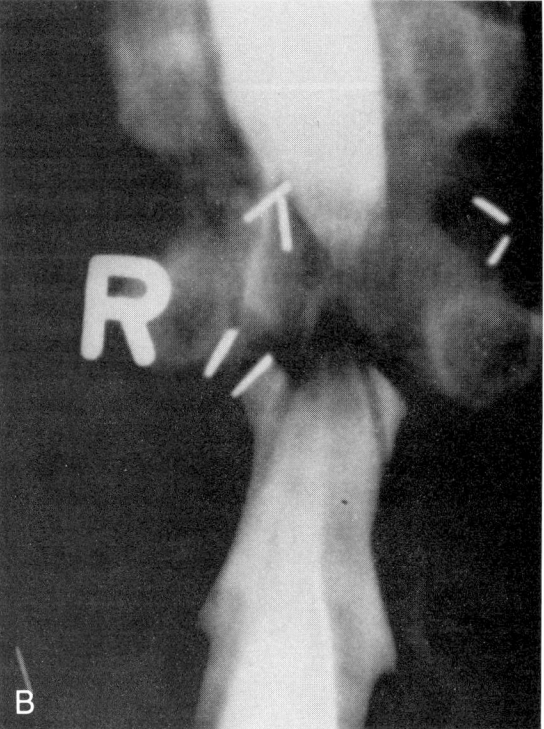

Fig. 8–3. Reactive tuberculous osteomyelitis in the spine. (A) Plain films show a destroyed disk space at L2–3 with reactive sclerosis in the surrounding vertebral bodies as well as a hint of soft tissue mass lying anteriorly. (B) A myelogram shows a virtually complete block at the same level. Note the surgical marker clips showing diagnostic excision of lymph nodes 6 years before. (C) A CT scan confirms the destruction of the vertebral body with a huge soft tissue abscess lying within the psoas muscle (arrow).

ern theories as to the cause of avascular necrosis. Depending on the age of the patient, radiation to the pelvis and hip may produce either a slipped capital femoral epiphysis in young children or avascular necrosis in adults. This is considered separately.

SLIPPED CAPITAL FEMORAL EPIPHYSIS

Characteristically, the epiphyseal slip in slipped capital femoral epiphysis, secondary to irradiation, occurs at an earlier age than the idiopathic type[28] and it has been described both in the hip and proximal humeral epiphysis following radiation for Hodgkin's disease and other tumors such as Ewing's sarcoma.[28-33] Slipped capital femoral epiphysis occurs in children irradiated for pelvic and lower adominal tumors whose hips were included in the field of irradiation.[21]

The most radiation sensitive regions of the growth plate are zones 1 (the resting zone) and 2 (the proliferating zone). If less than 1200 cGy are given, full recovery occurs. If 2400 cGy are used, there is cessation of chondrogenesis in these two zones, although there may eventually be some recovery. With over 3000 cGy, cessation of growth occurs with poor or no recovery.[30] The damaged growth plate is apparently unable to withstand the normal forces on the hip and hence the epiphysis slides off (Fig. 8–4).

Silverman[31] found eight epiphyseal plates in five children who developed slipped capital femoral epiphyses following irradiation therapy out of a total of 50 patients under the age of 15. A total of 83 plates were at risk, so the overall incidence of slipped capital femoral epiphysis is 9.6%. Of the eight plates, only four were asymptomatic and all eight were true examples of slipped capital femoral epiphysis. Three plates showed asymptomatic epiphyseal irregularity and widening; one patient had a slipped capital femoral epiphysis and was asymptomatic. In Silverman's review of these patients, no problems were encountered below a dose of 2500 cGy. The incidence of slipped capital femoral epiphysis was found to be dose related above this level. Children under 4 were at the highest risk (below 2 were most susceptible: 4 out of 8 plates, from 2 to 4: 3 out of 7 plates). The slip occurred at 8 to 10 years of age; this has also been described by other authors.[28-32] Botnick[33] described 52 children who received radiation therapy for Hodgkin's disease between 1969 and 1975 and found only one child with slipped capital femoral epiphysis. His paper, however, was written in 1976, which is too short a period for adequate follow-up. On the other hand, Wolf[32] described five patients who received radiation therapy between the ages of 3 and 10 who developed slipped capital femoral epiphysis at ages 9 to 11. Two of his patients had Hodgkin's disease; at age 9, one was treated with 3950 cGy given in 28 fractions over 49 days. This child developed slipped capital femoral epiphysis 2 years later. The other developed Hodgkin's disease at age 10, received 4000 cGy over 28 days, and developed slipped capital femoral epiphysis at age 14. Similarly, Ryan's two pa-

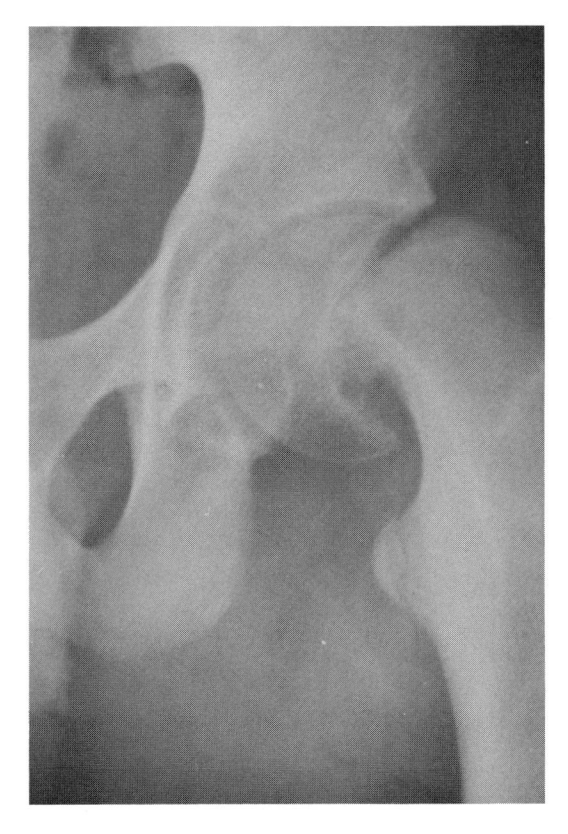

Fig. 8–4. A slipped capital femoral epiphysis, secondary to radiation therapy, is suggested by the magnitude of the slip, the rounding off of the femoral metaphysis, and the increased width of the physeal plate.

tients received pelvic irradiation for Hodgkin's disease, the first had it at 2 years (2850 cGy over 3 weeks) and developed a slip 5½ years later. The second was treated at age 6½ with 6000 cGy over 7 weeks and developed slipped capital femoral epiphysis at 9 years of age.[30]

To summarize these findings: Slipped capital femoral epiphysis following radiation therapy occurs as a result of radiation damage of the growth plate (zones 1 and 2: resting and proliferating zones); it often occurs earlier than the idiopathic variety and occurs if over 3000 cGy are given to the pelvis and hip; children under 4 (particularly those under 2) seem to be most at risk, but all children have some risk; the slip does not usually occur until age 8 to 10 and, although usually symptomatic, may not be (see Table 8–1).

Case History: Slipped Capital Femoral Epiphysis

Figure 8–4 shows an 11-year-old boy who had received radiation therapy for Hodgkin's disease 2 years before. He presents with a limp and an obvious slipped capital femoral epiphysis—an unusual condition in this age group. The radiographic appearance is rather strange for a conventional slipped capital femoral epiphysis.

AVASCULAR NECROSIS (OSTEONECROSIS)

As has been stated earlier, there are many causes of avascular necrosis (see Table 8–2) and various etiologic factors have been proposed (see Table 8–3).

Etiology

Avascular necrosis occurs in some patients with Hodgkin's disease either as a late complication of radiation or steroid therapy. In a 1981 review of 25 patients with osteonecrosis and malignant lymphoma, the common factor in all the patients was the administration of chemotherapy containing steroids.[34] However, 16 of 17 patients with Hodgkin's disease and five of eight nonHodgkin's disease lymphoma patients also received irradiation to the area that subsequently developed osteonecrosis (Fig. 8–5). Symptoms develop from 12 to 32 months following completion of either the irradiation therapy or the chemotherapy. Ihde and DeVita[35] reported four patients with Hodgkin's disease who developed avascular necrosis while receiving chemotherapy without radiation therapy. Since then, there have been several other reports of patients with Hodgkin's disease developing avascular necrosis, either following radiation therapy, chemotherapy, or both.[36-42]

In the 1970s, a number of authors have attempted to relate steroid dosage to the occurrence of avascular necrosis. Hancock[40] describes two patients with Hodgkin's disease who received high doses of prednisone and developed avascular necrosis 5 months and 1

Table 8–1. Radiation-Induced Slipped Capital Femoral Epiphysis

Author	Number of Patients	Incidence	Underlying Disease Process and Age	Radiation Dose	Slip Occurred Years Late	Comments
Silverman[31]	8	10%	Rhabdomyosarcoma	>2500 cGy	8–10	Diagnosis under age 4
	1 (of 8)		HD	2800 cGy (16 fractions)	3	
Botnick[33]	1	2%	HD	No details		
Wolf[32]	5	6% (?)				
	1 (of 5)		HD, age 9	3950 cGy (28 fractions, 49 days)	2	
	1 (of 5)		HD, age 10	4000 cGy (28 days)	4	
Ryan[30]	1		HD, age 2	2850 cGy (>3 weeks)	5½	
	1		HD, age 6	6000 cGy (7 weeks)	2½	
Libshitz[43]	1	5%	Rhabdomyosarcoma	4000 cGy	4½	
	1			3000 cGy	9	
Edeiden[28]	1		Ewings sarcoma	5500 cGy	1½	
Walker[29]	1	3%	HD, age 2½	2800 cGy	5½	
	1		HD, age 1½	6000 cGy	6	

Table 8-2. Conditions Associated with Avascular Necrosis

- Fractures
- Dislocations
- Microfractures
- Cushing's disease
- Steroid therapy
- Pancreatitis
- Alcoholism
- Caisson disease
- Decompression states
- Sickle-cell disease & traits
- Sickle-cell thalassemia
- Polyarteritis nodosa
- Systemic lupus erythematosis
- Giant-cell arteritis
- Fabry's disease
- Gaucher's disease
- Radiation therapy
- Burns
- Degenerative joint disease
- Pregnancy
- Cytotoxic drug therapy
- Hyperparathyroidism
- Familial
- Malignant infiltration

year later. Sweet[41] described four patients with Hodgkin's disease who developed avascular necrosis of their femoral heads following chemotherapy, including prednisone. The total steroid dose ranged from 3.5 to 5.7 g and the interval before avascular necrosis appeared varied from 9 to 24 months. Albala[42] also described three patients with Hodgkin's disease who received 6300, 10,280, and 13,200 mg prednisone and developed avascular necrosis 12 to 36 months later. Mould[37] attempted to discover whether the steroids or the radiation therapy caused the avascular necrosis in his seven patients. The overall incidence in his group of patients was 2.2%. All those patients received radiation therapy, but it was mainly to the neck and mediastinum and only three received radiation to the part that subsequently developed avascular necrosis. They were all young, fit, male manual workers; six of the seven developed avascular necrosis of the hip (three bilateral) and one of the humeral head. This highly supports the theory that steroids are the primary cause of avascular necrosis in these patients.

Thus, it appears that although high-dose steroid therapy is mainly to blame for osteonecrosis, radiation produces further damage to the area, thus predisposing the femoral or humeral head to osteonecrosis. Radiation itself is known to be a cause of osteonecrosis.

Table 8-3. Etiologic Factors Possibly Involved in Producing Avascular Necrosis

- Post-traumatic
- Embolic
- Small vessel disease and vasculitis
- Deposition of abnormal cells
- Unknown

This may also be seen in association with protrusio acetabuli, which occurs presumably as a result of bone atrophy.[43] Hence, avascular necrosis in long-term survivors of Hodgkin's disease is probably the result of steroid therapy, although radiation therapy may cause further damage and it is difficult if not impossible to separate the two etiologic factors.

Pathophysiology. Many mechanisms have been postulated for the cause of avascular necrosis following corticosteroid therapy. These include vasculitis, microfractures, fat embolism, abnormalities of coagulation, and capillary fragility.[44] Presumably, radiation therapy causes avascular necrosis in the femoral head by affecting the chondrogenesis, by causing microfractures, and by producing vascular changes that in turn lead to a vascular necrosis.[43]

Clinical Features. Most patients with avascular necrosis complain of a vague ache or pain in the affected joint. The pain is usually aggravated by weight bearing. Gait is affected, although the range of motion is usually normal.

Radiographic Findings. Once avascular necrosis has occurred, it is usually 6 to 9 months before any radiographic changes become visible.[44,45] Bone scanning is a more sensitive method for detecting early osteonecrosis, particularly using the vascular phase of the scan. The earliest radiographic finding in avascular necrosis of the femoral head is usually the presence of a "crescent sign," which is best seen on the "frog leg" view of the hip and represents a fracture through the subchondral trabecular bone (Fig. 8-6a). However a mixed sclerotic and lytic pattern in the central area of the femoral head may also be seen (Fig.

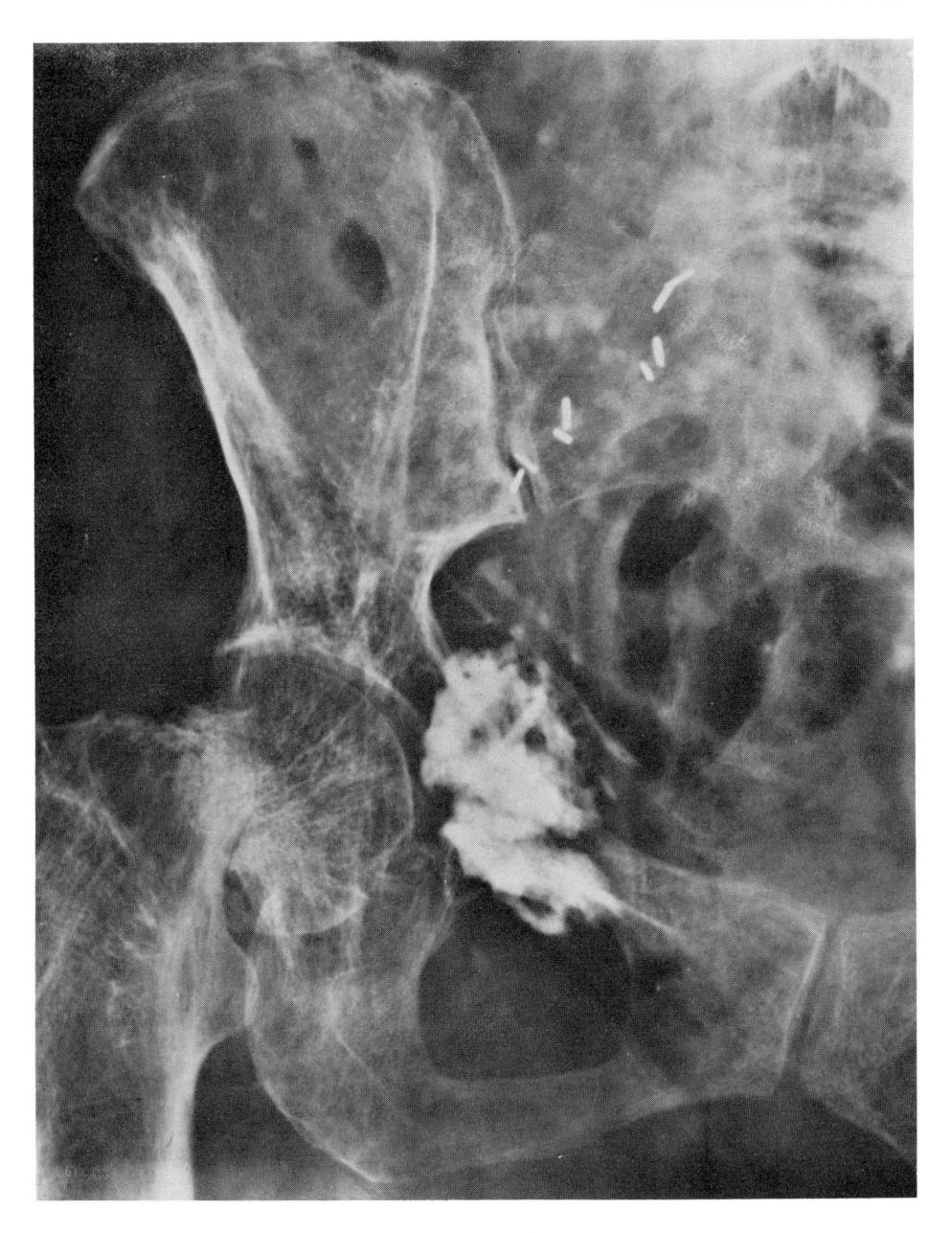

Fig. 8–5. Radiation osteitis in a patient with spindle cell sarcoma of the pelvis who had been heavily irradiated 30 years earlier. Note stress fracture associated with irradiation and the large mass of dystrophic calcification. These gross changes are rarely seen. (From Smith, J. Radiation-induced sarcoma. Clin. Radiol. 33:205, 1982.)

8–6b). As the osteonecrosis progresses, the subchondral bone collapses. This leads to the more characteristic findings of collapse of the femoral head with fragmentation and a clear-cut sclerotic margin between the dead bone and the normal bone (Fig. 8–6c). These findings can be seen in avascular necrosis of any etiology. Similar findings may also be seen in the humeral head. There are various methods of assessing moderate to severe avascular necrosis, including radiography, radionuclide studies, and CT scanning.[44] The early detection of avascular necrosis, however, has always been a radiographic problem since radiographs are usually negative and bone scans are only useful if the disease is unilat-

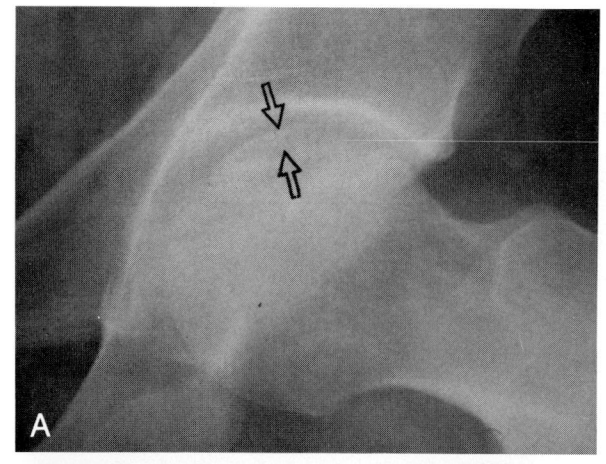

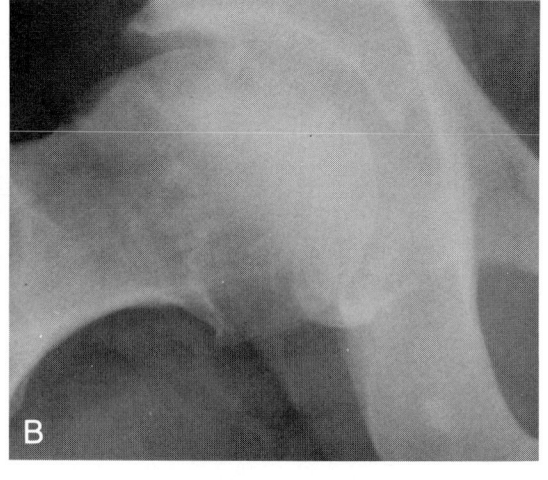

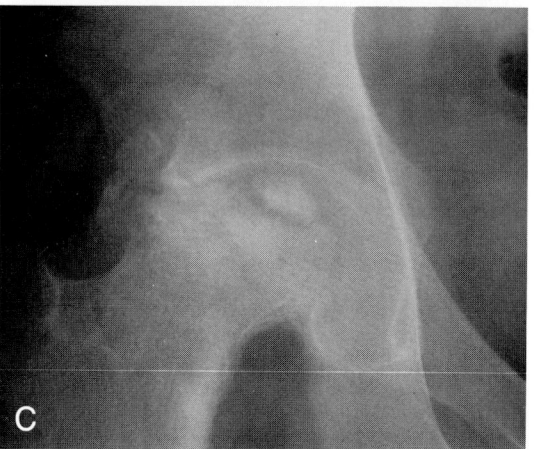

Fig. 8–6. Avascular Necrosis Following Radiation Therapy. (A) The earliest evidence of avascular necrosis in the hip is usually a "crescent sign" or a lucency seen just under the subchondral bone at the outer margin of the femoral head (arrows). (B) As the avascular necrosis progresses, further collapse with sclerosis in the center of the femoral head often occurs. Note the secondary degenerative arthritis with osteophytes in this patient who received radiation therapy for Hodgkin's disease five years earlier. (C) Without adequate treatment the femoral head will collapse further, frequently with fragmentation. This is associated with chondronecrosis and premature degenerative arthritis, which is well shown in this man of 22 less than three years after receiving radiation therapy for Hodgkin's disease.

eral (Figs. 8–7a and b). Recently, magnetic resonance imaging (MRI) has proven to be useful in the early diagnosis of avascular necrosis;[45,46,47] there are a number of characteristic patterns, depending on the stage of the disease, starting with a relatively well defined oblique area of decreased intensity running across the femoral head and neck that advances to total loss of signal in the infarcted femoral head.

Treatment and Prevention

The best treatment of avascular necrosis is prevention. Thus, the lower the dose of prednisone, the lower the risk of avascular necrosis. The use of a mantle, which excludes the femoral or humeral head, decreases the incidence of avascular necrosis following radiation therapy. Once early avascular necrosis has occurred and the patient is complaining of symptoms, prolonged nonweight bearing by using crutches often allows the femoral head to heal, although premature degenerative arthritis will almost certainly follow in 10 to 15 years. If the avascular necrosis progresses, either a femoral endoprosthesis or a total hip replacement will have to be performed.

RADIATION-INDUCED TUMORS

The occurrence of radiation-induced osteochondromas and osteosarcomas is well accepted. Rutherford[3] reviewed his own experience and described 35 cases of radiation-induced exostoses. The radiation dose ranged from 1600 to 6425 cGy and the exostoses occurred anywhere: ribs, ilium, clavicles, scapula, and vertebral bodies as well as long bones. Rutherford also reviewed the occurrence of postirradiation sarcomas; these were

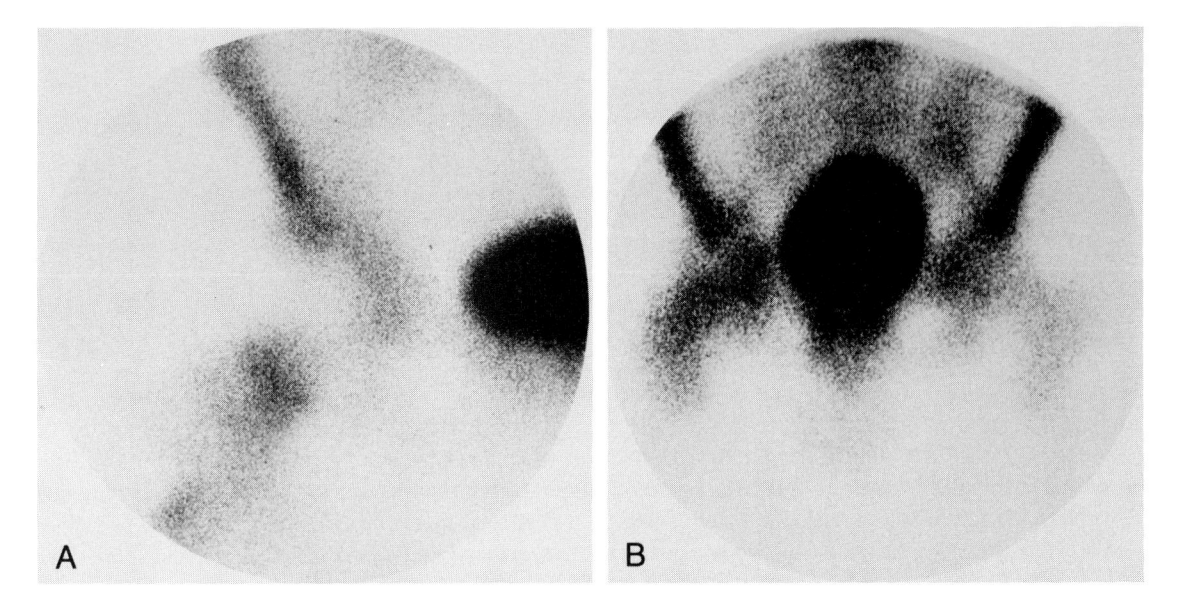

Fig. 8–7. (A) The initial bone scan of a patient with avascular necrosis shows a decrease in uptake in the region of the right femoral head—a cold or photopenic scan, although increased uptake is apparent in the intertrochanteric region on the same side. (B) A scan performed one month later shows increased uptake to the head and neck on the affected side.

mainly osteosarcomas, but fibrosarcomas and chondrosarcomas have also been described. The radiation dose varied from 1200 to 24,000 cGy and the sarcomas may appear up to 30 years after the irradiation. Parker[4] also considered radiation-induced tumors and found that osteosarcoma following radiation occurred in 1 of 3000 patients. These entities are considered separately.

RADIATION-INDUCED OSTEOCHONDROMA

Radiation-induced osteochondromas can develop in any irradiated enchondral bone in children until growth ceases.[24] The latent period between the appearance of an osteochondroma following radiation varies in different studies.[3,4,48,49] The majority of the exostoses develop within 5 years after irradiation, although they may occur as early as 3 years or as late as 7 years later. The tumor may occur following both supervoltage and orthovoltage treatment. In the study reported by Libshitz and Cohen, the lowest dose was 1200 cGy using 6 MEV irradiation and the lowest orthovoltage was 3000 cGy. Radiation-induced osteochondromas may grow just like the spontaneously occurring lesions, particularly at the time of the pubertal growth spurt (Fig. 8–8).

Radiation-induced osteochondromas are completely benign, and malignant change in these tumors is virtually undescribed, although Perez[50] reported that a low-grade chondrosarcoma occurred in a radiation-induced osteochondroma 12 years after radiotherapy. These lesions are usually asymptomatic and are often detected on routine radiographs of the chest or extremities. The incidence of radiation-induced osteochondroma is uncertain, but they appear to occur in about 1 to 5% of all irradiated bones. Jaffe[48] recently described 200 long-term survivors, of whom 6% developed osteochondromas; 47 of these children had Hodgkin's disease and two developed radiation-induced osteochondromas (an incidence of 4%). Of these lesions, the majority were single, but a few patients developed multiple osteochondromas.

Aggressive treatment of Hodgkin's disease with total-nodal irradiation and intensive chemotherapy has prolonged patient survival. At Memorial Sloan-Kettering Cancer Center (MSKCC), the average rate of survival between 1950 and 1954 was 45%. This rate increased to 80% between 1970 and 1974. In-

Table 8–4. Radiation-Induced Osteochondroma (RIO)

Author	Patient Population	Age at Diagnosis of HD	Radiation Dose	Number of Years Later RIO Occurred	Comments
Rutherford et al.[3]	35—Variety of tumors	1–9 years	1600–6425 cGy	5 years 3–7 years	RIO occurs anywhere in field
Lipschitz et al.[49]	14—4 had HD	5 years	1200–3000 cGy	3–16 years	
Perez et al.[50]	No details				1–5% incidence
Jaffe et al.[48]	200—47 had HD 2 had RIO	1–11½ years	1500–5500 cGy	3–13½ years	6% incidence
Nenhauser et al.[2]	General 5/34				14% incidence

creased survival has unfortunately led to the risk of new tumors, the best known being leukemia and nonHodgkin's lymphoma. Several other complications have been described.

Among the least common of these complications are sarcomas that arise within the irradiated field, either in bone or soft tissue.[51-55] Reports from some centers indicate that these soft tissue sarcomas are more common than primary sarcomas of bone. The histologic variety of soft tissue sarcomas exceeds that of bone. Soft tissue osteosarcoma, malignant fibrous histiocytoma, and fibrosarcoma may be found; however, liposarcoma, leiomyosarcoma, and neurogenic sarcoma have predominated.[56,57]

Reports of radiation-induced malignant tumors of bone date from the early 1920s. Beck was the first of several European physicians to report sarcomas in bone following radiation treatment of tuberculous arthritis. The exact doses were frequently unknown, but the reports suggested that excessive amounts were given at frequent intervals over a long period. When this danger was recognized, sarcoma as a complication of radiation therapy for tuberculous arthritis was no longer seen. Jaffe regarded this clinical experience as perhaps the best evidence that external irradiation could induce sarcomas of bone. In the United States, the experience with luminous dial painters who ingested ^{226}Ra while pointing

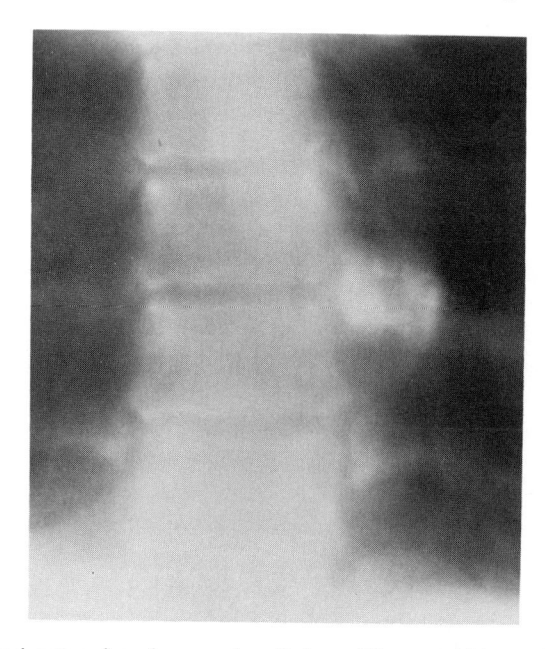

Fig. 8–8. Radiation-induced osteochondroma of a rib in a 17-year-old boy who had had radiation to the thoracic spine 10 years earlier for Hodgkin's disease, which was discovered incidentally on chest radiographs without any symptoms. (From Smith, J., O'Connell, R.S., Huvos, A.G. et al. Hodgkin's disease complicated by radiation sarcoma in bone. Br. J. Radiol. 53:314, 1980.)

their brushes received considerable publicity, and Martland and Humphries' study of these patients became widely known.

Beginning about 1965, many institutions began to treat patients with Hodgkin's disease more aggressively than before. In addition to therapeutic irradiation of active sites, extensive prophylactic radiation was given, and various chemotherapeutic regimens were often added to the protocol. As a result, there has been a significant improvement in the 5-year survival rate, with a consequent increase in the number of Hodgkin's patients who live past the minimum latent period (about 4 years) necessary for the development of radiation sarcomas. Although radiation-induced sarcomas from causes other than Hodgkin's disease have been regularly seen at MSKCC in small numbers over the years, the radiation sarcomas associated with Hodgkin's disease have dramatically increased since the 1970s.

From 1935 (when records were first kept of this condition) to 1974, only one patient had a radiation sarcoma secondary to Hodgkin's disease. Between 1974 and 1985, 15 cases have been well documented. Since 1974, 16 patients have had radiation sarcomas, which developed in normal bone following irradiation of a variety of tumors other than Hodgkin's disease. Thus, Hodgkin's disease constituted 48% of all cases of radiation-induced sarcomas seen at Memorial Sloan-Kettering Cancer Center in the last 12 years. This primary tumor is associated with radiation-induced sarcoma in approximately 70 patients. It has surpassed other more common cancers such as breast cancer, which was formerly the most common underlying cancer. We believe that this increased incidence in the different decades is significant and not related to selection factors.

The ages of the patients with Hodgkin's disease at the time of original diagnosis ranged from 11 to 48 years, with a median of 27 years and a mean of 25 years. The latent period varied from 4 to 31 years, with a median of 8 years and a mean of 11.5 years. The mean survival of this group was 12 months. Review of the 16 patients with the non-Hodgkin's group of sarcomas, seen since 1974, revealed a range of 4 months to 63 years of age, with a median of 38.5 years and a mean of 33 years. The median latent period was 12.5 years, with a mean of 13 years and a range of 4 to 23 years. There were four long-term survivors, but the mean survival for the group as a whole was only 18 months.

Twelve of the Hodgkin's disease patients received treatment with Co-60 gamma rays or with x-rays generated at 1 to 6-MEV. In 11 of the cases, the treatment was completed in one cycle lasting a few weeks. In five, it lasted up to 5 years. The median dose for Hodgkin's disease was 4000 cGy.

Radiation sarcomas most commonly involve the bones of the chest, wall, and shoulder, accounting for 12 of the 16 tumors in our series. There were three lesions in the upper humerus, two clavicular lesions, two sternal lesions, two lesions in the scapula, and two lesions in the spine. A single rib lesion occurred. Three lesions involved the pelvis and one involved the femur. This femoral lesion was unique because we believed it represented a primary Hodgkin's disease of the femur, an uncommon tumor. Despite the fact that all the tumors were secondary to Hodgkin's disease, the appearance of the tumor varied considerably. The largest of the tumors were those invading the pelvis. Two of these were truly huge and occupied almost the entire hemipelvis. One of the other lesions was much smaller. The bulky tumors were osteosarcomas, and the smaller lesion was a malignant fibrous histiocytoma. The unusual size of the pelvic lesions at the time of presentation is difficult to explain, but two other radiation sarcomas with huge pelvic lesions have also been seen related to other cancers. In three patients, the presenting symptom of the sarcomas was pathologic fracture. In one case particularly, an underlying sarcoma was totally unexpected, both clinically and radiographically. One of the clavicular lesions was bulky and involved the sternum as well. The other clavicular lesion was much smaller. The sternal lesions were relatively small, as were the scapular lesions. Soft tissue masses were frequently difficult to recognize. Radiation osteitis was relatively uncommon and was best recognized in patients with lytic lesions. It is frequently impossible to diagnose radiation osteitis before the histologic examination, and

Table 8-5. Postradiation Sarcoma of Bone in Hodgkin's Disease
Group I: Details of Clinical, Radiologic, and Radiation Therapy of 16 Cases. Lesions Involved Previously Normal Bone.
Group II: Sarcoma Developing in Primary Hodgkin's Disease of Bone.

	Case No. Initial Sex Age/Year at Irradiation	Bone Involved Year	Latent Period (Yrs)	Radiation Data	Histology of Sarcoma	Radiologic Appearance Radiation Osteitis	Sarcoma Treatment	Outcome	Comment
Group I	1 M.S. Male 28 1937	Left 1st rib, 1953.	16	Brachytherapy with Ra 226. Small doses of x-rays. Factors unknown. 1938, 1939–40, MSKCC.	Osteosarcoma	Films not available for review.	Radiation therapy	Died 14 mo later	
	2 J.S.B. Female 26 1966	Right upper humerus, 1974.	13	Co-60 R Neck; 3000 cGy in 21 days. Irradiated Elsewhere.	Osteosarcoma	Sclerotic with periosteal reaction. Soft tissue mass.	Resection	Died 1 yr later	14, 23
	3 H.S. Male 30 1970	Upper sternum, 1975.	8	Co-60 3600 cGy in 21 days. Irradiated Elsewhere.	Osteosarcoma	7cm mixed lytic & sclerotic changes. Expansile, partially eroded cortex. Radiation Osteitis.	Resection	Died 6 mo later	Bilateral hip replacements for AVN 1 yr prior to sarcoma. Chemotherapy.
	4 G.B. Male 34 1952	Scapula acromion, 1975.	5	250kv 05 Cu 70cm 18 × 18 field. Dose to scapula about 5000 cGy in 3 wks. Marked telangiectasia & fibrosis. Irradiated Elsewhere.	Malignant fibrous histiocytoma	3cm lytic lesion with pathologic fracture. Radiation Osteitis.	Resection	Died 6 mo later	
	5 A.S. Male 14 1972	Left humerus diaphysis (prox), 1976.	23	6 MeV x-rays 4000 cGy in 28 days MSKCC.	Fibrosarcoma	8cm pathologic fracture. Bulky, mixed pattern. Radiation Osteitis.	Palliative	Died 6 mo later	Chemotherapy
	6 A.Y. Female 36 1970	Scapula acromion, 1976.	4	Radiation to numerous fields 4 MeV x-rays 4000 cGy, 1972. Only 1 of mantle fields reached other scapula. Irradiated Elsewhere.	Malignant fibrous histiocytoma	5cm lytic lesion in scapula soft tissue mass. Radiation Osteitis.	Resection	Died 2½ yrs later	
	7 R.L. Male 29 1971	Sternum, 1977.	4	4050 cGy mantle 6 MEV Linac. MSKCC.	Osteosarcoma	7cm blastic lesion with soft tissue mass.	Resection Chemotherapy	Died 1 yr later	Chemotherapy
	8 D.F. Female 11 1968	Humerus upper, 1/3 1978.	6	Left spine & pelvis, March–June, 1968. 12-20-69-1-5-70 Co-60 3000 cGy to entire scapula including upper humerus. No details. MSKCC.	Osteosarcoma	10cm sclerotic mass with periosteal reaction and pathologic fracture.	Resection	Died 1 yr later	Developed leukemia terminally. Chemotherapy.

# / Patient	Site, year	Age	Irradiation details	Sarcoma type	Tumor description	Treatment	Outcome	Comments
9 G.C. Male 21 1971	Right hemipelvis (ilium & pubis), 1979	8	4000 cGy on linac, Aug-Oct 1972 to lumbar spine & pelvis. MSKCC	Osteosarcoma	15 cm (plus) tumor, blastic, involving right hemipelvis.	Chemotherapy	Died 6 mo later	Developed leukemia terminally. Chemotherapy.
10 D.C. Male 16 1953	Sternum, clavicle, 1980.	17	1963-5053 cGy to thymus CS 137. High voltage Photons 4400 cGy. Irradiated Elsewhere.	Malignant fibrous histiocytoma	Bulky tumor plus 8 cm soft tissue mass.	Chest wall resection	Died 1½ yr later	Calcified mediastinal nodes. Pulm. mets.
11 R.G. Female 13 1972	Right hemipelvis, ilium, pubis & ischium, 1980.	8	Co-60 10-11/72 3400 cGy to inverted Y plus 1000 cGy right iliac & femoral nodes. Irradiated Elsewhere.	Osteosarcoma	Massive tumor 25 cm. Soft tissue tumor. No radiation osteitis.	Right hemipelvectomy	Died 1 yr	Post-op complications.
Group I 12 D.C. Male 48 1971	10th dorsal vertebra, 1982.	10	Mantle field elsewhere in 1971. 3500 cGy inverted Y at MSKCC. 6 MEV 1971. 3550 cGy including 1500 cGy to para-aortic & spleen, 1972. Irradiated Elsewhere and MSKCC.	Chondrosarcoma	Mixed blastic & lytic disease. Soft tissue mass.	Resection	Died 1 yr	Lung mets
13 H.B. Female 31 1954	2nd thoracic vertebra, 1982.	31	Irradiated in 1954. Skin changes & radiographic changes. Irradiated Elsewhere.	Osteosarcoma	Osteoblastic Osteosarcoma 3cm.	Biopsy followed by resection surgery	Cardiac/arrest following definitive surgery.	Marked calcification in mediastinal nodes.
14 T.W. Female 24 1961	Clavicle medial, 1985	21	Irradiated in Cuba in 1961. Factors unknown but skin changes present in 1966. Irradiated at MSKCC Jan-Feb 1966. 1 MEV dose to mediastinum. 3700 cGy anterior & 1500 cGy to medial clavicle. Irradiated Elsewhere and MSKCC.	Malignant fibrous histiocytoma	5m mixed lytic & blastic lesion, soft tissue mass.	Resection	Alive NED	Alive NED marked nodal calcification in mediastinum.
15 J.W. Male 30 1972	Ilium & sacrum, 1985.	13 yrs	Total nodal irradiation with 6 MEV Aug 72–March 73. 4000 cGy reached the site of the subsequent sarcoma in 7 months. MSKCC.	Malignant fibrous histiocytoma	Mixed lytic-blastic lesion. Bulky soft tissue mass. Radiation osteitis.	Chemotherapy, hemipelvectomy.	Died 6 months later.	Treatment completed by protracted treatment. Patient failed to appear for appointments.
Group II 16 L.F. Male 13 1975	Lower femur, 1981.	6 4	Co-60 11/75-12/75 4570 cGy in 31 days. 8-3-23/77 1000 cGy 20 days. MSKCC.	Osteosarcoma	Very bulky sclerotic lesion with soft tissue mass. No radiation osteitis. Pathologic fracture.	Resection	Alive NED.	Unique case of RIS following primary HD. Chemotherapy.

even then it may be difficult. Recognition of skin fibrosis and telangiectasia, however, may lead one to suspect the diagnosis.

In three of the patients, prominent calcification in mediastinal nodes was noted and interpreted as a manifestation of radiation necrosis. The mediastinum was irradiated in 11 patients in this study. The occurrence of radiation necrosis with visible calcification in three of eleven patients is a higher percentage than is usually noted with plain films.

The histologic examination of these tumors revealed nine osteosarcomas, five malignant fibrous histiocytomas, one fibrosarcoma, and one chondrosarcoma.

The criteria established at Memorial Sloan-Kettering Cancer Center by Cahan et al. in 1948 has stood the test of time and are generally widely accepted:
1. The tumor must have occurred in an irradiated field.
2. There must have been a symptom-free interval of several years between the first irradiation and the diagnosis of bone tumor. The shortest latent period we have seen in this series is 4 years.
3. The diagnosis of the radiation tumor must be confirmed histologically.
4. Good evidence that the bone was not the site of the similar tumor at the time of irradiation must be present. In one of our cases, the Hodgkin's disease was primary in the bone, but the tumor that appeared after a 4-year, symptom-free period was an osteogenic sarcoma.

Chemotherapy has frequently been suggested as a factor in inducing radiation sarcomas; however, only six of the patients received chemotherapy at the time of initial therapy for Hodgkin's disease.

Patients with advanced Hodgkin's disease have impaired immunologic response, which may remain after remission. Immunosuppression, either inherent in the disease or subsequent to therapy, may have disrupted or altered the defense mechanisms of the host to oncogenic stimuli. It is becoming important to modify the intensity of therapy in cases of less advanced disease to avoid late neoplastic effects. Patients with disseminated disease, however, should not be denied optimal initial therapy for fear of late complications. It is important that all patients be observed for prolonged periods since secondary malignant neoplasms may occur. It is also important that all patients with Hodgkin's disease should have these neoplastic complications reported.

Another factor that may influence the possibility of carcinogenesis in bone is the volume of osseous tissue exposed. In patients with Hodgkin's disease who receive total-nodal radiation, about 25% of all the osseous tissue in the body is included in the fields. Other common treatment plans, such as those for carcinoma of the breast or cervix, involve only 3% and 9% of osseous tissue.[29] We have reviewed the literature on reported cases of Hodgkin's disease, and these total 12 cases. The fact that other authors have reported similar findings indicates that these patients are not limited to Memorial Sloan-Kettering Cancer Center.

Case History

Figure 8–9 shows mixed lytic and blastic changes in the upper humerus of an 18-year-old girl who presented with a backache and a nodal mass 9 years earlier. Radiographs revealed a destructive lesion in the lumbar spine. She was staged as IVB and given 3000 cGy on a 6-MEV linear accelerator. She later developed a right axillary node and was given further radiation of 3000 cGy. The right humerus was in the port. The patient presented in 1978 with a pathologic fracture. Histologic changes revealed osteosarcoma. She was treated with high-dose methotrexate protocol. She died one year after the diagnosis of radiation-induced sarcoma was made.

Case History

A 35-year-old woman presented with a mass in the left axilla (Fig. 8–10). Radiologic evaluation revealed hilar mediastinal adenopathy. She received 4000 cGy to the neck, both supraclavicular areas, and both axillae. She developed Hodgkin's disease of the right breast and was given 4000 cGy to the breast. One year later she developed enlargement of the right axillary nodes and 4000 cGy were given to the region. Four years after her initial presentation she developed destruction in her scapula (arrow) and soft tissue mass. Despite chemotherapy and amputation the patient

THE SKELETAL SYSTEM   199

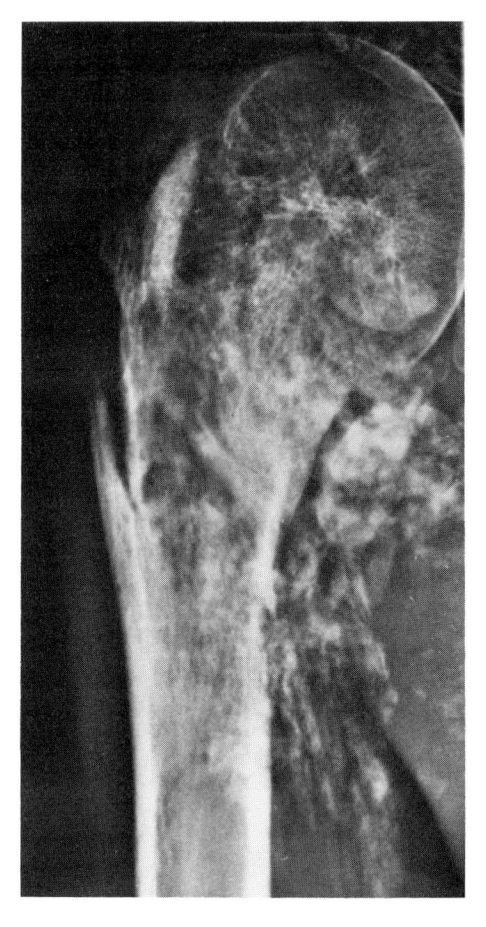

Fig. 8–9. Mixed lytic and blastic changes in the upper humerus.

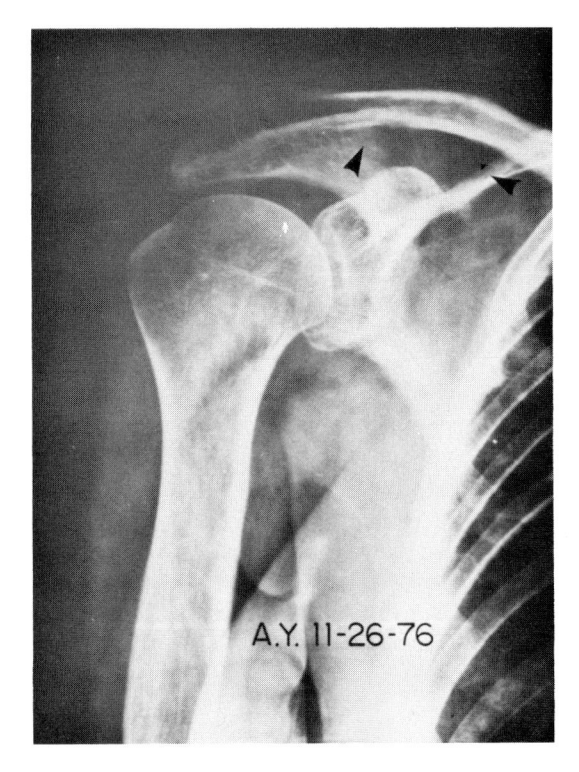

Fig. 8–10. Destruction in the scapula and soft tissue mass four years after initial treatment for Hodgkin's disease. (From Smith, J., O'Connell, R.S., Huvos, A.G. et al. Hodgkin's disease complicated by radiation sarcoma in bone. Br. J. Radiol. 53:314, 1980.)

died 2-and-a-half years after the initial diagnosis.

Case History

Figure 8–11 shows a predominantly blastic lesion involving the humeral head and metaphysis in a 56-year-old man who presented with a destructive lesion in his scapula 25 years earlier. He had a nodal mass excised from his axilla and was given 3000 cGy. He had no recurrence of disease until he fractured his right acromion process. A biopsy revealed malignant fibrous histiocytoma. Despite amputation and resection he died within nine months.

Case History

The 29-year-old man in Figure 8–12 presented with a left supraclavicular mass of short duration, which on biopsy revealed Hodgkin's disease. He received intensive chemotherapy for several courses. He was given 3000 cGy to the medastinum and an abdominal strip anteriorly and posteriorly. He developed enlarged para-aortic nodes and received several courses of chemotherapy. He developed bilateral osteonecrosis of the femoral heads. Four years following his initial presentation a mass of the sternum appeared, which revealed osteosarcoma after a biopsy was performed. The sternum was resected but the patient died six months later.

The radiation effects on the skeleton in long-term survivors of Hodgkin's disease are discussed with reference to the pathophysiology. Radiation-induced damage to the spine is now largely restricted to the presence of retarded growth in the irradiated vertebral bodies although scoliosis may still be seen occasionally. Other effects include both generalized and localized osteoporosis, bone atrophy and radiation osteitis, slipped capital femoral epiphysis, and avascular necrosis. Fi-

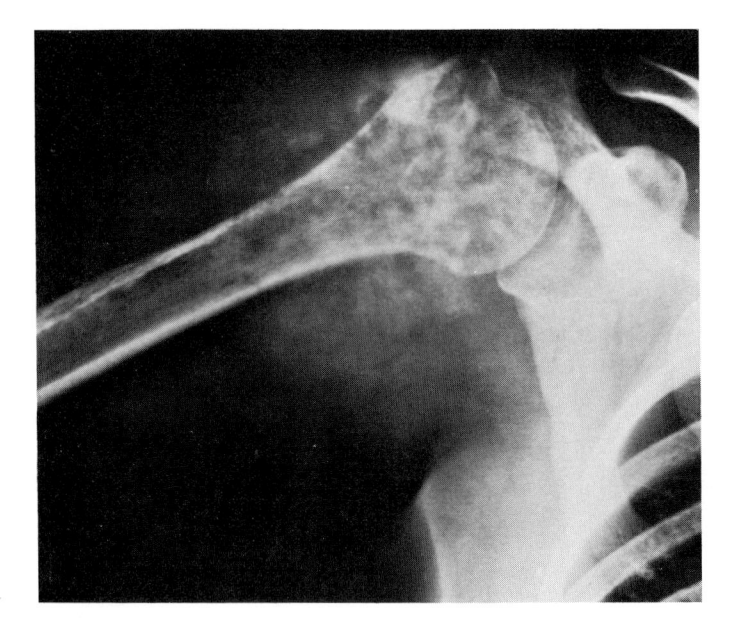

Fig. 8-11. A predominantly blastic lesion involving the humeral head and metaphysis. (From Smith, J., O'Connell, R.S., Huvos, A.G. et al. Hodgkin's disease complicated by radiation sarcoma in bone. Br. J. Radiol. 53:314, 1980.)

nally, radiation-induced osteochondromas and sarcomas are discussed. Many radiation effects do not appear until 3 to 5 years following irradiation, and they were never seen in those patients who died within 2 to 3 years of diagnosis. With longer survival rates, however, it is obvious that we shall be seeing more complications of radiation in the skeletons of patients with Hodgkin's disease in the future.

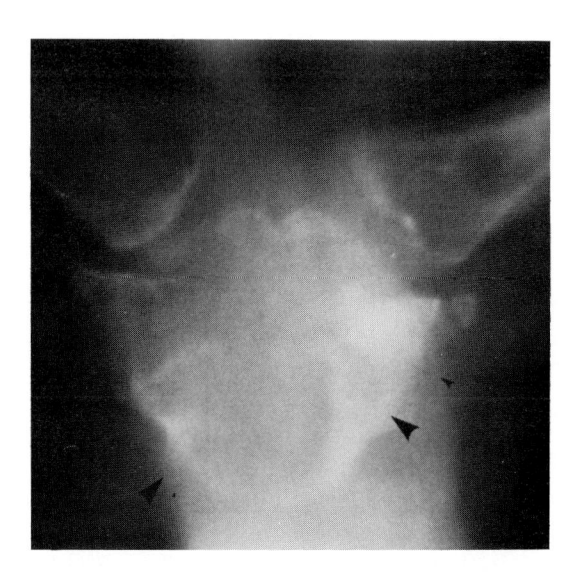

Fig. 8-12. Sclerotic changes on the periphery of the tumor (arrows) reveal osteoradionecrosis and not tumor. (From Smith, J., O'Connell, R.S., Huvos, A.G. et al. Hodgkin's disease complicated by radiation sarcoma in bone. Br. J. Radiol. 53:314, 1980.)

REFERENCES

1. Probert, J.C. and Parker, B.R. Effects of radiation therapy on bone growth. Radiology 114:155, 1975.
2. Neuhauser, E.B.D., Wittenborg, M.H., Beman, C.Z. et al. Irradiation effects of roentgen therapy on the growing spine. Radiology 59:637–650, 1952.
3. Rutherford, H. and Dodd, G.S. Complications of radiation therapy: growing bone. Semin. Roentgenol. 9:15, 1974.
4. Parker, R.G. and Berry, H.C. Later effects of therapeutic irradiation on the skeleton and bone marrow. Cancer 37:1162, 1976.
5. Dalinka, M.K., Edeiken, J., and Finkelstein, J.B. Complications of radiation therapy: adult bone. Semin. Roentgenol. 9:29, 1974.
6. Shimanovskaya, K. and Shirman, A.D. Radiation Injury of Bone. Elmsford, Pergamon Press Inc., 1983.
7. Probert, J.S., Parker, B.R., and Kaplan, H.S. Growth retardation in children after megavoltage irradiation of the spine. Cancer 32:634, 1973.
8. Marx, R.E. Osteonecrosis: a new concept of its pathophysiology. J. Oral Maxillofac. Surg. 41(5):283–288, 1983.
9. Ergun, H. and Howland, W.J. Postradiation atrophy of mature bone. CRC Crit. Rev. Diagn. Imaging 12(3):225–243, 1980.
10. Johnson, A.G., Lane, B., Harding Rains, A.J. et al. Large artery damage after x radiation. Br. J. Radiol. 42:937–939, 1969.
11. King, M.A., Casarett, G.W., and Wever, D.A. A study of irradiation bone: I. histopathologic and physiologic changes. J. Nucl. Med. 20(11):1142–1149, 1979.
12. Whitehouse, W.N. and Lampe, I. Osseous damage in irradiation of renal tumors in infancy and childhood. Am. J. Roentgenol. 70:721, 1953.
13. Roseborough E.J. Irradiation induced kyphosis. Clin. Orthop. 128:101, 1977.

14. Rubin, P., Duthie, R.B., and Young, L.W. The significance of scoliosis in postirradiated Wilm's tumor and neuroblastoma. Radiology 79:539, 1962.
15. Thomas, P.R.M. et al. Late effects of treatment of Wilm's tumor. Int. J. Radiat. Oncol. Biol. Phys. 9:651, 1983.
16. Heaston, D.K., Libshitz, H.I., and Chan, R.C. Skeletal effects of megavoltage irradiation in survivors of Wilm's tumor. A.J.R. 133(3):389–395, 1979.
17. Corticosteroid-induced bone collapse. B.M.J. 1:581–582, 1972.
18. Cruess, R.L. Cortisone-induced avascular necrosis of the femoral head. J. Bone Joint Surg. 59:308–317, 1977.
19. Kenzora, J.E. and Glimcher, M.J. The role of renal bone disease in the production of transplant osteonecrosis. Orthopaedics 4:303–313, 1981.
20. Schwartz, A.M. and Leonidas, J.C. Methotrexate osteopathy. Skeletal Radiol. 11:13–16, 1984.
21. Titterington, W.P. Osteomyelitis and osteoradionecrosis of the jaws. J. Oral Med. 26:7–16, 1971.
22. Bragg D.G., Shidnia, H., Chu, F.C.H. et al. The clinical and radiographic aspects of radiation osteitis. Radiology 97:103–111, 1970.
23. Howland, W.J., Loeffler, R.K., Starchman, D.E. et al. Postirradiation atrophic changes of bone and related complications. Radiology 117:677–685, 1975.
24. Bedwink, J.M., Shukowsky, L.J., Fletcher, G.H. et al. Osteoradionecrosis in patients treated with definitive radiotherapy for squamous cell carcinomas of the oral cavity and naso and oropharynx. Radiology 119:665, 1976.
25. Niebel, H.H. and Neenan, E.W. Dental aspects of osteoradionecrosis. Oral Surg. 10:1011–1024, 1957.
26. Hulth, A. The vessel anatomy of the upper femur end with special regard to the mechanism of origin of different vascular disorders. Acta. Orthop. Scand. Suppl. 27:192–209, 1958.
27. Dubois, E.L. and Cozen, L. Avascular (aseptic) bone necrosis associated with systemic lupus erythematosus. JAMA 174:966–971, 1960.
28. Edeiken, B.S., Libshitz, H.I., and Cohen, M.A. Slipped proximal humeral epiphysis: a complication of radiotherapy to the shoulder in children. Skeletal Radiol. 9(2):123–125, 1982.
29. Walker, S.J., Whiteside, L.A., McAlister, W.H. et al. Slipped capital femoral epiphysis following radiation and chemotherapy. Clin. Orthop. 159:186–193, 1981.
30. Ryan, B.R. and Walters, T.R. Slipped capital femoral epiphysis following radiotherapy and chemotherapy. Med. Pediatr. Oncol. 6:279–283, 1979.
31. Silverman, C.L., Thomas, P.R.M., McAlister, W.H. et al. Slipped femoral capital epiphyses in irradiated children: dose, volume and age relationships. Int. J. Radiat. Oncol. Biol. Phys. 7:1357–1363, 1981.
32. Wolf, E.L.M., Berdon, W.E., Cassady, J.R., et al. Slipped femoral capital epiphysis as a sequela to childhood irradiation for malignant tumors. Radiology 125:781–784, 1977.
33. Botnick, L.E., Goodman, R., Jaffe, N. et al. Stages I–III Hodgkin's disease in children. Results in staging and treatment. Cancer 39:599–603, 1977.
34. Engel, I.A., Straus, D.J., Lacher, M. et al. Osteonecrosis in patients with malignant lymphoma: A review of twenty-five cases. Cancer 48(5):1245–1250, 1981.
35. Ihde, D.C. and DeVita, V.T. Osteonecrosis of the femoral heads in patients with lymphoma treated with intermittent combination chemotherapy. Cancer 36:1585–1588, 1975.
36. Prosnitz, L.R., Lawson, J.P., Friedlaender, G.E. et al. Avascular necrosis of bone in Hodgkin's disease patients treated with combined modality therapy. Cancer 47(12):2793–2797, 1981.
37. Mould, J.J. and Adam, N.M. The problem of avascular necrosis of bone in patients treated for Hodgkin's disease. Clin. Radiol. 34(2):231–236, 1983.
38. Thorne, J.C., Evans, W.K., Alison, R.E. et al. Avascular necrosis of bone complicating treatment of malignant lymphoma. Am. J. Med. 71:(5):751–758, 1981.
39. Timothy, A.R., Tucker, A.K., Park, W.M. et al. Osteonecrosis in Hodgkin's disease. Br. J. Radiol. 51:328–332, 1978.
40. Hancock, B.W., Huck, P., and Ross, B. Avascular necrosis of the femoral head in patients receiving intermittent cytotoxic and corticosteroid therapy for Hodgkin's disease. Postgrad. Med. J. 54:545–546, 1978.
41. Sweet, D.L., Roth, D.G., Desser, R.K. et al. Avascular necrosis of the femoral head with combination therapy. Ann. Intern. Med. 85:67–68, 1976.
42. Albala, M.M., Steinfeld, A.D., and Khilnami, M.T. Osteonecrosis in patients with Hodgkin's disease following combination chemotherapy. Med. Pediatr. Oncol. 8:165–170, 1980.
43. Libshitz, H.I. and Edeiken, B.S. Radiotherapy changes of the pediatric hip. A.J.R. 137:585–588, 1981.
44. Griffiths, H.J. Etiology, pathogenesis, and early diagnosis of ischemic necrosis of the hip. JAMA 246:2615–2617, 1981.
45. Mitchell, D.G., Rao, V.M., Dalika, M.K. et al. Femoral head avascular necrosis: correlation of MR imaging, radiographic staging, radionuclide imaging, and clinical findings. Radiology 162:709–715, 1987.
46. Mitchell, M.D., Kundel, H.L., Steinberg, M.E. et al. Avascular necrosis of the hip: comparison of MR, CT and scintigraphy. A.J.R. 147:67–71, 1986.
47. Beltran, J., Herman, L.J., Burk, J.M. et al. Femoral Head Avascular Necrosis: MR imaging with clinical-pathologic and radionuclide correlation. Radiology 166:215–220, 1988.
48. Jaffe, N., Ried, H.L., Cohen, M. et al. Radiation induced osteochondroma in long-term survivors of childhood cancer. Int. J. Radiat. Oncol. Biol. Phys. 9:665–670, 1983.
49. Libschitz, H.L. and Cohen, M.A. Radiation-induced osteochondomas. Radiology 142:643–647, 1982.
50. Perez, C.A., Vietti, T., Ackerman, L.V. et al. Tumors of the sympathetic nervous system in children. An appraisal of treatment and results. Radiology 88:750–760, 1967.
51. Smith, J., O'Connell, R.S., Huvos, A.G. et al. Hodg-

kin's disease complicated by radiation sarcoma in bone. Br. J. Radiol. 53:314–321, 1980.

52. Smith, J. Radiation-induced sarcoma of bone: Clinical and radiographic findings in 43 patients irradiated for soft tissue neoplasms. Clin. Radiol. 33:205–221, 1982.

53. Kim, J.H., Chu, F.C., Woodard, H.Q. et al. Radiation-induced soft tissue sarcoma and bone sarcoma. Radiology 129:501–508, 1978.

54. Huvos, A.G., Woodard, H.Q., Cahan, W.G. et al. Postradiation osteogenic sarcoma of bone and soft tissues. A clinicopathologic study of 66 patients. Cancer 55:1244–1255, 1985.

55. Smith, J. Postradiation sarcoma of bone in Hodgkin's disease. Skeletal Radiol. 16:524–532, 1987.

56. Foley, K.M., Woodruff, J.M., Ellis, F.T. et al. Radiation induced malignant and atypical peripheral nerve sheath tumors. Ann. Neurol. 7:311–318, 1980.

57. Halperin, E.C., Greenberg, M.S., and Suit, D.H. Sarcoma of bone and soft tissue following treatment of Hodgkin's disease. Cancer 53:232–236, 1984.

CHAPTER 9

Late Neurologic Complications of Hodgkin's Disease Treatment*

TERRENCE L. CASCINO
BRIAN P. O'NEILL

The prognosis is good in Hodgkin's disease. Improvements in current diagnosis and treatment have been paralleled by an improvement in overall disease-free survival. Between 60% and 90% of patients with localized Hodgkin's disease may be cured after early radical radiation therapy, as may approximately half of patients with stage IV Hodgkin's disease treated with aggressive combined therapy.[1,2]

Unfortunately, the prolonged survival that the patient accrues by virtue of aggressive therapy exposes that patient to the side effects of such therapy. The "price" that one pays in acute and chronic toxicity is directly related to the therapeutic index of the particular agent or agents used and the sensitivity of tissues that are the target of action. Most (if not all) treatments (radiation and chemical) are cytotoxic to tumor cells, but they may also cause reversible or irreversible damage to normal tissues. Toxicity directed at these tissues is regarded as acceptable if the therapeutic effectiveness relative to the degree of toxicity ("therapeutic index") is sufficiently high.[3]

Fortunately, the clinical course of Hodgkin's disease determines which treatment to use and how and when it is to be given. Acute or chronic neurotoxicity occurs less often in Hodgkin's disease than in other lymphomas and leukemias for two main reasons. First, the central nervous system is only infrequently involved directly; thus, specific therapy (such as brain irradiation) directed against nerve tissue is not required. Second, unlike those used in nonHodgkin's lymphoma and leukemias, which are of significant neurotoxicity, the drugs used in treating Hodgkin's disease have, in general, a low order of neurotoxicity.

Still, there can be and is significant morbidity and sometimes mortality from the treatment of Hodgkin's disease. The neurotoxicity may be direct, such as the peripheral neuropathy associated with vincristine, or may be indirect, such as a metabolic encephalopathy from the inappropriate secretion of antidiuretic hormones.

Because patients with Hodgkin's disease live longer, it becomes increasingly important for both neurologists and oncologists to know

*Copyright 1987 Mayo Foundation.

the details of each other's field. The nervous system can respond only in a limited number of ways to injuries. The neurologist may be confronted with a patient who has undergone treatment for Hodgkin's disease and is now suffering from dysfunction of the central or peripheral nervous system. Investigation of this new neurologic disorder requires the astute and careful attention of both the neurologist and the oncologist to determine, at the earliest possible time, the cause of the neurologic disease. To do so requires knowledge of the natural course of the illness, the neurologic complications of the therapy the patient has received, and the particular disorders that the patient with Hodgkin's disease may be likely to develop.

In 1976, Somasundaram and Posner[4] reviewed the neurologic complications of Hodgkin's disease. Careful attention was given to the diagnosis of the panoply of conditions. Less attention was given to the late effects of therapy because of the fairly recent use of what are now accepted regimens of treatment. For example, MOPP (mechlorethamine, Oncovin, procarbazine, and prednisone) chemotherapy had been in use for approximately 10 years, and some of the long-term complications had not yet been recognized. Similarly, the late development of radiation-induced sarcoma as a complication of treatment had not yet been described.

The purpose of this chapter is to review the late neurologic complications of Hodgkin's disease therapy. Excellent reviews of complications of cancer treatment in general are available[5-8] and are not repeated here. We have arbitrarily selected those areas that we think are most pertinent to the oncologist caring for the patient with Hodgkin's disease and for the neurologist who may be asked to see such patients when they develop neurologic disease after the successful treatment of their disorder.

LONG-TERM RADIATION-ASSOCIATED SIDE EFFECTS

Radiation therapy is associated with toxicity to normal tissue, which is unavoidably included in the port of treatment. Fortunately, the disorders are rare, but they can be catastrophic. Often these syndromes are mistaken for recurrent tumor, which results in unnecessary testing.

Radiation damage to the nervous system occurs either by direct damage to nerve tissue or indirectly to supporting tissues, such as the carotid arteries. The syndromes can be classified by the anatomic area affected.

Brain. Radiation of the brain usually is not necessary in patients with Hodgkin's disease unless tumor to the meninges or other intracranial structures is demonstrated. The doses given for these complications are relatively low. Because of these factors, the frequency of radionecrosis of the brain in patients with Hodgkin's disease is extremely low.[4]

The clinical pattern of radiation damage to the brain is variable. Acute and subacute forms are well described and usually have their onset during or soon after radiation therapy.[9,10] Delayed radiation necrosis may present with a focal neurologic deficit and a computed tomographic (CT) scan demonstrating a contrast-enhancing mass that is indistinguishable from a recurrent tumor.[11-13] Controversy surrounds whether surgical resection is beneficial for the treatment of this disorder.[14-16] Many patients have a slowly progressive course despite treatment.[14]

A second syndrome is cerebral atrophy, which may be associated with a slowly progressive decline in intellectual capacity but with few other central nervous system findings. Findings on CT scan and magnetic resonance imaging (MRI) are variable and include those of cerebral atrophy[17] and cerebral demyelination.[18] There is no known treatment. The frequency of this disorder is unknown.

The latency of radionecrosis of the brain is approximately 4 months to 3 years. The incidence increases with increasing doses of radiation.[11] It has been estimated that a relatively safe dose of radiation is 1600 RET (radiation-equivalent therapy)[19] or 6000 cGy in 6 weeks.[11] The pathogenesis of radionecrosis is still unclear.

Spinal Cord. Radiation disorders of the spinal cord are more frequent in patients with Hodgkin's disease because the spinal cord is unavoidably included when many patients receive radiotherapy.

Two types of radiation-induced myelopathy have been reported. The first occurs within a few months of treatment and is manifested by the complaint of an electric shock-like sensation below the neck, precipitated by neck flexion (Lhermitte's sign).[20] The sensation is not accompanied by neurologic signs and is self-limiting. Usually, neurologic testing is not required. This syndrome probably represents reversible demyelination of sensory fibers in the cervical spinal cord.

Chronic progressive radiation myelopathy is a disabling disorder.[21-23] The usual setting is after mantle radiation therapy to primary head and neck tumors and for Hodgkin's disease.[21] The onset is insidious, with an initial slow progression and then often stabilization.

Symptoms of chronic progressive radiation myelopathy include paresthesias, weakness, and bowel/bladder dysfunction. The signs are frequently of hemicord dysfunction (Brown-Séquard syndrome) or a transverse myelopathy. The disorder may end in death or severe disability.

The latency from radiotherapy to onset of symptoms varies, but is usually between 5 and 30 months.[21] The incidence of radiation damage increases with increasing dose to the spinal cord. A relatively safe dose is believed to be 3000 cGy in 10 fractions.[24]

The diagnosis of chronic radiation myelopathy should be suspected in any patient whose previous radiation portals have included any part of the spinal cord and whose symptoms and signs are consistent with spinal cord damage in the irradiated segment. The differential diagnosis includes tumor that is intramedullary, meningeal, or epidural. Benign causes, such as degenerative disease, also can occur.

The diagnosis requires myelography to rule out other diseases. Myelography in patients with radiation myelopathy may reveal a normal, atrophic, or swollen spinal cord in a portal of previous radiation.[21] The roles of MRI or CT scans in this disorder are not fully clear. To rule out the possibility of meningeal seeding, the cerebrospinal fluid should be examined at the same time that myelography is done. The protein concentration in the spinal fluid may be increased in radiation myelopathy alone, however.

The cause of chronic radiation myelopathy is not fully established. Endothelial damage and demyelination likely have a role.[19] There is no proven treatment, but a trial of corticosteroids may be of benefit.[22]

Peripheral Nerve. Peripheral nerves also may be affected adversely by radiation therapy. Although unlikely to be fatal, radiation-induced neuropathy may be accompanied by severe neurologic disability. Areas adjacent to the spinal cord (brachial and lumbosacral plexuses) are most commonly involved. In addition, radiation to the neck or base of the skull may infrequently lead to radiation-induced cranial neuropathies.

Brachial Plexus. The brachial plexus is formed by the contributions of C-5 to T-1 roots. The area stretches from the base of the neck to the axilla. These areas frequently lie in portals of radiation that include cervical, supraclavicular, and axillary lymph nodes as well as the apex of the lung. Radiation-induced brachial plexopathy has been well described.[25-29]

The disorder usually begins with paresthesia or dysesthesia of the arm or hand, which is followed by weakness. Pain is usually not an early complaint and may not occur during the course of the disease. The onset is insidious and the course is slowly progressive.

On examination, unilateral arm weakness, sensory loss, and hyporeflexia are often seen. Lymphedema has been noted to be more common in radiation plexopathy,[25] whereas the presence of Horner's syndrome is suggestive of tumor plexopathy. Contralateral arm involvement or long-tract findings in the legs make intraspinal disease more likely and usually require myelography to determine the cause.

The course of radiation brachial plexopathy is usually a progressive one; sometimes there is a clinical plateau.

The differential diagnosis of brachial plexopathy includes tumor as well as other benign causes, such as inflammatory plexopathy. A tumor often presents initially with pain, followed by neurologic disability. Horner's syndrome, as noted above, is more common when a tumor is the cause.

In patients with previous radiation to the area, the diagnosis is sometimes difficult. The clinical findings are helpful, but are not always reliable. CT scanning through the area of the brachial plexus is frequently useful in demonstrating a tumor or in guiding a surgical biopsy.[29] Unfortunately, CT scanning does not always differentiate tumor from radiation damage; in fact, the CT scan may be normal in either radiation or tumor plexopathy.[29] Other studies, including cervical spine roentgenograms, chest roentgenograms, or bone scans, are unlikely to be helpful. Myelography is frequently performed to look for epidural extension of tumor from the laterally situated brachial plexus into the epidural canal. The presence of long-tract signs, indicating spinal cord compression, is a definite indication for myelography.

More recently, electromyography has been used in an attempt to differentiate tumor from radiation-induced brachial plexopathy. Either disorder is commonly associated with denervation in muscles innervated by the brachial plexus. Myokymia, a repetitive spontaneous motor discharge, seems to be more common in patients with radiation plexopathy.[30,31] The specificity of this finding is still open to debate.

The interval from the completion of radiation to the onset of symptoms of plexopathy varies. The median time in a large series of patients with radiation-induced plexopathy was 4 years, but the range was 3 months to 26 years.[21]

The dose of radiation to the brachial plexus that causes nerve injury shows high individual variability. In general, patients who have received more than 6000 cGy are more likely to suffer neurologic injury than those getting less than 6000 cGy.[25] Unfortunately, patients receiving far less than 6000 cGy have been reported to have suffered definite radiation plexopathy.[29]

Despite thorough investigation, the cause of the brachial plexopathy remains unclear at times. A thorough work-up should be conducted for systemic Hodgkin's disease. If a tumor is found, the cause of the brachial plexopathy becomes a secondary issue, and appropriate treatment for recurrent disease should be instituted. If no disease outside the brachial plexus is discovered, surgical biopsy is considered. Even a negative biopsy, however, does not entirely rule out tumor as the cause of the plexopathy.[21]

No known curative treatment for radiation-induced brachial plexopathy exists. Symptomatic treatment includes physical therapy and rehabilitation measures. If present secondary to radiation plexopathy, pain may be difficult to treat. The use of transcutaneous nerve stimulation or non-narcotic analgesics, such as aspirin or nonsteroidal anti-inflammatory agents, is reasonable. If these are ineffective, other potential treatments include tricyclic antidepressants, corticosteroids, or narcotics. Obviously, the long-term side effects of steroids or narcotics must be considered.

Lumbosacral Plexus. Lumbosacral plexopathy includes damage of the motor and sensory nerves to the legs. Most of the plexus lies in the pelvis, forming the named nerves. In patients with tumor, less information has been published concerning lumbosacral plexopathy than brachial plexopathy.[23-34]

Radiation-induced lumbosacral plexopathy has been associated with various conditions, including nonHodgkin's lymphoma and Hodgkin's disease. The median latency time of development of symptoms from radiation therapy is 5 years, with a range of 1 to 31 years.[32] The dose of radiation varies, and doses as little as 3000 cGy have been reported to cause radiation-induced lumbosacral plexopathy.[32] Fortunately, this is an apparently rare disorder, and there has been only one known case in approximately 9000 cases in which pelvic radiation was given at a single institution.[32]

The symptoms are those of painless weakness, numbness, and bowel/bladder dysfunction. The disorder is often bilateral but asymmetric. Pain may occur later in the course of the disease, but is usually not a prominent complaint. Neurologic findings include leg weakness, hypoactive reflexes, and impairment of sensation. Findings are commonly bilateral and asymmetric.

Roentgenograms and bone scans are helpful only in demonstrating diffuse metastatic disease. In patients with neoplastic lumbosacral plexopathy, CT scanning of the pelvis usually shows a mass in the area of the lumbosacral plexus, whereas patients with radiation injury usually have normal CT scans. Myelography is again helpful in demonstrating epidural extension of disease or in ruling out other spinal conditions as a cause of the symptoms. As in brachial plexopathy caused by radiation, electromyography may be helpful in demonstrating myokymia, which is suggestive of radiation damage.

The differential diagnosis includes tumor as well as benign causes secondary to diabetes or degenerative intraspinal disease. Tumor plexopathy is usually the most worrisome alternate diagnosis. This commonly presents with unilateral leg pain followed by neurologic deficit. Evidence of Hodgkin's disease elsewhere usually makes the cause of the plexopathy a moot point. Occasionally, a diagnosis cannot be made. If further treatment of Hodgkin's disease is predicated on the cause of the plexopathy, biopsy may be necessary.

The course in patients with radiation-induced lumbosacral plexopathy varies, with some patients showing a slow progression and others showing stabilization. Rarely patients have been reported who have shown improvement. No known treatment exists.

Cranial Neuropathy. Cranial nerves are unavoidably included in many radiation treatments to the head and neck. Attempts are made to shield certain areas (such as the optic nerves), but this is not always possible. Consequently, on rare occasions, radiation damage to cranial nerves occurs.[35]

Optic neuropathy is the most dramatic form of cranial neuropathy secondary to radiation therapy. The syndrome presents after many years of latency, with either a painless loss of vision leading to optic atrophy or a central retinal artery thrombois.[36] Other cranial neuropathies described secondary to radiation are those of cranial nerves XII, VIII, X, and V. The latency for these is also believed to be in years, with the differential diagnosis primarily being tumor recurrence.[35]

Radiation-Induced Carotid Artery Disease. In addition to nerve tissue being damaged, other structures that are included in the field of radiation may be injured. Carotid artery disease can develop and may lead to cerebral infarction.[37–39] Radiation can also accelerate atherosclerosis in an artery that has been included in the portal of previous radiation.[40] The latency varies from months to many years. Patients may be asymptomatic or have as their first symptom a transient ischemic attack or a cerebral infarction in the distribution of the affected artery. An asymptomatic bruit may be present before the onset of symptoms. Often radiation changes are seen in the skin of the neck overlying the artery.

Treatment for this disorder is usually the same as for any other atherosclerotic carotid artery disease. Antiplatelet agents, anticoagulants, and carotid endarterectomy are considered. The treatment of asymptomatic carotid artery disease, be it from radiation or not, is controversial.

In addition to the development of premature atherosclerosis, thrombotic disease may be found related to a carotid vasculopathy.[38] Subintimal and medial fibrosis may occur, with thinning and fragmentation of the internal elastic lamina. The clinical findings are similar to those of other carotid artery occlusive disorders, with risk of transient ischemic attack or stroke. The latency is months to years.

Radiation-Induced Nerve Tumors. Radiation-induced malignant tumors of the peripheral nerve sheath[33] are potentially the most serious complication of radiation-induced disorders of the nerve. The most common sites affected are nerve trunks, including the brachial plexus and lumbosacral plexus. The latency from radiation therapy to the development of tumor is many years (4 to 40 in one study).[41] Symptoms include a painful mass as well as a progressive neurologic deficit related to the nerve involved. Unfortunately, the prognosis is poor, especially if the pathologic changes are consistent with a malignant peripheral nerve-sheath tumor rather than the less commonly seen atypical benign neurofibroma.

LONG-TERM CHEMOTHERAPEUTIC SIDE EFFECTS

Chemotherapy of disseminated Hodgkin's disease is now considered standard care.

Also, chemotherapy is being added to the treatment of some patients who are at high risk of extranodal spread. The three most widely used chemotherapy regimens are MOPP, B-CUPP, and ABVD,[1,2] all multiagent programs sequentially administered. Other more experimental regimens are being tested for effectiveness and toxicity. The individual drugs in these newer programs, as well as those in present use, are summarized by category in Table 9–1.

Multiple-agent chemotherapy is now commonly used for several reasons. First, different drugs may act at different biochemical sites in the cell or at different stages of the cell cycle. Thus, the use of multiple therapeutic agents allows for attack on a single cell at different sites. Second, many tumors are mosaics of heterogeneous cell populations; one agent may be able to kill certain cells of a tumor but leave others to grow unchecked.

No definite evidence confirms that toxicity to the nervous system in Hodgkin's disease is enhanced by these combinations. Toxicity may be increased, however, when certain drugs are used in conjunction with radiation therapy. Table 9–2 lists the known neurotoxicity of the agents commonly used in the treatment of Hodgkin's disease. The drugs are listed by general category. Most of these agents produce toxicity that affects the nervous system only indirectly or not at all. Some drugs, however, possess toxicity specific to the nervous system (for example, vincristine), which is a dose-limiting side effect of the drug. Most neurotoxicity is reversible if discovered early, but in some patients, it may produce serious and irreversible damage and frequently does so if not recognized early.

Alkylating Agents. Alkylating agents are cell-cycle, nonspecific drugs that interfere with DNA synthesis by inducing cross links with DNA monoalkylating sites.[7,42,43] The alkylating agents used in Hodgkin's disease include nitrogen mustard (mechlorethamine, NH_2), chlorambucil (Leukeran), and cyclophosphamide (Cytoxan). Their systemic toxicity is directed mainly at bone marrow and the gastrointestinal tract. Little long-term chronic or late-onset toxicity to the nervous system occurs.

Newer synthetic agents that are cell-cycle, nonspecific alkylating agents (nitrosoureas, procarbazine) have structural differences that dictate water and lipid solubility.[7] These agents sensitize cells to the action of ionizing radiation; their cytostatic effect and their neurotoxicity are enhanced when used with radiotherapy.[44,45] Late-onset complications are not common, but they are seen more often in patients with primary brain tumors or lung cancer when combination therapy is used.

Nitrogen Mustard. Nitrogen mustard is mainly used to treat advanced Hodgkin's disease as part of the MOPP combination.[1,2,43] In customary doses late neurotoxicity does not occur. The drug is a powerful stimulant of the central nervous system.[42] Thus, nausea and vomiting are frequent, and sometimes the patient complains of headache and lassitude. Convulsions, progressive muscular paralysis, and cholinomimetic effects have occurred af-

Table 9–1. Chemotherapeutic Agents Used in the Treatment of Hodgkin's Disease

Category	Drug
Alkylating agents	Nitrogen mustard
	Chlorambucil
	Cyclophosphamide (Cytoxan)
	Carmustine (BCNU)
	Lomustine (CCNU)
Vinca alkaloids	Vincristine
	Vinblastine
Antibiotics	Doxorubicin (Adriamycin)
	Bleomycin
Others	Prednisone
	Procarbazine
	DTIC (dacarbazine)
	Methotrexate

Table 9–2. Neurotoxicity of Chemotherapeutic Agents Commonly Used in Treating Hodgkin's Disease

Drug	Mode of Administration	Common Systemic Side Effects	Brain/Cranial Nerves	Spinal Cord Roots/Meninges	Peripheral Nerve/Muscle
Alkylating agents					
Nitrogen mustard	IV, HD, IV, IA, IC	Gastrointestinal, Hematologic	Edema, neuritis (in HD intra-arterial)	—	Plexopathy/neuropathy (in HD pelvic perfusion)
Chlorambucil	PO	Gastrointestinal, Hematologic	—	—	—
Cyclophosphamide	IV, PO	Gastrointestinal, Hematologic, Neurologic	—	—	—
Vinca alkaloids					
Vincristine	IV	Gastrointestinal, Dermatologic	Seizures, cranial neuropathy, inappropriate ADH secretion	—	Peripheral neuropathy, autonomic neuropathy
Vinblastine	IV, IA	Gastrointestinal, Hematologic, Dermatologic	Depression, cranial neuropathy	—	Peripheral neuropathy, autonomic neuropathy
Antibiotics					
Adriamycin	IV	Gastrointestinal, Cardiac, Dermatologic, Hematologic	—	—	—
Bleomycin	IV, IM, REG	Gastrointestinal, Pulmonary, Dermatologic	Encephalopathy, cranial (ototoxicity) neuropathy	—	—
Others					
Prednisone	PO	Gastrointestinal, Endocrine	Depression, psychosis, seizures	—	Myopathy
Procarbazine	PO, IV	Gastrointestinal, Hematologic	Encephalopathy	—	Neuropathy
DTIC	IV	Gastrointestinal, Hematologic, Dermatitis	—	—	Neuropathy
Methotrexate	PO, IV, HD, IV, IT, IA	Gastrointestinal, Hematologic, Renal	Disseminated leukoencephaly	Acute myelopathy, aseptic meningitis, radiculopathy	—
BCNU	IV	Gastrointestinal, Hematologic	Leukoencephalopathy when used with RT	—	—
CCNU	PO	Gastrointestinal, Hematologic	—	—	—

Intravenous (IV); intra-arterial (IA); intrathecal (IT); high dose (HD); radiation therapy (RT); antidiuretic hormone (ADH); regional (REG); oral (PO); intracavity (IC). (Modified from Young and Posner[6] and Jellinger.[7])

ter standard use.[42] One patient with Hodgkin's disease experienced fever, hemiplegia, and coma after each of two conventional doses of nitrogen mustard.[46] At autopsy 4 years later, focal areas of neuronal loss and gliosis were found; no evidence of intracranial Hodgkin's disease was seen. The syndrome was indirectly related to nitrogen mustard as an idiosyncratic response.

Neurotoxicity has been more noticeable when the nervous system is exposed to higher concentrations of the drugs; these high levels are not being used as of 1988. Intracarotid infusion of nitrogen mustard has been associated with seizures, hemiplegia, coma, and death.[47] Similarly, high-dose intra-arterial infusions, which are used in the treatment of pelvic and limb tumors, have produced lumbosacral plexopathy.[48,49] In some studies,[50,51] high systemic concentrations from large intravenous doses or regional intra-arterial infusions have produced tinnitus and hearing loss and have damaged the auditory and vestibular portions of the eighth cranial nerve in all patients treated.

Chlorambucil. Chlorambucil is not recognized as neurotoxic. However, acute toxicity to the nervous system occurred in two children who ingested large quantities of the drug. In one child, repetitive seizures (refractory to anticonvulsant agents) and coma ensued;[52] ataxia and gross tremors occurred in the other patient.[53] Both patients recovered quickly without sequelae. As with nitrogen mustard, chlorambucil is a potent stimulator of the nervous system and nausea, vomiting, and headache may be seen acutely after its administration.[42] Seizures may be a problem when chlorambucil is given in conventional dosage to patients with the nephrotic syndrome.[54]

Cyclophosphamide. Cyclophosphamide has the widest therapeutic range of any of the alkylating agents. In addition to its use in the treatment of hematologic malignancies and solid tumors, cyclophosphamide is used as an immunosuppressive agent in the treatment of nonmalignant disease.[42] No significant long-term neurologic toxicity has resulted from standard oral or intravenous use of the drug. Like other alkylating agents, however, when infused it may be a potent stimulator of the central nervous system.[42] Nausea, vomiting, dizziness, visual blurring, headache, facial flushing, and a tingling sensation in the posterior pharynx may occur.[55-57] Inappropriate secretion of antidiuretic hormone has been linked to high dosages of cyclophosphamide; thus, metabolic encephalopathy with seizures can occur.[58]

Plant Alkaloids. Plant alkaloids include vincristine and vinblastine, the periwinkle (*Vinca rosea*) derivatives, and vindestine, the synthetic derivative of vinblastine. They are mitotic and microtubular poisons; they interfere with RNA and DNA synthesis and disrupt mitosis in metaphase.[6,7,59,60] Unlike other chemotherapeutic agents, the vinca alkaloids have neurotoxicity as their dose-limiting factor. Neurotoxicity presumably is caused by destruction of neurotubules, with accumulation of neurofilaments and subsequent disturbance in axoplasmic transport.[7]

Vincristine. Vincristine is toxic to the peripheral nervous system primarily, but it can also affect the central nervous system, the cranial nerves, and the autonomic nervous system. A mild peripheral neuropathy occurs in virtually every patient treated with repeated doses.[6] The severity of neurotoxicity is largely related to dose and dose frequency.[61] Vincristine is toxic primarily to the neuron and its axon, rather than to supportive tissues such as the Schwann cell.[62]

The brain and spinal cord are largely excluded from the neurotoxic effects of vincristine because it only minimally penetrates the intact blood/brain barrier. The inadvertent intrathecal injection of vincristine has caused ascending motor and sensory paralysis, leading to respiratory failure, coma, and death.[63] Children can have seizures when given conventional dosages.[64,65] Furthermore, seizures can be seen as part of the metabolic derangement caused by the inappropriate secretion of antidiuretic hormones.[66-68]

In children, myopathy, muscle tenderness, and pain of variable degree may develop within the first week or two after the administration of vincristine.[6,62] Usually, this syndrome is reversible, but severe autophagic degeneration of muscle fibers has been decribed.[69] Most reports indicate, however, that muscle atrophy, when it occurs, is of the denervation type.[69–71]

Various uncommon syndromes of the cranial nerves have been described. Mild bifacial paresis may occasionally occur, especially in children,[72] but this paresis may be part of a diffuse myopathy or motor neuropathy because it is almost always seen when there is significant peripheral weakness.[6] Paroxysmal jaw or throat pain may have its onset within hours after vincristine has been administered, and the pain subsides quickly and does not recur with repeated administration.[66] Some patients may develop diplopia caused by sixth-nerve palsy[72] and hoarseness as a result of paralysis of the vocal cords.[61,73] Vincristine has also been associated with an optic neuropathy in patients with Hodgkin's disease given multimodality treatment.[74,75]

Constipation, usually attributed to vincristine-induced autonomic neuropathy, occurs in about one-third of the patients.[61,72] Constipation may be prevented by a prophylactic regimen of laxative and hydrophilic agents. Paralytic ileus with abdominal pain and distention may ensue.[61,72] Bladder atony, impotence, and orthostatic hypotension have also been described as examples of the autonomic neuropathy associated with vincristine.[61,76,77] In the primary autonomic degeneration of vincristine, sphincter disturbances usually precede the other neurologic symptoms. Recovery may be incomplete, even after withdrawal of the drug.

Paresthesia is usually the first symptom of peripheral neuropathy caused by vincristine. Before that, however, depression of the ankle jerks may appear after one or two weekly treatments.[61,72] As the total dose increases, all reflexes may disappear. Even after treatment has ceased, complete areflexia is common.[78] Despite prominent symptoms, objective impairment of sensation is usually disproportionately mild, and sensory thresholds are only slightly increased.[61,72] Fortunately, sensory signs, when present, disappear when treatment is stopped. Only rarely does irreversible sensory loss occur.

Distal weakness may occur, usually after sensory complaints are prominent. The weakness of the hands and feet is usually mild, although more pronounced weakness is seen in children.[62] Weakness most typically affects the dorsiflexors of the toes and ankles.[61,78] In more severe disease, the extensors of the fingers and wrists also may be affected, but in almost all patients, the feet are the first and most severely affected. Weakness is usually reversible, but recovery frequently takes many months.[8] In some patients, however, motor deficits show little improvement and the patient has a chronic neuropathic disability.

The peripheral neuropathy of vincristine may make the patient more susceptible to compression or entrapment neuropathies and respond more dramatically to other neurotoxic factors.[62] Some patients may also be more sensitive than others to the effects of vincristine. For example, some patients with myotonic dystrophy[79] or mild Charcot-Marie-Tooth neuropathy have suffered profound neuropathy after only one or two doses.[62,80] It is not clear whether common neuropathies, such as those associated with diabetes and alcohol abuse, enhance the neuropathy caused by vincristine.

The most severe neurologic manifestations of vincristine use may be avoided or reversed by suspending therapy or reducing the dosage when the earliest symptoms are noted. Total doses greater than 2 mg are associated with progressive disability, particularly in older patients and those taking weekly treatments. Severe neuropathic effects are seen in overdoses.[5]

Vinblastine. The neurotoxicity of vinblastine is similar to that of vincristine, but it occurs much less frequently because hematologic toxicity (and not neurotoxicity) is the dose-limiting factor. Headache, peripheral neuropathy, psychosis, convulsions, depression, and photosensitivity have been associated with the use of this drug.[81,82] The more serious side effects have been partly explained by the presence of concurrent cerebral metastases.[81]

Antibiotic Agents. No significant neurotoxicity has been seen with antibiotics, two of which—doxorubicin and bleomycin—have substantial clinical use in Hodgkin's disease. The drugs do not cross the intact blood/brain barrier, which may account for the lack of neurotoxicity.

Other Drugs. Procarbazine is a monoamine oxidase inhibitor and may inhibit DNA, RNA, and protein synthesis.[6,83] Side effects are predominantly gastrointestinal and hematologic. Procarbazine can cause four types of neurologic toxicity: (1) Central, with alteration of alertness; (2) Ataxia; (3) Peripheral neuropathy, with myalgia, paresthesia, and loss of reflexes; and (4) Undue sensitivity to narcotics, phenothiazines, and catecholamines because of monoamine oxidase inhibition.[5]

When procarbazine is given intravenously (no longer generally used), somnolence, hallucinations, confusion, depression, and mania may occur.[84] In standard oral doses, 10 to 15% of patients have a transient cerebral disorder.[85,86] One study using higher doses, however, reported that nearly one-third of patients had significant central depression of the central nervous system.[87]

In addition to the effects on the central nervous system, peripheral neuropathy occurred in 10 to 15% of the patients treated with high oral doses.[6] When neuropathy occurs, it is usually manifested as depressed reflexes, ataxia, and distal weakness.[86,87] Paresthesia occurs after approximately 1 month of treatment.[87] Sometimes symptoms improve, despite continuation of the drug. Peripheral neuropathy is unusual at currently used dosages.[6]

Many reports urge caution in using procarbazine because of the possible side effects and drug interactions associated with monoamine oxidase inhibitors.[6,8,86,87] Orthostatic hypotension, as well as excessive sedation with phenothiazines, barbiturates, alcohol, and narcotics, has been described.[86-89]

Nitrosoureas. These agents are cell-cycle, nonspecific drugs that have been discussed in general terms with the alkylating agents. The compounds used in the therapy of Hodgkin's disease are BCNU (carmustine) and CCNU (lomustine).

BCNU. Systemic toxicity after drug infusion includes bone-marrow suppression and central nervous system stimulation associated with nausea and vomiting. High-dose regimens have produced pulmonary fibrosis and renal failure, which in turn can produce metabolic encephalopathies.[6,42,43]

Of itself, BCNU is probably not neurotoxic. When used in innovative ways, however, BCNU has produced a number of toxic effects. For example, the administration of BCNU in the carotid artery for the treatment of primary and metastatic tumors has been accompanied by orbital and neck pain at the time of injection.[3,90] Some patients have suffered seizures, encephalopathy, and visual loss.[91] Pathologic changes in the ipsilateral eye and cerebral hemisphere have been convincing evidence for chemical-induced toxicity.[92] Also, high-dose BCNU treatment accompanied by autologous bone-marrow rescue has been followed by multifocal neurologic abnormalities 3 to 12 weeks after treatment.[93]

BCNU may potentiate the side effects of high doses of radiation therapy to the brain. In patients receiving prophylactic cranial radiation after chemotherapy in an attempt to prevent brain metastasis in small-cell lung cancer, a slowly progressive disabling dementia is seen, along with a gait disorder involving apractic and ataxic elements.[94] The precise mechanism is not known, but BCNU probably is acting in a synergistic fashion with the brain irradiation to produce accelerated neurotoxicity.[7] A similar type of syndrome has been seen in several patients who have survived 2 or more years after BCNU and radiation therapy for malignant gliomas.[6] These complications have not been noted in Hodgkin's disease, probaby because the central nervous system is not irradiated and the dosages are well within conventional ranges.

CCNU. Like BCNU, CCNU probably carries the increased risk of neurotoxicity when used in conjunction with radiation therapy.

DTIC (Dacarbazine). DTIC is a cell-cycle, nonspecific agent that has alkylating and antimetabolic properties. It probably inhibits RNA and protein synthesis after the drug is activated in the liver.[5-7,42,43] Some of the drug crosses the intact blood/brain barrier, which probably explains the nausea and vomiting seen soon after its administration.

There is no clear-cut evidence of neurotoxicity. Acute side effects that may have a neurologic basis include jaw pain, facial burning, paresthesia with facial flushing (when the drug is used in high dosage), and hypotension.[95] A single report of delayed neurotoxicity associated with dementia and hemiparesis seems reasonable to ascribe to DTIC because autopsy showed no evidence of a neuropathologic process that could have accounted for the clinical findings.[96]

Methotrexate. Methotrexate (MTX) is the only chemotherapeutic agent that has a significant potential for causing serious structural damage of the brain.[3] In Hodgkin's disease, MTX was used in the mid-1970s in an attempt to find alternative treatment for patients who failed on MOPP therapy. MTX is now excluded from all the first- and second-order combination chemotherapy regimens for advanced Hodgkin's disease.[2] The reader is referred to reviews for descriptions of MTX neurotoxicity seen in the treatment of other malignancies.[5-7]

CENTRAL NERVOUS SYSTEM INFECTIONS

The increased risk of infection in patients with Hodgkin's disease is well known.[97-100] Infection accounts for approximately 20% of deaths. Infections of the central nervous system are not uncommon and are a potential cause of significant morbidity and mortality. Defects in cellular immunity in patients with Hodgkin's disease predispose the patient to infection by unusual pathogens.[99,100] In addition, some patients have neutropenia, which in turn further predisposes the patient to infection of the central nervous system.[99,101] Finally, splenectomy is associated with increased risks of infection.

Fortunately, patients with Hodgkin's disease who are in remission and who have survived treatment seem to be at less risk for these infections.[102,103] Prolonged neutropenia secondary to treatment or splenectomy (or both) still represents an increased risk.

In patients with Hodgkin's disease who have symptoms of unexplained fever or alteration of mental status (or both), an investigation for central nervous system infections should be made. The usual signs of headache and meningismus may not be present, especially in patients with neutropenia.[101]

The infecting organism often can be predicted if the host-defense abnormality is known. Cellular immune system disorders such as those seen in lymphoma, Hodgkin's disease, and organ transplantation, predispose patients to different pathogens than those seen with neutropenia, immunoglobulin deficiencies, and splenectomy associated with other disorders.

Bacterial Infections. The most common cause of meningitis in patients with abnormal cellular immunity is Listeria monocytogenes.[100] This is a gram-positive bacillus that may be mistaken for a diphtheroid organism on Gram's stain and may take several days to grow in culture. Treatment is usually with penicillin or ampicillin.

Other common causes of bacterial meningitis include Streptococcus pneumoniae and Nocardia asteroides. Nocardia infection may present as a single or multiple brain abscess rather than as meningitis.

Patients with neutropenia are much more likely to develop gram-negative meningitis than infections from any of the above organisms. The most common pathogens are Pseudomonas aeruginosa and Escherichia coli.[100,101] If neutropenia is present, the cerebrospinal-fluid-cell count may be normal in overt meningitis, even when the culture is positive.

Splenectomized patients seem to be at greatest risk of developing Streptococcus pneumonia, Neisseria meningitis, or Haemophilus influenza.

Fungal Infections. The most common fungal infection of the central nervous system in Hodgkin's disease is caused by Cryptococcus neoformans. This infection is a meningitis that occurs in patients with altered cellular immunity. The infection usually presents as meningitis, although fever and stiff neck may be absent. Change in mental status is common. Testing for a cryptococcal antigen in cerebrospinal fluid is an easy, rapid method of making a diagnosis.

Less common fungal infections, especially in neutropenic patients, are candidiasis and aspergillosis. These infections usually are part of a disseminated process in a seriously ill patient. Aspergillus infection may present as an abscess or as a necrotizing meningoencephalitis.

Parasitic Infections. Toxoplasma gondii infections occur in patients with altered cellular immunity.[104] Presentations include multiple parenchymal masses and encephalitis. Toxoplasmosis is one of the most common causes of intracranial masses in patients with Hodgkin's disease and is at least as common as intraparenchymal tumor in these patients. Cerebrospinal fluid may show pleocytosis or be entirely normal. Findings on CT scans are nonspecific, but often include multiple, small, contrast-enhancing lesions. Serologic tests, such as the Sabin-Feldman dye test, are not always useful. Biopsy of intracranial lesions is often necessary to differentiate toxoplasmosis from intracranial Hodgkin's disease or from tumors.

Viral Infections. Viral infections of the central nervous system are rarely diagnosed in patients with cancer. Diseases include viruses that cause similar diseases in normal hosts, but cause disease of increasing severity in immunocompromised patients (such as those with herpes zoster), infections with unusual manifestations caused by viruses that also cause disease in normal hosts (measles), and infection by viruses that rarely cause central-nervous-system infection in normal hosts (progressive multifocal leukoencephalopathy).

Varicella-Zoster. The virus that causes either chickenpox as a primary infection or shingles (herpes zoster) as a secondary infection is varicella-zoster. Herpes zoster may occur any time during the course of Hodgkin's disease. It occurs in as many as 30% of patients with Hodgkin's disease,[105] but in only 0.2% of the normal population.[106] The neurologic complications include a radicular-type pattern of sensory loss. The lesion may occur in areas of spinal tumor or previous radiation. Less frequent complications include weakness,[107] cranial neuropathy, myelopathy,[108] cerebrovasculitis,[109] and encephalitis.[110] Postherpetic neuralgia is an uncommon but extremely painful sequela.

Dissemination of herpes zoster occurs more commonly in patients with Hodgkin's disease than in the normal population. The virus may spread to other skin areas or visceral organs, and the mortality rate is 6% to 17%.[111] Recent studies indicate that the administration of acyclovir reduces the likelihood of dissemination and shortens the period of culture positivity for virus in severely immunocompromised patients.[111]

Herpes Simplex Virus. Herpes simplex encephalitis is a rare complication in patients with decreased cell-mediated immunity.[112] Systemic disease is diagnosed more commonly. This central-nervous-system disorder presents as a subacute encephalitis with seizures and focal findings, but the clinical findings are nonspecific. The virus infection occurs when there is a defect in cell-mediated immunity.

Measles. In persons with intact immune systems, measles is usually a benign disorder. Rarely, a parainfectious, immune-mediated, central-nervous-system disease occurs. Defects in cell-mediated immunity may lead to more severe infections. Encephalitis with seizures, coma, and death has been reported.[113]

Cytomegalovirus. Cytomegalovirus infections occur when cell-mediated immunity is depressed. Systemic disease is diagnosed more commonly than central-nervous-system disease. Encephalitis does occur, athough the clinical findings are nonspecific.[114,115]

Progressive Multifocal Leukoencephalopathy. Progressive multifocal leukoencephalopathy is a widespread, multifocal, demyelinating disease of the cerebral hemispheres, brainstem, cerebellum, or spinal cord secondary to a papovavirus infection of the nervous system. The disorder occurs most commonly in immunocompromised patients with Hodgkin's disease, chronic lymphocytic leukemia, and autoimmune deficiency syndrome.[116] The disorder is characterized by generalized and multifocal findings in the central nervous system, such as dementia, hemiparesis, hemisensory defects, and aphasia. The course is progressive, and most patients die within a year. Findings on cerebrospinal-fluid examination, electroencephalography, and angiography are nonspecific. The antibody to the virus is present in 40 to 60% of normal patients by the age of 10 years. An increase in antibody during the course of the illness is rare.

A CT scan may show areas of multifocal low density, suggestive of the diagnosis. Magnetic resonance imaging scans may show defects throughout the central nervous system, consistent with multifocal demyelination. Brain biopsy, is the only dependable way to make an accurate diagnosis. No treatment is available, though patients are reported who have responded to cytosine arabinoside.[117,118]

NEUROLOGIC PARANEOPLASTIC SYNDROMES

Paraneoplastic syndromes are neurologic disorders not caused by direct invasion of nerve tissue by the neoplasm or by other conditions, such as metabolic derangements or antineoplastic therapy. The association is statistical; these disorders, also referred to as "remote effect syndromes," occur more frequently in patients with cancer than can be accounted for by chance alone.[60] The cause of these disorders is unknown. Each of the neurologic paraneoplastic conditions has been seen as a sporadic event; thus, the presence of a neoplasm is not essential for the expression of a syndrome. Furthermore, no convincing evidence suggests that treatment of Hodgkin's disease (or any other cancer) in itself predisposes a patient to develop these disorders. However, there is likely a mechanism common to these disorders that is uncovered or enhanced by a number of factors, including the presence of a neoplasm. Theories that are currently advanced include circulating antibodies against nerve tissue,[119,120] viral infections in immunosuppressed hosts,[121] and disordered thyrogastric immunity.[122]

These disorders are rare. In a series reported from the London Hospital, the incidence of paraneoplastic conditions was 2.5% of 210 patients with Hodgkin's disease seen during a 10-year period.[123] The disorders may precede or herald evidence of the cancer or they may occur when the tumor is quiescent. Some of the disorders are nonspecific and give no clue as to the presence of any underlying neoplasm.[4] Others occur with unusual frequency, such as the myasthenic syndrome with small-cell cancer of the lung,[124] the POEMS (polyneuropathy-organomegaly-endocrinopathy-M-protein-skin changes) syndrome with osteosclerotic myeloma,[125] and subacute cerebellar degeneration seen in cancer of the ovary.[119] The presence of these disorders should alert the physician to search carefully for the cancer and, if not found, to keep the patient under close surveillance.

Most of these syndromes do not respond to treatment. Several of them are self-limited or respond to treatment of the primary tumor.[126-128] Because a putative immune condition is implicated in many of these disorders, scattered reports have described at least partial success in the treatment of the neurologic condition itself.[129,130]

Patients tend to have a simultaneous occurrence or the subsequent development of more than one type of disorder. Within each cancer type, no single factor can predict which patient will develop the disorder. The disorders that are relatively specific for Hodgkin's disease include subacute sensory neuropathy, chronic motor neuropathy, and subacute cerebellar degeneration. For a discussion of the other paraneoplastic disorders not seen in Hodgkin's disease, the reader is referred to several excellent reviews.[131,132]

Encephalomyelitis. Patients with encephalomyelitis have clinical signs of damage to different parts of the nervous system, and postmortem signs of inflammation within the brain, brainstem, spinal cord, posterior root ganglia, and the nerve roots are present.[60] The largest group of such disorders is seen in small-cell carcinoma of the lung; several examples of the syndrome identical to this have been described in Hodgkin's disease. The main pathologic feature that characterizes this group is a prominent inflammatory reaction associated with neuronal damage. It is primarily a polioencephalitis—that is, an inflammation of the gray matter. The distribution of lesions is variable but tends to predominate in one particular part of the nervous system.

Henson and Urich[60] have divided this group of disorders into five subcategories emphasizing the frequent overlap: (1) a limbic encephalitis, which is mainly expressed as an amnestic dementia with disordered mood and affect; (2) a bulbar encephalitis, which is usually a medullary syndrome with vertigo, ataxia, nystagmus, or progressive bulbar palsy, sometimes with ascending and eventual involvement of the midbrain; (3) a cerebellar encephalitis in which cerebellar signs predominate; (4) a myelitis with muscular wasting and weakness, with or without fasciculations, predominantly involving the upper limbs, sometimes asymmetrically; and (5) a posterior root ganglionitis, expressed as a subacute sensory syndrome with paresthesia, pain, and sensory ataxia, quickly progressing to a severe and unremitting state.

In all patients, the cerebrospinal fluid may be abnormal in the early stages. It can display a mild pleocytosis and an increase in the total protein value. All patients do not have these findings, however, and the findings do not reflect the intense histopathologic changes seen at autopsy. In amost all patients, the syndrome develops several years before or after the diagnosis of the primary lesion. The condition tends to stabilize but not improve.

The mechanism is not known, but convincing evidence is accumulating that points to antibodies directed specifically at target cells as being important for the causation of the diseases. For example, reports from several laboratories have described antiPurkinje cell antibodies, the level of which may sometimes be correlated with the degree of clinical involvement.[133,134] Furthermore, similar antibodies have been described in dorsal root ganglionitis (subacute sensory neuropathy) and in optic neuropathy, a condition not described in Hodgkin's disease.[135,136]

Corticocerebellar Degeneration. This is a purely degenerative process largely confined to the cerebellar cortex. Patients with Hodgkin's disease who have this disorder, but have no inflammation, have been described sporadically. Although this condition may be a "burnt out" example of the inflammatory cerebellar encephalitis described previously, many authors consider this a separate disorder. In Henson and Urich's series, 4 of 27 patients with this condition also had Hodgkin's disease. In these four patients, the illness preceded the diagnosis of Hodgkin's disease by as much as 8 years.

The pathologic hallmark is the loss of neurons in the Purkinje cell layer—the loss occurs evenly throughout the cerebellum. Associated lesions in other parts of the neuraxis are not usually seen, although one patient with Hodgkin's disease also had a remitting demyelinating peripheral neuropathy.[137] The mechanism is not known, although one report refers to the "Gordon" phenomenon (that is, the effect of degenerating eosinophils on the cerebellum).[138]

As in the former group, corticocerebellar degeneration can precede or follow the onset of Hodgkin's disease. Most patients develop a pancerebellar deficit acutely or subacutely, but in some, a deficit may slowly evolve. Most patients are significantly disabled, having severe truncal and limb ataxia, and sometimes also having nystagmus, myoclonus, and mental symptoms.

Peripheral Neuropathy. Acute, subacute, and chronic forms of sensorimotor neuropathy occur. No clinical features distinguish the neuropathy seen in Hodgkin's disease from neuropathies of other causes.[4] The primary disease may be active or quiescent, but in general, the Hodgkin's disease has already been diagnosed. This is in contradistinction to the other disorders, in which the neurologic condition sometimes predates the diagnosis of Hodgkin's disease by days to years. Again, in many patients, a mixed clinical pattern occurs, associated with cerebellar disorder, dementia, or both. These unique combinations should draw attention to the possible association with malignancy.[4,60,130]

Mixed peripheral neuropathy occurs relatively infrequently in Hodgkin's disease. Currie et al.[123] described an incidence of 1.4% of neuropathy in Hodgkin's disease, lower than in other lymphomas. Asymptomatic involvement of the peripheral nerve is, however, far more common. Six of 20 patients had decreased motor conduction velocities when Hodgkin's disease, without clinical neurologic manifestations, was initially diagnosed.[60] In another series of 20 patients, only one patient had clinical signs of mild peripheral neuropathy, whereas four others had generalized impairment of nerve conduction unrelated to the clinical stage of the malignancy.[139] In their experience at the London Hospital, Henson and Urich estimated that the incidence of clinically apparent neuropathy was less than 5% of patients with Hodgkin's disease.

Croft et al.[140] divided patients into three main groups according to the clinical course:

(1) a group with mild symmetric peripheral neuropathy occurring in the terminal stage of the disease; (2) subacute or occasionally acute neuropathy that is similar to the Guillain-Barré syndrome, usually preceding the diagnosis of malignancy; and (3) relapsing or remitting sensorimotor peripheral neuropathy. All the disorders seem to be of the demyelinating type when studied pathologically, although the mechanism is not known.[140] Several patients with Guillain-Barré syndrome have been described, some having full or partial recovery.[141,142] Recently, we found a demyelinating bilateral, though asymmetric, brachial plexopathy in a young man with stage IIA Hodgkin's disease who has shown a convincing response to corticosteroid usage.

A disorder unique to lymphomas is usually classified under the peripheral nerve paraneoplastic conditions, although it may be a form of poliomyelitis.[143,144] Five patients with Hodgkin's disease who were in clinical remission and had received therapeutic radiation, which included that to the spinal cord, suffered a progressive, predominantly motor neuropathy. Wasting and weakness, often asymmetric, were present and affected the upper and lower limbs in three patients and the lower limbs in the other two patients. Distal sensory changes were minor. The clinical course was one of slow progression, stabilization, and sometimes improvement. One patient died of Hodgkin's disease relapse. The autopsy findings consisted of loss of anterior horn cells with axonal degeneration of the anterior roots of the motor nerves. They concluded, on the basis of their experience, that these pathologic changes were the most common remote effects on the nervous system seen in Hodgkin's disease.[143]

REFERENCES

1. Wiernik, P.H. Hodgkin disease. In Clinical Medicine. Vol. 5. Edited by J.A. Spittell. Philadelphia, Harper & Row, 1985.
2. Bakemeier, R.F., Zagars, G., Cooper, R.A. et al. The malignant lymphomas: Hodgkin's disease and non-Hodgkin's lymphoma, multiple myeloma, and macroglobulinemia. In Clinical Oncology for Medical Students and Physicians: A Multidisciplinary Approach. Edited by P. Rubin. American Cancer Society, 1983.
3. Young, D.F. Neurological complications of cancer chemotherapy. In Neurological Complications of Therapy. Edited by A. Silverstein. Mount Kisco, Futura Publishing Company, 1982.
4. Somasundaram, M. and Posner, J.B. Neurological complications of Hodgkin's disease. In Hodgkin's Disease. Edited by M.J. Lacher. New York, John Wiley & Sons, 1976.
5. Sawicka, J., Dawson, D.M., and Blum, R. Neurologic aspects of the treatment of cancer. In Current Neurology. Vol 1. Edited by H.R. Tyler. Boston, Houghton Mifflin, 1977.
6. Young, D.F. and Posner, J.B. Nervous system toxicity of chemotherapy agents. In Handbook of Clinical Neurology. Vol. 39. Edited by P.J. Vinken and G.W Bruyn. Amsterdam, North-Holland Publishing Company, 1980.
7. Jellinger, K. Pathologic effects of chemotherapy. In Oncology of the Nervous System. Edited by M.D. Walker. Boston, Martinus Nijhoff, 1983, p. 416.
8. Weiss, H.D., Walker, M.D., and Wiernik, P.H. Neurotoxicity of commonly used antineoplastic agents. N. Engl. J. Med. 291:127–133, 1974.
9. Rider, W.D. Radiation damage to the brain—a new syndrome. J. Can. Assoc. Radiol. 14:67, 1963.
10. Chu, F.C.H. and Hilaris, B.B. Value of radiation therapy in the management of intracranial metastases. Cancer 14:577, 1961.
11. Rottenberg, D.A. et al. Cerebral necrosis following radiotherapy of extracranial neoplasms. Ann. Neurol. 1:339, 1977.
12. Brismar, J., Roberson, G.H., and Davis, K.R. Radiation necrosis of the brain: Neuroradiological considerations with computed tomography. Neuroradiology 12:109, 1976.
13. Mikhael M.A. Radiation necrosis of the brain: Correlation between computed tomography, pathology, and dose distribution. J. Comput. Assist. Tomogr. 2:71, 1978.
14. Rottenberg, D.A. Horten, B., Kim, J-H. et al. Progressive white matter destruction following irradiation of an extracranial neoplasm. Ann. Neurol. 8:76, 1980.
15. Glass, J.P., Hwang T-L., Leavens, M.E. et al. Cerebral radiation necrosis following treatment of extracranial malignancies. Cancer 54:1966, 1984.
16. Shaw, P.J. and Bates, D. Conservative treatment of delayed cerebral radiation necrosis. J. Neurol. Neurosurg. Psychiatry 47:1338, 1984.
17. Wilson, G.H., Byfield, J., and Hanafee, W.N. Atrophy following radiation therapy for central nervous system neoplasms. Acta Radiol. (Suppl) 11:361, 1972.
18. Frytak, S. et al. Magnetic resonance imaging for neurotoxicity in long-term survivors of carcinoma. Mayo Clin. Proc. 60:803, 1985.
19. Ellis, F. Nominal standard dose and the ret. Br. J. Radiol. 44:101, 1971.

20. Jones, A. Transient radiation myelopathy. Br. J. Radiol. 37:727, 1964.
21. Reagan, T.J., Thomas, J.E., and Colby, M.Y., Jr. Chronic progressive radiation myelopathy: Its clinical aspects and differential diagnosis. JAMA 203:128, 1968.
22. Jellinger, K. and Strum, K.W. Delayed radiation myelopathy in man: Report of twelve necropsy cases. J. Neurol. Sci. 14:389, 1971.
23. Godwin-Austen, R.B., Howell, D.A., and Worthington, B. Observations on radiation myelopathy. Brain 98:557, 1975.
24. Wara, W.M., Phillips, T.L., Sheline, G.E. et al. Radiation tolerance of the spinal cord. Cancer 35:1558, 1975.
25. Kori, S.H., Foley, K.M., and Posner, J.B. Brachial plexus lesions in patients with cancer: 100 cases. Neurology 31:45, 1981.
26. Stoll, B.A. and Andrews, J.T. Radiation-induced peripheral neuropathy. Br. Med. J. [Clin. Res.] 1:834, 1966.
27. Thomas, J.E. and Colby, M.Y., Jr. Radiation-induced or metastatic brachial plexopathy? A diagnostic dilemma. JAMA 222:1392, 1972.
28. Bagley, F.H. et al. Carcinomatous versus radiation-induced brachial plexus neuropathy in breast cancer. Cancer 41:2154, 1978.
29. Cascino, T.L., Kori, S., Krol, G. et al. CT of the brachial plexus in patients with cancer. Neurology 33:1553, 1983.
30. Albers, J.W., Allen, A.A., II, Bastron, J.A. et al. Limb myokymia. Muscle Nerve 4:494, 1981.
31. Lederman, R.J. and Wilbourn, A.J. Brachial plexoppathy: Recurrent cancer of radiation? Neurology 34:1331, 1984.
32. Thomas, J.E., Cascino, T.L., and Earle, J.D. Differential diagnosis between radiation and tumor plexopathy of the pelvis. Neurology 35:1, 1985.
33. Jaekle, K.A., Young, D.F., and Foley, K.M. Lumbosacral plexopathy in cancer. Neurology 35:8, 1985.
34. Aho, K. and Sainio, K. Late irradiation-induced lesions of the lumbosacral plexus. Neurology 33:953, 1983.
35. Berger, P.S. and Bataini, J.P. Radiation-induced cranial nerve palsy. Cancer 40:152, 1977.
36. Shukovsky, L.J. and Fletcher, G.H. Retinal and optic nerve complications in a high dose irradiation technique of ethmoid sinus and nasal cavity. Radiology 104:629, 1972.
37. Nardelli, E., Fiaschi, A., and Ferrari, G. Delayed cerebrovascular consequences of radiation to the neck. Arch. Neurol. 35:538, 1978.
38. Conomy, J.P. and Kellermeyer, R.W. Delayed cerebrovascular consequences of therapeutic radiation: A clinicopathologic study of a stroke associated with radiation-related carotid arteriopathy. Cancer 36:1702, 1975.
39. Glick, B. Bilateral carotid occlusive disease. Arch. Pathol. Lab. Med. 93:352, 1972.
40. Cascino, T.L., Dale, A.J.D., Sundt, T.M. et al. Radiation-induced carotid artery disease. Stroke 11:135, 1980.
41. Foley, K.M., Woodruff, J.M., Ellis, F.T. et al. Radiation-induced malignant and atypical peripheral nerve sheath tumors. Ann. Neurol. 7:311, 1980.
42. Calabresi, P. and Parks, R.E., Jr. Chemotherapy of neoplastic diseases. In The Pharmacological Basis of Therapeutics. 6th Ed. Edited by A.G. Gilman, L.S. Goodman, and A. Gilman. New York, MacMillan Publishing Co., 1980, p. 1249.
43. Chabner, B.A. and Myers, C.E. Clinical pharmacology of cancer chemotherapy. In Cancer: Principles and Practice of Oncology. Edited by V.T. DeVita, Jr., S. Hellman, and S.A. Rosenberg. Philadelphia, Lippincott, 1982.
44. Byfield, J.E. Central nervous system toxicities from combined therapies. Front. Radiat. Ther. Oncol. 13:228, 1979.
45. Leenhonts, H.P., Chadwick, K.H., and Deen, D.F. An analysis of the interaction between two nitrosourea compounds and x-radiation in rat brain tumour cells. Int. J. Radiat. Biol. 37:169, 1980.
46. Bethlenfalvay, N.C. and Bergin, J.J. Severe cerebral toxicity after intravenous nitrogen mustard therapy. Cancer 29:366, 1972.
47. French, J.D., West, P.M., von Amerongen, F.K. et al. Effects of intracarotid administration of nitrogen mustard: On normal brain and brain tumors. J. Neurosurg. 9:378, 1952.
48. Woodhall, B., Mahaley, S., Jr., Boone, S. et al. The effect of chemotherapeutic agents upon peripheral nerves. J. Surg. Res. 2:373, 1962.
49. Sholes, D.M., Jr. Pelvic perfusion with nitrogen mustard for cancer: A neurologic complication. Am. J. Obstet. Gynecol. 80:481, 1960.
50. Lawrence, W., Jr., Kuehn, P., Masle, E.T. et al. An abdominal tourniquet for regional chemotherapy. J. Surg. Res. 1:142, 1961.
51. Conrad, M.E. and Crosby, W.H. Massive nitrogen mustard therapy in Hodgkin's disease with protection of bone marrow by tourniquet. Blood 16:1089, 1960.
52. Wolfson, S. and Olney, M.B. Accidental ingestion of a toxic dose of chlorambucil: Report of a case in a child. JAMA 165:239, 1957.
53. Green, A.A. and Naiman, J.L. Chlorambucil poisoning. Am. J. Dis. Child. 116:190, 1968.
54. Williams, S.A., Makker, S.P., and Grupe, W.E. Seizures: A significant side effect of chlorambucil therapy in children. J. Pediatr. 93:516, 1978.
55. Arena, P.J. Oropharyngeal sensation associated with rapid intravenous administration of cyclophosphamide (NSC-26271). Cancer Chemother. Rep. 56:779, 1972.
56. Tashima, C.K. Immediate cerebral symptoms during rapid intravenous administration of cyclophosphamide (NSC-26271). Cancer Chemother. Rep. 59:441, 1975.
57. Kende, G., Sirkin, S.R., Thomas, P.R.M. et al. Blurring of vision. A previously undescribed complication of cyclophosphamide therapy. Cancer 44:69, 1979.
58. DeFronzo, R.A., Braine, H., Colvin, O.M. et al. Water intoxication in man after cyclophosphamide

therapy: Time course and relation to drug activation. Ann. Intern. Med. *78*:861, 1973.
59. Sullivan, M.P. Symposium on vincristine. Cancer Chemother. Rep. *52*:453, 1968.
60. Henson, R.A. and Urich, H. Cancer and the Nervous System: The Neurological Manifestations of Systemic Malignant Disease. Boston, Blackwell Scientific Publications, 1982.
61. Holland, J.F. et al. Vincristine treatment of advanced cancer: A cooperative study of 392 cases. Cancer Res. *33*:1258, 1973.
62. Allen, J.C. The effects of cancer therapy on the nervous system. J. Pediatr. *93*:903, 1978.
63. Schochet, S.S., Jr., Lampert, P.W., and Earle, K.M. Neuronal changes induced by intrathecal vincristine sulfate. J. Neuropathol. Exp. Neurol. *27*:645, 1968.
64. Hardisty, R.M., McElwain, T.J., and Darby, C.W. Vincristine and prednisone for the induction of remissions in acute childhood leukemia. Br. Med. J. *2*:662, 1969.
65. Johnson, F.L., Bernstein, I.D., Hartmann, J.R. et al. Seizures associated with vincristine sulfate therapy. J. Pediatr. *82*:699, 1973.
66. Rosenthal, S. and Kaufman, S. Vincristine neurotoxicity. Ann. Intern. Med. *80*:733, 1974.
67. Cutting, H.O. Inappropriate secretion of antidiuretic hormone secondary to vincristine therapy. Am. J. Med. *51*:269, 1971.
68. Robertson, G.L., Bhoopalam, N., and Zelkowitz, L.J. Vincristine neurotoxicity and abnormal secretion of antidiuretic hormone. Arch. Intern. Med. *132*:717, 1973.
69. Bradley, W.G., Lassman, L.P., Pearce, G.W. et al. The neuromyopathy of vincristine in man: Clinical electrophysiological and pathological studies. J. Neurol. Sci. *10*:107, 1970.
70. Bradley, W.G. The neuromyopathy of vincristine in the guinea pig: An electrophysiological and pathological study. J. Neurol. Sci. *10*:133, 1970.
71. Slotwiner, P., Song, S.K., and Anderson, P.J. Spheromembranous degeneration of muscle induced by vincristine. Arch. Neurol. *15*:172, 1966.
72. Sandler, S.G., Tobin, W., and Henderson, E.S. Vincristine-induced neuropathy: A clinical study of fifty leukemic patients. Neurology *19*:367, 1969.
73. Whittaker, J.A. and Griffith, I.P. Recurrent laryngeal nerve paralysis in patients receiving vincristine and vinblastine. Br. Med. J. [Clin. Res.] *1*:1251, 1977.
74. Sanderson, P.A., Kuwabara T., and Cogan, D.G. Optic neuropathy presumably caused by vincristine therapy. Am. J. Ophthalmol. *81*:146, 1976.
75. Vecchi, V. et al. Transient optic neuropathy secondary to MOPP chemotherapy in Hodgkin's disease: Report of a case. Tumori *70*:571, 1984.
76. Gottlieb, R.J. and Cuttner, J. Vincristine-induced bladder atony. Cancer *28*:674, 1971.
77. Carmichael, S.M., Eagleton, L., Ayers, C.R. et al. Orthostatic hypotension during vincristine therapy. Arch. Intern. Med. *126*:290, 1970.
78. Casey, E.B., Jellife, A.M., Le Quesne, P.M. et al. Vincristine neuropathy: Clinical and electrophysiological observations. Brain *96*:69, 1973.
79. Michalak, J.C. and Dibella, N.J. Exacerbation of myotonia dystrophica by vincristine (letter to the editor). N. Engl. J. Med. *295*:283, 1976.
80. Weider, R.L. and Wright, S.E. Vincristine neurotoxicity (letter to the editor). N. Engl. J. Med. *286*:1369, 1972.
81. Frei, E. III et al. Clinical studies of vinblastine. Cancer Chemother. Rep. *12*:125, 1961.
82. Breza, T.S., Halprin, K.M., and Taylor, J.R. Photosensitivity reaction to vinblastine. Arch. Dermatol. *111*:1168, 1975.
83. Oliverio, V.T., Denham, C., DeVita, V.T. et al. Some pharmacologic properties of a new anti-tumor agent. N-isopropyl-α-(2-methylhydrazino)-p-toluamide, hydrochloride (NSC-77213). Cancer Chemother. Rep. *42*:1, 1964.
84. Chabner, B.A. et al. High-dose intermittent intravenous infusion of procarbazine (NSC-77213). Cancer Chemother. Rep. *57*:361, 1973.
85. Stolinsky, D.C. et al. Clinical experience with procarbazine in Hodgkin's disease, reticulum cell sarcoma, and lymphosarcoma. Cancer *29*:984, 1970.
86. Samuels, M.L. et al. Clinical trials with N-isoprophyl-α-(2-methylhydrazino)-p-toluamide hydrochloride in malignant lymphoma and other disseminated neoplasia. Cancer *20*:1187, 1967.
87. Brunner, K.W. and Young, C.W. A methylhydrazine derivative in Hodgkin's disease and other malignant neoplasms: Therapeutic and toxic effects studied in 51 patients. Ann. Intern. Med. *63*:69, 1965.
88. De Vita, V.T., Hahn, M.A., and Oliverio, V.T. Monoamine oxidase inhibition by a new carcinostatic agent, N-isoprophyl-α-(2-methylhydrazino)-p-toluamide (MIH). Proc. Soc. Exp. Biol. Med. *120*:561, 1965.
89. Billmeier, G.J. and Holton, C.P. Procarbazine hydrochloride in childhood cancer. J. Pediatr. *75*:892, 1969.
90. Yamada, K. et al. Intra-arterial BCNU therapy in the treatment of metastatic brain tumor from lung carcinoma. Cancer *44*:2000, 1979.
91. Kupersmith, M.J. et al. Visual dysfunction related to intra-arterial chemotherapy for gliomas (abstract). Neurology *35* (Suppl 1):114, 1985.
92. Foo, S-H. et al. Experience with supraophthalmic intra-arterial BCNU infusion in malignant glioma (abstract). Neurology *35* (Suppl 1):114, 1985.
93. Schold, S.C. and Fay, J.W. Central nervous system toxicity from high-dose BCNU treatment of systemic cancer. Neurology *30*:429, 1980.
94. So, N.K., O'Neill, B.P., Frytak, S., et al. Delayed leukoencephalopathy in survivors with small cell lung cancer. Neurology *37*:1198, 1987.
95. Moertel, C.G., Reitemeier, R.J., Hahn, R.G. et al. Study of 5-(3,3-dimethyl-1-triazeno) imidazole-4-carboxamide (NSC-45388) in patients with gastrointestinal carcinoma. Cancer Chemother. Rep. *54*:471, 1970.
96. Paterson, A.H.G. and McPherson, T.A. A possible

neurologic complication of DTIC. Cancer Treat. Rep. 61:105, 1977.
97. Donaldson, S.S. and Kaplan, H.S. Complications of treatment of Hodgkin's disease in children. Cancer Treat. Rep. 66:977, 1982.
98. Donaldson, S.S., Glatstein, E. and Vosti, K.L. Bacterial infections in pediatric Hodgkin's disease. Cancer 41:1949, 1978.
99. Chernik, N.L., Armstrong, D., and Posner, J.B. Central nervous system infections in patients with cancer. Medicine 52:563.
100. Chernik, N.L., Amstrong, D., and Posner, J.B. Central nervous system infections in patients with cancer: Changing patterns. Cancer 40:268, 1977.
101. Lukes, S.A., Posner, J.B., Nielsen, S. et al. Bacterial infections of the CNS in neutropenic patients. Neurology 34:269, 1984.
102. Casazza, A.R., Duvall, C.P., Carbone, P.P. Infection in lymphoma. Histology, treatment and duration in relation to incidence and survival. JAMA 197:710, 1966.
103. Schimpff, S.C., O'Connell, M.J., Greene, W.H. et al. Infections in 92 splenectomized patients with Hodgkin's disease. Am. J. Med. 59:695, 1975.
104. Ruskin, J. and Remington, J.S. Toxoplasmosis in the compromised host. Ann. Intern. Med. 84:193, 1976.
105. Skovby, F. and Sullivan, M.P. Herpes zoster and varicella in children with Hodgkin's disease. Acta Paediatr. Scand. 71:269, 1982.
106. Schimpff, S., Rumack, B., and Block, J. Varicella-zoster infection in patients with cancer. Ann. Intern. Med. 76:241, 1972.
107. Thomas, J.E. and Howard, F.M., Jr. Segmental zoster paresis—a disease profile. Neurology 22:459, 1972.
108. Hogan, E.L. and Krigman, M.R. Herpes zoster myelitis. Evidence for viral invasion of spinal cord. Arch. Neurol. 29:309, 1973.
109. Gilbert, G.J. Herpes zoster ophthalmicus and delayed contralateral hemiparesis: Relationship of the syndrome to central nervous system granulomatous angiitis. JAMA 229:302, 1974.
110. McCormick, W.F., Rodnitzsky, R.L., Schochet, S.S., Jr. et al. Varicella-zoster encephalomyelitis: A morphologic and virologic study. Arch. Neurol. 21:559, 1969.
111. Shepp, D.H., Dandliker, P.S., and Meyers, J.D. Treatment of varicella-zoster virus infection in severely immunocompromised patients. A randomized comparison of acyclovir and vidarabine. N. Engl. J. Med. 314:208, 1986.
112. Price, R., Chernik, N.L., Horta-Barbosa, L. et al. Herpes simplex encephalitis in an anergic patient. Am. J. Med. 54:222, 1973.
113. Wolinsky, J.S., Swoveland, P., Johnson, K.P. et al. Subacute measles encephalitis complicating Hodgkin's disease in an adult. Ann. Neurol. 1:452, 1977.
114. Dorfman, L.J. Cytomegalovirus encephalitis in adults. Neurology 23:136, 1973.
115. Snider, W.D. et al. Neurological complications of acquired immune deficiency syndrome: analysis of 50 patients. Ann. Neurol. 14:403, 1983.
116. Brooks, B.R. and Walker, D.L. Progressive multifocal leukoencephalopathy. Neurol. Clin. 2:299, 1984.
117. Bauer, W.R., Turel, A.P., Jr., and Johnson, K.P. Progressive multifocal leukoencephalopathy and cytarabine. Remission with treatment. JAMA 226:174, 1973.
118. Marriot, P.J., O'Brien, M.D., MacKenzie, I.C.K. et al. Progressive multifocal leucoencephalopathy: Remission with cytarabine. J. Neurol. Neurosurg. Psychiatry 38:205, 1975.
119. Greenlee, J.E. and Brashear, H.R. Antibodies to cerebellar Purkinje cells in patients with paraneoplastic cerebellar degeneration and ovarian carcinoma. Ann. Neurol. 14:609, 1983.
120. Trotter, J.L., Hendin, B.A., and Osterland, C.K. Cerebellar degeneration with Hodgkin's disease: An immunological study. Arch. Neurol. 33:660, 1976.
121. Walton, J.N., Tomlinson, B.E., and Pearce, G.W. Subacute "poliomyelitis" and Hodgkin's disease. J. Neurol. Sci. 6:435, 1968.
122. Lennon, V.A. Unpublished observations.
123. Currie, S., Henson, R.A., Morgan, H.G. et al. The incidence of the non-metastatic neurological syndromes of obscure origin in the reticuloses. Brain 93:629, 1970.
124. Elmqvist, D. and Lambert, E.H. Detailed analysis of neuromuscular transmission in a patient with the myasthenic syndrome sometimes associated with bronchogenic carcinoma. Mayo Clin. Proc. 43:689, 1968.
125. Kelly, J.J., Jr., Kyle, R.A., Miles, J.M. et al. Osteosclerotic myeloma and peripheral neuropathy. Neurology 33:202, 1983.
126. Carr, I. The Ophelia syndrome: Memory loss in Hodgkin's disease. Lancet 1:844, 1982.
127. Rewcastle, N.B. Subacute cerebellar degeneration with Hodgkin's disease. Arch. Neurol. 9:407, 1963.
128. Patten, J.P. Remittent peripheral neuropathy and cerebellar degeneration complicating lymphosarcoma. Neurology 21:189, 1971.
129. Streib, E.W. and Rothner, A.D. Eaton-Lambert myasthenic syndrome: Long-term treatment of three patients with prednisone. Ann. Neurol. 10:448, 1981.
130. Dau, P.C. and Denys, E.H. Plasmapheresis and immunosuppressive drug therapy in the Eaton-Lambert syndrome. Ann. Neurol. 11:570, 1982.
131. Palma, G. Paraneoplastic syndromes of the nervous system. West J. Med. 142:787, 1985.
132. Posner, J.B. Neurological complications of systemic cancer. DM 25:1, 1978.
133. Rodriguez, M., Trul, L., O'Neill, B.P. et al. Autoimmune cerebellar degeneration associated with cancer: Localization of Purkinje cytoplasmic antigen by immuno-electron microscopy. Neurology 38:1380, 1988.
134. Greenlee, J.E., Brashear, H.R., and Herndon, R.M. Anticerebellar antibodies in patients with cancer and paraneoplastic cerebellar degeneration (abstract). J. Neurol. 232 Suppl:530, 1985.

135. Croft, P.B., Henson, R.A., Urich, H. et al. Sensory neuropathy with bronchial carcinoma: A study of four cases showing serologic abnormalities. Brain 88:501, 1965.
136. Grunwald, G.B., Simmonds, M.A., Klein, R. et al. Autoimmune basis for visual paraneoplastic syndrome in patients with small-cell lung carcinoma. Lancet 1:658, 1985.
137. Brain, L. and Wilkinson, M. Subacute cerebellar degeneration associated with neoplasms. Brain 88:465, 1965.
138. Meyer, J.S. and Foley, J.M. The encephalopathy produced by extracts of eosinophils and bone marrow. J. Neuropathol. Exp. Neurol. 12:349, 1953.
139. Walsh, J.C. Neuropathy associated with lymphoma. J. Neurol. Neurosurg. Psychiatry 34:42, 1971.
140. Croft, P.B., Urich, H., and Wilkinson, M. Peripheral neuropathy of sensorimotor type associated with malignant disease. Brain 90:31, 1967.
141. Klingon, G.H. The Guillain-Barré syndrome associated with cancer. Cancer 18:157, 1965.
142. Lisak, R.P. et al. Guillain-Barré syndrome and Hodgkin's disease: Three cases with immunological studies. Ann. Neurol. 1:72, 1977.
143. Somasundaram, M., Cho, E-S., and Posner, J.B. Anterior horn cell degeneration as a "remote effect" of lymphoma. Trans. Am. Neurol. Assoc. 100:144, 1975.
144. Schold, S.C., Cho, E-S., Somasundaram, M. et al. Subacute motor neuronopathy: A remote effect of lymphoma. Ann. Neurol. 5:271, 1979.

CHAPTER 10

Therapy-Related Thyroid and Parathyroid Dysfunction in Patients with Hodgkin's Disease

JOHN R. REDMAN
DAIVA R. BAJORUNAS

One of the most common complications in the treatment of Hodgkin's disease is radiation-induced thyroid dysfunction, notably hypothyroidism. Fortunately, this complication causes only limited morbidity, especially with early recognition and treatment. This chapter reviews the problem of treatment-induced hypothyroidism, including its incidence, potential causative factors, clinical presentation, treatment, and prevention. Less common complications such as hyperthyroidism and ophthalmopathy, thyroid carcinoma, and radiation-induced parathyroid disease are also discussed.

HYPOTHYROIDISM

HISTORY

Until the last two decades, hypothyroidism, as a consequence of radiation to the normal thyroid gland, was considered a rare complication of treatment. Studies on the effects of thyroid irradiation had suggested that the gland was relatively radio-resistant.[1] In the early 1950s, however, it was recognized that external radiation to the human thyroid, in doses of 225 to 4300 cGy, could result in histopathologic changes of atrophy and fibrosis.[2] With the increasing use of ^{131}I therapy for Graves' disease, radiation-induced clinical hypothyroidism became more frequently diagnosed;[3,4] its incidence was noted to be as high as 29% with a follow-up of 10 years in one representative series.[5]

The first case of hypothyroidism after incidental thyroidal irradiation in patients with malignancy was reported in 1961, following therapy for carcinoma of the larynx.[6] Several further cases, including patients with lymphoma, were reported in 1965.[7,8] In 1966, irradiation for Hodgkin's disease was first associated with this complication.[9] In these earlier studies, the diagnosis of hypothyroidism was generally made clinically, since the available thyroid function tests, such as protein bound iodine (PBI) and radioactive iodine uptake (RAIU), were subject to iodine contamination in patients who had undergone prior lymphangiography. In the 1960s, the introduction of specific assays for serum concentrations of thyroxine (T_4), triiodothyronine (T_3), thyroid-stimulating hormone (TSH), and estimates of thyroid-binding capacity (RT_3U) made it possible to appreciate subtle as well as overt thyroidal dysfunction. Using these methods Glatstein et al. found that 44% of 74 patients with Hodgkin's disease or non-Hodgkin's lymphoma who had received neck irradiation developed elevated serum TSH levels,[10] with primary thyroid failure (depressed T_4 and elevated TSH) occurring in 11%. These investigators later extended their observations to a larger series (N = 297) and found 44% of the irradiated patients with lymphoma to have compensated hypothyroidism (increased TSH, normal T_4) and 19% to be hypothyroid (increased TSH, decreased T_4), a 63% incidence of thyroidal dysfunction overall.[11]

INCIDENCE

The incidence of hypothyroidism following irradiation for Hodgkin's disease depends on multiple factors, the most important being the rigor of the search and the sensitivity of the testing procedures. When no routine laboratory thyroid function testing has been done and the diagnosis of hypothyroidism has been made clinically, the incidence has been reported to be 3 to 6%,[12-13] presumably an underestimate of the thyroid dysfunction actually present. At the other extreme has been the inclusion of a particularly sensitive testing procedure (the TRH stimulation test), with which 91% of patients tested have been shown to have abnormal responses.[14] Clinically, the most useful indicators of thyroid function have been the measurement of serum T_4 and TSH levels. In patients with Hodgkin's disease, a depressed serum T_4 level has been found in 0 to 25% of patients and an elevated serum TSH level has been found in 20 to 80% (Table 10-1).[10-33]

PRETREATMENT THYROID FUNCTION

Studies of thyroid function in patients with Hodgkin's disease, prior to treatment, have found no significant preexisting thyroid dysfunction. In one series of 48 patients evaluated pretherapy by thyroid function testing, only one patient had abnormal function and this was longstanding.[10] We have noted similar pretreatment findings in a series of 114 patients with Hodgkin's disease studied prospectively. None had abnormal T_4 or TSH levels at the time of diagnosis, although two patients were receiving chronic thyroxine replacement therapy.[34] However, in one subgroup of patients, those with stage IVB lymphoma, pretreatment thyroid dysfunction has been described.[35] These patients had thyroid function tests consistent with reduced peripheral conversion of T_4 to T_3, the "euthyroid sick syndrome." This condition has been reported in other patients with significant acute and chronic medical illness, and is an index of the severity of the underlying disease.[36]

Involvement of the thyroid gland by malignant lymphoma at the time of diagnosis is an uncommon occurrence, with approximately 250 cases reported through 1979;[37-39] however, it may be increasing in incidence.[40] Hodgkin's disease infiltrating the thyroid gland at diagnosis is an even rarer finding, with less than forty cases reported in the literature.[41-48] NonHodgkin's lymphomas of the thyroid gland, arising in the setting of preexisting Hashimoto's thyroiditis, have been recognized for many years;[39,49-52] in a 1985 investigation of patients with chronic lymphocytic thyroiditis, a 67-fold increase in the incidence of thyroid lymphoma was found.[53] In 1984, a relationship of Hashimoto's thyroiditis to thyroidal Hodgkin's disease was suggested as well.[48]

POTENTIAL FACTORS LEADING TO THE DEVELOPMENT OF HYPOTHYROIDISM FOLLOWING TREATMENT OF HODGKIN'S DISEASE

Radiation Dose

Experimental models in animals provide good evidence that radiation-induced changes in the thyroid are dose-dependent.[54,55] Cumulative evidence suggests that this is also true in humans. A linear correlation between the radiation dose to the thyroid

Table 10–1. Incidence of Hypothyroidism After Neck Irradiation for Hodgkin's Disease (HD) and NonHodgkin's Lymphoma

Reference Authors/Year of Study	Number of Patients Studied	Primary Thyroid Failure (%) (Increased TSH, Decreased T_4)	Compensated Hypothyroidism (%) (Increased TSH, Normal T_4)	Total Thyroidal Dysfunction (%) (Increased TSH, Normal or Decreased T_4)
Glatstein et al. 1971[10]				
HD	162	—	—	44
NHL	63	—	—	17
Prager et al. 1972[15]	23	22	—	—
Fuks et al. 1976[11]				
HD	235	20	44	64
NHL	62	15	43	58
Carmel et al. 1976[16]	377	—	—	13*
Donaldson et al. 1976[17]	79	15	19	34
Johnson et al. 1976[13]	136	—	—	4‡
Shalet et al. 1977[14]	32	16	53	69 (91)†
Slanina et al. 1977[18]	78	—	—	17
Nelson et al. 1978[19]	50	—	—	20‡
Poussin-Rosillo et al. 1978[12]	127	—	—	2‡
Schimpff et al. 1980[20]	169	25	41	66
Kim et al. 1980[21]				
(HD & NHL)	70	14	19	33
Green et al. 1980[22]	27	0	37	37
Tamura et al. 1981[23]	48	8	40	48
Smith et al. 1981[24]	64	6	31	38
Sutcliffe et al. 1981[25]	60	10	70	80 (100)†
Mauch et al. 1983[26]	37	5	52	57
Holt et al. 1983[27]	62	10	27	37
Farley 1983[28]	32	12	31	43
Constine et al. 1984[29]	119	—	—	63
Devney et al. 1984[30]	24	21	67	88
Nair et al. 1984[31]	63	8	29	37
Fleming et al. 1985[32]	118	3	13	16
Morgan et al. 1985[33]	25	8	44	52 (92)†

*Not all patients were tested
†Percentage of patients with abnormal testing when TRH stimulation is included (in parentheses).
‡Clinical diagnoses of hypothyroidism; systematic testing not done.

from radioiodine-131 and development of hypothyroidism has been demonstrated after treatment of Graves' disease.[56] Hypothyroidism induced by external irradiation is also likely to be dose-dependent: low doses used for therapy of benign conditions of childhood fail to induce hypothyroidism, while high doses used for therapeutic irradiation result in a significant incidence of thyroid dysfunction.[56] In the specific example of Hodgkin's disease, most studies are not able to assess a dose relationship because of the narrow dose range therapeutically employed, usually 35 to 45 Gy. Two studies, however, have recorded a wider variation in therapeutic dosage and have been able to document a dose effect. In one investigation, elevated TSH levels were found in 41% of patients (N=196) who received 40 to 50 Gy versus 0% in those who received 15 Gy (N=7).[10] Another good demonstration of a dose effect is from a pediatric series where 17% of children who received less than 26 Gy (N=24) developed elevated TSH levels compared to 75% who received a larger dose (N = 95).[29] Radiation dose to the thyroid is, therefore, one factor predictive of subsequent thyroid dysfunction.

Lymphangiography

Rogoway was the first to point out the possible relationship of lymphangiography to subsequent thyroid dysfunction.[9] When the incidence of thyroid dysfunction after irradiation for lymphoma was compared to that following irradiation for head and neck cancer, it was found that the former group of patients had a higher incidence despite receiving a lower dose of radiation.[10] It was postulated that iodide loading from the lymphangiography was the critical difference. The lymphangiographic dye, ethiodol, is fat soluble and is excreted slowly from the lymphatic system. An estimated 2 g of iodine persists in the body after lymphangiography and is gradually released over the ensuing months. The adverse effects of iodides on thyroid function have been well recognized,[57] particularly the acute inhibitory effect of large doses of iodides (Wolff-Chaikoff effect), which results in decreased T_3 and T_4 formation.[57–59] It should be noted that the administration of pharmacologic doses of iodine can result in goiter or hyperthyroidism as well as hypothyroidism. Preexisting thyroid pathology may render patients more susceptible to iodine-induced thyroidal abnormalities: hypothyroidism has been reported to develop after iodine exposure in euthyroid patients with Hashimoto's thyroiditis,[131]I or surgically treated Graves' disease, or following hemithyroidectomy. Conversely, hyperthyroidism may be a consequence of iodine administration to euthyroid patients with iodine-deficient goiter, autonomous nodules, or nontoxic nodular goiter; it also occurs in patients treated for Graves' disease with antithyroid drugs or in patients without previous thyroid disease.[57,60]

What are the results of investigations comparing the effects of irradiation with or without lymphangiography on subsequent thyroid function? In a study by Glatstein and coworkers, patients with Hodgkin's disease or nonHodgkin's lymphoma who received both lymphangiography and radiation had a higher incidence of increased serum TSH levels than patients with head and neck cancer receiving radiation alone.[10] A subsequent report by the same investigators confirmed these results.[11] These two studies, however, compared a group with a different diagnosis in which other concomitant factors (e.g., age or median time of follow-up) may have played a role in lessening the thyroidal risk. Because of the routine use of lymphangiography in the staging of Hodgkin's disease, it is difficult to obtain an adequate comparison group of patients who did not have pretreatment lymphangiography. Several investigators have been able to make this comparison, however (Table 10–2), and have noted an increased,[14,31,61] a similar,[20,23,30,32,33] or a decreased[8] incidence of thyroid dysfunction following lymphangiography. In evaluating such comparisons, one has to consider that patients who did not receive lymphangiography pretreatment, nevertheless may have been exposed to a significant iodine load from diagnostic contrast studies employed, such as intravenous pyelography and computerized tomography.

The length of time between lymphangiography and irradiation has also been examined in relation to the incidence of thyroid dysfunction. Smith and colleagues found the severity of thyroid disease and the level of TSH to be inversely proportional to the length of time between lymphangiography and radiation.[24] Others too have found this same relationship; with an interval of less than 30 days, a 77% and 44% incidence of increased TSH was noted, in contrast to a 53% and 29% incidence, respectively, if the interval was greater than 30 days.[20,23] Later analyses, however, have not confirmed these findings.[29,30,33]

How important a factor is the lymphangiogram in producing thyroid dysfunction in patients who do not receive any neck irradiation? In one series, 14% of patients who had lymphangiography without radiation developed increased TSH levels.[11] Similarly, others have noted a 6% incidence of thyroidal dysfunction after lymphangiography, a rate not statistically different from an incidence of 8% seen in control patients receiving neither lymphangiography nor radiation.[20] While the above cited studies evaluated thyroid func-

Table 10-2. Effect of Lymphangiography on Postirradiation Thyroid Function

Reference	Subjects	Incidence of Elevated TSH	
		LAG Done	LAG Not Done
Deleterious Effect			
Shalet 1977[14]	Pediatric HD	11/12 (92%)	9/20 (45%)
Kaplan 1983*[61]	Childhood cancer (44 HD patients)	30/41 (73%)	10/50 (20%)
Nair 1984[31]	HD	16/26 (62%)	11/37 (30%)
No Effect			
Schimpff 1975[20]	HD	103/156 (66%)	6/9 (66%)
Tamura 1981[23]	HD and NHL	21/51 (41%)	10/23 (43%)
Devney 1984[30]	Pediatric HD	18/21 (86%)	3/3 (100%)
Fleming 1985[32]	Pediatric HD	7/65 (11%)	12/88 (14%)
Morgan 1985[33]	HD	No difference	
Protective Effect			
Green 1980[22]	Pediatric HD	3/4 (21%)	7/13 (54%)

*Patients who had a prior LAG tended to have a higher radiation dose; however, even when logistic regression analysis was done to account for this, lymphangiography was still associated with an increased risk of developing an elevated TSH ($p = 0.01$).

tion after therapy for Hodgkin's disease, other investigators have examined the effect of lymphangiography prior to therapy. TSH was found to be elevated in 77% of 17 patients following lymphangiography, with the earliest elevation seen 24 hours following the contrast study. Repeat testing during chemotherapy showed that these TSH elevations generally normalized spontaneously.[25]

If lymphangiography does result in an increased incidence of thyroid dysfunction, what might be the mechanism? The Wolff-Chaikoff effect of iodides previously mentioned may be a significant factor. The finding of elevated TSH levels following lymphangiography, but prior to treatment, is consistent with this hypothesis. TSH-induced thyroidal stimulation may result in increased thyroid cellular division during the period of radiation with resultant increased cellular damage. The finding of an increased incidence of thyroid dysfunction when the interval from lymphangiography to radiation is short also supports this hypothesis.

One cannot, however, dismiss the evidence that lymphangiography does not result in an increased incidence of thyroid dysfunction, or that it may even lessen the risk. The investigators who found a protective effect of lymphangiography postulated that another mechanism might be operative.[22] Iodine administration can acutely decrease thyroidal vascularity and cause involution of the gland. The resultant compromise in tissue oxygenation may potentially diminish the cell kill from radiation, as has been shown to occur in other experimental situations,[62] thereby decreasing the incidence of thyroid dysfunction.

In summary, investigators have disagreed on whether lymphangiography leads to a greater, a similar, or a lesser incidence of thyroid dysfunction. The data relating the interval between lymphangiography and radiation administration to the incidence/severity of thyroid dysfunction are also conflicting. It does seem clear that lymphangiography alone does not result in a high incidence of hypothyroidism.[11,20] The accumulated evidence suggests that lymphangiography, while not a major factor in radiation-induced thyroid dysfunction, may enhance the occurrence of iatrogenic hypothyroidism.

Age

Several groups have examined the effect of age at time of irradiation on the subsequent incidence of hypothyroidism. Glatstein and coworkers found that, of those patients less than 20 years of age, 48% had elevated TSH levels, while those older than 20 years had an incidence of 33%.[10] While this was statistically significant ($p < .05$), the population included patients with both Hodgkin's disease and nonHodgkin's lymphoma. Because in this study there was a much greater incidence of thyroid dysfunction in patients with Hodgkin's disease and because these patients were younger than those with nonHodgkin's lymphoma, it is possible that the apparent effect was related to the underlying disease itself. A similar trend, albeit not statistically significant, has been reported in children where those younger than 13 years of age had a 47% incidence of elevated TSH levels, compared to an incidence half that in children older than 13 years.[22] The majority of investigations, however, have not found age to be a significant factor.[19,20,29,31]

Gender

Where gender has been evaluated as a risk factor, no difference between males and females in the incidence of thyroid dysfunction following treatment for Hodgkin's disease has been found.[10,20,29]

Stage/Histologic Subtype

No effect of either stage or histologic subtype of Hodgkin's disease has been found in the single study where they have been evaluated.[20]

Extent of Radiation Portal

It has been shown that bilateral neck irradiation results in a significantly higher incidence of compensated hypothyroidism than unilateral neck irradiation.[10,23]

Previous Hemithyroidectomy

In head and neck cancer, it seems clear that the addition of hemithyroidectomy to primary irradiation results in a three- to fourfold higher incidence of thyroid dysfunction.[63,64] In Hodgkin's disease, hemithyroidectomy is rarely, if ever, performed and therefore does not constitute a major consideration.

Time Interval After Radiation

As expected, the prevalence of radiation-induced hypothyroidism increases with the duration of follow-up, as found by Schimpff et al.[20] In this study, a plateau was reached at five years post-therapy, despite an additional 48 patients being tested.[20] Others, however, have noted a progressive occurrence of thyroidal dysfunction with up to 16 years of patient follow-up.[23,32]

Effect of Chemotherapy

Only limited information is available regarding the effect of chemotherapy alone on thyroid function. The incidence of increased TSH has been 7% and 44% in two studies that have addressed this question.[20,25] The latter figure is higher than expected and needs to be confirmed. The risk of thyroid dysfunction following the administration of both radiation and chemotherapy, in comparison to that with neck irradiation alone, has been reported to be the same[20,29,33] or lower.[23] In the latter study, the lower incidence was hypothesized to be the result of prednisone and/or alkylating agents suppressing the development of chronic autoimmune thyroiditis.

Compared to the effects of chemotherapy alone, when both neck irradiation and chemotherapy are given, an increased incidence of TSH elevation has been noted.[20,25] However, Nelson and colleagues, using a different endpoint (the detection of an elevated TSH level or the appearance of thyroid nodules), found the same incidence of abnormalities in patients receiving combined modality therapy (4 of 8) as in the entire group studied (25 of 50).[19]

In general, the effects of individual chemotherapeutic agents on thyroid function have not been well studied. In 1965, Blomgren and colleagues found that no significant effect of long-term 5-fluorouracil therapy could be demonstrated.[65] In 1977, however, fluorouracil was reported to cause an elevation in serum T_4 and T_3 levels in patients with breast carcinoma. In this series, serum-free T_4 levels were normal and there was no clinical evidence of hyperthyroidism, leading the authors to suggest that the elevated total T_4 levels were caused by increased serum binding of T_4.[66] Conversely, asparaginase therapy has been reported to cause an acute decrease in serum thyroxine binding globulin (TBG) levels, which were shown to revert to normal within four weeks after completion of treatment. While the serum total T_4 concentrations in this setting were lowered due to the decrease in TBG levels, normal serum-free T_4 and TSH levels confirmed euthyroidism.[67] Others have also noted TBG deficiency occurring following asparaginase therapy; however, free T_4 levels were also found to be low in more than half the patients studied. Blunted TSH release after TRH stimulation suggested secondary hypothyroidism, postulated by the authors to be caused by inhibition of protein synthesis by L-asparaginase.[68] The concomitant use of steroids, however, with their known suppressive effect on the hypothalamic-pituitary-thyroid axis, makes the results difficult to interpret. Platinum therapy has also been postulated to result in alterations in thyroid hormone metabolism.[69] In a group of patients with testicular carcinoma, serum concentrations of T_3, reverse T_3 and T_4 were found to rise during treatment with cisplatin, vinblastine, and bleomycin, while TSH levels decreased. The authors proposed that the interaction of platinum with the sulfhydryl groups of the deiodinating enzyme resulted in diminished conversion of T_4, T_3, and rT_3.

Similarly, data derived from animal experimentation give limited information on the effects of chemotherapeutic agents on the thyroid. While one study suggested that 5FU and actinomycin D stimulated ^{131}I uptake in the mouse thyroid,[70] in a later report these same investigators concluded that the findings were the result of decreased food intake and subsequent iodine deficiency.[71] In a rat model, 5FU had no effect on thyroid weight or ^{131}I uptake[72] and no effect on the thyroid/serum iodide concentration ratio;[73] this ratio was increased, however, in the presence of propylthiouracil blockage.[74] Lastly, vinblastine has been shown to inhibit thyroid hormone secretion in the mouse by interfering with microtubular action.[75] Nevertheless, the relevance of data obtained in animals to the use of these chemotherapeutic agents in humans remains unclear.

Autoimmune Disease

Markson and Flatman were among the first to suggest that autoimmune disease might be responsible for the hypothyroidism seen after external irradiation, as thyroid autoantibodies were present in all five of their reported patients with various nonthyroidal malignancies and hypothyroidism.[8] Others have also speculated that thyroidal antigens released from a damaged thyroid gland during radiation could ultimately result in autoimmune thyroid disease.[23,76-78] In one study, an index case had exophthalmos, hypothyroidism, and elevated antimicrosomal and antithyroglobulin antibody titers; the subsequent 51 patients evaluated, however, did not.[20] While Tamura et al. found 31% of 74 patients who received neck irradiation for Hodgkin's disease to have positive thyroid autoantibodies, 21% of the 52 control patients who did not receive neck irradiation also had a measurable antibody titer, a difference that was not statistically significant.[23] Patients receiving chemotherapy as part of their treatment regimen, however, had a significantly lower incidence of thyroid autoantibodies (17% versus 48%, $p<0.01$) and elevated serum TSH levels (29% versus 58%, $p<0.025$) than those who were treated with radiation alone. The authors postulated that chemotherapy may have prevented the occurrence of radiation-induced autoimmune thyroiditis, thereby lessening the incidence of hypothyroidism. This hypothesis is supported by experiments where simultaneous injections of cyclophosphamide and bovine thyroglobulin given to adult rabbits have resulted in an acquired unresponsiveness to bovine thyroglobulin.[79] Also, experimental allergic thyroiditis in Wistar rats has been shown to be reversed with a 10-day course of cyclophosphamide.[80] Because the study of Tamura and coworkers was retrospective, however, there may have been other factors playing a role, such as chemotherapy-treated patients receiving a lesser dose of neck irradiation and therefore having a lower risk of developing thyroid antibodies and elevated TSH levels.

One other large-scale study has investigated the incidence of antithyroglobulin antibodies after neck irradiation for Hodgkin's disease.[27] An 8% incidence in 62 patients was found, despite an overall 37% incidence of thyroidal dysfunction. On the basis of the above-cited studies, it appears that thyroid autoantibodies play a limited role (if any) in the pathogenesis of radiation-induced hypothyroidism.

CLINICAL PRESENTATION

Patients who develop thyroid dysfunction following radiation typically present with nonspecific symptoms: chronic fatigue, cold intolerance, bloating, and edema have all been described. Usually, these nonspecific complaints have been attributed by the patients to the after-effects of the Hodgkin's disease treatment and thus are often not even mentioned to the physician. Certain clues on physical examination may be ascribed to the treatment as well, such as hyporeflexia following vincristine therapy, and so they too are overlooked. Theoretically, any of the presenting signs and symptoms of hypothyroidism could be found in these patients. We have seen several patients presenting with myopathy, sometimes severe and disabling.[81] Galactorrhea has also been noted as the presenting symptom of hypothyroidism in our patient population, and when galactorrhea is associated with amenorrhea and hyperprolactinemia, thyroid replacement may reverse all of these findings.[82]

POTENTIAL RELATIONSHIP OF HYPOTHYROIDISM TO OTHER CLINICAL SETTINGS

Pericardial Effusion

A possible relationship between hypothyroidism and radiation-induced pericarditis has been noted in the early studies of thyroid dysfunction after treatment for Hodgkin's disease.[10] Of 19 patients with Hodgkin's disease who had radiation-induced pericarditis, 84% were found to have elevated serum TSH levels, compared to an incidence of 44% seen in the entire patient population studied. Although pericardial effusions can accompany hypothyroidism,[83] it is possible that both of these problems occur as independent radiation-induced dose-related complications. Further studies are needed to examine this relationship.

Infertility in Women

Because many of the women treated for Hodgkin's disease are young and fertility is of concern, it is important to examine whether therapy-related thyroid dysfunction can affect their subsequent child-bearing potential. By far the most important threat to fertility in these women is primary ovarian failure, occurring as a consequence of cytotoxic drugs and/or radiation. Hypothyroidism alone, however, has been shown to have an effect on fertility in otherwise normal women. In long-standing, untreated hypothyroidism, amenorrhea or oligomenorrhea can occur, generally accompanied by anovulation. Because thyroid replacement therapy has been shown to result in an ovulatory cycle within 1 to 2 months,[84] evaluation of thyroid function should be performed in every infertile woman with Hodgkin's disease so that this less common, but potentially remediable, cause of infertility may be detected without delay.

Pregnancy

A second mechanism of infertility is found in women with mild hypothyroidism who conceive, but then are faced with an increased risk of abortion, prematurity, and stillbirth.[85,86] Fetal loss in the first trimester of the hypothyroid mother is on the order of 50% or more. Whether this is the result of altered ovarian function, altered placental development, or abnormal embryogenesis is not clear, but it does appear that the fetal loss can be prevented by thyroid replacement.[84] Even if hypothyroid women continue their pregnancy to term, there is a 20% perinatal mortality, a 10 to 20% risk of congenital malformations, and a 50 to 60% rate of impaired mental and somatic development in the surviving children.[85,87,88] In a 1981 report, with the hypothyroid mothers generally receiving thyroid replacement, the latter complication has not been described.[89] It has been recommended that pregnant women who have an enlarging goiter or a history of previous thyroid surgery or radioiodine treatment for hyperthyroidism have thyroid function testing done both early in pregnancy and in the second trimester.[84] Because of the high risk of hypothyroidism, women who have received neck irradiation for Hodgkin's disease should receive similar surveillance.

TREATMENT

Treatment of the clinically or biochemically hypothyroid patient is standard. Most physicians would agree that thyroid hormone replacement should be initiated with synthetic thyroxine. Guidelines for treatment can be reviewed in a separate text.[90]

Some controversy arises, however, when one considers therapy for the patient with compensated hypothyroidism. Issues requiring analysis are: (1) Whether patients with this biochemical profile suffer any clinically deleterious effects and (2) Whether post-therapy abnormalities in thyroid function revert to normal with time.

Potential adverse effects of compensated hypothyroidism include an increased susceptibility to the development of cardiac disease and thyroid carcinoma. Previous investigations of compensated hypothyroidism have both favored and refuted its relationship to cardiac disease.[91-93] In 1981, it was suggested that patients with elevated TSH levels but normal T_4 levels have a mild but significant form of hypothyroidism, rather than just a biochemical abnormality.[94] In this study, cardiac systolic time intervals, found to be correlated with serum T_4 and TSH levels, were significantly decreased with thyroxine therapy. In a double-blind, randomized trial, these same investigators compared the effects of thyroxine therapy versus placebo in patients with compensated hypothyroidism.[95] While thyroxine administration had no measurable effect on the mean serum-lipid levels or systolic time intervals, the latter parameter normalized in the five patients with the most abnormal values. In patients who were symptomatic, significant improvement occurred in those treated with thyroxine as compared to those receiving placebo. The authors concluded that thyroxine therapy may be useful in compensated hypothyroidism in patients who are symptomatic or who have abnormal myocardial contractility.

Experimentally, in animals, elevated TSH has been shown to lead to an increased incidence of thyroid carcinoma in the setting of prior thyroid irradiation.[96] The possible carcinogenic effect of thyroidal stimulation by TSH has been advanced as a reason to give thyroxine to these patients.[10,20] Although there have been many case reports of thyroid carcinoma occurring following treatment of Hodgkin's disease, it is only recently that epidemiologic evidence suggests that the incidence is increased above that seen in the normal population.

In patients with radiation-induced thyroid dysfunction, recovery of euthyroid function apparently occurs, although the actual probability is not currently defined. In a series of reports from the University of Minnesota, 21 of 24 children who had received neck irradiation developed elevated serum TSH levels post-therapy.[30,97,98] Of the five patients with depressed T_4 levels, one patient had recovery of euthyroid function; the other four were started on thyroid replacement therapy. Of the 16 patients with normal T_4 levels, three patients had normalization of TSH levels, six were placed on thyroxine therapy, three had continued compensated hypothyroidism, and four progressed to frank hypothyroidism. Two reports from Stanford University have also documented this spontaneous normalization of thyroid function tests in a pediatric population.[29,99] Of 119 children who received neck irradiation, 63% developed elevated TSH levels. In 20 of these children, TSH levels normalized, and in seven others a greater than 50% decline in TSH levels occurred. Therefore, at least 27% had spontaneous normalization. In fact, these data may underestimate the recovery rate, as many of these patients did not have repeat TSH determinations performed or were receiving continued thyroxine replacement therapy. One study examining this question in a predominantly adult population found that of 25 patients with abnormal testing, seven patients had reversion to normal after one to two years of follow-up.[31] In contrast, however, Schimpff and colleagues have reported that, post-therapy, none of the 79 adult patients with Hodgkin's disease who had repeated thyroid function testing recovered euthyroid function.[20]

In summary, controversy exists whether

therapy should be instituted in the patient with Hodgkin's disease who has compensated hypothyroidism. Data have been presented to suggest that physiologic changes of hypothyroidism may occur, despite a normal T_4 level, when TSH levels are elevated. There is also experimental evidence that TSH may act as a co-carcinogen in the setting of prior thyroid irradiation, although limited data exist supporting this hypothesis in patients treated for Hodgkin's disease. Recovery of normal thyroid function has been reported, but its frequency needs to be better defined. Until further data are available and because thyroxine replacement carries few risks, we have adopted the policy of treating all patients who maintain an elevated serum TSH level during a 3 to 6 month observation period.

PREVENTION

Possible preventive measures, such as omitting the lymphangiogram or radiation therapy, or lengthening the interval from lymphangiography to radiation, are not generally feasible. One potential approach currently being evaluated is the administration of thyroxine, prior to lymphangiography, for the duration of radiation therapy.[24,100] Theoretically, this would serve to decrease TSH levels, suppress thyroidal uptake of exogenous iodine, and minimize thyroid cellular proliferation during the period of radiation. An initial nonrandomized trial to test this hypothesis compared eventual thyroid dysfunction in 20 patients who received thyroxine during radiation therapy to 20 patients who served as controls.[101] The similar incidence of thyroid dysfunction in the two groups in the early follow-up makes it unlikely that early administration of thyroxine during neck radiation will have a role in preventing subsequent thyroid dysfunction.

HYPERTHYROIDISM AND OPHTHALMOPATHY FOLLOWING NECK IRRADIATION FOR HODGKIN'S DISEASE

Hyperthyroidism and/or ophthalmopathy have been increasingly reported after radiation therapy for Hodgkin's disease (see Table 10–3),[19,20,27,29,30,77,78,102–114] and available evidence suggests a causal relationship. In the greater than 37 cases reported, there has been a consistent relationship between radiation and hyperthyroidism or ophthalmopathy, occurring a median time of 3.5 years after radiation, with a female preponderance of 3:2. Hyperthyroidism and ophthalmopathy have not been reported in most series of Hodgkin's disease patients examined for thyroid dysfunction,[14,15,22–26,31,61] however, in some series the prevalence of these disorders has been significantly increased. This prevalence has varied from 1.4 to 7%[109–111] and when compared to the expected prevalence of hyperthyroidism in the general population (0.3%)[115] by Mortimer et al., there was a significant increase ($p<0.0001$).[110] Loeffler et al. ascertained a 2% actuarial risk of developing Graves' disease 10 years following mantle radiation, and this risk also was found to exceed that of the general population.[111] It has been postulated that thyroidal irradiation results in damage to the gland, with subsequent release of thyroid antigens and a triggered immunologic reaction leading to the occurrence of Graves' disease. Antithyroglobulin and antimicrosomal antibodies and long-acting thyroid stimulator (LATS) immunoglobulin have frequently been present, which supports this contention. Absence of HLA-B8 positivity in patients postirradiation has also been proposed as being consistent with a radiation-induced complication rather than being genetic in nature, because 50% of patients with spontaneous Graves' disease have this finding.[102] Another mechanism proposed to explain the radiation induction of hyperthyroidism is that suppressor lymphocytes are more sensitive to irradiation than helper lymphocytes and thyroid autoantibodies are therefore stimulated similar to in vitro experiments with irradiated lymphocytes from patients with Hashimoto's disease.[116] In summary, these recent reports support the contention that hyperthyroidism and ophthalmopathy are radiation-induced complications of the treatment of Hodgkin's disease, although their occurrence remains uncommon. At this time the mechanism is speculative, but current evidence implicates radiation-induced

Table 10–3. Hyperthyroidism and Ophthalmopathy Following Treatment for Hodgkin's Disease

Reference/Year	Age (at HD dx)	Sex	Thyroid Function	Time after RT (months)	Ophthalmopathy
Wasnich 1973[102]	39	M	Euthyroid	18	+
Wasnich 1973[102]	41	M	Euthyroid	60	+
Nelson 1978[19]	NS	M	Euthyroid	42	+
Pilepich 1978[103]	16	F	Hyperthyroid	48	+
Jackson 1979[77]	28	F	Hyperthyroid	24	+
Jackson 1979[77]	63	F	Hypothyroid	156	+
Schimpff 1980[20]	NS	NS	Hypothyroid	NS	+
Schimpff 1980[20]	NS	M	Hyperthyroid	5	None
Tamura 1981[104]	22	F	Hypo- later hyperthyroid	41	+
Willimze 1982[105]	21	M	Hyperthyroid	8	NS
Constine 1982[78]	18	F	Hypo- later hyperthyroid	40	NS
Slavin 1982[106]	34	F	Hypothyroid	48	+
Jacobson 1984[107]	31	M	Hyperthyroid	108	+
Devney 1984[30]	Child	F	Hyper- later euthyroid	No RT	NS
Devney 1984[30]	Child	NS	Hyper- later hypothyroid	NS	NS
Constine 1984[29]	16	M	Hypo- later hyperthyroid	NS	NS
Blitzer 1985[108]	35	F	Hyperthyroid	6	None
Blitzer 1985[108]	39	M	Hyperthyroid	<1	None
Ghandour 1985[109]	21	F	Hyperthyroid	43	None
Ghandour 1985[109]	36	F	Hyperthyroid	35	None
Ghandour 1985[109]	19	F	Hyperthyroid	6	None
Ghandour 1985[109]	20	F	Hyperthyroid	3	None
Ghandour 1985[109]	26	M	Hyperthyroid	7	None
Ghandour 1985[109]	27	M	Hyperthyroid	4	None
Mortimer 1986[110]	35	F	Hyperthyroid	84	NS
Mortimer 1986[110]	19	M	Hyperthyroid	72	NS
Mortimer 1986[110]	29	F	Euthyroid, later hyper-thyroid	60	NS
Mortimer 1986[110]	25	F	Euthyroid	36	+
Mortimer 1986*[110]	28	M	Euthyroid, Graves'	72	NS
Loeffler 1988[111]	20	F	Hyperthyroid	53	+
Loeffler 1988[111]	27	F	Hyperthyroid	39	+
Loeffler 1988[111]	24	F	Hyperthyroid	12	+
Loeffler 1988[111]	20	M	Hyperthyroid	48	+
Loeffler 1988[111]	30	F	Hyperthyroid	93	+
Loeffler 1988[111]	23	F	Hyperthyroid	10	+
Loeffler 1988†[111]	36	M	Hyperthyroid	71	+
Porter 1988[114]	33	M	Hypo- later hyperthyroid	96	+

NS = Not Stated
*Original three patients reported by Holt, 1983[27]
†Partial reports by Loeffler, 1985[112] and Leslie, 1983[113]

release of thyroidal antigens together with immunologic alterations secondary to the treatment and/or Hodgkin's disease.

RADIATION-INDUCED THYROID NODULES AND THYROID CANCER

A larger body of information implicates radiation as a cause of both benign and malignant thyroid nodules.[56,117] Beginning in the 1920s, low-dose external radiation was commonly used for almost four decades as treatment for enlarged thymus, acne, cervical adenitis, or tonsillitis. In 1950, Duffy and Fitzgerald first called attention to the association of low-dose thyroid irradiation with the subsequent development of thyroid carcinoma.[118] Further reports confirmed this association, demonstrating a long latent period of 5 to 30 years.[119–121] In humans, an increased risk of thyroid neoplasia has also been demonstrated after fallout containing radioactive iodine in the Marshall Islands[122] and in the irradiated survivors of Hiroshima and Nagasaki.[123] Researchers have also been concerned that radioactive-iodine treatment of thyrotoxicosis might lead to thyroid neoplasia; although individual cases have occurred,[124] no increased risk has been demonstrated.[125–127]

The previously cited studies share several features in common: irradiation during childhood, low-dose radiation, and a long latency period. The thyroid undergoes a growth spurt from 1 to 2 g at birth to 15 to 25 g by puberty.[128] This increased growth rate may result in a greater sensitivity to the carcinogenic action of radiation, rendering the childhood thyroid at special risk. While adults were not usually exposed to the low-dose radiation that children frequently received for benign diseases such as acne or an enlarged thymus, in the Marshall Islands both adults and children were exposed to low-dose irradiation and only the children had a higher incidence of thyroid nodules.[122] However, while the bulk of evidence favors the conclusion that children are more susceptible to radiation-induced thyroid neoplasia, reports of thyroid carcinoma arising after irradiation of the adult thyroid can be found in the literature.[129–131]

Low-dose (opposed to high-dose) radiation is a second factor postulated to be important in the genesis of postradiation thyroid carcinoma. A linear dose-response curve has been constructed for doses less than 1500 rem.[56] Higher doses have not resulted in an increased incidence of thyroid neoplasia in several earlier series,[130,132,133] and the commonly held view is that high doses (greater than 20 Gy) cause thyroid-cell death, whereas the lower dose allows chromosomal injury without cell death, subsequently leading to mutant cell proliferation and malignancy. However, increasing numbers of cases of thyroid cancer seen after high-dose radiation, as well as new epidemiologic data, is leading to re-evaluation of this concept.

The latent period between the time of irradiation and the time of diagnosis of thyroid carcinoma has been examined for 660 cases in two series.[132,134] Combining the data for individual patients, a mean latent period of 10.5 years was found,[56] although others have reported this risk remains even after 30 years.[135–137]

EXPERIMENTAL RADIATION CARCINOGENESIS OF THE THYROID

In rats, both radioactive iodine and external thyroidal irradiation were shown to result in the development of thyroid adenomas and/or carcinomas, the optimal radiation dose being 10 to 20 Gy.[128–138] With the addition of goitrogenic drugs, tumors appeared in greater number.[96,139] If radiation acts as the initiator of malignancy, an elevated TSH may act as a promoter by increasing proliferation of thyroid cells. With regard to radiation-induced damage to the thyroid, radiation may be acting as both initiator and promoter. Suppressing serum TSH levels by adding T_4 to the diet of irradiated animals has been shown to reduce the development of thyroid tumors.[55,140]

THYROID CARCINOMA AFTER TREATMENT OF HODGKIN'S DISEASE

The occurrence of secondary neoplasia after treatment of Hodgkin's disease is an important concern. A large number of reports have documented that the incidence is increased,

Table 10-4. Thyroid Carcinoma Subsequent to Hodgkin's Disease and NonHodgkin's Lymphoma

Reference	Sex	Age at Diagnosis of Thyroid Cancer	Latent Interval (years)	Pathology	Neck Irradiation Dose
Hodgkin's Disease					
Morris 1964*[141]	M	28	20	papillary/follic	20 Gy
Hynes 1964[142]	M	25	10	papillary	1600 cGy
Moon 1968[143]	F	25	6	papillary	3000 cGy to supraclavicular area
Meyer 1971[144]	M	37	30	follicular	14 Gy
Glatstein 1971[10] Fuks 1976[11]	F	NS	9	papillary/follic	33 Gy
Jacquillat 1973[145]	M	47	2	papillary	+ (dose not stated)
Hempelmann 1975*[136]	F	37	36	spindle cell	2931 cGy
Weshler 1978[146]	M	22	16	papillary/follic	20 Gy
Getaz 1979[147,148] Shimaoka 1979[149]	M	49	44	anaplastic	2.9 Gy plus 12 more treatments
Getaz 1979[147,148] Shimaoka 1979[149]	M	66	31	anaplastic	46 Gy
Chase 1980[150]	F	26	10	follicular	NS
McDougall 1980[151]	M	39	10	papillary	40 Gy
McDougall 1980[151]	F	36	13	papillary	51 Gy
McDougall 1980[151]	F	41	9	papillary/follic	40 Gy
Frank 1980[152]	NS	34	15	papillary/follic	30 Gy
Frank 1980[152]	NS	22	14	papillary/follic	22 Gy
Bryda 1980[153]	M	37	13	papillary/follic	38 Gy
Valagussa 1980[154]	NS	NS	2.5	NS	+
Baccarani 1980[155]	M	52	1	adenocarcinoma	+
Palmer 1980[156]	NS	40–52	18	NS	30 Gy
Palmer 1980[156]	NS	40–52	18–24	NS	30 Gy
Palmer 1980[156]	NS	40–52	24	NS	30 Gy
Smallridge 1981[157]	M	64	10	papillary	3700 cGy
Smallridge 1981[157]	M	46	8	papillary	none
Sutcliffe 1981[157]	NS	NS	NS	NS (metastatic)	NS
Mazzaferri 1981[15]	NS	NS	NS	papillary	+
Pretorius 1982[159]	F	25	7	papillary	40 Gy
Pretorius 1982[159]	M	33	21	papillary/follic	30 Gy
Nicol 1982[160]	M	21	17	follicular	30 Gy
Glicksman 1982[161]	NS	NS	NS	NS	NS
Glicksman 1982[161]	NS	NS	NS	NS	NS
Coeur 1982[162]	F	29	17	follicular	20 Gy
Simone 1982[163]	NS	19	10	papillary	+
Najean 1982[164]	F	25	17	papillary	2500 cGy
Amin 1983[165]	F	55	25	follicular	17 Gy
Bakri 1983[166]	M	61	48	adenosquamous	2 Gy
Friedman 1983[167]	F	38	12	follicular	NS
Friedman 1983[167]	M	54	7	follicular	NS
Hamburger 1983[168]	F	21	9	papillary	40 Gy
Constine 1984[29]	F	14	10	NS	+
Tester 1984[169]	F	26	8	papillary	+
Boivin 1984[170]	F	37	14	papillary/follic	+
Rosen 1984[171]	M	34	16	papillary	25 Gy
Rosen 1984[171]	M	35	10	papillary	25 Gy

Table 10–4. Thyroid Carcinoma Subsequent to Hodgkin's Disease and NonHodgkin's Lymphoma
Continued

Reference	Sex	Age at Diagnosis of Thyroid Cancer	Latent Interval (years)	Pathology	Neck Irradiation Dose
Naunheim 1984[172]	F	17	6	papillary	50 Gy
Turrin 1985[173]	F	16	10	papillary	+
Turrin 1985[173]	F	21	3	papillary	+
Moroff 1986[174]	M	44	15	follicular	40 Gy
Jenkin 1987[175]	NS	NS	NS	carcinoma	+
Jenkin 1987[175]	NS	NS	NS	carcinoma	+
Jenkin 1987[175]	NS	NS	NS	carcinoma	+
McHenry 1987[176]	NS	22	9	papillary	44 Gy
McHenry 1987[176]	NS	39	16	papillary	>40 Gy
McHenry 1987[176]	NS	35	8	papillary	39 Gy
MSKCC[34]	F	34	17	follicular	2000 cGy
MSKCC[34]	M	26	7	follicular	1584 cGy
MSKCC[34]	M	24	5	papillary/follic	47 Gy
NonHodgkin's Lymphomas					
Rabinowitz 1958[177]	F	12	7	papillary	2000 cGy
Raventos 1964[134]	NS	NS	NS	NS	+
Raventos 1964[134]	NS	NS	NS	NS	+
Voisin 1975[178]	F	54	6	anaplastic	40 Gy
Satran 1983[179]	F	21	8	papillary/follic	43.5 Gy

*Diagnosis of Hodgkin's disease not confirmed

Table 10–5. Incidence of Thyroid Carcinoma After Treatment of Hodgkin's Disease

Reference	Cases of Thyroid Cancer	Patients With Hodgkin's Disease	Incidence (%)
Greene 1985[180]	Not Stated	3211	NS (RR=6.7)
McDougal 1980[151]	3	544	0.55
Weshler 1978[146]	1	207	0.48
Tucker 1984[181]	5	1036	0.48 (RR=68)
Getaz 1979[148]	2	494	0.40
Frank 1980[152]	2	631	0.32
Tester 1984[169]	1	473	0.21
Baccarani 1980[155]	1	613	0.16
Glicksman 1982[161]	2	1332	0.15
Valagussa 1980[154]	1	764	0.13
Tucker 1988[182]	1	1507	0.07 (RR=NS)
Boivin 1984[170]	1	2591	0.04
Kaldor 1987[183]	8	28462	0.02 (RR=2.5)
Newfeld 1978[184]	0	232	0
Toland 1978[185]	0	643	0
Coltman 1982[186]	0	659	0
Coleman 1982[187]	0	1222	0
Henry-Amar 1983[188]	0	334	0

RR = relative risk
NS = not significant

especially that of leukemia. Given the previously mentioned relationship of low-dose radiation to the development of thyroid carcinoma, it is important to evaluate whether thyroid carcinoma is a consequence of mantle radiation for Hodgkin's disease. More than 50 cases of thyroid carcinoma have been reported after primary therapy for Hodgkin's disease (Tables 10–4 and 5),[10,11,29,34,134,136,141–188] but these cases have generally been anecdotal reports or cases from investigations of second malignancies in Hodgkin's disease populations with an intermediate follow-up of less than 10 years. Less information has been available, however, from epidemiologic investigations of long-term Hodgkin's survivors. One study of 355 patients with non-Hodgkin's lymphoma treated from 1910 to 1960 found not even a single case of thyroid carcinoma.[189] More recently, however, three reports have investigated second malignancies in large Hodgkin's disease populations with long follow-up and have found an increased incidence of thyroid carcinoma.[180–183] The Connecticut Tumor Registry included 3211 people who developed Hodgkin's disease between 1935 and 1982.[180] A significant excess of subsequent thyroid cancer was found (relative risk = 6.7; 95% confidence interval = 1.8–17.1) and this was especially significant beyond 10 years of follow-up. An international collaborative study also investigated the incidence of second malignancies in 28,462 patients treated for Hodgkin's disease between 1945 and 1984.[183] An elevated relative risk was found for subsequent thyroid carcinoma (RR=2.5, p=NS) that was most striking after 10 or more years of follow up (RR=6.2; P<0.01). The Late Effects Study Group has also found a significantly increased rate of thyroid cancer in children treated for Hodgkin's disease (relative risk = 68).[181] The mean latent interval for thyroid cancer occurring after low-dose radiation has been estimated to be 10.5 years,[56] and these recent studies suggest the same holds true after high-dose, therapeutic radiation in Hodgkin's disease. The increasing reports of thyroid cancer after high-dose radiation together with the epidemiologic data mentioned above have led to re-examination of the concept that high-dose radiation is not associated with an increased risk of thyroid cancer.[61,171,190] This positive dose-response relationship above 20 Gy has also been seen in patients who received x-ray treatment for cervical tuberculosis adenitis[137] and also in children (including patients with Hodgkin's disease) following cancer treatment.[191] To date, the cumulative evidence favors a conclusion that there is a slightly increased risk of thyroid cancer in the long-term survivors of Hodgkin's disease.

RADIATION-INDUCED PARATHYROID DISEASE

Hypoparathyroidism and hyperparathyroidism have both been reported to occur infrequently following neck irradiation. While hypoparathyroidism has been noted within months after the use of ^{131}I in the treatment of thyrotoxicosis,[192–197] in a systematic study of this relationship, no decrease in parathyroid function was found in 1070 cardiac patients given ^{131}I.[198] Also, while seven of 60 patients were reported to develop "partial parathyroid insufficiency" after ^{131}I therapy for hyperthyroidism, the clinical significance of this is unclear.[199] To date, no cases have been reported to occur after therapy for thyroid carcinoma.[200] At present, therefore, the evidence that irradiation is causally related to the occurrence of hypoparathyroidism is not convincing.

Hyperparathyroidism, on the other hand, does seem to be related to previous neck irradiation. This association was first noted by Rosen in a case report that appeared in 1975.[201] Subsequently, a number of reports have confirmed this relationship. In patients found to have hyperparathyroidism, 11 to 30% have had a history of prior, low-dose external radiation for benign disease,[156,202–208] an incidence of radiation significantly greater than that seen in control patients.[207–208] Conversely, in patients who have received neck irradiation for benign disease, 5 to 14% have been reported to ultimately develop hyperparathyroidism.[204–208,209] In analyzing risk factors for the development of hyperparathyroidism in irradiated patients, a significant factor has been dose of radiation, with a 12%

incidence at less than 14 Gy and a 29% incidence at more than 14 Gy.[209] Pathologically, adenomas are found in 75% of the cases, with hyperplasia in the remainder.[210] While some investigators have found an increased incidence of associated thyroid abnormalities (68 to 80%), presumably also radiation-induced,[207–210] others have not.[208,211] A mean latent period of 30 to 47 years following low-dose external radiation has been reported,[202–204,206–208,210,212] a period even longer than that found with thyroid carcinoma.

In contrast to radiation for benign disease, high-dose external radiation for malignancy has not been associated with an increased risk of parathyroid dysfunction. In 35 patients with head and neck malignancies, external radiation with 58 to 66 Gy did not acutely change serum calcium, phosphorus, or parathyroid hormone levels.[213] Similarly, in a follow-up of 95 patients who had received high-dose neck irradiation for childhood cancer 5 to 34 years prior, Kaplan and colleagues could not detect a single case of hyperparathyroidism.[61] Given the long latency period found after low-dose radiation, it is possible that the follow-up of these patients was not long enough to see dysfunction. At least three patients with parathyroid adenomas have been reported after treatment for Hodgkin's disease,[159,214,215] occurring 13, 15, and 21 years following neck irradiation. In the single systematic study of this relationship, 220 patients treated for Hodgkin's disease with neck irradiation were followed with serum calcium determinations two to 22 years later, and only one patient was found to have hyperparathyroidism.[215] This incidence is not significantly different from that seen in the normal population, but the follow-up is short compared to the 30 to 47-year latent interval previously mentioned. It would not be surprising to see further cases accrue with the prolonged observation of patients treated with neck radiation for malignancies.

CONCLUSION

The improved survival of patients with Hodgkin's disease has led to the realization that hypothyroidism is a common iatrogenic complication. A major causative factor appears to be the dose of radiation delivered to the thyroid gland; other factors, such as the use of contrast studies, are not clearly documented to be of importance. Because of the high incidence of this complication and the paucity of specific symptoms in patients with treatment-induced hypothyroidism, routine thyroid function testing is indicated in all Hodgkin's disease patients following the completion of neck irradiation therapy. Testing is particularly necessary in patients presenting with myopathy, galactorrhea, or a pericardial effusion, and in pregnant or infertile women with Hodgkin's disease. Treatment of primary thyroid failure should be instituted with synthetic thyroxine. The issue of replacement therapy in patients with compensated hypothyroidism is more controversial. Arguments in support of replacement therapy in this situation have been presented: studies suggest that compensated hypothyroidism is a mild form of clinical hypothyroidism rather than merely a biochemical abnormality; experimental animal data demonstrate that an elevated TSH level can act as a co-carcinogen in the setting of prior thyroidal irradiation; a lack of risk is associated with thyroxine replacement therapy; and lastly, evidence shows the persistence of the abnormally elevated TSH over time. However, reports finding the significant occurrence of spontaneous normalization of TSH levels in children with time post-therapy, argue that, in fact, some patients with Hodgkin's disease may be receiving lifelong thyroid hormone therapy needlessly. Further studies regarding the reversibility of therapy-induced thyroid dysfunction should help resolve this question. The prevention of post-treatment hypothyroidism is an even more desirable, albeit elusive, goal. Although unsuccessful, the use of thyroxine administration to decrease thyroidal cell proliferation during the period of radiation treatment has been one such attempt.

While hypothyroidism is clearly a treatment-related complication of Hodgkin's disease, the occurrence of several other thyroid and parathyroid disorders following treatment has been noted. Evidence has been presented that hyperthyroidism, ophthalmopathy, and thyroid carcinoma occur in patients after treatment, and recent population-based studies suggest that the frequency is higher than that seen in the general population. Continued surveillance of cohorts of patients treated for Hodgkin's disease will be necessary to define the actual long-term risk of developing these therapy-related endocrine complications.

REFERENCES

1. Warren, S. Effects of radiation on normal tissues. Arch. Pathol. 35:304, 1943.
2. Lindsay, S., Dailey, M.E., and Jones, M.D. Histologic effects of various types of ionizing radiation on normal and hyperplastic human thyroid gland. J. Clin. Endocrinol. 14:1179, 1954.
3. Beling, U. and Einhorn, J. Incidence of hypothyroidism and recurrences following I[131] treatment of hyperthyroidism. Acta. Radiol. 56:275, 1961.
4. Goolden, A.W.G. and Cavey, J.B. The ablation of normal thyroid tissue with iodine-131. Br. J. Radiol. 36:340, 1963.
5. Green, M. and Wilson, G.M. Thyrotoxicosis treated by surgery or iodine-131. With special reference to the development of hypothyroidism. Brit. Med. J. 1:1005, 1964.
6. Felix, H., Dupre, N., Dupre, M. et al. Incidence a long terme d'une radiothérapie pour cancer du larynx, sur l'apprition d'un myxoedeme. Lyon Med. 206:1043, 1961.
7. Logan, J. Thyroid hypofunction in patients with lymphomatous tumours. N.Z. Med. J. 64:135, 1965.
8. Markson, J.L. and Flatman, G.E. Myxoedema after deep x-ray therapy to the neck. Br. Med. J. 1:1228, 1965.
9. Rogoway, W.M., Finkelstein, S., Rosenberg, S.A. et al. Myxedema developing after lymphangiography and neck irradiation. Clin. Res. 14:133, 1966 (abstract).
10. Glatstein, E. et al. Alterations in serum thyrotropin (TSH) and thyroid function following radiotherapy in patients with malignant lymphoma. J. Clin. Endocrinol. Metab. 32:833, 1971.
11. Fuks, Z. et al. Long term effects of external radiation on the pituitary and thyroid glands. Cancer 37:1152, 1976.
12. Poussin-Rosillo, H., Nisce, L.Z., and Lee, B.J. Complications of total nodal irradiation of Hodgkin's disease stages III and IV. Cancer 42:437, 1978.
13. Johnson, R.E., Ruhl, U., Johnson, S. et al. Split course radiotherapy of Hodgkin's disease. Cancer 37:1713, 1976.
14. Shalet, S.M. et al. Thyroid dysfunction following external irradiation to the neck for Hodgkin's disease in childhood. Clin. Radiol. 28:511, 1977.
15. Prager, D., Sembrot, J.T., and Southard, M. Cobalt-60 therapy of Hodgkin's disease and the subsequent development of hypothyroidism. Cancer 29:458, 1972.
16. Carmel, R.J. and Kaplan, H.S. Mantle irradiation in Hodgkin's disease. An analysis of technique, tumor eradication, and complications. Cancer 37:2813, 1976.
17. Donaldson, S.S., Glatstein, E., Rosenberg, S.A. et al. Pediatric Hodgkin's disease. II. Results of therapy. Cancer 37:2436, 1976.
18. Slanina, J. et al. Long-term side effects in irradiated patients with Hodgkin's disease. Int. J. Radiat. Oncol. Biol. Phys. 2:1, 1977.
19. Nelson, D.F., Reddy, K.V., O'Mara, R.E. et al. Thyroid abnormalities following neck irradiation for Hodgkin's disease. Cancer 42:2553, 1978.
20. Schimpff, S.C. et al. Radiation related thyroid dysfunction: Implications for the treatment of Hodgkin's disease. Ann. Intern. Med. 92:91, 1980.
21. Kim, Y.H., Fagos, J.V., and Sisson, J.C. Thyroid function following neck irradiation for malignant lymphoma. Radiology 134:205, 1980.
22. Green, D.M. et al. Thyroid function in pediatric patients after neck irradiation for Hodgkin's disease. Med. Ped. Oncol. 8:127, 1980.
23. Tamura, K., Shimaoka, K., and Friedman, M. Thyroid abnormalities associated with treatment of malignant lymphoma. Cancer 47:2704, 1981.
24. Smith, R.E. et al. Thyroid function after mantle irradiation in Hodgkin's disease. JAMA 245:46, 1981.
25. Sutcliffe, S.B., Chapman, R., and Wrigley, P.F.M. Cyclical combination chemotherapy and thyroid function in patients with advanced Hodgkin's disease. Med. Ped. Oncol. 9:439, 1981.
26. Mauch, P.M. et al. An evaluation of long term survival and treatment complications in children with Hodgkin's disease. Cancer 51:925, 1983.
27. Holt, G. et al. Serum thyroglobulin after mantle irradiation for Hodgkin's disease. Clin. Endocrinol. 18:605, 1983.
28. Farley, P.C. Thyroid dysfunction following radiation therapy for lymphoma in the military population. Milit. Med. 148:740, 1983.
29. Constine, L.S. et al. Thyroid dysfunction after radiotherapy in children with Hodgkin's disease. Cancer 53:878, 1984.
30. Devney, R.B. et al. Serial thyroid function measurements in children with Hodgkin's disease. J. Pediatr. 105:223, 1984.
31. Nair, N., Advani, S.H., and Dinshaw, K.A. Thyroid dysfunction following mantle radiotherapy for Hodgkin's disease. Int. J. Nucl. Med. Biol. 11:175, 1984.
32. Fleming, I.D. et al. Thyroid dysfunction and neoplasia in children receiving neck irradiation for cancer. Cancer 55:1190, 1985.
33. Morgan, G.W., Freeman, A.P., McLean, R.G. et al. Late cardiac, thyroid and pulmonary sequelae of mantle radiotherapy for Hodgkin's disease. Int. J. Radiat. Oncol. Biol. Phys. 11:1925, 1985.

34. Redman, J.R. and Bajorunas, D.R. Unpublished data.
35. Brinckmeyer, L.M., Worm, A.M., and Nissen, N.I. Thyroid function in malignant lymphoma. Acta. Med. Scand. 202:475, 1977.
36. Wartofsky, L. and Burman, K.D. Alterations in thyroid function in patients with systemic illness: "The euthyroid sick syndrome." Endocr. Rev. 3:164, 1982.
37. Burke, J.S., Butler, J.J., and Fuller, L.M. Malignant lymphoma of the thyroid. Cancer 39:1587, 1977.
38. Sirota, D.K. and Segal, R.L. Primary lymphomas of the thyroid gland. JAMA 242:1743, 1979.
39. Hamburger, J.I., Miller, J.M., and Kini, S.R. Lymphoma of the thyroid. Ann. Intern. Med. 99:685, 1983.
40. Miller, J.M., Kini, S.R., Rebuck, J., and Hamburger, J.I. Is lymphoma of the thyroid a disease which is increasing in frequency? In Controversies in Clinical Thyroidology. Edited by J.I. Hamburger and J.M. Miller. New York, Springer-Verlag, 1981, p. 267.
41. Rupp, J.J., Moran, J.J., and Griffith, J.R. Goiter as an initial manifestation of Hodgkin's disease. Arch. Intern. Med. 110:386, 1962.
42. Roberts, T.W. and Howard, R.G. Primary Hodgkin's disease of the thyroid: report of one case and review of the literature. Ann. Surg. 157:625, 1963.
43. Gibson, J.M. and Prinn, M.G. Hodgkin's disease involving the thyroid gland. Br. J. Surg. 55:236, 1968.
44. Abel, W.G. and Finnerty, J. Primary Hodgkin's disease of the thyroid. N.Y. State J. Med. 69:314, 1969.
45. Wood, N.L. and Coltman, C.A. Localized primary extranodal Hodgkin's disease. Ann. Intern. Med. 78:113, 1973.
46. Compagno, J. and Oertel, J.E. Malignant lymphoma and other lymphoproliferative disorders of the thyroid gland: a clinicopathologic study of 245 cases. Am. J. Clin. Pathol. 74:1, 1980.
47. Kugler, J.W., Armitage, J.O., and Dick, F.R. Hodgkin's disease presenting as a thyroid mass. Postgrad. Med. 72:243, 1982.
48. Mate, T.P. and Chen, M.G. Hodgkin's disease manifesting as Hashimoto's thyroiditis. Arch. Intern. Med. 144:1473, 1984.
49. Mikal, S. Primary lymphomas of the thyroid gland. Surgery 55:233, 1963.
50. Crile, G. Lymphosarcoma and reticulum cell sarcoma of the thyroid. Surg. Gynecol. Obstet. 116:449, 1963.
51. Woolner, L.B. et al. Primary malignant lymphoma of the thyroid: review of 46 cases. Am. J. Surg. 111:502, 1966.
52. Shimkin, P.M. and Sagerman, R.H. Lymphoma of the thyroid gland. Radiology 92:812, 1969.
53. Holm, L.E., Blomgren, H., and Lowhagen, T. Cancer risks in patients with chronic lymphocytic thyroiditis. N. Engl. J. Med. 312:601, 1985.
54. Greig, W.R., Boyle, J.A., Buchanan, W.W. et al. Clinical and radiobiological observations on latent effects of X-irradiation on the thyroid gland. J. Clin. Endocrinol. 25:1009, 1965.
55. Doniach, I. Experimental evidence of etiology of thyroid cancer. Proc. R. Soc. Med. 67:1103, 1974.
56. Maxon, H.R. et al. Ionizing irradiation and the induction of clinically significant disease in the human thyroid gland. Am. J. Med. 63:967, 1977.
57. Vagenakis, A.G. and Braverman, L.E. Adverse effects of iodides on thyroid function. Med. Clin. N. Am. 59:1075, 1975.
58. Wolff, J. Iodide goiter and the pharmacologic effects of excess iodide. Am. J. Med. 47:101, 1969.
59. Vagenakis, A.G. et al. Control of thyroid hormone secretion in normal subjects receiving iodides. J. Clin. Invest. 52:528, 1973.
60. Fradkin, J.E. and Wolff, J. Iodine-induced thyrotoxicosis. Medicine 62:1, 1983.
61. Kaplan, M.M. et al. Risk factors for thyroid abnormalities after neck irradiation for childhood cancer. Am. J. Med. 74:272, 1983.
62. Perez, C.A. Basic concepts and clinical implications of radiation therapy. In Clinical Pediatric Oncology. 2nd Ed. Edited by W.W. Sutow, T.J. Vietti, and D.J. Fernbach. St. Louis, C.V. Mosby, 1977, p. 149.
63. Shafer, R.B., Nuttal, F.Q., Pollak, K. et al. Thyroid function after radiation and surgery for head and neck cancer. Arch. Intern. Med. 135:843, 1975.
64. Murken, R.E. and Duvall, A.J. Hypothyroidism following combined therapy in carcinoma of the laryngopharynx. Laryngoscope 82:1306, 1972.
65. Blomgren, S.E. and Ansfield, F.J. Thyroid status following prolonged therapy with fluoropyrimidines. JAMA 193:51, 1965.
66. Beex, L., Ross, A., Smals, A. et al. 5 fluorouracil-induced increase of total serum thyroxine and triiodothyronine. Cancer Treat. Rep. 61:1291, 1977.
67. Garnick, M.B. and Larsen, P.R. Acute deficiency of thyroxine-binding globulin during L-asparagine therapy. N. Engl. J. Med. 301:252, 1979.
68. Heidemann, P.H., Stubbe, P., and Beck, W. Transient secondary hypothyroidism and thyroxine binding globulin deficiency in leukemic children during polychemotherapy: an effect of L-asparaginase. Eur. J. Pediatr. 136:291, 1981.
69. Willemse, P.H.B. et al. Alterations in thyroid hormone metabolism during chemotherapy in patients with testicular carcinoma. Clin. Endocrinol. 16:303, 1982.
70. Dumont, J.E., Rodesch, F.R., and Rocmans, P. Stimulation of thyroidal radioiodine uptake by actinomycin and fluorouracil. Biochem. Pharmacol. 13:935, 1964.
71. Rodesch, F., Rocmans, P., and Dumont, J.E. Stimulation of thyroidal radioiodine uptake by actinomycin D and fluorouracil—an indirect effect. Biochem. Pharmacol. 16:907, 1967.
72. Curti, J.T., Rupp, J.J., and Cantarow, A. Influence of 5-fluorouracil on thyroid function. Proc. Soc. Exp. Biol. Med. 125:1125, 1967.
73. Halmi, N.S., Gifford, T.H., and Glesne, R.E. Further observations concerning the effect of actinomycin D on thyroidal iodide transport in rats. Endocrinology 81:893, 1967.
74. Vagenakis, A.G. et al. Stimulatory effect of 5-fluo-

rouracil on thyroid/serum iodide concentration ratios in the rat. Endocrinology 88:1250, 1971.
75. Williams, J.A. In vitro studies on the nature of vinblastine inhibition of thyroid secretion. Endocrinology 98:1351, 1976.
76. Adler, R.A., Corrigan, D.F., and Wartofsky, L. Hypothyroidism after X-irradiation to the neck: Three case reports and a brief review of the literature. Johns Hopkins Med. J. 138:180, 1976.
77. Jackson, R. et al. Ophthalmopathy following neck irradiation therapy for Hodgkin's disease. Cancer Treat. Rep. 63:1393, 1979.
78. Constine, L.S. et al. Radiation therapy for Hodgkin's disease followed by hypothyroidism and then Graves' hyperthyroidism. Clin. Nucl. Med. 7:69, 1982.
79. Nakamura, R.M. and Weigle, W.O. Suppression of thyroid lesions in rabbits by treatment with cyclophosphamide after the induction of thyroiditis. Clin. Exp. Immunol. 7:541, 1970.
80. Paterson, P.Y. and Drobuish, D.G. Reversal of experimental allergic thyroiditis in cyclophosphamide-treated rats. Clin. Exp. Immunol. 20:125, 1975.
81. Schnipper, E.F., Malamet, R.L., and Arlin, Z.A. "Polymyositis"-like syndrome resulting from hypothyroidism in a patient with a nodular lymphoma. Clin. Bull. 11:34, 1981.
82. Grubb, M.R., Chakeres, D., and Malarkey, W.B. Patients with primary hypothyroidism presenting as prolactinomas. Am. J. Med. 83:765, 1987.
83. Klein, I. and Levey, G.S. Unusual manifestations of hypothyroidism. Arch. Intern. Med. 144:123, 1984.
84. Hembree, W.C. and VanderWiele, R.L. Female reproductive system. In The Thyroid. 4th Ed. Edited by S.C. Werner and S.H. Ingbar. Maryland, Harper & Row, 1978, 914.
85. Greenman, G.W., Gabrielson, M.O., Howard-Flanders, J. et al. Thyroid dysfunction in pregnancy. Fetal loss and follow-up evaluation of surviving infants. N. Engl. J. Med. 267:426, 1962.
86. Niswander, K.R., Gordon, M., and Berendes H.W. The Women and Their Pregnancies. Philadelphia, W.B. Saunders, 1972.
87. Man, E.B. Maternal hypothyroxinemia, development of 4 and 7 year old offspring. In Perinatal Thyroid Physiology and Disease. Edited by D.A. Fisher and G.N. Burrow. New York, Raven Press, 1975, 117.
88. Jones, W.S. and Man, E.B. Thyroid function in human pregnancy: VI. Premature deliveries and reproductive failures of pregnant women with low serum butanol extractable iodines. Am. J. Obstet. Gynecol. 104:909, 1969.
89. Montoro, M., Colea, J.V., Frasier, S.D. et al. Successful outcome of pregnancy in women with hypothyroidism. Ann. Intern. Med. 94:31, 1981.
90. Werner, S.C. Treatment. In The Thyroid. 4th Ed. Edited by S.C. Werner and S.M. Ingbar. Maryland, Harper & Row, 1978, 965.
91. Bastenie, P.A. et al. Preclinical hypothyroidism: A risk factor for coronary heart disease. Lancet 1:203, 1971.
92. Nilsson, G., Nordlander, S., and Levin, K. Studies on subclinical hypothyroidism with special reference to the serum lipid pattern. Acta. Med. Scand. 200:63, 1976.
93. Fowler, P.B.S. Premyxoedema—a cause of preventable coronary heart disease. Proc. R. Soc. Med. 70:297, 1977.
94. Ridgeway, E.C. et al. Peripheral responses to thyroid hormone before and after L-thyroxine therapy in patients with subclinical hypothyroidism. J. Clin. Endocrinol. Metab. 53:1238, 1981.
95. Cooper, D.S. et al. L-thyroxine therapy in subclinical hypothyroidism. A double-blind, placebo controlled trial. Ann. Intern. Med. 101:18, 1984.
96. Doniach, I. The effect of radioactive iodine alone and in combination with methylthiouracil upon tumour production in the rat's thyroid gland. Br. J. Cancer 7:181, 1953.
97. Ramsay, N. et al. Thyroid dysfunction in pediatric patients after mantle field radiation therapy for Hodgkin's disease. Proc. Am. Assoc. Cancer Res. 19:389, 1979 (abstract).
98. Devney R.B. et al. Thyroid function in children treated for Hodgkin's disease. Pediatr. Res. 15:507, 1981 (abstract).
99. McDougall, I.R. et al. Thyroid dysfunction after radiotherapy in children with Hodgkin's disease. Clin. Nucl. Med. 5:S22, 1980.
100. Fisher, R.I., Portlock, C.S., and Longo, D.L. Hodgkin's disease. In American Society of Hematology, Educational Program, 24, 1983.
101. Bantle, J.P., Lee, C.K.K., and Levitt, S.H. Thyroxine administration during radiation therapy to the neck does not prevent subsequent thyroid dysfunction. Int. J. Radiat. Oncol. Biol. Phys. 11:1999, 1985.
102. Wasnick, R.D. et al. Graves' ophthalmopathy following external neck irradiation for nonthyroidal neoplastic disease. J. Clin. Endocrinol. Metab. 37:703, 1973.
103. Pilepich, M.V., Jackson, I., Munzenrider, J.E. et al. Graves' disease following irradiation for Hodgkin's disease. JAMA 240:1381, 1978.
104. Tamura, K. and Shimaoka, K. Hodgkin's disease: thyroid dysfunction following external irradiation. N.Y. State J. Med. 81:69, 1981.
105. Willemze, R. et al. Hyperthyroidism following mantle field irradiation for Hodgkin's disease. Acta. Hematol. (Basel) 67:225, 1982.
106. Slavin, M.L. and Glaser, J.S. Idiopathic orbital myositis. Arch. Ophthalmol. 100:1261, 1982.
107. Jacobson, D.R. and Fleming, B.J. Case report: Graves' disease with ophthalmopathy following radiotherapy for Hodgkin's disease. Am. J. Med. Sci. 288:217, 1984.
108. Blitzer, J.B., Paolozzi, F.P., Gottlieb, A.J. et al. Thyrotoxic thyroiditis after radiotherapy for Hodgkin's disease. Arch. Intern. Med. 145:1734, 1985.
109. Ghandour, C., LePrise, P-Y, and Hespel, J-P. Hodg-

110. Mortimer, R.H., Hill, G.E., Galligan, J.P. et al. Hypothyroidism and Graves' disease after mantle irradiation: a follow-up study. Aust. N.Z. J. Med. 16:347, 1986.
111. Loeffler, J.S., Tarbell, N.J., Garber, J.R. et al. The development of Graves' disease following radiation therapy in Hodgkin's disease. Int. J. Radiat. Oncol. Biol. Phys. 14:175, 1988.
112. Loeffler, J.S., Mauch, P.M., Leslie, N.T. et al. The development of Graves' disease following radiation therapy in Hodgkin's disease. Int. J. Radiat. Oncol. Biol. Phys. 11:156, 1985 (abstract).
113. Leslie, N.T., Mauch, P.M., and Hellman, S. Evaluation of long term survival and treatment complications in patients with stage IA–IIB Hodgkin's disease. Int. J. Radiat. Oncol. Biol. Phys. 9(suppl. 1):127, 1983 (abstract).
114. Porter, A.T. and Ostrowski, M.J. Fluctuating thyroid dysfunction following irradiation of the neck for the treatment of Hodgkin's disease. J. R. Soc. Med. 81:45, 1988.
115. Tunbridge, W.M.G. et al. The spectrum of thyroid disease in a community: the Whickham survey. Clin. Endocrinol. 7:481, 1977.
116. McGregor, A.M., McLachlan, S.M., Smith, B.R. et al. Effect of irradiation on thyroid autoantibody production. Lancet 2:442, 1979.
117. Doniach, I. Biologic effects of radiation on the thyroid. In The Thyroid. 4th Ed. Edited by S.C. Werner and S.H. Ingbar. Maryland, Harper and Row, 1978, p. 274.
118. Duffy, B.J. and Fitzgerald, P.J. Thyroid cancer in children and adolescence. A report on twenty-eight cases. Cancer 3:1018, 1950.
119. Clark, D.E. Association of irradiation with cancer of the thyroid in children and adolescents. JAMA 159:1007, 1955.
120. Simpson, C.L. and Hempelmann, L.H. Association of tumours and roentgen-ray treatment of the thorax in infancy. Cancer 10:42, 1957.
121. Wilson, G.M., et al. Thyroid neoplasms following irradiation. Br. Med. J. 2:929, 1958.
122. Conard, R.A., Rall, J.E., and Sutow, W.W. Thyroid nodules as a late sequela of radioactive fallout in a Marshall Island population exposed in 1954. N. Engl. J. Med. 274:1391, 1966.
123. Socolow, E.L., Hashizume, A., Neriishi, S. et al. Thyroid carcinoma in man after exposure to ionizing radiation. A summary of the findings of Hiroshima and Nagasaki. N. Engl. J. Med. 268:406, 1963.
124. Gossage, A.A.R. et al. Cases of carcinoma of thyroid following iodine-131 therapy for hyperthyroidism. Oncology 41:8, 1984.
125. Dobyns, B.M. et al. Malignant and benign neoplasms of the thyroid in patients treated for hyperthyroidism: A report of the co-operative thyrotoxicosis therapy follow-up study. J. Clin. Endocrinol. Metab. 38:976, 1974.
126. Safa, A., Schumacher, P. and Rodriguez-Antunez, A. Long term follow up results in children and adolescents treated with radioactive iodine (^{131}I) for hyperthyroidism. N. Engl. J. Med. 292:167, 1975.
127. Holm, L.E., Dahlqvist, I., Israelsson, A. et al. Malignant thyroid tumors after iodine-131 therapy. A retrospective cohort study. N. Engl. J. Med. 303:188, 1980.
128. Doniach, I. Experimental induction of tumours of the thyroid by irradiation. Brit. Med. Bull. 14:181, 1958.
129. Jelliffe, A.M. and Jones, K.M. Thyroid cancer after irradiation in adult life. Clin. Radiol. 11:162, 1960.
130. Hanford, J.M., Quimby, E.M., and Frantz, V.K. Cancer arising many years after radiation therapy: incidence after irradiation of benign lesions in the neck. JAMA 181:404, 1962.
131. Block, M.A., Miller, M.J., and Horn, R.C. Carcinoma of the thyroid after external radiation to the neck in adults. Am. J. Surg. 118:764, 1969.
132. Beach, S.A. and Dolphin, G.W. A study of the relationship between x-ray dose delivered to the thyroids of children and the subsequent development of malignant tumours. Phys. Med. Biol. 6:583, 1962.
133. DeLawter, D.S. and Winship, T. Follow up of adults treated with roentgen rays for thyroid disease. Cancer 16:1028, 1963.
134. Raventos, A. and Winship, T. The latent interval for thyroid cancer following irradiation. Radiology 83:501, 1964.
135. Colman, M. et al. Thyroid cancer associated with radiation exposure: dose effect relationships. Proceedings of Symposium on Biological Effects of Low Level Radiation Pertinent to Protection of Man and his Environment (IAEA SM 202), Vol. 2. Vienna, International Atomic Energy Agency, 285, 1976.
136. Hempelmann, L.H. et al. Neoplasms in persons treated with x-ray in infancy: fourth survey in 20 years. J. Natl. Cancer Inst. 55:519, 1975.
137. Fjalling, M., Tisell, L.-E., Carlson, S. et al. Benign and malignant thyroid nodules after neck irradiation. Cancer 58:1219, 1986.
138. Lindsay, S. and Charkoff, I.L. The effects of irradiation on the thyroid gland with particular reference to the induction of thyroid neoplasms: a review. Cancer Res. 24:1099–1107, 1964.
139. Lindsay, S., Nichols, C.W., and Charkoff, I.L. Induction of benign and malignant thyroid neoplasms in the rat. Induction of thyroid neoplasms by injection of ^{131}I with or without the feeding of diets containing propylthiouracil and/or desiccated thyroid. Arch. Pathol. 81:308, 1966.
140. Nichols, C.N., Lindsay, S., Sheline, G.E. et al. Induction of neoplasms in rat thyroid glands by x-irradiation of a single lobe. Arch. Pathol. 80:177, 1965.
141. Morris, J.H. and Hardin, C.A. Thyroid cancer in adults following external radiation. Arch. Intern. Med. 113:99, 1964.
142. Hynes, J.F. Thyroid cancer developing after irradiation of the adult. Del. Med. J. 36:124, 1964.
143. Moon, J.H. and Hudson, P. Recurrent neck mass following irradiation of Hodgkin's disease. Va. Med. Mon. 95:31, 1968.

144. Meyer, O.O. Carcinoma of the thyroid following ionizing radiation for Hodgkin's disease. Wis. Med. J. 70:129, 1971.
145. Jacquillat, C.L. et al. Les neoplasies simultanees et successives. Nouv. Presse Med. 2:3089, 1973.
146. Weshler, A. et al. Thyroid carcinoma induced by irradiation for Hodgkin's disease. Report of a case. Acta. Radiol. Oncol. Radiat. Phys. Biol. 17:383, 1978.
147. Getaz, E.P., Shimaoka, K., and Rao, U. Anaplastic carcinoma of the thyroid following external irradiation. Cancer 43:2248, 1979.
148. Getaz, E.P. and Shimaoka, K. Anaplastic carcinoma of the thyroid in a population irradiated for Hodgkin's disease 1910–1960. J. Surg. Oncol. 12:181, 1979.
149. Shimaoka, K., Getaz, E.P., and Rao, U. Anaplastic carcinoma of the thyroid: radiation associated. N.Y. State J. Med. 79:874, 1979.
150. Chase, L. et al. A functioning thyroid nodule in a patient previously treated with irradiation for Hodgkin's disease. Am. J. Med. 68:429, 1980.
151. McDougall, I.R. et al. Thyroid carcinoma after high dose external radiotherapy for Hodgkin's disease. Report of three cases. Cancer 45:2056, 1980.
152. Frank, H.J.L. and Ashcraft, M.W. Thyroid carcinoma after radiation for Hodgkin's disease. Ann. Intern. Med. 93:145, 1980 (letter).
153. Bryda, S. and Ward, J.A. Thyroid carcinoma after radiation for Hodgkin's disease. Ann. Intern. Med. 93:145, 1980 (letter).
154. Valagussa, P. et al. Second malignancies in Hodgkin's disease: a complication of certain forms of treatment. Br. Med. J. 280:216, 1980.
155. Baccarani, M., Bosi, A., and Papa, G. Second malignancy in patients treated for Hodgkin's disease. Cancer 46:1735, 1980.
156. Palmer, J.A., Mustard, R.A., and Simpson, W.J. Irradiation as an etiologic factor in tumors of the thyroid, parathyroid and salivary glands. Can. J. Surg. 23:39, 1980.
157. Smallridge, R.C., Wartofsky, L., and Burman, K.D. Thyroid carcinoma and Hodgkin's disease. Ann. Intern. Med. 94:412, 1981.
158. Mazzaferri, E.L. Thyroid carcinoma following therapeutic and accidental radiation exposure. Spec. Top. Endocrinol. Metab. 2:103, 1981.
159. Pretorius, H.T. et al. Thyroid nodules after high dose external radiotherapy. Fine needle aspiration cytology in diagnosis and management. JAMA 247:3217, 1982.
160. Nicol, F., McLaren, K.M., and Toft, A.D. Multifocal follicular carcinoma of thyroid following radiotherapy for Hodgkin's disease. Postgrad. Med. J. 58:180, 1982.
161. Glicksman, A.S. et al. Second malignant neoplasms in patients successfully treated for Hodgkin's disease: A Cancer and Leukemia Group B study. Cancer Treat. Rep. 66:1035, 1982.
162. Coeur, P., Berthezene, F., Berger-Dutrieux, N. et al. Cancer vesiculaire du corps thyroide 17 ans apres irradiation cervicale pour maladie de Hodgkin. Lyon Med. 247:53, 1982.
163. Simone, J.V. Late complications of treatment of children with leukemia and lymphoma. In Malignant Lymphoma: Etiology, Immunology, Pathology, Treatment. Edited by S.A. Rosenberg, H.S. Kaplan. New York, Academic Press, 1982, p. 665.
164. Najean, Y. and Messian, O. Cancer de la thyroide survenu 15 ans apres guerison d'une maladie de Hodgkin traitee par irradiation cervicale; puis chimiotherapie. La Nouv. Presse Medicale 11:2851, 1982.
165. Amin, R. Follicular carcinoma of the thyroid following radiotherapy for Hodgkin's disease. Br. J. Radiol. 56:768, 1983.
166. Bakri, K., Shimaoka, K., Rao, U. et al. Adenosquamous carcinoma of the thyroid after radiotherapy for Hodgkin's disease. A case report and review. Cancer 52:465, 1983.
167. Friedman, M., Shimaoka, K., Fox, S. et al. Second malignant tumours detected by needle aspiration cytology. Cancer 52:699, 1983.
168. Hamburger, S., Stoffer, S.S., and Swamy, N. Thyroid cancer following higher dose radiation therapy. Postgrad. Med. 73:111, 1983.
169. Tester, W.J. et al. Second malignant neoplasms complicating Hodgkin's disease: The National Cancer Institute Experience. J. Clin. Oncol. 2:762, 1984.
170. Boivin, J.F. et al. Second primary cancers following treatment of Hodgkin's disease. J. Natl. Cancer Inst. 72:233, 1984.
171. Rosen, I.B., Simpson, J.A., Sutcliffe, S. et al. High-dose radiation and the emergence of thyroid nodular disease. Surgery 96:988, 1984.
172. Naunheim, K.S. et al. High-dose external radiation to the neck and subsequent thyroid carcinoma. In Surgery of the thyroid and parathyroid gland. Edited by E.L Kaplan. New York, Churchill Livingstone, Inc., 1983, p. 51.
173. Turrin, A., Pilotti, S., and Ricci, S.B. Characteristics of thyroid cancer following irradiation. Int. J. Radiat. Oncol. Biol. Phys. 11:2149, 1985.
174. Moroff, S.V. and Fuks, J.Z. Thyroid cancer following radiotherapy for Hodgkin's disease: a case report and review of the literature. Med. Ped. Oncol. 14:216, 1986.
175. Jenkin, D. and Doyle, J. Paediatric Hodgkin's disease—late results and toxicity. Radiat. Oncol. Biol. Phys. 13(Suppl. 1):92, 1987 (abstract).
176. McHenry, C., Jarosz, H., Calandra, D. et al. Thyroid neoplasia following radiation therapy for Hodgkin's lymphoma. Arch. Surg. 122:684, 1987.
177. Rabinowitz, D. and Katz, J. Carcinoma of the thyroid following irradiation of the neck. S. Afr. Med. J. 32:723, 1958.
178. Voisin, M. et al. Epithelioma anaplastique de la thyroide 6 ans apres irradiation cervicale pour lymphome malin. Can. Med. Assoc. J. 113:648, 1975.
179. Satran, L. et al. Thyroid neoplasm after high-dose radiotherapy. Am. J. Ped. Hem. Oncol. 5:307, 1983.
180. Greene, M.H. and Wilson, J. Second cancer following lymphatic and hematopoietic cancers in Con-

necticut, 1935–82. Natl. Cancer Inst. Monogr. 68:191, 1985.
181. Tucker, M.A., Meadows, A.T., Boice, J.P. Cancer risk following treatment of childhood cancer. In Radiation Carcinogenesis: Epidemiology and Biological Significance. Edited by J.D. Boice and J.F. Fraumeni. New York, Raven Press, 1984, p. 211.
182. Tucker, M.A., Coleman, C.N., Cox, R.S. et al. Risk of second cancers after treatment for Hodgkin's disease. N. Engl. J. Med. 318:76, 1988.
183. Kaldor, J.M. et al. Second malignancies following testicular cancer, ovarian cancer and Hodgkin's disease: an international collaborative study among cancer registries. Int. J. Cancer 39:571, 1987.
184. Newfeld, H., Weinerman, B.H., and Kemal, S. Secondary malignant neoplasms in patients with Hodgkin's disease. JAMA 239:2470, 1978.
185. Toland, D.M., Coltman, C.A., and Moon, T.E. Second malignancies complicating Hodgkin's disease: the Southwest Oncology Group experience. Cancer Clin. Trials 1:21, 1978.
186. Coltman, C.A. and Dixon, D.O. Second malignancies complicating Hodgkin's disease: A Southwest Oncology Group 10 year follow up. Cancer Treat. Rep. 66:1023, 1982.
187. Coleman, C.N. et al. Secondary leukemia and non-Hodgkin's lymphoma in patients treated for Hodgkin's disease. In Advances in Malignant Lymphomas. Etiology, Immunology, Pathology and Treatment. Edited by H.S. Kaplan and S.A. Rosenberg. New York, Academic Press, 1982.
188. Henry-Amar, M. Second cancers after radiotherapy and chemotherapy for early stages of Hodgkin's disease. J. Natl. Cancer Inst. 71:911, 1983.
189. Bakri, K. et al. Thyroid abnormalities and carcinoma of the thyroid in a population irradiated for non-Hodgkin's lymphoma 1910–1960. Proc. Am. Soc. Clin. Oncol. 22:C-716, 1981 (abstract).
190. Doniach, I., Kingston, J.E., Plowman, P.N. et al. The association of post-radiation thyroid nodular disease with compensated hypothyroidism. Br. J. Radiol. 60:1223, 1987.
191. Tucker, M.A., Meadows, A.T., Morris-Jones, P. et al. Therapeutic radiation at young age linked to secondary thyroid cancer (TC). Proc. Am. Soc. Clin. Oncol. 5:211, 1986 (abstract).
192. Tighe, W.J. Temporary hypoparathyroidism following radioactive iodine treatment for thyrotoxicosis. J. Clin. Endocrinol. 12:1220, 1952.
193. Gilbert-Dreyfus, Zara, M., and Gali, P. Cataract due to tetany following radioactive iodine therapy. Sem. Hop. Paris 34:1301, 1958.
194. Townsend, J.D. Hypoparathyroidism following radioactive iodine therapy for intractable angina pectoris. Ann. Intern. Med. 55:662, 1961.
195. Helou, A., Tyan, E., and Zara, M. A new case of tetany following the treatment of thyrotoxicosis with radioactive iodine. Ann. Endocrinol. 25:238, 1964.
196. Eipe, J. et al. Hypoparathyroidism following ^{131}I therapy for hyperthyroidism. Arch. Intern. Med. 111:270, 1968.
197. Orme, M.E. and Conolly, M.E. Hypoparathyroidism after iodine-131 treatment of thyrotoxicosis. Ann. Intern. Med. 75:136, 1971.
198. Blumgart, H.L., Freedberg, A.S., and Hurland, E.S. Treatment of incapacitated euthyroid cardiac patients with radioactive iodine. JAMA 157:1, 1955.
199. Adams, P.M. and Chalmers, T.M. Parathyroid function after ^{131}I therapy for hyperthyroidism. Clin. Sci. 29:391, 1965.
200. de Deuxchaisnes, C.N. and Krane, S.M. Hypoparathyroidism. In Metabolic Bone Disease. Edited by L.V. Avioli and S.M. Krane. Vol. 2. New York, Academic Press, 1978, p. 217.
201. Rosen, I.B., Strawbridge, H.G., and Barn, J. A case of hyperparathyroidism associated with radiation to the head and neck area. Cancer 36:1111, 1975.
202. Prinz, P.A. et al. Radiation-associated hyperparathyroidism: a new syndrome? Surgery 82:296, 1977.
203. Tisell, L-E., Carlsson, S., Lindberg, S. et al. Autonomous hyperparathyroidism: A possible late complication of neck radiotherapy. Acta. Chir. Scand. 142:367, 1976.
204. Tisell, L-E. et al. Hyperparathyroidism in persons treated with x-rays for tuberculosis cervical adenitis. Cancer 40:846, 1977.
205. Block, M.A. Discussion of radiation associated hyperparathyroidism: a new syndrome? Surgery 82:300, 1977.
206. Christensson, T. Hyperparathyroidism and radiation therapy. Ann. Intern. Med. 89:216, 1978.
207. Russ, J.E., Scanlon, E.F., and Sener, S.F. Parathyroid adenomas following irradiation. Cancer 43:1078, 1979.
208. Rao, S.D. et al. Hyperparathyroidism following head and neck irradiation. Arch. Intern. Med. 140:205, 1980.
209. Tisell, L-E. et al. Hyperparathyroidism subsequent to neck irradiation. Risk factors. Cancer 56:1529, 1985.
210. Katz, A. and Braunstein, G.D. Clinical, biochemical and pathologic features of radiation-associated hyperparathyroidism. Arch. Intern. Med. 143:79, 1983.
211. Livolsi, V.A., LoGerfo, P., and Feind, C.R. Coexistent parathyroid adenomas and thyroid carcinoma. Can radiation be blamed? Arch. Surg. 113:585, 1978.
212. Swelstad, J.A. et al. Irradiation-induced polyglandular neoplasia of the head and neck area. Am. J. Surg. 135:820, 1978.
213. Holten, I. and Christiansen, C. Unchanged parathyroid function following irradiation for malignancies of the head and neck. Cancer 53:874, 1984.
214. Karstrup, S., Hegedus, L., and Sehested, M. Hyperparathyroidism after neck irradiation for Hodgkin's disease. Acta. Med. Scand. 215:287, 1984.
215. Nader, S., Schultz, P.N., Fuller, L.M. et al. Calcium status following neck radiation therapy in Hodgkin's disease. Arch. Intern. Med. 144:1577, 1984.

CHAPTER 11

Hodgkin's Disease: Pregnancy and Progeny

JOHN R. REDMAN
DAIVA R. BAJORUNAS
MORTIMER J. LACHER

Two major stresses on the female patient, pregnancy and the discovery of Hodgkin's disease, pose difficult decisions for both patient and physician. Will continuation of the pregnancy have a detrimental effect on the patient? Should a therapeutic abortion be performed? What are the potential fetal side effects of radiation and chemotherapy? These questions all have to be considered when these dual diagnoses are made, and the decisions affect not only the patient, but also the fetus. Potential outcomes for the fetus include abortion (spontaneous or therapeutic), congenital defect, or normal life expectancy without disability. Proper weighing of risks and benefits in the management of the pregnant woman with Hodgkin's disease is therefore essential.

Increasingly, patients with malignancies are being cured and living to conceive children after the treatment has been completed. This is true not only of Hodgkin's disease but also of other malignancies, including leukemia, nonHodgkin's lymphomas, testicular cancer, trophoblastic tumors, and Wilm's tumor. It has been estimated that there are more than 45,000 survivors of childhood cancer now alive.[1] In addition, many patients treated in their early adult years will be in remission during their reproductive period. Some of these patients will have been rendered sterile by the treatment, but many will be capable of having children. Are these children at a higher risk of having congenital defects? Will the gene pool be affected by treatment? In the case of survivors of Hodgkin's disease, will their children have an increased risk of developing Hodgkin's disease or other malignancies?

CANCER IN PREGNANCY

The special problems of malignant disease in the pregnant woman have been discussed in several recent reviews.[2-5] This association of controlled growth (pregnancy) and uncontrolled growth (malignancy) is fortunately rare. Reports of the incidence of this occurrence are biased by referral patterns and small numbers of cases and probably overestimate the incidence. One large-scale study, not hav-

*The authors wish to thank Sandra Reyes for her excellent secretarial assistance.

ing these biases, found an incidence of 17 cases of invasive malignancy per 100,000 pregnancies.[6] The most frequently diagnosed malignancies in women are the following: *Under 15 years old:* leukemia, brain and central nervous system, kidney, bone and connective tissue; *15 to 34 years old:* leukemia, breast, brain and central nervous system, uterus, and Hodgkin's disease; *35 to 54 years old:* breast, lung, colon and rectum, uterus, and ovary.

The most frequent malignancies associated with pregnancy roughly follow this same pattern and are as follows: cervix, breast, ovary, lymphoma, melanoma, brain, and leukemia.[6] The incidence of malignancy increases dramatically with the age of the mother, from 1.96 per 100,000 live births among 15 to 19-year-old women, up to 232.4 per 100,000 live births in the 40 to 44-year-old age groups.[6] With the societal trend toward delaying childbearing, we may see an increased occurrence of this association of malignancy and pregnancy.

HODGKIN'S DISEASE ASSOCIATED WITH PREGNANCY

Hodgkin's disease occurring in the pregnant woman is rare. The ratio of cases of Hodgkin's disease associated with pregnancy to the number of pregnancies in the population has been reported at different times as follows: 5 of 30,000 in 1945,[7] 3 of 18,509 in 1952,[8] 8 of 7822 in 1953,[9] and 3 of 16,000 in 1976.[10]

Converse figures (prior to the combination chemotherapy era) show that approximately 30% of premenopausal women with Hodgkin's disease became pregnant during the course of their disease.[11-13] Hodgkin's disease has changed from a chronic relapsing disease to one in which cure is accomplished in the majority of patients. Today, therefore, the occurrence of pregnancy is typically in the cured patient rather than in women with active Hodgkin's disease.

EFFECT OF PREGNANCY ON HODGKIN'S DISEASE

Prior to the era of potentially curative chemotherapy and megavoltage radiation therapy, controversy settled on the issue of the influence of pregnancy on the course of Hodgkin's disease. Analysis of this question was limited by the scarcity of cases available for evaluation. Most case reports and small series found no significant effect of pregnancy on the course of Hodgkin's disease,[8,9,14-20] although some reports suggested a detrimental influence of pregnancy.[21-24]

At Memorial Hospital, early impressions suggested that pregnancy did have an unfavorable influence.[22-24] Southam found that there was a shorter mean survival if the Hodgkin's disease occurred during pregnancy (46 months) compared to the Hodgkin's disease occurring prior to conception (91 months).[24] This comparison had a significant selection bias, however, because the second group had already survived from diagnosis of Hodgkin's disease to the time of pregnancy, and patients were healthy enough to become pregnant. When the same investigators later compared the pregnant women to a group of nonpregnant women with Hodgkin's disease, no adverse effect of pregnancy was found.[12] The influence of pregnancy on Hodgkin's disease has not attracted as much attention over the last two decades; however, when studied, no detrimental effect on maternal survival was found[25,26] (with the possible exception in one series of women diagnosed in late pregnancy or shortly after delivery).[27] Similarly, women in complete remission who became pregnant had no increased risk of relapse.[26,27]

EFFECT OF HODGKIN'S DISEASE ON THE FETUS

Theoretically, Hodgkin's disease can directly affect the fetus in at least two ways: (1) it can metastasize directly to the fetus to cause Hodgkin's disease; (2) it can influence the pregnancy to result in a miscarriage. Neither of these mechanisms occurs to a significant extent and the more common influence of Hodgkin's disease on the fetus is an indirect one: the physician is influenced to do a therapeutic abortion or to use radiation or chemotherapy during the pregnancy.

Metastasis of maternal cancer to the placenta and/or fetus is rare, but has been reported in a number of malignancies, most commonly malignant melanoma.[28] Direct passage of Hodgkin's disease to the fetus is not well documented, but is suggested to have occurred in six cases.[29-32] This rare event should have no influence on the therapeutic decisions involved in the management of pregnant women with Hodgkin's disease.

The direct influence of Hodgkin's disease on pregnancy outcome is also an issue more closely scrutinized in the decades prior to the 1960s. These early reports were generally flawed by the lack of adequate control populations, but researchers concluded that there was no increased risk of spontaneous abortion or stillbirths.[8,11,12,16,18,23,33] One report did note, however, that spontaneous abortion was more common in patients with active disease and in those with intra-abdominal or disseminated disease.[24] More recent analyses have few patients who are untreated during pregnancy, but these pregnancies generally have normal outcomes.[25]

EFFECT OF RADIATION ON THE EMBRYO AND FETUS

Evidence from several sources has led to the conclusion that radiation can exert a deleterious effect on the embryo and fetus.[34] These sources have included studies of animals irradiated in utero, follow-up of people exposed in utero to atomic bomb radiation at Nagasaki and Hiroshima, and studies of humans exposed during fetal life to diagnostic and therapeutic radiation. Depending on the radiation dose, rate of administration, and the stage of embryonic/fetal development, several consequences may occur: (1) growth retardation, (2) embryonic, fetal, or perinatal death, and/or (3) congenital malformations.[35] There is also some evidence that humans exposed in utero may have an increased risk of childhood malignancy.

ANIMAL STUDIES

While the death of a few cells in the adult has little effect, the death of a few cells in the fetus may be lethal. Mouse experiments have shown that the developmental stage of the embryo at the time of irradiation is important in determining outcome.[36] Prenatal death is a frequent result when the mouse is radiated prior to implantation. Even a dose of 10 cGy reduces litter size if the radiation is given preimplantation.[37] As the embryo matures, however, it can survive higher doses of radiation until finally the lethal dose is the same as that for adults.

The dose as well as the timing of radiation exposure is also important in determining the frequency and type of congenital defect.[37] Irradiation using doses greater than 25 cGy during the early phase of organogenesis in mice and rats leads to the highest incidence of fetal malformation. (This early period of organogenesis corresponds to the twelfth to fiftieth day of a human pregnancy.) As the dose increases, the incidence of malformation increases, the most common abnormalities being central-nervous-system damage, sense organ damage, and stunted growth.

EXPOSURE IN UTERO TO ATOMIC BOMB RADIATION AT HIROSHIMA AND NAGASAKI

Exposure of pregnant women to the radiation from the atomic bombs in 1945 resulted in mortality for many of the women and fetuses and also morbidity for many of the surviving offspring. Of those women who were exposed within two kilometers of the hypocenter and had symptoms of acute radiation illness, an overall morbidity and mortality of 60% was found for their offspring, which included mental retardation, fetal death, and neonatal death.[38] One of the most striking outcomes of the exposure in utero was microcephaly (head circumference less than two standard deviations below the age and sex-specific mean head size), which was usually associated with mental retardation.[38] The frequency of microcephaly was correlated with radiation dose and time of exposure prior to the eighteenth week of pregnancy (especially 3 to 17 weeks). The minimum fetal radiation dose producing microcephaly was 10 to 19 cGy in Hiroshima versus 150 cGy in Nagasaki, the difference presumably being secondary to the different neutron exposure in the two cities.[39] Besides an increased mortality and an increased incidence of microcephaly, other outcomes of in utero exposure included an increased incidence of retarded growth and development, a temporary fall of antibody production,[40] and an increased frequency of chromosomal abnormalities in peripheral lymphocytes.[41] However, the long-term consequences of in utero exposure were not found to include an increased risk of leukemia or cancer[42] or infertility[43] in the offspring.

EXPOSURE IN UTERO TO DIAGNOSTIC AND THERAPEUTIC RADIATION

Since the 1920s it has been recognized that therapeutic irradiation given during pregnancy can result in a high frequency of malformations, particularly microcephaly and mental retardation.[44] Although the early use of ionizing radiation was indiscriminate, once these consequences were recognized the use of radiation was avoided in pregnant women. Despite this, occasional reports of children born after therapeutic radiation in utero continued to appear, and this information led to a tentative timetable of abnormalities induced by irradiation during various stages of gestation.[45] These findings in humans are similar to the data derived from animal studies, which demonstrated that the period of organogenesis is the most sensitive to radiation. The most frequent abnormalities noted were (1) growth retardation, (2) microcephaly, (3) mental retardation, (4) microphthalmus, (5) pigmentary degeneration of the retina, (6) genital and skeletal malformation, and (7) cataracts. It is important to point out that, in these studies, when pregnant women were radiated after the twentieth week of gestation, no severe abnormalities were noted.

Diagnostic irradiation of the pregnant woman results in exposure of the embryo to less than 2 cGy (Table 11–1).[35] In contrast to therapeutic irradiation, the lower doses used in diagnostic imaging have not been shown to confer an increased risk of significant congenital malformations,[46] although heterochromia of the iris is a minor abnormality that may be increased in frequency.[47]

Controversy exists regarding the relationship of prenatal radiation exposure to a subsequent increased risk of childhood malignancy. This association has been noted for 30 years[48] and has been supported by several studies examining the incidence of malignancy in children who had obstetrical roentgenograms done while in utero.[49–51] These studies have been criticized because the mothers were selected for obstetrical radiography secondary to an underlying medical condition and therefore a factor other than the roentgenogram exposure may be causal. Twin studies potentially avoid the confounding influence of the underlying disease process, as the radiation is typically given solely because of the suspicion of a twin pregnancy, a factor not known to be related to risk of subsequent malignancy.[52] When twins have been studied, the association of incidental in utero irradiation with subsequent development of childhood malignancy has been significant.[52,53] Negative twin studies,[54] which found no association between routine pelvimetry during pregnancy[55] and a risk of malignancy for the offspring, refute this data. Furthermore, there was no increase in malignancy among the children exposed in utero to the atomic bombs of Hiroshima and Nagasaki.[42] Because the practice of irradiating the pregnant woman for diagnostic reasons has been replaced by more modern techniques, such as sonography, the question of this relationship is less important and is unlikely to be resolved now that these superior methods avoid radiation exposure to the mother and fetus.[56]

Table 11–1. Embryonic/Fetal Dose Estimates for Radiologic Procedures*

Dose	Procedure
1–2 cGy	Barium enema (with fluoroscopy)
0.5–1.0 cGy	Upper GI series (with fluoroscopy)
	Intravenous pyelography
	Lumbosacral spine roentgenograms
0.1–0.5 cGy	Cholecystography
	Flat plate of the abdomen (KUB)
<0.1 cGy	Skull roentgenogram
	Chest roentgenogram
	Cervical and thoracic spine roentgenograms

*Adapted from Pizzarello, 1982[35]

Table 11–2. Radiation Therapy for Hodgkin's Disease During Pregnancy

Reference	Gestational Age at Treatment	Radiation Portal	Tumor Dose	Estimated Fetal Dose	Outcome of Pregnancy	Outcome for Mother
Jacobs 1981[25]	Conception	Mantle (+MOPP)	2000 cGy	—	Therapeutic abortion	NED × 4.5 years
Jacobs 1981[25]	Conception	Mantle	4000 cGy	—	Therapeutic abortion	NED × 13 years
Jacobs 1981[25]	Conception	L breast	4435 cGy	—	Spontaneous abortion	Relapse NED × 5 years
McSwain 1951[57]	Conception	L neck and L axilla	1900 R	—	Normal female	AWD 2 years
Smith 1978[58]	1 week	Upper mantle Paraaortic	4000 cGy 4000 cGy	—	Normal male	NED postpartum
Mulvihill 1987[59] (also McKeen 1979)[60]	3 weeks	Mantle	NS	—	Inner-ear defect	NS
Becker 1965[61]	1 month	Upper abdomen	600 R	4 R	Normal female, 2 weeks premature	NED 20 years
Nisce 1986[62]	6 weeks	Mantle (also prior MOPP)	1000 cGy	7 cGy	Normal infant at C-section	NED 32 months
Stewart 1952[8]	2 months	R neck	NS	—	Normal female	DOD 4.5 years
McDonald 1956[63]	2 months	Thorax and neck	NS	—	Therapeutic abortion	DOD 6 weeks
Thomas 1976[64]	10 weeks	Neck and R axilla	2550 cGy	2.5 R	Normal infant	Relapse 2.5 years
Jacobs 1981[25]	12 weeks	Mantle Paraaortic Spleen	4400 cGy 1150 cGy 1200 cGy	—	Therapeutic abortion	Alive 12 years
Nisce 1986[62]	12 weeks	Mediastinum	3000 cGy	30 cGy	Normal infant	DOD 4 years
Tawil 1985[65]	1st trimester	L neck	4000 cGy	—	Normal infant	Relapse 2 years NED at 14 years
Kushner 1941[66]	1st trimester	Neck and chest	1200 R	—	Normal female	DOD 2 years
Kasdon 1949[31]	1st trimester	Chest	11,000 R	—	Male expired at 4 days of massive atelectasis	Expired 8 days postpartum
Becker 1965[61]	3 months	Mediastinum	4000 cGy	0.1 R	Normal male	NED 7 years
Covington 1969[67]	3 months	Mantle	3500 cGy	7.9 cGy	Normal infant	AWD 1 year
Hennessy 1963[18]	"Early pregnancy"	NS	NS	—	Normal infant (×8)	NS
Thomas 1976[64]	15 weeks	Axilla	4000 cGy	4.4 cGy	Normal male	NED 1 year
Thomas 1976[64]	16 weeks	Mantle	3600 cGy	10.4 cGy	Normal infant	NED 4 years
Jacobs 1981[25]	16 weeks	Mantle	3300 cGy	—	Normal infant	NED 12 years
Nisce 1986[62]	16 weeks	Supraclavicular mediastinum	2000 cGy	4 cGy	Normal infant	NED 2 years
Tenenblatt 1951[68]	4 months	Cervical mediastinum	900 R	—	Normal male	AWD 1 year

Reference	Gestational age	Site	Dose	Additional dose	Infant	Maternal outcome
Harris 1949[69]	4 months	Mediastinum Chest	900 R 900 R + 800 R	—	Expired 4 days postpartum	DOD 1 month
Thomas 1976[64]	20 weeks	Mediastinum	3000 cGy	—	Normal infant	NS
Nisce 1986[62]	20 weeks	Neck, mediastinum	2000 cGy	15 cGy	Normal infant	NED 11 years
Jacobs 1981[25]	22 weeks	Mantle	1500 cGy	—	Normal infant	NED 3.5 years
Brougher 1949[70]	5 months	Mediastinum, neck, lung	864 R	—	Normal infant	AWD 2 years
Riva 1953[9]	After 5th month	NS	NS	—	Normal infant	NS
Hartvigsen 1955[71]	5–6 months	Neck	NS	—	Normal infant	AWD 2 years
Nisce 1986[62]	24 weeks	Mantle	2000 cGy	13 cGy	Normal infant	NED 6 years
Nisce 1986[62]	24 weeks	Neck	2500 cGy	2 cGy	Normal infant	NED 9 years
Nisce 1986[62]	24 weeks	Neck + Mediastinum	2500 cGy	17 cGy	Normal infant	NED 10 years
Thomas 1976[64]	24 weeks	R neck and mediastinum	3500 cGy	—	Normal infant	DOD 2 years
Thomas 1976[64]	25 weeks	Mantle	3660 cGy	30 cGy	Normal female	NED 5.5 years
Tawil 1985[65]	2nd trimester	Mantle	4000 cGy	—	Normal infant	DOD 1.5 years
Becker 1965[61]	6 months	Axilla	2500 R	3 R	Normal male	DOD 1.5 years
Riva 1953[9]	6 months	Thyroid, supraclavicular mediastinum	2400 cGy	—	Normal female	NS
Conley 1977[72]	6 months	Upper mediastinum	1000 cGy	6 cGy	Normal infant	NED 2 years
Brent 1972[73]	6 months	Cervical	3200 cGy	25 cGy	Normal infant	NS
Boes 1982[74]	27 weeks	Mantle	4050 cGy	—	Normal female	NED 2 years
Jacobs 1981[25]	28 weeks	Mantle	1500 cGy	—	Normal infant	NED × 2 years
Mulvihill 1987[59] (also McKeen 1979)	28 weeks	Mediastinum	4000 cGy	—	Slow learner, scoliosis	NS
Becker 1965[61]	7 months	Mediastinum	2000 R	0.1 R	Normal male	DOD 1 year
Riva 1953[9]	7 months +	NS	NS	—	Normal infant (×2)	NS
Thomas 1976[64]	30 weeks	R hilum	3100 cGy	100 cGy	Normal infant	Relapse 2 years then NED
Jacobs 1981[25]	32 weeks	L neck	1600 cGy	—	Normal infant	Relapse NED × 3.5 years
Nisce 1986[62]	32 weeks	Neck, mediastinum	1600 cGy	50 cGy	Normal infant	DOD 19 months
Jacobs 1981[25]	33 weeks	Neck and mediastinum	1000 cGy	—	Normal infant	NED × 2.5 years
Riva 1953[9]	NS	NS	NS	—	Normal infant (×2)	NS

L = left; R = right; NS = not stated; cGy = centiGrays; R = roentgen; NED = no evidence of disease; AWD = alive with disease; DOD = dead of disease

EFFECT OF RADIATION ON THE FETUS OF THE WOMAN WITH HODGKIN'S DISEASE

Despite the clear evidence of radiation's adverse effect on the fetus, the experience in Hodgkin's disease has not corroborated this. Table 11-2 is a summary of more than 50 patients with Hodgkin's disease who had radiation therapy as the primary treatment modality.[8,9,25,31,57-74] Adverse outcomes for the fetuses were rare, with only two neonates who expired several days postpartum and two infants with congenital defects. In the majority of these cases, patients to be irradiated were carefully selected and, therefore, the trend was towards irradiating upper body portals (with resultant lower fetal doses) and irradiating women later in pregnancy (with lower risk of congenital defect). Fetal doses were typically less than 10 cGy, although some fetuses were exposed to 100 cGy[64] or even higher.[58]

Fetal radiation dose has been estimated in several investigations (Table 11-3).[61,67,75-78] Using a phantom, a mediastinal dose of 3500 cGy gave a fetal dose of 3.5 to 14 cGy in early pregnancy, 31 to 49 cGy in midpregnancy, and 129 to 248 cGy in late pregnancy.[67] The increased radiation exposure as the pregnancy progresses corresponds to the decreased distance from the radiation therapy portal to the fetus. A similar study estimated the fetal dose in the midpelvis 20 cm below the lower edge of the mediastinal treatment field.[61] For each 1000 cGy tissue dose, the fetal dose was estimated to be 2.9 cGy for 22.5 MEV betatron generating x-rays, 4.2 cGy for a cobalt 60 unit, and 12.9 cGy for a 250 kV x-ray unit. The internal scatter was least for the 22.5 MEV unit and this most penetrating equipment was therefore recommended whenever radiation therapy is given during pregnancy. More recently, this reduction of scattered dose was also seen comparing cobalt therapy (4.5 to 9.1 cGy) to the linear accelerator (3.5 to 6.3 cGy), confirming this advantage for the more penetrating equipment.[76] Use of a shielding apron over the abdomen has been reported to significantly reduce the fetal dose in one investigation[77] but not in a second.[78]

EFFECT OF CYTOTOXIC DRUGS ON THE EMBRYO AND FETUS

Cytotoxic drug exposure during pregnancy has been associated with a variety of adverse outcomes. Abortion,[79] fetal death,[79] growth retardation,[80] and malformation[80] may occur secondary to administration of these drugs. Principles of teratology that are true for radiation exposure during pregnancy also appear to be true for the use of anticancer drugs. The first trimester is the critical period for organogenesis and therefore the trimester when the highest incidence of congenital malformations is found.[81] Drug dose, similar to radiation dose, also appears to be directly related to the incidence of congenital malformations.

Pregnant experimental animals have amply demonstrated the fetal toxicity associated with cytotoxic drugs.[82] These observations, as well as the accumulated anecdotal human reports, have shown that teratologic complications are a danger, but not of the magnitude as was previously thought. In one review, when cases treated with aminopterin were excluded, only 5% of infants had congenital defects, which is no different than the incidence

Table 11-3. Phantom Estimates of Radiation Dose to the Fetus From Mantle Field Irradiation (as a Percentage of Total Dose)*

Reference	Source	First Trimester	Second Trimester	Third Trimester
Covington 1969[67]	6 MEV	0.1	0.9	3.7
	250 kv	0.4	1.4	7.1
Zucali 1981[76]	6 MEV	0.15	0.34	2.0
	^{60}Co	0.21	0.45	3.0
Sharma 1981[77]	10 MEV	0.8(0.4)	1.1(0.6)	2.2(1.2)
Wong 1985[78]	10 MEV	1.4(1.3)	2.0(1.9)	5.0(4.3)

*Percent of radiation dose after shielding noted in parentheses.

expected in the normal population. Of the 76 children who received cytotoxic drugs in the second or third trimester, no congenital defects were seen.[34] Other reports, however, have concluded that the risk of teratogenesis is real in the first trimester, with an incidence of 16%.[80]

ALKYLATING AGENTS

Nitrogen mustard, rarely used in malignancies other than Hodgkin's disease, has not been associated with congenital defects when used as a single agent[80] but has been associated with anomalies when used in the first trimester with other drugs.[64,83] Cyclophosphamide is a potent teratogen in experimental animals[84] and has been associated with hemangiomas, toe and extremity defects, and hernias when used in the first trimester.[80] Similarly chlorambucil and busulfan have been associated with anomalies after first trimester usage. Thiotepa and triethylenemelamine, however, have not been associated with malformation, perhaps as a result of limited use.[80]

ANTIMETABOLITES

One of the antimetabolites, aminopterin, has most consistently been demonstrated to be teratogenic. Used investigationally in humans as abortifacients in the 1950s, aminopterin frequently caused abortion as well as deformities, including neural-tube defects, craniofacial anomalies, hydrocephalus, and cleft palate.[79,85] Methotrexate, cytosine arabinoside, 6-thioguanine, 6-mercaptopurine, and 5-fluorouracil have all been associated with congenital defects in experimental animals and occasionally in humans when used in the first trimester.[80]

ANTIBIOTICS

Adriamycin and daunomycin, while resulting in animal teratogenesis, have not been associated with malformations in the 24 infants reported with in utero exposure.[86] In one of the few studies of drug levels in amniotic fluid, adriamycin was not found after previous intravenous administration, suggesting that there is a placental barrier to at least this particular drug.[87] Bleomycin, actinomycin D, and mithramycin have infrequently been used during pregnancy.

CORTICOSTEROIDS

Glucocorticoids given chronically have been reported to cause intrauterine growth retardation in both rats and humans.[88] The frequency of cleft palate has been increased in mice given corticosteroids, but only five cases were seen in infants born to more than 300 women receiving steroids for asthma during pregnancy.[89] Another study of patients receiving steroids for asthma during pregnancy found no congenital growth abnormalities,[90] so the magnitude of any effect appears small.

MISCELLANEOUS DRUGS

Vinblastine and vincristine have not been associated with congenital defects when used as single agents in pregnancy,[91,93] but have been associated with defects when used in combination chemotherapy programs in the first trimester.[64,83] Procarbazine is a known teratogen in animals and has been associated with malformations when used in combination chemotherapy protocols.[64,83] Several reviews have summarized the experience with antineoplastic drugs.[2,80,94,96]

CHEMOTHERAPY IN THE TREATMENT OF HODGKIN'S DISEASE DURING PREGNANCY

The effects of chemotherapy for Hodgkin's disease during pregnancy (Table 11–4)[9,11,12,18,25,27,59,60,62,64,83,91–93,97–115] are similar to the effects of chemotherapy for other malignancies. Nearly all of the offspring who had congenital malformations were exposed to cytotoxic drugs in utero during the first trimester. Nearly one third of the offspring reported to have been exposed during the first trimester in Table 11–4 were found to have congenital anomalies. This figure, however, is likely to overestimate the incidence secondary to a reporting bias. In contrast none of the infants exposed to drugs in the second or third trimesters had congenital anomalies.

Use of antineoplastic drugs in pregnancy requires careful assessment of risk versus

Table 11-4. Chemotherapy for Hodgkin's Disease During Pregnancy

Reference	Gestational Age at Treatment	Drug(s)	Outcome of Pregnancy	Maternal Outcome
Riva 1953[9]	Conception	NM	Normal infant	AWD 6 months
Garrett 1974[83]	Conception	NM, VLB, PCZ	Male with four toes on each foot	NS
Thomas 1976[64]	Conception	VLB, VCR, PCZ	Premature male expired due to acute respiratory distress syndrome, small atrial septal defect at autopsy	Relapse 3 months NED 3 years
Thomas 1976[64]	Conception	VLB, PCZ	Therapeutic abortion	NED 1.5 years
Armstrong 1964[91]	Conception to delivery	VLB (p.o.)	Spontaneous delivery, normal male	NS
Rosenzweig 1964[93]	Conception	VLB	Spontaneous delivery, normal female	NS
Greenberg 1964[97]	Conception	Cyclophosphamide (and radiation therapy)	Male with bilateral inguinal hernias and four toes on each foot	DOD 10 months
Wells 1968[98]	Conception	PCZ	Normal male except several hemangiomas	AWD 1 year
Sinkovics 1969[99]	Conception to delivery	Cyclophosphamide	Normal infant	DOD 1 year
Jacobs 1981[25]	Conception	MOPP (and radiation therapy)	Therapeutic abortion	NED 4.5 years
Mulvihill 1987[59] (also McKeen 1979)[60]	Conception	VLB	Spontaneous abortion at 6 weeks	NED 3 years
Jacobs 1981[25]	Conception to delivery	Chlorambucil	Normal infant	NED × 8 years
Mulvihill 1987[59]	1 week to term	Chlorambucil, VLB	Normal infant	NS
Mulvihill 1987[59] (also McKeen 1979)[60]	1 week	Lomustine, OPP, then VLB	Cleft lip and palate	NS
Rugh 1965[100]	3 weeks	Chlorambucil	Therapeutic abortion (histologic retinal damage)	NS
Mulvihill 1987[59]	3 weeks	VLB	Hydrocephalus	NED 4 years
Zoet 1950[101]	1st month	NM (and radiation therapy)	Cesarean section at 8½ months, normal male	AWD 8 months
Smith 1958[11]	1st month	Triethylenemelamine	Normal infant	AWD 8 months
Mennuti 1975[102]	1 month	MOPP	Therapeutic abortion at 3 months; reduced size and malposition of kidneys	NS
Nisce 1986[62]	4 weeks to term (twice)	VLB (twice)	Normal infant (×2)	NED 14 years
Shotton 1963[103]	1 month	Chlorambucil	Absent left kidney and ureter	NS
Toledo 1971[104]	6 weeks	Cyclophosphamide (and diagnostic roentgenogram)	Absence of all toes, single left coronary artery	NS
Barry 1962[12]	2 months	NM	Normal infant	NS
Wright 1955[105]	1st trimester	Triethylenemelamine	Spontaneous abortion (×2)	DOD 2 years
McKeen 1979[60]	1st trimester	Chemotherapy	Hydrocephalus	NS
Blatt 1980[106]	1st trimester	MOPP	Normal male	NS
Carcassonne 1981[107]	1st trimester	VLB	Normal infant	NS

Table 11-4. Chemotherapy for Hodgkin's Disease During Pregnancy Continued

Reference	Gestational Age at Treatment	Drug(s)	Outcome of Pregnancy	Maternal Outcome
Goguel 1970[108]	1st trimester (×8)	VLB	8 Normal infants	NS
Boland 1951[109]	3 months	NM	Therapeutic abortion (no congenital defects)	NS
Deutschle 1953[110]	4 months	NM	Cesarean section, normal male	DOD 7 months
Deutschle 1953[110]	4 months	NM	Premature labor at 7 months, normal female	Died 2 days postpartum
Lacher 1966[111]	18 weeks	VLB Cyclophosphamide	Cesarean section, normal male	DOD 2 months
Daly 1980[112]	18 weeks	COPP	Low birth weight, otherwise normal female	Relapse 1 year
Nisce 1986[62]	18 weeks to delivery	VLB	Normal infant	NED 6 years
Smith 1958[11]	4½ months	NM Chlorambucil	Normal delivery, normal female	DOD 1 month
McKeen 1979[60]	2nd trimester	Chemotherapy	Normal infant	NS
Jouet 1988[27]	2nd trimester	MOPP	Normal infant	NED 12 years
Jouet 1988[27]	2nd trimester	MOPP	Normal infant	DOD 5.5 years
Carcassonne 1981[107]	6 months	MOPP	Premature delivery, normal infant	NS
Jones 1979[113]	26 weeks	MOPP	Labor induced at 38 weeks, normal male	NS
Johnson 1977[114]	28 weeks	MVPP	Premature, but otherwise normal infant	NED 1 year
Smith 1958[11]	7 months	Chlorambucil	Normal infant	AWD 10 months
Lacher 1964[92]	7 months	VLB (and radiation therapy)	Normal labor, normal male	AWD 1 month
Nordlund 1968[115]	32 weeks	VLB	Normal female	NS
McKeen 1979[60]	3rd trimester	Chemotherapy	Normal infant	NS
Jouet 1988[27]	3rd trimester	MOPP	Normal infant	DOD 3.5 years
Hennessy 1963[18]	NS	Triethylenemelamine	Normal infant	NS
Carcassonne 1981[107]	NS	NS	Premature delivery. One twin died of malformation at 27 days old	NS

MOPP = Nitrogen mustard, vincristine (oncovin), procarbazine, prednisone; COPP = Cyclophosphamide, vincristine (oncovin), procarbazine, prednisone; MVPP = Nitrogen mustard, vinblastine, procarbazine, prednisolone; PCZ = procarbazine; NM = nitrogen mustard; VLB = vinblastine; VCR = vincristine; AWD = alive with disease; NED = no evidence of disease; DOD = dead of disease; NS = not stated

benefit for the individual patient. First trimester use appears to be associated with some increased risk of congenital defect, but the risk is not of a great magnitude. Second and third trimester usage, on the other hand, may not be associated with any increased risk to the fetus. Several problems remain as a result of inadequate information. One is that we cannot appropriately assess the incidence of malformations with a specific agent at a specific time of pregnancy. Too few reports are available, and the cases have been reported often because of their uniqueness (i.e., malformation). Broader investigations of all women receiving anticancer agents during pregnancy at a given institution(s) would give us a better grasp of the frequency of these complications. A second problem is that little is known regarding the results of pregnancies occurring in the wives of men receiving chemotherapy. Many men will become azoospermic during treatment and are unable to father children, but there are some men who do father children while they are receiving anticancer drugs. Thalidomide has been reported to result in malformation even when only the father was taking the drug.[116] Malformation and growth retardation can occur in the offspring of male rats receiving chronic cyclophosphamide.[117] Only anecdotes exist of men receiving chemotherapy who have malformed[118] or normal[119] offspring, and more information is needed. Finally, what is the longer term effect on the offspring conceived while their mothers received cytotoxic drugs? Will the future fertility of these offspring be affected? Chemotherapy has been causally associated with the development of secondary malignancies, especially leukemia in Hodgkin's disease patients. Can in utero exposure to these agents also lead to an increased incidence of malignancy?

MANAGEMENT OF THE PREGNANT WOMAN WITH HODGKIN'S DISEASE

Care of the pregnant woman with Hodgkin's disease often involves a compromise. Optimal therapy for the mother usually provides a risk to the fetus. The best care of the fetus precludes cytotoxic agents and radiation therapy. An optimal risk/benefit ratio involves a clinical judgment, in part based on the mother's wishes. While the following guidelines are useful, individualized management is necessary.

An initial problem is staging of the pregnant patient with newly diagnosed Hodgkin's disease. History (A or B symptoms), physical examination, serologic studies, chest roentgenography, and bone-marrow aspiration/biopsy provide a good assessment of stage short of abdominal evaluation. If continuation of pregnancy is intended, then staging laparotomy would be a risk to the fetus and is therefore avoided. Likewise, radioisotopic studies are relatively contraindicated. A modified lymphangiogram with a single abdominal radiograph at 24 hours has been reported to provide useful information on three patients in one series.[64] In another report, however, three patients had lymphangiography done before they were known to be pregnant and all of them had a subsequent abortion or miscarriage.[25] While the use of modified lymphangiography in the second or third trimester exposes the fetus to less than 1 cGy, its safety has not been adequately assessed and it should only be done if the information will lead to a change in management. Computed tomography of the abdomen is relatively contraindicated because of the radiation exposure, but ultrasonography may provide useful information in some circumstances and with little risk.

FIRST HALF OF PREGNANCY

Generally, therapeutic abortion has been recommended for patients presenting with Hodgkin's disease during the first trimester and first half of the second trimester.[25,65] An exception to this may be the woman with asymptomatic disease localized to the neck or axilla where local radiation with abdominal shielding could be used.[25,65]

SECOND HALF OF PREGNANCY

For patients with stage IA, IB, IIA, or IIB supradiaphragmatic disease, one recommendation has been to postpone treatment until after delivery. Induction of delivery is suggested as soon as possible, usually at 32 to 34 weeks.[25,65] In women with rapid progression of disease, supradiaphragmatic radiation has been recommended with lead shielding of the abdomen.[25,65] If the disease of concern is infradiaphragmatic or if there is stage IV disease, systemic chemotherapy should be used and vinblastine has been suggested as the drug of choice by some since fetal abnormalities have not been reported when it it used as a single agent.[25,65] In view of the data on cytotoxic drugs reviewed previously, which indicate that fetal abnormalities are not increased with second or third trimester usage, and the superior effectiveness of combination chemotherapy programs, multiple drug regimens should be considered in these circumstances.

DIAGNOSIS OF PREGNANCY DURING CHEMOTHERAPY OF HODGKIN'S DISEASE

With effective pretreatment counseling regarding the importance of contraception during treatment, the complication of pregnancy should be avoided. If it occurs, however, therapeutic abortion should be encouraged.

MATERNAL OUTCOME ACCORDING TO TREATMENT CHOICE

Because of small numbers of patients, individualized choice of management, and occurrence of case reports over a timespan where the treatment and prognosis of the disease has changed, it is difficult to compare the management options for the pregnant woman with Hodgkin's disease. One attempt to do so, however, has found no difference in the proportion of women who were in remission according to the treatment choice: observation until delivery (75%), therapeutic abortion (83%), and radiation therapy (74%).[120] Maternal outcome after chemotherapy was not analyzed in this series, but one would expect these women to have the worst prognosis since chemotherapy would be chosen for more advanced disease. This outcome varies enormously as to whether they were treated prior to the mid-1960s when chemotherapy was usually palliative versus a more recent year when chemotherapy has had a higher curative potential.

PREGNANCY AFTER COMPLETION OF TREATMENT

Completion of treatment for Hodgkin's disease brings with it a new set of questions from the woman who desires children. Will my child have an increased risk of developing Hodgkin's disease? How long should I wait before becoming pregnant? Will the radiation and chemotherapy I have had cause congenital defects in my child? None of the answers to these questions are absolute, but the available medical literature on Hodgkin's disease and other malignancies provides us with some guidelines.

FAMILIAL HODGKIN'S DISEASE AND THE RISK OF HODGKIN'S DISEASE IN OFFSPRING

Despite a great effort in the epidemiologic investigation of Hodgkin's disease, the etiology remains unknown. Both environmental and genetic influences have been supported by different studies but with more support for environmental influences.[121] A large number of families have been reported to have multiple occurrences of Hodgkin's disease.[122-128] The risk of a patient's first-order relatives developing Hodgkin's disease has been estimated as threefold[123] to ninefold.[127] A relative risk of 7.1 was found for siblings in another study.[129] A recent analysis in Scotland found a fourfold increase in deaths due to Hodgkin's disease among first- and second-degree relatives of patients.[128]

Though the incidence of Hodgkin's disease does appear to be increased in relatives, this does not necessarily argue for a genetic basis of the disease; common environmental exposures are usually also shared. Histocompatibility testing, however, does give further support for a limited genetic basis for Hodgkin's disease. Since Amiel first pointed out the association of the antigen 4c (later split into four subspecificities B5, B15, B18, and BW 35) with Hodgkin's disease, there have been a large number of investigations into this association.[130-137] When HLA types of Hodgkin's disease patients have been compared to controls, there has generally been an increased frequency but the antigens involved have been inconsistent. When the results of 1500 patients were reviewed in 1975, A1, B5, and B18 were found to be significantly increased.[138] Inconsistencies among reports can in part be explained by differing populations being studied: some patients are newly diagnosed; some are long-term survivors. These two groups of patients could have different HLA types with some types being important prognostically. DR typing has only been included in a few studies but the results have been negative[135,139,140] except for one group of investigators who found an increased incidence of DR5.[141,142] Another approach has been to study concordance in the families with multiple cases of Hodgkin's disease and a significant concordance has been found.[140,143]

Based on the above information, one reaches the conclusion that there is a genetic basis for Hodgkin's disease but the magnitude is not great. This is illustrated by the fact that in a 1977 review there had been a total of 53 sibling pairs and 32 parent-child pairs with Hodgkin's disease.[126] This limited genetic influence should not dissuade the woman in remission after treatment of Hodgkin's disease from childbearing.

EFFECT OF PRECONCEPTION CHEMOTHERAPY AND RADIATION THERAPY ON PROGENY

A major concern of patients treated for Hodgkin's disease is whether chemotherapy or radiation will have any effect on future pregnancies or offspring. Many women and men will have treatment-induced sterility and will be unable to have children. In the remaining patients, however, treatment-induced congenital defects in the offspring have been an important theoretical possibility. Besides congenital defects in the offspring, other outcomes of concern include spontaneous abortion, stillbirths, premature births and future malignancies in the offspring. Accumulating information is finally allowing us to address whether or not these possible adverse outcomes are real risks.

A significant body of information exists on the effects of radiation and cytotoxic drugs for nonmalignant conditions on offspring when exposed in utero. For exposure to these agents prior to conception, however, only limited information is available of the effects on future offspring. Several studies suggest that preconception diagnostic radiation of the mother and/or father result in an increased risk of childhood malignancy[144-145] or leukemia.[51] Because there was a medical indication for the diagnostic radiation, however, the findings may simply be an association and not causal in nature. In contrast, after parental exposure to atomic bomb radiation at Hiroshima and Nagasaki, no increase in leukemia incidence[146] or shortening of survival[147] was seen in the offspring. Similarly no increased rate of deaths or cancer was seen in the offspring of patients treated with ^{131}I therapy for hyperthyroidism.[148]

The ability of chemotherapy and/or radiation to cure an increasing proportion of patients with cancer has led to concerns about potential teratogenesis in the offspring of survivors after therapy has been completed. Accumulating information from investigations of progeny over the last decade, however, have led to a reassurance that congenital defects are not significantly increased (Table 11–5).[59,106,149-171] In a review of the published series, approximately 4% had major birth defects,[172] which is similar to the expected frequency in the general population.[173] Additional investigations listed in Table 11–5 have also confirmed this conclusion. Of more than 3000 pregnancies reported in these series, approximately 100 congenital defects occurred (approximately 3%). There may be a subset of patients, however, who do have an adverse outcome of their pregnancies. Among the women treated for Wilm's tumor with abdominal radiation, nearly one-third of pregnancies ended in perinatal death or low-birth-weight infants.[160,170] The pathogenesis of this problem is unclear, but is likely to be the result of radiation-induced damage to abdominopelvic structures.

Besides the concern about congenital defects in the offspring of cancer survivors, researchers have also been concerned that there may be an increased risk of malignancy in the progeny. Several investigations involving more than 3000 offspring have helped to allay these worries.[59,154,170,172] The largest of these investigations involved 2308 offspring of pediatric and adolescent cancer survivors as well as 4719 offspring of patient sibling controls; and no excess cancer risk was found (0.3% versus 0.23% respectively).[174] Again there may be a caveat, however, because there are known cancers that have familial clusters such as medullary thyroid cancer, retinoblastoma, and Wilm's tumor, and therefore, the offspring of patients with these rare tumors may have an increased risk of cancer.

Over the last decade, the outcome of pregnancies occurring after the treatment of

Hodgkin's disease has been frequently investigated.[27,59,60,106,175-186] Similar to the findings in other malignancies, no significant increase in congenital defects in the offspring has been found. One possible exception did report an increased rate of congenital defects in the offspring born to the subset of patients who received both chemotherapy and radiation;[177] however, the statistical methods used to reach this conclusion have been criticized.[187] Aside from this one study, if one assesses the 14 other studies of progeny in Hodgkin's disease, no increase in congenital defects is found. Together with the studies of progeny in other malignancies there is good information to reassure the patient contemplating pregnancy after successful treatment of Hodgkin's disease.

BREASTFEEDING

The infrequent occurrence of lactation in women receiving chemotherapy has led to measurement of milk-drug levels in several patients.[188-191] Cyclophosphamide,[188] methotrexate,[189] doxorubicin,[190] and hydroxyurea[191] have all been measurable in the milk of lactating mothers receiving these drugs, although cisplatin[190] was not measurable in the single patient where it was investigated. In separate reports the nursing infants of two women receiving cyclophosphamide were noted to have blood-count depression, presumably related to ingestion of cyclophosphamide from the mothers' milk.[192,193] Based on this limited information it would appear reasonable for women receiving cytotoxic drugs to avoid breastfeeding.

PATIENT EDUCATION AND COUNSELING

Patient education regarding the interaction between pregnancy and treatment for Hodgkin's disease is essential at the time of diagnosis. In the case of a pregnant woman with recently diagnosed Hodgkin's disease, it is obvious that information about possible teratogenic effects of cytotoxic drugs and radiation is necessary in making the decision whether to proceed with anticancer therapy, not treat until after delivery, or have a therapeutic abortion. In the case of nonpregnant women with Hodgkin's disease in the reproductive years, patient education about pregnancy is not as obvious and is often neglected. It is in these women that a few words about the risks of pregnancy and the need for effective contraception can have its greatest preventive benefit. Advising the patient to report missed menses is also important in order to make a diagnosis (pregnancy, ovarian dysfunction, or other cause) and take appropriate action.

Post-treatment counseling is mainly related to possible teratogenc effects and the previously mentioned evidence leads us to conclude that no increase in congenital defects after cancer therapy has been demonstrated. We emphasize to patients that the risk of malformations in their future offspring is no different from that of the general population where it is 3 to 6%.[173] While amniocentesis has demonstrated its utility in screening for many genetic and metabolic diseases, it does not appear to have a general role in screening pregnancies that occur subsequent to cancer therapy, particularly in view of the lack of any documented teratogenic increase.

How long to wait after therapy before becoming pregnant is a frequently asked question. The general practice has been to wait 1 or 2 years following completion of therapy before recommending that pregnancy is appropriate. The rationale for a 2-year recommendation in one report was that 85% of relapses occur within the first two years[64] and, therefore, it is better to avoid pregnancy in this period of highest risk. An individualized approach for each patient would be better, considering patient preference, prognostic factors, and past results with the treatment regimen used. There are no data to suggest an increased risk of malformation or other adverse outcome in those pregnancies in the early post-treatment period.

In summary, the concurrent diagnoses of Hodgkin's disease and pregnancy can lead to emotional decisions for both the patient and physician. Weighing of benefits and risks involves primarily the patient but the fetus

Table 11–5. Outcome of Pregnancies After Treatment of Malignancy

Reference	Malignancy	Treatment	Women with Pregnancy*	Number of Pregnancies	Births Term	Premature & Low Birth Weight (Stillbirths)	Congenital Defects
Sandeman 1966[149]	Testis Ca	Unilateral orchiectomy and RT	15 M	24	21	NS(1)	0
Van Thiel 1970[150]	Gestational trophoblastic tumors (GTT)	Chemotherapy	50 F	88	71	NS	NS
Amelar 1971[151]	Testis Ca	Unilateral orchiectomy and RT	3 M	4	4	0	0
Pastorfide 1973[152]	GTT	Chemotherapy = 38 No chemotherapy = 44	82 F	118	73	11(1)	4/85
Smithers 1973[153]	Testis Ca	Unilateral orchiectomy and RT	34 M	54	52	NS	0
Li 1974[154]	Pediatric Ca	Various	29 F 17 M	64 43	44 39	8 1	14
Ross 1976[155]	GTT	Chemotherapy	58 F	96	— 78 —		3
Sarkar 1976[156]	Thyroid cancer	[131]I	18 F 11 M	43 27	43 22	0 6	1 0
Moe 1979[157]	Leukemia	Chemotherapy	5 F & 1 M	10	9	0	0
Li 1979[158]	Pediatric Ca	Various	84 F 62 M	159 134	242	NS(1)	24
Walden 1979[159]	GTT	Chemotherapy	159 F	218	156	6	7
Blatt 1980[106]	Misc.	Chemotherapy	20 F 5 M	25 10	15 7	0	0

Study	Tumor	Treatment	Patients				
Green 1982[160]	Unilateral Wilm's tumor	Various	27 F and 9 M	81	51	7	5
Carroll 1982[161]	Misc.	Chemotherapy	5 F and 8 M	13	15	NS	0
Bundy 1982[162]	Neurol. tumors	Various	27 F and M	NS	45	NS	2
Rustin 1984[163]	GTT	Chemotherapy	187 F	368	——273——	(8)	7
Li 1984[164]	Brain tumors	Various	21 F and M	41	NS	NS	0
Goldstein 1984[165] (update of Pastorfide 1973[152])	GTT	Surgery ± chemotherapy	NS, F	929	626	79(4)	32
Senturia 1985[166]	Testis Ca	Chemotherapy	25 M	NS	30	NS	4
		RT	27 M		40		3
Rockicka-Milewska 1986[167]	ALL	Chemotherapy ± RT	4 F and 3 M	7	7	0	1
Fossa 1986[168]	Testis Ca	Unilateral orchiectomy & RT	69 M	95+	95	NS	2
Gulati 1986[169]	Misc.	Chemotherapy + or RT	6 F and 3 M	13	11	0(1)	1
Li 1987[170]	Wilm's Tumor	Abdominal RT	60 F	114	80	22 (+12 Fetal and neonatal deaths)	0
		No Abdominal RT	5 F	13	13	0	0
		Abdominal RT	34 M	64	62	2	0
Mulvihill 1987[59]	Misc.	Various	40 F	58	30	7(2)	6
Nijman 1987[171]	Testis Ca	Unilateral orchiectomy ± Chemotherapy	8 M	8	7	0	0

NS = Not Stated
*F indicates the patient had the pregnancy; M indicates the wife of a male patient had the pregnancy

Table 11–6. Outcome of Pregnancies After Treatment of Hodgkin's Disease

Reference	Treatment	Women With Pregnancies*	Number of Pregnancies	Term Births	Premature and Low Birth Weight (Stillbirths)	Congenital Defects
Baker 1972[175]	RT	5 F	5	5	0	0
LaFloch 1976[176]	RT	9 F	11	8	0	0
Holmes 1978[177]	Various	29 F	55	84	2(2)	6
		19 M	38			
McKeen 1979[60]	Various	19 F	44	23	6(2)	3
Johnson 1979[178]	RT + chemotherapy	2 F	2	2	0	0
Blatt 1980[106]	MOPP ± RT	5 F	7	7	0	0
Schilsky 1981[179]	MOPP	7 F	15	13	0	0
Horning 1981[180]	Various	20 F	28	21	3	0
Andrieu 1983[181]	MOPP	22 F	30	21	1	1
Whitehead 1983[182]	MVPP	12 F	17	9	0	0
Specht 1984[183]	RT ± MOPP	8 F	11	9	0	0
Slanina 1985[184]	RT	39	63	41	3	2
Green 1986[185]	Various	14 F	28	22	0(2)	3
	Various	3 M	7	5	0	
Lacher 1986[186]	TVPP/RT	12 F	17	12	0	0
Mulvihill 1987[59] (update of McKeen 1979)	Various	(NS) F	NS	NS	4(2)	5
Jouet 1988[27]	Various	11 F	16	16	0	0

*F indicates the patient had the pregnancy; M indicates the wife of a male patient had the pregnancy. NS = not stated.

must also be considered; this judgment is influenced by the social and religious convictions of patient and physician. The choice of management is therefore not absolute, but frequently involves therapeutic abortion for patients with first trimester pregnancies and observation for third trimester pregnancies. Congenital defects are a potential concern after radiation or chemotherapy, but appear uncommon except after chemotherapy is given in the first trimester. Individualized management is essential in this situation.

For the man or woman in remission after treatment of Hodgkin's disease, the outlook is more reassuring. In the woman with intact gonadal function, a subsequent pregnancy does not appear to increase the risk of relapse. Offspring of either men or women with prior Hodgkin's disease have a slight but negligible increased risk of developing Hodgkin's disease. Importantly the rate of congenital defects and malignancy in the offspring is similar to that of the general population. For the survivor of Hodgkin's disease emerging from the tribulations of treatment, there can be optimism for future progeny.

REFERENCES

1. Mandelson, M.T. and Li, F.P. Survival of children with cancer. JAMA 225:1572, 1986 (letter).
2. Barber, H.R.K.: Malignant disease in the pregnant woman. In Gynecologic Oncology. Edited by M. Coppleson. Edinburgh, Churchill Livingstone, 1981, p. 795.
3. Orr, J.W. and Singleton, H.M. Cancer in pregnancy. Curr. Probl. Cancer 8(1):1–50, 1983.
4. Disaia, P.J. and Creasman, W.T. Cancer in pregnancy. In Clinical Gynecologic Oncology. 2nd Ed. St. Louis, C.V. Mosby Co., 1984, p. 428.
5. Disaia, P.J. and Berman, M.L. Cancer in pregnancy. In Maternal-Fetal Medicine. Edited by R.K. Creasy and R. Resnik. Philadelphia, W.B. Saunders, 1984, p. 1063.
6. Haas, J.F. Pregnancy in association with a newly diagnosed cancer: a population-based epidemiologic assessment. Int. J. Cancer 34:229, 1984.
7. Palacios, Costa N., Chavanne, F.C., and Zebel Ternandez, O. An de ateneo, Buenos Aires, 127, 1945.
8. Stewart, H.L. and Monto, R.W. Hodgkin's disease and pregnancy. Am. J. Obstet. Gyncecol. 63:570, 1952.
9. Riva, H.L., Anderson, P.S., and O'Grady, J.W. Pregnancy and Hodgkin's disease. Am. J. Obstet. Gynecol. 66:866, 1953.
10. Morgan, O.S., Hall, J.S., and Gibbs, W.N. Hodgkin's disease in pregnancy; a report of three cases. West Indian Med. J. 25:121, 1976.
11. Smith, R.B.W., Sheehy, T.W., and Rothberg, H. Hodgkin's disease and pregnancy. Arch. Intern. Med. 102:777, 1958.
12. Barry, R.M., Diamond, H.D., and Craver, L.F. Influence of pregnancy on course of Hodgkin's disease. Am. J. Obstet. Gynecol. 84:445, 1962.
13. Stutzman, L. and Sohal, J. Use of anticancer drugs in pregnancy. Clin. Obstet. Gynecol. 11:416, 1968.
14. Goldman, L.B. and Victor, A.W. Hodgkin's disease. N.Y. J. Med. 45:1313, 1945.
15. Portmann, W.V. and Mulvey, B.E. Hodgkin's disease and pregnancy. Cleve. Clin. Quart. 17:149, 1950.
16. Bichel, J. Hodgkin's disease and pregnancy. Acta. Radiol. 33:427, 1950.
17. Hennessy, J.P. and Rottino, A. Hodgkin's disease in pregnancy with a report of twelve cases. Amer. J. Obstet. Gynecol. 63:756, 1952.
18. Hennessy, J.P. and Rottino, A.: Hodgkin's disease and pregnancy. Amer. J. Obstet. Gynecol. 87:851, 1963.
19. Frank, H.G.: The effect of Hodgkin's disease on pregnancy and fertility. J. Obst. Gynaec. Brit. Emp. 62:266, 1955.
20. Peters, M.V. and Middlemiss, K.C.H. A study of Hodgkin's disease treated by irradiation. Am. J. Roentgenol. 79:114, 1958.
21. Gemmel, A.A. Menstruation and pregnancy in Hodgkin's disease. J. Obstet. Gynaecol. Br. Emp. 30:373, 1923.
22. Craver, L.F. Some aspects of the treatment of Hodgkin's disease. Cancer 7:927, 1954.
23. Myles, T.J.M. Hodgkin's disease and pregnancy. J. Obstet. Gynaecol. Brit. Comm. 62:884, 1955.
24. Southam, C.M., Diamond, H.D., and Craver, L.F. Hodgkin's disease in pregnancy. Cancer 9:1141, 1956.
25. Jacobs, C., Donaldson, S.S., Rosenberg, S.A. et al. Management of the pregnant patient with Hodgkin's disease. Ann. Int. Med. 95:669, 1981.
26. Gobbi, P.G. et al. Hodgkin's disease and pregnancy. Haematologia 69:336, 1984.
27. Jouet, J.P. et al. Influence de la grossesse sur l'evolutivite de la maladie de Hodgkin? La Presse Med. 17:423, 1988.
28. Potter, J.F. and Schoeneman, M. Metastasis of maternal cancer to the placenta and fetus. Cancer 25:38, 1970.
29. Priesel, A and Winkelbauer, A. Placentare Ubertragung des Lymphogranulms Virchows Arch. F. Path. Anat. 262:749, 1926.
30. Branch, C.F. A case of congenital lymphoblastoma. Amer. J. Pathol. 9:777, 1933.
31. Kasdon, S.C. Pregnancy and Hodgkin's disease. Am. J. Obstet. Gynecol. 57:282, 1949.
32. Mazar, S.A. and Straus, B. Marital Hodgkin's disease. Arch. Int. Med. 88:819, 1951.
33. Greenspan, E.M. and Lesnick, G.J. Pregnancy and cancer. In Medical, surgical and gynecological com-

plications of pregnancy. Edited by A.F. Guttmacher and J.J. Rovinsky. Baltimore, Williams and Wilkins, 1960, p. 555.
34. Sweet, D.L. and Kinzie, J. Consequences of radiotherapy and antineoplastic therapy for the fetus. J. Reprod. Med. 17:241, 1976.
35. Pizzarello, D.J. and Witcofski, R.L. Effects of radiation on embryonic and fetal development. In Medical Radiation Biology. 2nd Ed. Philadelphia, Lea & Febiger, 1983, p. 65.
36. Russell, L J. and Russell, W.L. An analysis of the changing radiation response of the developing mouse embryo. J. Cell Physiol. 1:103, 1954.
37. Rugh, R. and Grupp, E. Exencephaly following x-irradiation of the preimplantation mammalian embryo. J. Neuropathol. Exp. Neurol. 18:468, 1959.
38. Committee for the compilation of materials on damage caused by the atomic bombs in Hiroshima and Nagasaki: Hiroshima and Nagasaki. The Physical, Medical and Social Effects of the Atomic Bombings. New York, Basic Books Inc., 1981, p. 217.
39. Miller, R.W. and Blot, W.J. Small head size after in utero exposure to atomic radiation. Lancet 2:784, 1972.
40. Kanamitsu, M. et al. Serologic response of atomic bomb survivors following Asian influenza vaccination. Jpn. J. Med. Sci. Biol. 19:73, 1966.
41. Bloom, A.D., Nerlishi, S., and Archer, P.G. Cytogenetics of the in-utero exposed of Hiroshima and Nagasaki. Lancet 2:10, 1968.
42. Jablon, S. and Kato, H. Childhood cancer in relation to prenatal exposure to atomic bomb radiation. Lancet 2:1000, 1970.
43. Blot, W.J., Smimizu, Y., Kato, H. et al. Frequency of marriage and live birth among survivors prenatally exposed to the atomic bomb. Atomic Bomb Casualty Commission Technical Report, p. 2–75, 1975.
44. Murphy, D.P. and Goldstein, L. Etiology of the ill-health of children born after maternal pelvic irradiation. Part 1. Unhealthy children born after preconception pelvic irradiation. Am. J. Roentgenol. 22:207, 1929.
45. Dekaban, A. Abnormalities in children exposed to x-irradiation injury to the human fetus. J. Nucl. Med. 9:471, 1968.
46. Kinlen, L.J. and Acheson, E.D. Diagnostic irradiation congenital malformations and spontaneous abortion. Br. J. Radiol. 41:648, 1968.
47. Lejuene, J., Turpin, A., Rethore, M.O. et al. Resultats d'une premiere enquete sur les effets somatiques de l'irradiation foeto-embryonnaire in utero. Revue Fr. Etud. Clin. Biol. 5:982, 1960.
48. Stewart, A., Webb, J., Giles, D. et al. Malignant disease in childhood and diagnostic irradiation in utero. Lancet 2:447, 1956.
49. MacMahon, B. Prenatal x-ray exposure and childhood cancer. J. Natl. Cancer Inst. 28:1173, 1962.
50. Ford, D.D., Paterson, J.C.S., and Treuting, W.L. Fetal exposure to diagnostic x-rays and leukemia and other malignant diseases in childhood. J. Natl. Cancer Inst. 22:1093, 1959.
51. Graham, S. et al. Preconception, intrauterine, and postnatal irradiation as related to leukemia. Natl. Cancer Inst. Monogr. 19:347, 1966.
52. Mole, R.H. Antenatal irradiation and childhood cancer: causation or coincidence? Br. J. Cancer 30:199, 1974.
53. Harvey, E.B., Boice, J.D., Honeyman, M. et al. Prenatal x-ray exposure and childhood cancer in twins. N. Engl. J. Med. 312:541, 1985.
54. Court-Brown, W.M., Soll, R., and Hill, R.B. Incidence of leukemia after exposure to diagnostic radiation in utero. Br. Med. J. 2:1539, 1960.
55. Oppenheim, B.E., Griem, M.L., and Meier, P. Effects of low-dose prenatal irradiation in humans: analysis of Chicago Lying-In data and comparison with other studies. Radiat. Res. 57:508, 1974.
56. MacMahon, B. Prenatal x-ray exposure and twins. N. Engl. J. Med. 312:376, 1985.
57. McSwain, B. and Haber, A. Hodgkin's disease complicated by pregnancy. South. Med. J. 44:105, 1951.
58. Smith, H.N. and Spaulding, L. Hodgkin's disease in pregnancy. South. Med. J. 71:374, 1978.
59. Mulvihill, J.J., McKeen, E.A., Rosner, F. et al. Pregnancy outcome in cancer patients. Experience in a large cooperative group. Cancer 60:1143, 1987.
60. McKeen, E.A., Mulvihill, J.J., Rosner, F. et al. Pregnancy outcome in Hodgkin's disease. Lancet 2:590, 1979.
61. Becker, M.H. and Hyman, G.A. Management of Hodgkin's disease coexistent with pregnancy. Radiology 85:725, 1965.
62. Nisce, L.Z., Tome, M.A., He, S. et al. Management of coexisting Hodgkin's disease and pregnancy. Am. J. Clin. Oncol. 9:146, 1986.
63. McDonald, I. Hodgkin's disease in pregnancy. J. Obstet. Gynaec. Brit. Emp. 63:931, 1956.
64. Thomas, P.R.M. and Peckham, M.J. The investigation and management of Hodgkin's disease in the pregnant patient. Cancer 38:1443, 1976.
65. Tawil, E., Mercier, J.P., and Dandavino, A. Hodgkin's disease complicating pregnancy. J. Canad. Assoc. Radiol. 36:133, 1985.
66. Kushner, J.I. Pregnancy complicating Hodgkin's disease (Lymphogranuloma malignum). Am. J. Obstet. Gynec. 42:536, 1941.
67. Covington, E.E. and Baker, A.S. Dosimetry of scattered radiation to the fetus. JAMA 209:414, 1969.
68. Tenenblatt, W. and Horton, C.E. Hodgkin's disease and pregnancy: review of the literature and report of a case. West. J. Surg. 59:120, 1951.
69. Harris, W.H. Pregnancy in Hodgkin's disease: a case report. Bull. McGuire Clin. 13:53, 1949.
70. Brougher, J.C. Pregnancy in Hodgkin's disease. West. J. Surg. 57:430, 1949.
71. Hartvigsen, B. Hodgkin's disease and pregnancy. Acta. Radiol. 44:317, 1955.
72. Conley, J.G. and Jacobson, A. Modified radiation therapy regimen for Hodgkin's disease in the third trimester of pregnancy. Am. J. Roentgenol. 128:666, 1977.
73. Brent, R.L. and Gorson, R.O. Radiation exposure in pregnancy. Curr. Prob. Radiol. 11:1, 1972.

74. Boes, D.J. Hodgkin's disease: diagnosis and management during the reproductive years and pregnancy. J. Am. Osteopath. Assoc. 82:261, 1982.
75. Kartha, P. et al. Fetus dose from mantle field treatment for Hodgkin's disease. Med. Phys. 5:327, 1978 (abstract).
76. Zucali, R. et al. Abdominal dosimetry for supradiaphragmatic irradiation of Hodgkin's disease in pregnancy. Experimental data and clinical considerations. Tumori 67:203, 1981.
77. Sharma, S.C., Williamson, J.F., Khan, F.M. et al. Measurement and calculation of ovary and fetus dose in extended field radiotherapy for 10 MV x-rays. Int. J. Radiat. Oncol. Biol. Phys. 7:843, 1981.
78. Wong, P.S., Rosemark, P.J., Wexler, M.C. et al. Doses to organs at risk from mantle field radiation therapy using 10 MV x-rays. Mt. Sinai J. Med. 52:216, 1985.
79. Thiersch, J.B.: Therapeutic abortions with a folic acid antagonist, 4-aminopterolyglutamic acid administered by the oral route. Am. J. Obstet. Gynecol. 63:1298, 1952.
80. Stern, J.L. and Johnson, T.R.B. Antineoplastic drugs and pregnancy. In Drug Use in Pregnancy, edited by J.R. Niebyl. Philadelphia, Lea & Febiger, 1982, p. 67.
81. Bender, R.A. and Young, R.C. Effects of cancer treatment on individual and generational genetics. Semin. Oncol. 5:47, 1978.
82. Chaube, S. and Murphy, M.L. The teratogenic effects of the recent drugs active in cancer chemotherapy. In Advances in Teratology. Edited by D.H.M. Woollam. New York, Academic Press, 1968, p. 181.
83. Garrett, M.J. Teratogenic effects of combination chemotherapy. Ann. Intern. Med. 80:667, 1974 (letter).
84. Mirkes, P.E. Cyclophosphamide teratogenesis: a review. Teratogenesis, Carcinog. Mutagen. 5:75, 1985.
85. Shaw, E.B. and Steinbach, H.L. Aminopterin induced fetal malformation. Am. J. Dis. Child. 155:477, 1968.
86. Turchi, J.J. and Villasis, C. Anthracyclenes in the treatment of malignancy in pregnancy. Cancer 61:435, 1988.
87. Roboz, J. et al. Does doxorubicin cross the placenta? Lancet 2:1382, 1979 (letter).
88. Reinisch, J.M., Simon, N.G., Karow, W.G. et al. Prenatal exposure to prednisone in humans and animals retards intrauterine growth. Science 202:436, 1978.
89. Bongiovanni, A.M. and McFadden, A.J. Steroids during pregnancy and possible fetal consequences. Fertil. Steril. 11:181, 1960.
90. Snyder, R.D. and Snyder, D. Corticosteroids for asthma during pregnancy. Allergy 41:340, 1978.
91. Armstrong, J.G., Dyke, R.W., Fouis, P.J. et al. Delivery of a normal infant during the course of oral vinblastine sulfate therapy for Hodgkin's disease. Ann. Intern. Med. 61:106, 1964.
92. Lacher, M.J. Use of vinblastine sulfate to treat Hodgkin's disease during pregnancy. Ann. Intern. Med. 61:113, 1964.
93. Rosenzweig, A.I., Crews, Q.E., and Hopwood, H.G. Vinblastine sulfate in Hodgkin's disease in pregnancy. Ann. Intern. Med. 60:108, 1964.
94. Sokal, J.E. and Lessman, E.M. Effects of cancer chemotherapy agents on the human fetus. JAMA 172:1765, 1960.
95. Nicholson, H.O. Cytotoxic drugs in pregnancy. Br. J. Obstet. Gynaecol. 75:307, 1968.
96. Gililland, J. and Weinstein, L. The effects of cancer chemotherapeutic agents on the developing fetus. Obstet. Gynecol. Surv. 38:6, 1983.
97. Greenberg, L.H. and Tanaka, K.R. Congenital anomalies probably induced by cyclophosphamide. JAMA 188:423, 1964.
98. Wells, J.H., Marshall, J.R., and Carbone, P.P. Procarbazine therapy for Hodgkin's disease in early pregnancy. JAMA 205:935, 1968.
99. Sinkovics, J.G. and Shullenberger, C.C. Pregnancy and systemic malignant disease. Cancer Chemother. Rep. 53:94, 1969 (abstract).
100. Rugh, R. and Skaredoff, L. Radiation and radiomietic chlorambucil and the fetal retina. Arch. Ophthal. 74:382, 1965.
101. Zoet, A.G. Pregnancy complicating Hodgkin's disease. Northwest Med. 49:373, 1950.
102. Mennuti, M.R., Shepard, T.H., and Mellman, W.J. Fetal renal malformations following Hodgkin's disease during pregnancy. Obstet. Gynecol. 46:194, 1975.
103. Shotton, D. and Monie, I.W. Possible teratogenic effect of chlorambucil on a human fetus. JAMA 186:74, 1963.
104. Toledo, T.M., Harper, R.C., and Moser, R.H. Fetal effects during cyclophosphamide and irradiation therapy. Ann. Intern. Med. 74:87, 1971.
105. Wright, J.C. The effect of tri-ethylene melamine and of tri-ethylene phosphoramide on human neoplastic disease. Acta. Unio. Internat. Cancer 11:220, 1955.
106. Blatt, J., Mulvihill, J.J., Ziegler, J.L. et al. Pregnancy outcome following cancer chemotherapy. Am. J. Med. 69:828, 1980.
107. Carcassonne, Y., Dodemant, P., and Favre, R. Hodgkin's disease and pregnancy. Acta. Haemat. 66:67, 1981.
108. Goguel, A. Etude de l'influence de la grossesse sur le pronostic et le traitement de la maladie de Hodgkin. La Presse Med. 78:1507, 1970.
109. Boland, J. Clinical experience with nitrogen mustard in Hodgkin's disease. Br. J. Radiol. 24:513, 1951.
110. Deuschle, K.W. and Wiggins, W.S. The use of nitrogen mustard in the management of two pregnant lymphoma patients. Blood 8:576, 1953.
111. Lacher, M.J. and Geller, W. Cyclophosphamide and vinblastine sulfate in Hodgkin's disease during pregnancy. JAMA 195:486, 1966.
112. Daly, H., McCann, S.R., Hanratty, T.D. et al. Successful pregnancy during combination chemotherapy for Hodgkin's disease. Acta. Haematol. 64:154, 1980.
113. Jones, R.T. and Weinerman, B.H. MOPP (nitrogen

113. ...mustard, vincristine, procarbazine and prednisone) given during pregnancy. Obstet. Gynecol. 54:477, 1979.
114. Johnson, I.R. and Filshie, G.M. Hodgkin's disease diagnosed in pregnancy. Br. J. Ob. Gynaeol. 84:791, 1977.
115. Nordlund, J.J., DeVita, V.T., and Carbone, P.P. Severe vinblastine-induced leukopenia during late pregnancy with delivery of a normal infant. Ann. Intern. Med. 69:581, 1968.
116. Editorial. The drugged sperm. Br. Med. J. 1:1063, 1964.
117. Trasler, J.M., Hales, B.F., and Robaire, B.: Paternal cyclophosphamide treatment of rats causes fetal loss and malformations without affecting male fertility. Nature 316:144, 1985.
118. Russell, J.A., Powles, R.L., and Oliver, R.T.D. Conception and congenital abnormalities after chemotherapy of acute myelogenous leukaemia in two men. Br. Med. J. 1:1508, 1976.
119. Kroner, T.H. and Tschuma, A. Conception of a normal child during chemotherapy of acute lymphoblastic leukaemia in the father. Br. Med. J. 1:1322, 1977.
120. Yahalom, J. Management of lymphoma associated with pregnancy. In Radiation Therapy of Gynecological Cancer. Edited by D. Nori and B.S. Hilaris. New York, Alan R. Liss, Inc., 1987, p. 345.
121. Grufferman, S. Hodgkin's disease. In Cancer Epidemiology and Prevention. Edited by D. Schottenfeld and J.F. Fraumeni. Saunders, Philadelphia, 1982, p. 739.
122. DeVore, J.W. and Doan, C.A. Studies in Hodgkin's disease. XII. Hereditary and epidemiologic aspects. Ann. Intern. Med. 47:300, 1957.
123. Razis, D.V., Diamond, H.D., and Craver, L.F. Familial Hodgkin's disease: its significance and implications. Ann. Intern. Med. 51:933, 1959.
124. Perlin, E. et al. Hodgkin's disease in siblings: a family study. Oncology 33:116, 1976.
125. Lynch, H.T. et al. Familial Hodgkin's disease and associated cancer. Cancer 38:2033, 1976.
126. Grufferman, S. Clustering and aggregation of exposures in Hodgkin's disease. Cancer 39:1829, 1977.
127. Haim, N., Cohen, Y., and Robinson, E. Malignant lymphoma in first-degree blood relatives. Cancer 49:2197, 1982.
128. Kerzin-Storrar, L., Faed, M.J.W., MacGillvary, J.B. et al. Incidence of familial Hodgkin's disease. Br. J. Cancer 47:707, 1983.
129. Grufferman, S., Cole, P., Smith, P.G. et al. Hodgkin's disease in siblings. N. Eng. J. Med. 296:248, 1977.
130. Amiel, J.L. Study of the leucocyte phenotypes in Hodgkin's disease. In Histocompatibility Testing, 1967. Report of a Conference and Workshop, Torino and Saint-Vincent, 14–24 June 1967. Edited by E.S. Curtoni, P.L. Mattiuz and R.M. Tosi. Munksgaard, Copenhagen, 79, 1967.
131. Forbes, J.F. and Morris, P.J. Analysis of HL-A antigens in patients with Hodgkin's disease and their families. J. Clin. Invest. 51:1156, 1972.
132. Falk, J.A. and Osoba, D. The association of the human histocompatibility system with Hodgkin's disease. J. Immunogenet. 1:53, 1974.
133. Kissmeyer-Nielsen, F., Kjerbye, K.E., and Lamm, L.U. HL-A in Hodgkin's disease. III. A prospective study. Transpl. Rev. 22:168, 1975.
134. Marshall, W.H., Bernard, J.M., Buehler, S.K. et al. HLA in familial Hodgkin's disease. Results and a new hypothesis. Int. J. Cancer 19:450, 1977.
135. Hansen, J.A. et al. HLA and MLC typing in patients with Hodgkin's disease. In HLA and Malignancy. Edited by G.P. Murphy. New York, A.R. Liss, 1977, p. 217.
136. Greene, M.H. et al. HLA antigens in familial Hodgkin's disease. Intern. J. Cancer 23:777, 1979.
137. Dausset, J., Colombani, J., and Hors, J. Major histocompatibility complex and cancer, with special reference to human familial tumours (Hodgkin's disease and other malignancies). Cancer Surveys 1:119, 1982.
138. Svejgaard, A. et al. HLA and disease associations—a survey. Transplant. Rev. 22:3, 1975.
139. Welsh, K.J., Amlot, P., and Batchelor, J.R. Do alleles in linkage disequilibrium compensate for each other's disadvantageous effects? Tissue Antigens 17:91, 1981.
140. Hors, J. and Dausset, J. HLA and susceptibility to Hodgkin's disease. Immunol. Rev. 70:167, 1983.
141. Winchester, R. et al. Association of susceptibility to certain hematopoietic malignancies with the presence of Ia alloderminants distinct from the DR series; utility of monoclonal antibody reagents. Immunol. Rev. 70:155, 1983.
142. Logalbo, P., Nunez-Roldan, A., Cuttner, J. et al. Association of HLA-DR5 with the occurrence of Hodgkin's disease in a New York City population. Disease Markers, 3:39, 1985.
143. Berberich, F.R. et al. Hodgkin's disease susceptibility: linkage to the HLA locus demonstrated by a new concordance method. Human Immunol. 6:207, 1983.
144. Stewart, A., Webb, J., and Hewitt, D. A survey of childhood malignancies. Br. Med. J. 1:1495, 1958.
145. Shiono, P.G., Chung, C.S., and Myrianthopoulos, N.C. Preconception radiation, intrauterine diagnostic radiation and childhood neoplasia. J. Natl. Cancer Inst. 65:681, 1980.
146. Hoshino, T. et al. Leukemia in offspring of atomic bomb survivors. Blood 30:719, 1967.
147. Neel, J.V., Kato, H.K., and Schull, W.J. Mortality in children of atomic bomb survivors and control. Genetics 76:311, 1974.
148. Safa, A.M., Schumacher, O.P., and Rodriguez-Antunez, A. Long term followup results in children and adolescents treated with radioactive iodine (^{131}I) for hyperthyroidism. N. Eng. J. Med. 292:167, 1975.
149. Sandeman, T.F. The effects of x irradiation on male human fertility. Br. J. Radiol. 39:901, 1966.
150. Van Thiel, D., Ross, G.T., and Lipsett, M.B. Pregnancies after chemotherapy of trophoblastic neoplasms. Science 169:1326, 1970.
151. Amelar, R.D., Dubin, L., and Hotchkiss, R.S. Res-

151. ...toration of fertility following unilateral orchiectomy and radiation therapy for testicular tumors. J. Urol. 106:714, 1971.
152. Pastorfide, G.B. and Goldstein, D.P. Pregnancy after hydatidiform mole. Obstet. Gynecol. 42:67, 1973.
153. Smithers, D.W., Wallace, D.M., and Austin, D.E. Fertility after unilateral orchidectomy and radiotherapy for patients with malignant tumours of the testis. Br. Med. J. 4:77, 1973.
154. Li, F.P. and Jaffe, N. Progeny of childhood cancer survivors. Lancet 2:707, 1974.
155. Ross, G.T. Congenital anomalies among children born of mothers receiving chemotherapy for gestational trophoblastic neoplasms. Cancer 37:1043, 1976.
156. Sarkar, S.D., Beierwaltes, W.H., Gill, S.P. et al. Subsequent fertility and birth histories of children and adolescents treated with ^{131}I for thyroid cancer. J. Nucl. Med. 17:460, 1976.
157. Moe, P.J., Lethinen, M., Wegelius, R. et al. Progeny of survivors of acute lymphocytic leukemia. Acta. Paediatr. Scand. 68:301, 1979.
158. Li, F.P., Fine, W., Jaffe, N. et al. Offspring of patients treated for cancer in childhood. J. Natl. Cancer Inst. 62:1193, 1979.
159. Walden, P.A.M. and Bagshawe, K.D. Pregnancies after chemotherapy for gestational trophoblastic tumours. Lancet 2:1241, 1979.
160. Green, D.M., Fine, W.E., and Li, F.P. Offspring of patients treated for unilateral Wilm's tumor in childhood. Cancer 49:2285, 1982.
161. Carroll, R.J. and Case, D.C. Fertility after chemotherapy for malignant diseases. Proc. Am. Soc. Cl. Oncol. 1:54, 1982 (abstract)
162. Bundy, S. and Evans, K. Survivors of neuroblastoma and ganglioneuroma and their families. J. Med. Genet. 19:16, 1982.
163. Rustin, G.J.S. et al. Pregnancy after cytotoxic chemotherapy for gestational trophoblastic tumours. Br. Med. J. 288:103, 1984.
164. Li, F.P., Winston, K.R., and Gimbrere, K. Follow-up of children with brain tumors. Cancer 54:135, 1984.
165. Goldstein, D.P., Berkowitz, R.S., and Bernstein, M.R. Reproductive performance after molar pregnancy and gestational trophoblastic tumors. Clin. Obstet. Gynecol. 27:221, 1984.
166. Senturia, Y.D., Peckham, C.S., and Peckham, M.J. Children fathered by men treated for testicular cancer. Lancet 2:766, 1985.
167. Rockicka-Milewska, R. et al. Children cured of acute lymphoid leukemia. Long-term follow-up studies, including progeny. Am. J. Pediatr. Hematol. Oncol. 8:208, 1986.
168. Fossa, S.D., Almaas, B., Jetne, V. et al. Paternity after irradiation for testicular cancer. Acta. Radiol. Oncol. 25(Fasc. I):33–36, 1986.
169. Gulati, S.C., Vega, R., Gee, T., et al. Growth and development of children born to patients after cancer therapy. Cancer Invest. 4:197, 1986.
170. Li, F.P. et al. Outcome of pregnancy in survivors of Wilm's tumor. JAMA 257:216, 1987.
171. Nijman, J.M., Kopps, H.S., Kremer, J. et al. Gonadal function after surgery and chemotherapy in men with stage II and III nonseminomatous testicular tumors. J. Clin. Oncol. 5:651–656, 1987.
172. Mulvihill, J.J. and Byrne, J. Offspring of long-term survivors of childhood cancer. Clin. Oncol. 4:333–343, 1985.
173. Kalter, H. and Warkany, J. Congenital malformations. N. Engl. J. Med. 308:424 & 491, 1983.
174. Mulvihill, J.J. et al. Cancer in offspring of long-term survivors of childhood and adolescent cancer. Lancet 2:813, 1987.
175. Baker, J.W., Peckham, M.J., Morgan, R.L. et al. Preservation of ovarian function in patients requiring radiotherapy for para-aortic and pelvic Hodgkin's disease. Lancet 1:1307, 1972.
176. Le Floch, O., Donaldson, S.S., and Kaplan, H.S. Pregnancy following oophoropexy and total nodal irradiation in women with Hodgkin's disease. Cancer 38:2263, 1976.
177. Holmes, G.E. and Holmes, F.F. Pregnancy outcome of patients treated for Hodgkin's disease: A controlled study. Cancer 41:1317, 1978.
178. Johnson, S.A., Goldman, J.M., and Hawkins, D.F. Pregnancy after chemotherapy for Hodgkin's disease. Lancet 2:93, 1979.
179. Schilsky, R.L., Sherins, R.J., Hubbard, S.M. et al. Long-term follow-up of ovarian function in women treated with MOPP chemotherapy for Hodgkin's disease. Am. J. Med. 71:552, 1981.
180. Horning, S.J., Hoppe, R.T., Kaplan, H.S. et al. Female reproductive potential after treatment for Hodgkin's disease. N. Engl. J. Med. 304:1377, 1981.
181. Andrieu, J.M. and Ochoa-Molina, M.E. Menstrual cycle, pregnancies and offspring before and after MOPP therapy for Hodgkin's disease. Cancer 52:435, 1983.
182. Whitehead, E., Shalet, S.M., Blackledge, G. et al. The effect of combination chemotherapy on ovarian function in women treated for Hodgkin's disease. Cancer 52:988, 1983.
183. Specht, L., Hansen, M.M., and Geisler, C. Ovarian function in young women in long-term remission after treatment for Hodgkin's disease stage I or II. Scand. Haematol. 32:265, 1984.
184. Slanina, J., Wannenmacher, M., and Spratler, J. Shwangerschaft und kindesentwicklung nach therapie des Morbus Hodgkin. Strahlentherapie 161:558, 1985.
185. Green, D.M. Pregnancy outcome following treatment during childhood and adolescence for Hodgkin's disease. Blood 67 (Suppl. 1):210a, 1986 (abstract).
186. Lacher, M.J. and Toner, K. Pregnancies and menstrual function before and after combined radiation (RT) and chemotherapy (TVPP) for Hodgkin's disease. Cancer Invest. 4:93, 1986.
187. Simon, R. Statistical methods for evaluating pregnancy outcomes in patients with Hodgkin's disease. Cancer 45:2890, 1980.
188. Wiernik, P.H. and Duncan, J.H. Cyclophosphamide in human milk. Lancet 1:912, 1971 (letter).

189. Johns, D.G., Rutherford, L.D., Leighton, P.C. et al. Secretion of methotrexate into human milk. Am. J. Obstet. Gynecol. 112:978, 1972.
190. Egan, P.C., Costanza, M.E., Dodion, P. et al. Doxorubicin and cisplatin excretion into human milk. Cancer Treat. Rep. 69:1387, 1985.
191. Sylvester, R.K., Lobell, M., Teresi, M.E. et al. Excretion of hydroxyurea into milk. Cancer 60:2177, 1987.
192. Amato, D. and Niblett, J.S. Neutropenia from cyclophosphamide in breast milk. Med. J. Aust. 1:383, 1977.
193. Durodola, J.I. Administration of cyclophosphamide during late pregnancy and early lactation: a case report. J. Natl. Med. Assoc. 71:165, 1979.

CHAPTER 12

Cardiovascular Complications of the Treatment of Hodgkin's Disease

BARBARA GERLING
JOHN GOTTDIENER
JEFFREY S. BORER

The successful therapy of Hodgkin's disease has been one of the hallmarks of twentieth century medicine. It represents one of the few instances in oncology where a relatively common neoplastic malignant disease with a previously dismal prognosis can be medically cured. The use first of radiation therapy, and subsequently, of successful chemotherapy regimens, has permitted physicians to think not merely in terms of five-year survival, but to look forward to complete resolution of disease in a high proportion of patients. This has been especially gratifying considering the young age of many Hodgkin's patients who, as a result of successful therapy, are able to resume active and productive lives. Not unexpectedly, however, this therapeutic success has not been unqualified. In addition to noncardiovascular organ toxicity discussed elsewhere in this monograph, both radiation and chemotherapy used in the treatment of Hodgkin's disease have had toxic effects on the heart and peripheral vessels. While experience with radiation and drug dosage has diminished the frequency of acute toxicity, cardiovascular complications of therapy remain a problem. In addition, the continued survival of patients treated 10 to 20 years ago is only now allowing us to see the late consequences of treatment. Given the fact that many patients are treated for Hodgkin's in the second to fourth decades of life, delayed manifestations of cardiovascular toxicity are of particular importance as survivors approach the age when degenerative cardiovascular disease is usually first noted. In a curious way, to have the luxury of determining the delayed cardiovascular effects of Hodgkin's therapy highlights the remarkable success that has been achieved in the treatment of this disease. The purpose of this chapter shall be to examine the history, frequency, and clinical manifestations of cardiovascular toxicity of radiotherapy and chemotherapy used in the treatment of Hodgkin's disease. Mechanisms of injury will be discussed relative to an understanding of prevention and treatment of toxicity. Finally, the data that are emerging on the delayed clinical and subclinical cardiovascular toxicity of Hodgkin's therapy will be presented.

ADVERSE CARDIOVASCULAR EFFECTS OF RADIATION THERAPY

HISTORY OF CARDIOVASCULAR INJURY FROM ROENTGEN THERAPY

Adverse effects of radiation on blood vessels have been appreciated since the discovery of radiation, when early workers noted skin erythema within 2 weeks of handling radium. Subsequently, histologic studies established the presence of endothelial swelling and proliferation.[1] In 1899, Gassman suggested that radiation-induced vascular changes could account for organ injury by interfering with tissue perfusion and causing "starvation of the surrounding tissues." Later studies conducted by the same investigator demonstrated that, in addition to vascular endothelial swelling and smooth muscle proliferation, radiation produced lymphatic obliteration in rabbits. Human studies have shown similar vascular effects of radiation. Linser documented in 1904 that low doses of cutaneous radiation resulted in perivascular round-cell infiltration with thrombotic vascular occlusion.

Despite the sensitivity of vascular endothelium to radiation, early experience[1] with therapeutic radiation delivered to the thorax failed to disclose frequent, obvious cardiac toxicity. In 17 cases receiving thoracic radiation for cancer, Emery and Gordon found no clinical or autopsy evidence of cardiac injury.[2] Even in patients receiving thoracic radiotherapy for cardiac disease (rheumatic fever, angina pectoris, luetic aortitis, and myocarditis), adverse cardiac effects were not generally appreciated.[2-4] Nonetheless, Granzow noted severe damage to the myocardium following irradiation,[1] and Hartman and associates in 1927 described three cases where autopsy documented cardiac injury from radiation.[5] One of these was a 36-year-old woman who died 6 months after receiving radiation for lymphosarcoma. Histologic examination of the myocardium disclosed atrophy of muscle fibers, brown pigmentation, and vacuolization. In another patient, loss of cardiac muscle striations and thickening of the arteriolar walls of the myocardium were described. In contrast to uncertainty on the cardiac effects of external thoracic radiation, radium implants to the breast,[3,7] stomach,[8] and esophagus[3] caused clear and remarkable instances of cardiac injury, including pericardial perforation with pneumopericardium. Thus, it is likely that the failure to observe cardiac injury with early radiotherapeutic regimens was related to the limited dose capacity of x-ray generators available at that time. This may have led Emery and Gordon to conclude in 1925 that "until more intensive treatments could be given without damage to the skin there should be no reason to feel that serious injury to the myocardium may be produced through irradiation of the chest."[2]

In the first quarter of the twentieth century, several investigators sought to develop an experimental model for radiation-induced cardiac injury. An extensive review of animal experimental data written by Desjardins in 1932 noted diverse results based on differences in species and dose and type of radiation. While it was initially suggested that the apparent resistance of the heart to radiation was due to nonregeneration of cardiac muscle and conduction tissue, it has become apparent that radiation injury of vascular endothelium with consequent impairment of the microcirculation causes ischemic damage to even nonregenerative tissues. Hartman and associates[5] demonstrated pericardial effusion, right atrial and right ventricular enlargement with swelling of right ventricular muscle fibers, and increased thickness of the left ventricular wall within thirty days of chest-wall irradiation of sheep and dogs. After 30 days they observed thinning of the right ventricular walls with hyaline degeneration of the atria and hemorrhagic infiltration of the myocardium. Emery and Gordon, however, were able to produce only isolated areas of apparently nonspecific necrosis in rabbits.[2] In contrast, Warren and Whipple,[9] as well as Warthin and

Pohle,[10] found little effects of radiation on the hearts of dogs, though doses of radiation one to three times that necessary to produce skin erythema did produce cardiac damage in dogs in a study by Karlin and Mogilhitsky.[1] Atrophy of cardiac muscle fibers and increased hyalinization of pericardial connective tissue was described.

Thus, historically, experimental and clinical radiation injury to the heart was marked by rare, clinically overt evidence of cardiac damage and varying experimental results. In the early years of radiation therapy, failure of patients receiving thoracic radiation to survive long enough to manifest cardiac abnormality, as well as dosage limits of then available equipment, may account in part for these observations.

However, with the introduction of megavoltage therapy in the 1950s, permitting higher doses of deep radiation without limitation by skin injury, instances of adverse cardiac effects became more common in patients treated with a variety of intrathoracic neoplasms. Furthermore, the design of effective radiotherapy for Hodgkin's disease in the 1960s resulted in disease-free survival of patients in whom only palliation was previously possible. Hence, higher doses of radiation necessary to produce cardiac injury were being administered, and patients now free of their intrathoracic cancer were living long enough to manifest evidence of cardiac injury both acutely and chronically.

MECHANISMS OF RADIATION INJURY TO THE CARDIOVASCULAR SYSTEM

Early clinical and experimental data suggesting that the heart was radioresistant were supported theoretically by biologic considerations. In contrast to tissues that remain mitotically active, such as skin, bone marrow, and gut mucosa, the heart does not require continued cellular proliferation for organ function. Since a major effect of radiation on tissue is interference with reproductive viability of cells, the low proliferative rate of the myocardium could thus be considered to confer "radioresistance." However, indirect effects of radiation may have an important role in producing injury even in nonregenerative tissues. One of the effects of ionizing radiation is the generation of high energy-free radicals in intra- and extracellular water.[11] These short-lived particles are capable of causing substantial membrane injury, particularly in high oxygen tension environments, such as that found in vascular endothelium. Hence, ischemia resulting from radiation injury of microvasculature endothelium may be an important mechanism of radiation injury to tissues without proliferative requirement.

Of note, anthracycline antibiotics may have a similar mechanism of toxicity. Both doxorubicin (Adriamycin) and radiation generate high energy-free radicals, which damage lipid membranes, perhaps accounting for the phenomenon of "radiation recall" seen in some patients receiving doxorubicin, even many years after radiation therapy has been completed.[12] Also, loss of corticosteroid effects in stabilizing cell membranes and preventing lipid peroxidation may be related to reactivation of radiation injury on withdrawal of corticosteroid medication.[13]

Pathologic studies of the irradiated rabbit model have documented in detail the early ultrastructural alterations that occur in the microvasculature of the heart. Following a single dose of 2000 cGy to the heart using a 6-MEV linear accelerator, Fajardo and Stewart noted a number of abnormalities of the capillary endothelium on electron microscopy.[14] The abnormalities were apparent at a time when light microscopy revealed no evidence of injury ("latent" stage). This latent stage occurred 2 to 70 days following radiation. Shortly after irradiation, focal thinning of endothelial cytoplasm was noted, followed by projection of cytoplasm into the capillary lumen. Electron-dense bodies, thought to represent lysosomes, increased in number and in size within capillary endothelial cells. At the peak of endothelial damage (approximately day 20), broken capillary walls resulted from disruption of the basement membrane and the cytoplasm of the endothelial cell. Obstruction of the capillary was occasionally caused by protrusion of endothelial cytoplasm into the lumen and more often by platelet and fibrin thrombi. Damaged endothelial cells were removed by macrophages, accompanied by a decrease in the number of capillaries and increase in intercapillary distance. There was a 45% decrease in the ratio of capillaries to myocytes. Microcirculatory ischemia, from obstruction and loss of capillaries, resulted in collagen bands filling the spaces previously occupied by capillaries and eventually in grossly apparent fibrous replacement of myocardium.

While morphologic alterations described are likely a direct consequence of radiation, inflammatory and immune mechanisms may play a role in the pathogenesis of radiation injury to the heart.[15,16] Thus, it has been noted that lymphopenia, occurring prior to radiation therapy in humans, may protect from the occurrence of pericarditis.[16] This observation suggests that radiation pericarditis may in part represent an autoimmune reaction to tissue antigens altered by radiation.[17-19] In addition, intercurrent viral infection has been suggested as a possible contributing factor to radiation pericarditis.[16]

Besides capillary endothelial damage, radiation may directly injure lymphatics draining the epicardial surface of the heart, or the epipericardial fibrous reaction following irradiation can disrupt lymphatic drainage. In either case, lymphatic obstruction may contribute to formation and maintenance of pericardial effusion in patients with radiation pericarditis.

An additional mechanism by which radiation may injure the heart may involve radiation-induced decrease in vascular prostacyclin (PGI_2). Thus, after irradiation (200 cGy) of human umbilical artery, Allen and associates showed a decrease in vascular prostacyclin that was not accompanied by concomitant compensatory decrease in platelet-thromboxane production.[20] The investigators showed that this was not the result of a decrease in metabolic precursors. It was speculated that radiation-induced liberation of lipid peroxidases inhibited prostacyclin synthetase and cyclo-oxygenase. The physiologic effect of a decrease in prostacyclin is an increase in platelet aggregation and vasoconstriction, leading to a reduction in blood flow through the microcirculation. Again, the consequent myocardial ischemia would be followed by fibrous replacement of myocardial tissue and cardiac conduction tissue.

In addition to compromise of the microcirculation of the heart, radiation may accelerate atherosclerosis in the large epicardial coronary arteries. While numerous reports[21-29] have described epicardial coronary obstruction, often with myocardial infarction, it remains somewhat uncertain whether this represents chance occurrence or radiation acceleration of coronary artery atherosclerosis.

EVIDENT RESULTS OF CLINICAL RADIATION-INDUCED CARDIOVASCULAR INJURY

Pericardial Disease

The anterior pericardium lies within 6 cm of the chest wall surface. Hence, before incident radiation reaches the pericardium, relatively little is absorbed by noncardiac tissues. As a result, substantial pericardial absorption can be expected, particularly in patients receiving radiation therapy to the chest via an anterior port only (a dose regimen no longer employed).

The incidence of both acute and chronic pericardial disease is related to the amount of radiation delivered to the pericardium. The effects of radiation on the pericardium, however, appear to be modulated by a variety of technical and clinical variables. Stewart[28] proposed the concept of pericardial tolerance to define the amount and method of irradiation that would result in an incidence of less than 5% of mild late pericarditis. Three technical variables were found to contribute to pericardial radiation tolerance: total dose, fractionation, and the heart volume irradiated. Thus, a comparison of the incidence of pericardial disease at two institutions using different radiotherapeutic techniques revealed a greater than twofold higher incidence of pericardial disease in the patients who underwent a treatment regimen involving relatively shorter treatment times and fewer fractions, despite the fact that total radiation dose in cGy was only 9% greater in this group than in the less diseased group. This retrospective study suggests that a longer treatment course with more fractions may diminish the incidence of radiation-induced pericardial disease. In addition, a comparison of patients with Hodgkin's disease who received mantle radiotherapy with patients with breast cancer who received only internal mammary radiation suggested to Stewart that reduction of the volume of cardiac tissue irradiated also could reduce the incidence of pericarditis. Byhardt[30] was unable to confirm the correlation of radiation dose to the incidence of pericardial disease, but suggested that the development of pericarditis depends on pre- and postirradiation clinical factors. Consistently, Ruckdeschel[16] identified four pretreatment parameters that correlated with an increased risk of the development of radiation-induced pericardial disease: increased erythrocyte sedimentation rate (ESR), normal absolute lymphocyte count, chemotherapy, and bulky mediastinal lymphoma involvement. As noted earlier, a low absolute lymphocyte count may limit the inflammatory response to injury and consequently protect the pericardium from possible autoimmune processes. Ruckdeschel found that the addition of chemotherapy to the treatment regimen did not influence the incidence of pericardial disease after irradiation, but was associated with an increased likelihood of persistent effusions; 9 of 11 (81%) persistent effusions occurred in those patients who received chemotherapy as well as radiotherapy. The magnitude of mediastinal involvement by lymphoma resulted in a trend toward a higher incidence of pericardial effusions after irradiation, though this trend did not reach statistical significance. Bulky mediastinal involvement not only dictates larger fields of irradiation, but also is likely to be associated with a greater area of pericardium in close proximity to tumor. Those patients exhibiting all four characteristics had an 86% chance of developing a pericardial effusion after radiation therapy for Hodgkin's disease.

Techniques used to detect pericardial injury following radiation undoubtedly have a major effect on the reported incidence of radiation pericarditis. Studies that rely on autopsy data, on increases in cardiothoracic ratio on chest roentgenogram, or on clinical or electrocardiographic findings, are likely to underestimate the frequency of pericardial effusion. Unfortunately, many of the available clinical studies regarding the effects of radiation on the heart have employed such relatively insensitive indices. In contrast, newer diagnostic modalities, such as echocardiography have permitted greater sensitivity in detection of pericardial effusion. Since echocardiography is noninvasive and is performed relatively easily, its serial application may enhance detection of cardiac abnormalities not previously apparent from clinical exam, roentgenogram, or electrocardiogram. As yet, however, few data regarding the effects of radiation have been generated with echocardiographic mediation.

Histopathologic description of radiation-induced pericardial changes originate from surgical resections of pericardium or autopsy materials.[16,28,29,31] Early changes are primarily related to the microvasculature. Capillary dilatation and congestion is followed by endothelial edema, resulting in transudation of fluids into the interstitial tissues. In addition, the mesothelial membrane cells demonstrate morphologic changes suggestive of early degeneration. The pathologic findings may include increasing pericardial edema. Later, the mesothelial lining may be denuded and replaced by atypical and regenerating cells. The pericardium becomes increasingly thickened by interstitial edema and deposition of fibrin with an increase in fibrocyte population and collagen. Neovascularization of the pericardium with capillary proliferation extending into the organizing exudate occurs. The late endothelial response is limited to occasional thrombosed and necrotic capillaries. The fibrinous exudate adheres closely to the pericardial lining, becoming organized and eventually being replaced by fibrous adhesions. Throughout this course, little inflammatory infiltrate, other than increased numbers of macrophages, is present.

Pericardial injury from radiation may manifest itself in three forms: acute radiation pericarditis, chronic pericarditis, and constrictive pericarditis. While overlap is often present, any form may occur without being preceded by earlier manifestations, or followed by later sequelae.

Acute Radiation Pericarditis. Acute pericarditis may be the manifestation of two distinct clinical syndromes occurring in patients treated with radiation therapy for Hodgkin's disease. Acute pericarditis occurring during the initial course of radiation therapy seems to be the consequence of radiation-induced necrosis of contiguous mediastinal tumor masses.[28,29] Cohn noted the development of early acute pericarditis in 2 of 21 patients, both of whom had Hodgkin's disease with massive mediastinal involvement. Similarly, Stewart described 3 of 59 patients with mediastinal malignancies treated with radiotherapy who developed this syndrome. All of these patients continued their radiotherapy course with prompt resolution of the clinical pericarditis. However, acute pericarditis precipitated by direct effects of radiation on the pericardium clearly cannot be confidently excluded in these situations without pathologic examination.

In contrast to pericarditis occurring during the initial course of therapy, delayed acute pericarditis, a more common syndrome, is more likely to be a direct toxic manifestation of radiation on the pericardium. Cohn described 11 of 21 patients treated with mediastinal irradiation who developed acute pericarditis with a delayed onset.[29] Stewart noted 23 of 59 patients in this series with this syndrome.[28] It generally presents within 12 months of the completion of mediastinal radiotherapy, though intervals up to several years have been observed.[28]

The clinical picture is indistinguishable from acute pericarditis of any etiology. Patients may present with fever, pleuritic chest pain, and pericardial friction rubs. Pericardial effusions are frequently present, and if large or rapidly progressive, may result in mild to severe cardiac tamponade. These patients with hemodynamic compromise from pericardial fluid may present with dyspnea at rest or with exertion, orthopnea, cough, syncope, or fatigue in association with tachycardia, hypotension, significant paradoxical pulse, increased jugular venous pressure, orthostatic hypotension, edema, hepatosplenomegaly, ascites, and distant heart sounds.

The laboratory evaluation of pericarditis in patients with Hodgkin's disease treated with radiotherapy is particularly important in establishing the etiology and directing therapy. Radiation pericarditis must be distinguished from malignant, viral, bacterial, fungal, drug induced, autoimmune, and hypothyroid pericarditis, all potentially associated with the underlying disease, its sequelae, or its treatment. Radiation pericarditis must also be distinguished from idiopathic pericarditis because the therapeutic options may vary widely with etiology. The initial laboratory evaluation of the patient with suspected pericardial disease should include electrocardiography, chest roentgenography, and echocardiography. These studies may demonstrate the presence of pericardial masses, thickening, or fluid, and can serve as a baseline for evaluating the efficacy of therapy. The typical electrocardiographic findings of pericarditis of low QRS voltage, abnormal T waves, and ST-segment elevation were commonly present in patients with radiation pericarditis studied by Cohn and Stewart. Pericardial effusions may be appreciated as an enlarged cardiac silhouette on routine chest radiography or as fluid surrounding the heart on echocardiography. In cases in which hemodynamic compromise leading to tamponade has occurred, echocardiography may reveal compression of right-sided chambers and paradoxical septal motion. Right heart catheterization can document the diagnosis of tamponade, though in rapidly developing cases where accurate serial observations of neck veins and blood pressure are available and effusion is documented by echocardiography, catheterization is not required prior to institution of therapeutic pericardiocentesis. Pericardiocentesis or pericardial biopsy through a minithoracotomy may be required for definitive determination of etiology.[32] If radiation alone is the cause of pericardial effusion, the pericardial fluid may appear serous, serosanguinous, or sanguinous, with high protein content; cell count typically is relatively low, and both lymphocyte and polymorphonuclear cells are present. By definition, culture and cytologic examination are negative. If pericardial biopsy is performed, pericardial tissue may reveal only minimal thickening of the parietal pericardium, or may be more severely involved, with findings up to and including gross thickening of all layers with adhesion to the epicardial surface of the heart.

The natural history of acute radiation pericarditis is unpredictable. Nearly 60% of patients demonstrate spontaneous improvement, although some require pericardiocentesis for tamponade. Others, however, progress to develop chronic pericardial processes or may expire, frequently of cardiac disease. Of the 23 patients in Stewart's series, five developed pericardial constriction, and five had either pericardial fibrosis or pancarditis at necropsy.[28] Cohn reported similar findings in his series of 11 patients.[29]

Chronic Pericardial Disease. Clinically, chronic pericardial injury from radiation may manifest in either of two forms, chronic pericardial effusions and chronic constrictive pericarditis. The temporal appearance of pericardial disease after completion of course of radiation may vary considerably in each of these forms. Early reports of radiation-induced pericardial disease emphasized a relatively short interval of up to 48 months between radiotherapy and the onset of pericardial disease. The late appearance (later than 48 months), however, of chronic pericardial disease in patients treated with mediastinal irradiation is becoming increasingly recognized as a significant consequence of therapy for Hodgkin's disease. While Ruckdeschel has reported the incidence of early onset of chronic pericardial disease to be nearly 14%,[16] more recent reports of late onset of chronic pericardial disease have estimated the incidence to be from 11 to 50%.[33-35] The pathophysiologic processes that result in early acute pericarditis in some patients and late chronic pericardial disease in others are not clearly understood. The different clinical and pathologic syndromes suggest that several different pathophysiologic mechanisms may be contributing to the spectrum of radiation-induced pericardial disease. Moreover, many patients with these entities are asymptomatic and consequently are not recognized unless physicians caring for them maintain a high index of suspicion. In view of the potential sequellae of either form, early recognition and treatment would seem a highly appropriate goal.

Uncomplicated chronic pericardial effusions are frequently persistently asymptomatic and consequently often are not recognized. Stewart[28] identified 26 patients with chronic pericardial effusions, most of whom were asymptomatic when a routine follow-up chest roentgenogram revealed an enlarging cardiac silhouette. The interval between the course of radiation therapy and the onset of detectable pericardial disease was less than 12 months in most of these patients, although several patients were identified who developed effusions 2 to 5 years after therapy. In 14 of these 26 cases, the effusion cleared spontaneously, sometimes after persisting for longer than 2 years. Several patients, however, developed cardiac tamponade requiring pericardiocentesis. Of the remaining patients, five developed constrictive physiology requiring pericardiectomy and seven had evidence of either pericarditis or pancarditis on necropsy. Gottdiener used noninvasive techniques to document the frequency of cardiac abnormalities in 25 patients who had no evidence of cardiac disease before mediastinal irradiation for Hodgkin's disease 5 to 15 (mean 10.9) years earlier.[33] Pericardial effusion was present in 7 of 18 patients (39%) who did not have evidence of pericardial effusions within 2 years after irradiation, and in four of seven patients who did have effusions within 2 years of radiation. These late pericardial effusions usually were of no apparent clinical consequence. One patient did, however, progress to cardiac tamponade. Although the majority of uncomplicated radiation-induced pericardial effusions appear to resolve spontaneously, clearly they cannot be assumed to be innocuous, and these patients must be recognized and monitored closely, and on occasion, perhaps treated "prophylactically" with pericardiocentesis or pericardiectomy. The benefit of prophylactic anti-inflammatory agents in preventing development of later constriction in patients with chronic effusions is not known.

Chronic constrictive pericarditis is a more serious consequence of radiation therapy. Constriction with ("effusive-constrictive pericarditis") or without effusions is associated not only with a significantly higher incidence of morbidity than is effusion alone, but also requires more invasive and aggressive therapy than does effusion alone. As with chronic radiation-induced pericardial effusions, the temporal relationship of the clinical presentation to irradiation may be relatively early (less than 48 months) or late. Cohn reported six patients with chronic effusion-constrictive pericarditis, all presenting within 36 months of completion of radiation therapy.[29] Each of these patients demonstrated evidence of antecedent transient pericardial disease prior to the diagnosis of constriction (acute pericarditis in four and uncomplicated pericardial effusions in two). Applefeld reported a study of nine patients, a subset of 81 patients who received radiation therapy for Hodgkin's disease, who manifested constrictive pericarditis 53 to 124 months (mean 88 months) after irradiation.[34] Seven of these patients had prior documentation of pericardial effusions. Four had uncomplicated effusions 6 to 120 months after irradiation and three had pericardial effusions progressing to cardiac tamponade 12 to 79 months after irradiation. Four patients underwent anterior pericardiectomy for incapacitating dyspnea or refractory hepatomegaly. Two patients manifested excellent symptomatic relief; one patient with initial therapeutic amelioration of symptoms died 3 months after operation from chemotherapy-induced granulocytopenia and progressive Hodgkin's disease; one patient did not achieve symptomatic relief from pericardiectomy, apparently because of intractable visceral pericardial constriction. Because this series included only those patients referred for cardiac evaluation, the actual prevalence of late radiation-induced constrictive pericarditis may be greater than the 11% (9/81) suggested by this report. These studies suggest that the syndrome of chronic radiation-induced constrictive pericarditis is frequently preceded by other pericardial pathologic processes. Because as previously noted, however, chronic pericardial effusions are commonly asymptomatic and unrecognized; the true frequency of progression to constriction is not clear.

The clinical manifestations of chronic pericardial disease resulting from therapeutic mediastinal irradiation constitute a spectrum ranging from asymptomatic effusions to severely debilitating dyspnea and edema. This range is directly related to the variability in pathologic processes discussed above. Thus, while accumulation of pericardial fluid within the pericardial sac eventually may increase intrapericardial pressure sufficiently to produce cardiac compression, the development of such significantly increased intrapericardial pressure depends on the absolute volume of pericardial fluid, the rate of accumulation of fluid, and the physical characteristics of the pericardium itself. If fluid is accumulated slowly, the normal pericardium can alter its compliance to accommodate 1 to 2 L without an untoward increase in intrapericardial pressure. If the fluid is produced rapidly, however, the normal pericardial sac will accommodate only 80 to 200 ml before an increase in intrapericardial pressure develops. Moreover, fibrosis or infiltration of the pericardium diminishes pericardial compliance and increases the incremental pressure resulting from additional fluid accumulation. While intrapericardial pressure normally is similar to intrapleural pressure and lower than intracardiac pressures, fluid can accumulate in the pericardial sac sufficiently to increase intrapericardial pressure to the level of the right atrial and right ventricular end diastolic pressures. At that point, the transmural pressure gradient across the right heart is virtually obliterated, and limitation of right ventricular filling occurs. Further increase in fluid accumulation raises not only the intrapericardial pressure, but also the right ventricular end diastolic pressure and eventually the left ventricular end diastolic pressure to the point that left ventricular filling is impaired and systemic blood pressure falls (cardiac tamponade). While such accumulation is readily reversible with pericardiocentesis, pericardial fibrosis, with loss of compliance, is relatively irreversible. As fibrosis progresses, the pericardium acts as an inflexible limit to cardiac filling and expansion, necessarily limiting cardiac output reserve and ultimately even resting cardiac output (constrictive pericarditis). The two processes may be distinguished by the pattern of atrial emptying and ventricular filling noted at catheterization. However, when both pericardial effusion and pericardial fibrosis and thickening occur together, as in effusive-constrictive pericarditis, it may be difficult to distinguish the relative importance of these two processes without removing the pericardial fluid.

With either form of chronic pericarditis, increased systemic venous pressure, pulmonary vascular pressure, and decreased systemic blood pressure produce the signs and symptoms observed by the clinician in patients with chronic pericardial disease. The clinical presentation of patients with chronic radiation-induced pericardial disease is the same as that produced by pericardial effusion or constriction of any etiology. Dyspnea is clearly the most common presenting complaint. However, it is frequently attributed to other noncardiac causes such as mediastinal or pulmonary fibrosis, obesity, or sedentary lifestyle.[6] Fever and chest pain occur less frequently than noted in cases of acute pericarditis. Physical findings, if present, are similar to those described earlier with cardiac tamponade. Chest roentgenography and particularly echocardiography are invaluable in the evaluation of chronic pericardial disease. Of note is the usual absence of pericardial calcification found in other forms of constrictive pericarditis. The definitive diagnosis of tamponade and constriction depends on the demonstration of equalization of diastolic pressures among all cardiac chambers on cardiac catheterization.

The therapeutic approach to radiation-induced pericardial disease depends on the clinical status and the pathophysiologic process. In light of the high incidence of spontaneous resolution, patients with asymptomatic uncomplicated pericardial effusions after radiation generally do not require intervention other than frequent clinical and echocardiographic or roentgenographic monitoring. In patients with acute pericarditis and chest pain, anti-inflammatory agents such as aspirin or indomethacin provide symptomatic relief. Patients with hemodynamic compromise from pericardial fluid, or a combination of fluid and constriction, require more invasive measures. Percutaneous pericardiocentesis with a cannula allows rapid drainage of pericardial fluid and significant hemodynamic and symptomatic improvement in patients with cardiac tamponade. Since the fluid in radiation-induced effusions may be quite viscous, however, some investigators advocate a procedure consisting of a small subxiphoid incision with visualization of the pericardium and insertion of a large catheter. Alternatively, a pericardial window may be created through a thoracotomy, allowing drainage of the intrapericardial fluid into the pleural space, with subsequent resorption. In some cases, the improvement is only temporary and the effusion recurs once the catheter is removed or the window closes. The treatment for constrictive pericarditis and refractory pericardial effusions is removal of the pericardium. Pericardiectomy requires median sternotomy, cardiopulmonary bypass, and a long postoperative convalescence period with considerable incisional pain. It is generally recommended that this procedure be reserved for patients with disabling symptoms or refractory hepatomegaly,[6,34] although some recommend pericardiectomy solely on the basis of persistent effusions or hemodynamic evidence of constriction.[36,37]

Radiation-Induced Cardiomyopathy

Although pericardial injury is the most frequently encountered cardiovascular complication of therapeutic radiation, the occurrence of myocardial damage is becoming more frequently recognized. As with pericardial disease, the increasing recognition of radiation-induced myocardial disease is facilitated by the availability of noninvasive diagnostic techniques, such as echocardiography and radionuclide cineangiography. Several mechanisms have been proposed that may contribute to the development of radiation cardiomyopathy. These include vascular and microvascular insufficiency, degradation of DNA and disturbance of RNA transcription in myocytes, interstitial cell damage, neural damage, depletion of endogenous catecholamines, and autoimmune response to radiation-induced alteration in tissue antigens. Several lines of evidence suggest, however, that microvascular disruption leading to myocardial fibrosis is the predominant process resulting in radiation-induced cardiomyopathy. As will be discussed, ischemia from large epicardial vessel narrowing may also contribute to myocardial pathology.

Histologic evidence, obtained from surgical and autopsy specimens and experimental studies, has suggested that the blood capillaries are the primary myocardial structures affected by irradiation. Fajardo and Stewart studied the myocardial alterations observed by light and electron microscopy and radioautography and tritiated thymidine in rabbits irradiated with a single dose of 2000 cGy (Figure 12–1).[14] Light microscopy identified three phases in the morphologic evolution of radiation-induced myocardial alterations. The acute stage was characterized by an exudate of segmented heterophils (the rabbit granulocyte) in all layers of the heart occurring between 6 and 48 hours after irradiation. The latent stage was identified by the absence of any significant lesions by light microscopy during the period of 2 to 70 days after irradiation. The late stage was characterized by progressive myocardial fibrosis without significant inflammation. Collagen bands of variable thickness could be identified surrounding individual myocytes or groups of myocytes. On the other hand, the important ultrastructural manifestations of irradiation were especially prominent and severe during the latent stage. During this period, minimal myocyte alterations were observed; rather, the major ultrastructural changes were observed in the endothelial cells of the blood capillaries. Focal endothelial cytoplasmic degeneration occurred, which became more generalized, eventually causing capillary lumen obliteration by endothelial cytoplasm swelling, thrombosis, or rupture of the capillary walls, despite apparent recruitment of regenerative processes. The peak capillary damage occurred between 20 and 70 days after irradiation. This process results in a relatively diminished capillary bed, insufficient microcirculation, and diffuse myocardial ischemia. Ultimately, the diffuse fibrosis, seen during the late stage, develops.

These morphologic alterations seen in the rabbit model are identical to changes observed at necropsy in patients who have ra-

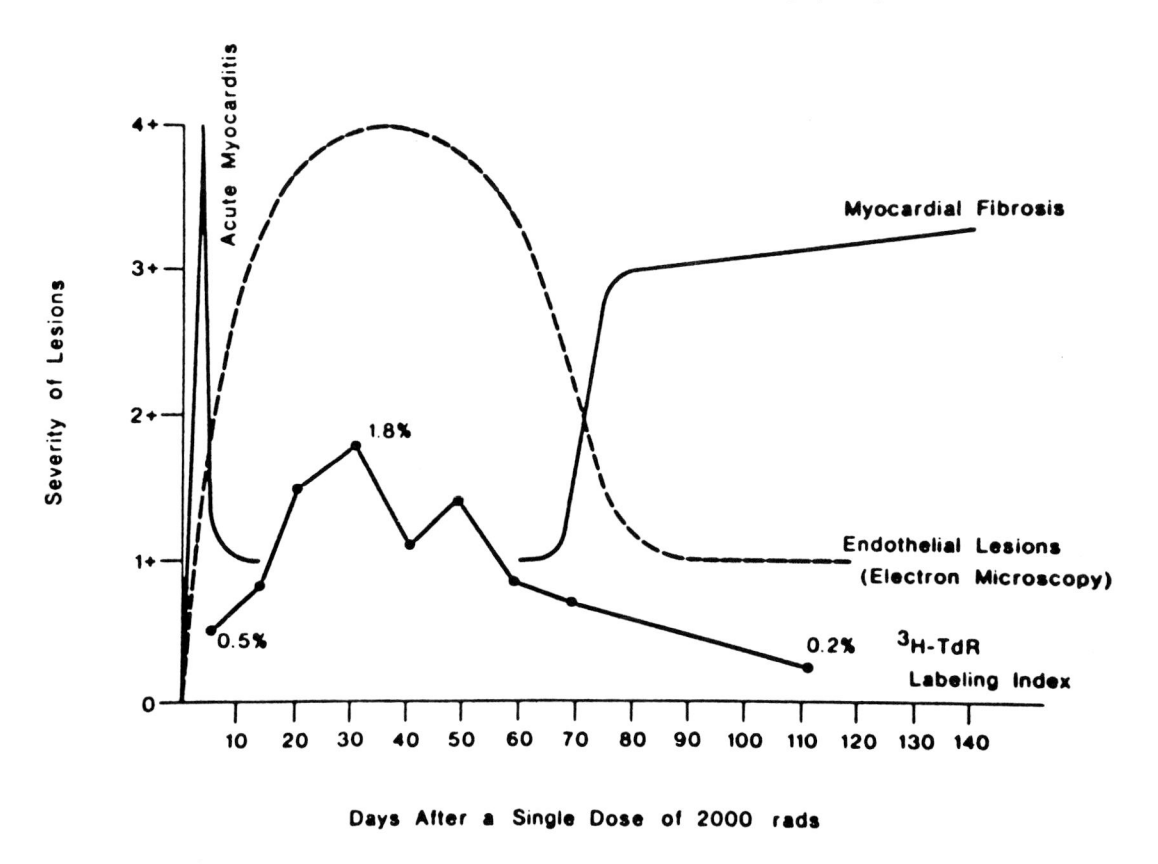

Fig. 12–1. Myocardial alterations observed by light and microscopy and radioautography of tritiated thymidine in rabbits irradiated with 2000 cGy. (From Fajardo, L.F. and Stewart, Jr. Pathogenesis of radiation-induced myocardial fibrosis. Lab. Invest. 29:244, 1973.)

diation-induced heart disease. Stewart[28] and Fajardo[38] described diffuse interstitial fibrosis as the predominant myocardial lesion in their series of patients who received radiation therapy. The fibrosis may be so extensive that the myocardial fibers are separated singly. There may be swelling of the myocardial fibers with separation of the myofibrils and an increase in chromatin. Some cells have bizarre or multiple nuclei that may be vacuolated. Only one specimen revealed myocardial necrosis and this was in the patient with thrombosis of a major coronary artery. Brosius described the necropsy findings in 16 patients who had received greater than 3500 cGy to the heart.[39] Interstitial fibrosis occurred in the right ventricular free wall in eight patients, in the left ventricular free wall in three patients, and in the interventricular septum in two patients. Proliferation of fibrous tissue with some elastic fibers resulted in thickening of the mural endocardium of one or more chambers in 12 patients, right atrium in 8, right ventricle in 10, left ventricle in 3, and left atrium in none. These pathologic findings were more frequently observed and were more extensive in the right ventricle than in the left ventricle, presumably because of greater radiation doses to the anterior surface of the heart.

The clinical manifestations of radiation-induced cardiomyopathies are frequently subtle. Most reports of clinical and pathologic myocardial lesions in patients undergoing radiotherapy are limited to the late fibrotic stage described earlier. Acute myocardial damage has been observed following radiation accidents or atomic warfare. However, the acute myocardial inflammation that results is thought to be less significant than the associated vascular lesions. Recent reports have indicated that the late fibrotic myocardial injury may be considerably more frequent and clinically significant than previous estimations had suggested. Burns evaluated 21 asymptomatic patients with rest and stress radionuclide cineangiography 7 to 20 years after receiving mediastinal radiotherapy (2000 to 7600 cGy) for Hodgkin's disease.[40] Abnormal left or right ventricular ejection fractions at rest or exercise, were identified in 57% of these patients. Gomez evaluated 55 patients with first-pass left ventricular ejection fractions 30 to 120 months after mediastinal irradiation for Hodgkin's disease.[41] Of these patients, all of whom were without any clinical signs of cardiovascular disease, 51% had reduced left ventricular ejection fractions at rest. Brosius has provided pathologic evidence supporting these clinical studies.[39] He reported the necropsy findings in 16 young (15 to 33 years) patients who received greater than 3500 cGy to the heart 5 to 144 months before death. None of these patients had clinical evidence of heart failure. In this series 8 of the 16 patients had evidence of myocardial fibrosis, especially in the right ventricle, and 12 had mural endocardial thickening.

The clinical manifestations of myocardial disease resulting from therapeutic mediastinal irradiation constitutes a spectrum from asymptomatic ventricular dysfunction to severe limitation of exercise tolerance with dyspnea and edema. The pathologic and hemodynamic processes exhibited by patients with radiation-induced myocardial disease are characteristic of the functional class of cardiomyopathies labeled restrictive. The major pathophysiologic manifestation of restrictive cardiomyopathy is subnormal diastolic function. The interstitial myocardial fibrosis results in relative ventricular wall stiffening with loss of compliance. Thus, as in constrictive pericarditis, ventricular filling is limited by the inability of the ventricle to dilate. The rigid nature of the ventricles results in elevated ventricular filling pressures and therefore increased systemic and pulmonary venous pressures. Contractile function of the ventricles is relatively spared, with preservation of normal or near normal ventricular ejection fractions. The impairment to ventricular filling and the resulting elevated systemic venous pressure and pulmonary vascular pressure produce the signs and symptoms observed by the clinician in patients with radiation-induced restrictive cardiomyopathy.

The clinical presentation of patients with myocardial disease after irradiation can be similar to the clinical features of chronic constrictive pericarditis. Dyspnea with orthopnea and paroxysmal nocturnal dyspnea may be present. Exercise intolerance also is common because of the inability of patients to increase their cardiac output by tachycardia without further limiting ventricular filling. Physical examination may reveal elevated jugular venous pressure, an S3 or S4 gallop, and, occasionally, systolic murmurs of atrioventricular valvular regurgitation. An inspiratory increase in jugular venous pressure (Kussmaul's sign) may be present. Peripheral edema with hepatomegaly, ascites, or anasarca may be observed in advanced cases. In contrast to constrictive pericarditis, the apical impulse usually is readily palpable. Recent evidence suggests that many patients with histologic evidence of myocardial disease do not have any important physical or symptomatic limitations many years after treatment with radiation; consequently, the recognition and diagnosis of radiation-induced cardiomyopathy depends on noninvasive and invasive laboratory evaluation. Chest roentgenography may demonstrate a decrease in transverse heart diameter and cardiothoracic ratio. Echocardiography (Figure 12–2) may reveal a subnormal left ventricular end-diastolic dimension, with variable degree of thinning of the ventricular walls.[33] Left atrial dimension may be decreased or increased. A decrease in mitral-valve-closure velocity suggests abnormal left ventricular pressure-volume relations. Left ventricular fractional shortening may be reduced. Radionuclide cineangiography (Figure 12–3) may reveal significant ventricular performance abnormalities at rest or, particularly, with exercise. Both Gottdiener[33] and Burns[40] have demonstrated subnormal left ventricular ejection fraction in patients treated with mediastinal radiation when compared to normal subjects. This is particularly evident when the functional reserve is compared in terms of left ventricular ejection fraction response during exercise. Burns also noted that there is often selective impairment of the right ventricle, which may be attributed to its relative proximity to the anterior chest wall. The definitive diagnosis of cardiomyopathy resulting from mediastinal radiation rests on specific hemodynamic observations from cardiac catheterization and on the demonstration of characteristic pathologic findings on examination of myocardial tissue. The role of endomyocardial biopsy in the diagnosis and determination of prognosis in radiation-induced myocardial disease remains to be investigated.

The clinical and hemodynamic features of both radiation-induced cardiomyopathy and constrictive pericarditis result from the limitation of filling of the ventricles and consequently may be difficult to distinguish. However, the differentiation between constrictive and restrictive physiology in a clinically deteriorating patient is essential in guiding further therapeutic approaches. If the patient has constrictive pericarditis, then pericardiotomy is likely to result in considerable relief of symptoms. If the patient has a restrictive cardiomyopathy, however, pericardial stripping exposes the patient to a dangerous and extensive procedure without significant potential for improvement. Several clinical features are useful in distinguishing myocardial from pericardial disease. An individual with restrictive myocardial disease is more likely to have associated impairment in left ventricular contractility and therefore may have a subnormal ejection fraction on radionuclide cineangiography or evidence of decreased systolic function on echocardiography. Right ventricular end-diastolic pressure is elevated, but it is usually less than one-third of the systolic pressure. Finally, endomyocardial biopsy may show interstitial myocardial fibrosis. Conversely, a patient with constrictive pericardial disease is more likely to have preserved systolic function on radionuclide cineangiography or echocardiography; right ventricular end-diastolic pressure greater than one-third of the systolic pressure; and, in pure constriction, the endomyocardial biopsy should be normal. Because both restrictive and constrictive cardiac diseases are relatively common complications of therapeutic mediastinal radiation, the concomitant occurrence of both processes is not unexpected. Separation of the relative contribution of each of the pathophysiologic processes may only be made after pericardiectomy and postoperative clinical and hemodynamic monitoring.

Coronary Artery Disease

Since 1957, a number of case reports have described accelerated coronary atherosclero-

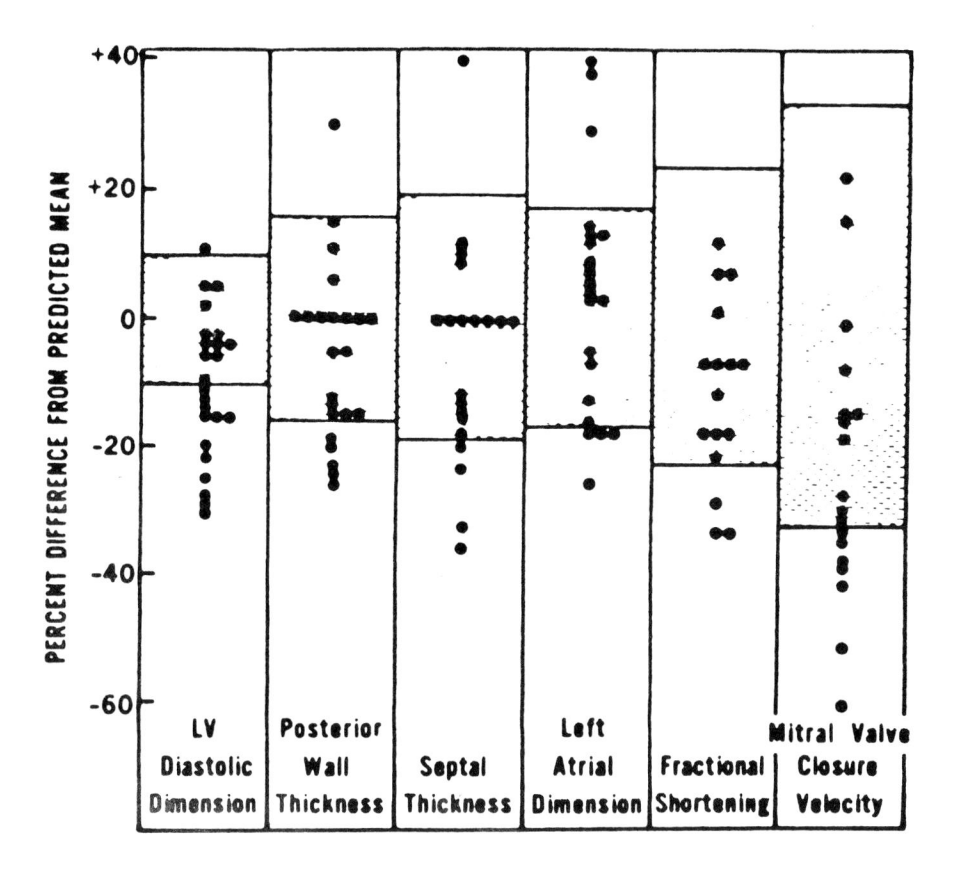

Fig. 12–2. Echocardiographic dimensions plotted as percentage differences from mean values predicted from body surface area. Stippled area represents the 95% predictive limits of normal values. Note the decreased left ventricular (LV) diastolic dimension in 12 of 24 patients (50%) and the decreased mitral-valve closure velocity in 7 of 18 patients (39%). Decreased left ventricular cavity size and abnormal left ventricular pressure-volume relations (suggested by decreased velocity of mitral closure) are consistent with left ventricular restriction. (From Gottdiener, J.S., Katin, M.J., Borer, J.S., Bacharach, S.L., and Green, M.V. Late cardiac effects of therapeutic mediastinal irradiation. N. Engl. J. Med. 308:567, 1983.)

sis after therapeutic mediastinal irradiation. Many of these reports are difficult to interpret because many patients were over the age of 40 or had evidence of other clinical, metabolic, or familial risk factors known to be related to the development of atherosclerosis. Investigators attempting to relate cancer and atherosclerotic coronary artery disease have suggested that the occurrence of coronary artery disease is less common in autopsied cancer patients than in noncancer hospitalized age- and sex-matched controls. However, another study that eliminated the bias resulting from the relatively high incidence of coronary artery disease in hospitalized patients failed to demonstrate this reduction in coronary artery disease, except in a few small subgroups.[42] Nonetheless, in one series of patients with Hodgkin's disease followed for 2 to 10 years after radiotherapy, only 1 of 377 patients developed a myocardial infarction.[43] In another series of similar patients followed for 6 years, only 1 of 467 individuals suffered a myocardial infarction.[44] Finally, Boivin and Hutchinson described 957 patients treated for Hodgkin's disease during the period from 1942 to 1975 with follow-up through 1977.[45] There were 25 deaths attributed to coronary heart disease. Fourteen of these deaths occurred in the 678 irradiated patients and 11 occurred in the 279 nonirradiated patients. Corrected for duration of follow-up, the coronary heart disease mortality of patients treated with mediastinal irradiation relative to those who did not receive radiation was 1.5 to 1. This estimate was considered suggestive, but not sig-

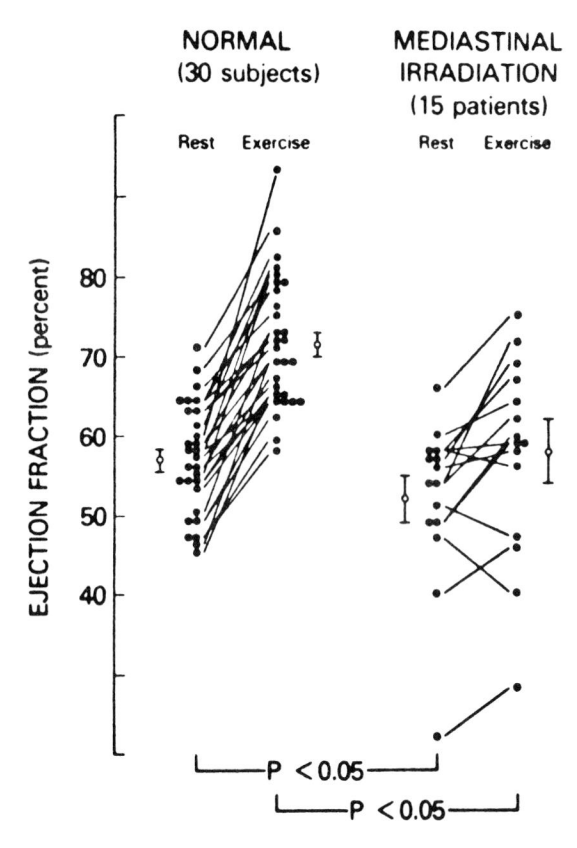

Fig. 12–3. Ejection fraction at rest and during exercise in 15 patients after mediastinal irradiation (right panel) and 30 normal subjects (left panel). The mean ejection fraction at rest of 52% in the patients was significantly lower than the value of 57% in the normal subjects. Although only 2 of 15 patients had resting ejection fractions that were below normal limits, 5 patients had decreased ejection fractions with exercise. (From Gottdiener, J.S., Katin, M.J., Borer, J.S., Bacharach, S.L. and Green, M.V. Late cardiac effects of therapeutic mediastinal irradiation. N. Engl. J. Med. 308:567, 1983.)

nificant, evidence that coronary heart disease mortality was increased after mediastinal radiation therapy for Hodgkin's disease. However, none of these studies evaluated either the incidence of angina or the autopsy incidence of coronary artery disease. In fact, the clinical incidence of ischemic heart disease in patients who have undergone radiation therapy for Hodgkin's disease is still undetermined. Moreover, reports of patients who have experienced myocardial infarctions, angina, positive stress tests, or electrocardiographic changes do not clearly demonstrate a causative role of radiation in inducing coronary artery disease because coincidental typical atherosclerotic coronary artery disease is not uncommon and distinguishing histologic features were not reported.[21–24,26,29,43,46–51]

Nonetheless, recent pathologic studies have provided strong evidence for the occurrence of radiation-induced coronary artery disease. McReynolds has described the necropsy findings in a 33-year-old patient who died suddenly after a presumed myocardial infarction.[23] Histologic examination of the coronary arteries revealed obstructive lesions atypical for usual atherosclerotic coronary disease. These was severe coronary adventitial fibrosis in continuity with overlying epicardial fibrous tissue and little lipid within the intimal lesions. In addition, a relatively large collection of plasma cells and fewer lymphocytes were present in the adventitia. In contrast, the usual pathologic findings in typical atherosclerotic coronary artery disease include a larger extracellular lipid content within the fibrotic plaque as well as many lymphocytes and few plasma cells. Brosius described the necropsy findings in 16 young (15 to 33 years) patients who received greater than 3500 cGy to the heart 5 to 144 months before death.[39] In these patients, 16 of the 64 major coronary arteries (left main, left anterior descending, left circumflex, and right) were narrowed by greater than 75% in cross-sectional area, primarily by fibrous plaques. In contrast, only one of the 40 major arteries in the 10 control subjects was similarly narrowed. The primary component of the atherosclerotic plaques in both groups of patients was fibrous tissue with little lipid. The study patients, however, had a remarkable loss of smooth muscle cells from the media and more adventitial fibrosis when compared to the control group. The proximal portions of the coronary arteries were more frequently involved in the irradiated patients. In this study, 40% of the patients who received radiation therapy had proliferation of fibrous tissue within the epicardial coronary arteries. It must be noted that a number of these patients received irradiation by techniques considered unacceptable by most radiation therapists today (anterior-only ports, tumor doses greater than 4000 cGy, two megavoltage radiation sources, and multiple courses of radiotherapy); therefore, the radiation effects described may be considerably diminished in severity or incidence in patients treated currently.

The occurrence and clinical importance of radiation-induced coronary artery obstruction continues to be a widely debated issue. Despite clinical and pathologic data supporting the existence of radiation-related coronary artery disease in humans, experimental models have generally failed to document that radiation alone can cause coronary-artery obstruction.[52-54] Studies in both New Zealand rabbits and Wistar rats have documented a synergistic effect of radiation, in combination with high fat diets, in producing coronary atherosclerosis of a greater degree than could be caused by diet alone. Total body or thoracic radiation, in the absence of an atherogenic diet, resulted in only a nonspecific coronary abnormality not thought to be of pathophysiologic importance. In addition, although atherosclerosis has been observed in irradiated systemic arteries, many reports are in patients who were at risk for spontaneous development of atherosclerotic changes. Finally, the occurrence of clinically important coronary-artery obstruction in several large studies is relatively infrequent considering the number of individuals at risk. On the other hand, considerable evidence supports the association between radiation and accelerated coronary atherosclerosis as a clinical entity. The premature occurrence of atherosclerotic changes has been reported in a number of individuals without the concomitant presence of other commonly accepted risk factors. Also, instances of advanced lesions limited to exposed coronary and noncoronary vessels with relatively minor lesions elsewhere have been reported. The most frequently described histologic changes in both experimental animal models and in man are atypical for spontaneous atherosclerosis. Finally, severe changes in the coronary arteries are commonly associated with characteristic radiation-induced pericardial and myocardial injuries.

The clinician caring for patients with Hodgkin's disease must be aware of the possibility of both radiation-induced and spontaneously occurring atherosclerosis, as well as other causes of myocardial infarction that may not be directly related to radiation therapy. In a patient presenting with a myocardial infarction or anginal syndrome, other possible mechanisms, such as marantic endocarditis with coronary emboli, tumor emboli, coronary ostial obstruction by tumor, and extrinsic compression of the coronary arteries by infiltrating tumor, must be considered. In addition, patients with pericardial or myocardial injury resulting from tumor, chemotherapy, and radiation may present with a clinical syndrome and electrocardiographic changes nearly indistinguishable from coronary artery occlusions. Echocardiography, radionuclide cineangiography, and cardiac catheterization with coronary angiography and endomyocardial biopsy supply helpful information in planning the therapeutic approach to patients with possible coronary artery disease. Not only will these examinations confirm or exclude the presence of coronary artery narrowing, but also they will establish the presence or absence of concomitant pericardial and myocardial disease, which may limit the utility of coronary artery bypass procedures or balloon dilatation.

Conduction System Disease

Conduction system disease is a rare complication of therapeutic radiation. Although atrial dysrhythmias, transient ST-T wave changes, and QRS complex changes simulating myocardial infarction may occur in patients with radiation-induced cardiomyopathy; documented cases of conduction system disease have been unusual. There have been five cases of complete heart block attributed to radiotherapy occurring 5 to 23 years after treatment and requiring pacemaker placement.[55-58] In the large Stanford series only one case of conduction system disease was reported: a 20-year-old patient developed significant myocardial fibrosis and a left bundle-branch block 11 years after receiving an estimated 4700 cGy to the heart.[29]

Radiotherapy can lead to conduction system disease by two different mechanisms. Diffuse myocardial fibrosis is a well-known complication of irradiation. This fibrotic process might easily extend to the conduction system. Cohen has clearly documented this with electrophysiologic and histopathologic examination of a 31-year-old individual with complete heart block 11 years after radiotherapy for Hodgkin's disease.[56] At autopsy, there was significant fibrosis of the conduction system leading to the atrioventricular node, as well as in the AV node, AV bundle, and right and left bundle branches. Coronary artery narrowing has also been described as a complication of radiotherapy. Limitation of the arterial supply to the sinus node, AV node, and conduction pathways may lead to ischemia or infarction and, consequently, may cause conduction system disease.

Electronic pacemaker implantation is the treatment of choice for clinically important conduction system defects. Walz examined the effects of direct radiation and scattered radiation on cardiac pacemaker function and discovered no clinically important alteration or inhibition of electronic pacemaker activity.[59] Case reports suggest, however, that the newer, more advanced, programmable pacemakers (AV sequential) using complementary metal oxide semiconductor circuitry may be more susceptible to radiation-induced malfunction.[60]

Valvular Disease

The occurrence of valvular heart disease after radiotherapy is extremely infrequent and rarely clinically important. In fact, there are only 16 reported cases of valvular injury after irradiation; 13 of these were incidental findings at autopsy. In Brosius' review of the necropsy findings of 16 young patients examined after greater than 3500 cGy to the heart 5 to 144 months before death, 13 patients had one or more cardiac valves thickened by fibrous tissue: tricuspid in eight, pulmonic in two, mitral in thirteen, an aortic valve in eight.[39] The thickening in all patients was noted to be relatively mild and not sufficiently severe to produce clinically evident valvular dysfunction. Morton and associates have reported two patients with aortic regurgitation at the time of cardiac catheterization after pericardial stripping.[36] Neither patient had a history of heart disease prior to radiation therapy for Hodgkin's disease, nor were heart murmurs noted prior to radiation or at the time of catheterization before the pericardial surgery. Cohn reported a case of a 20-year-old youth who developed mitral regurgitation and a left bundle-branch block after large doses of mediastinal therapy for a round-cell tumor of the left thorax.[29] He had pansystolic and short diastolic apical murmurs on physical examination and findings suggestive of mitral regurgitation on cardiac catheterization. The authors concluded that radiation fibrosis was the cause of both the conduction system defect and papillary muscle dysfunction, resulting in mitral regurgitation. Because no autopsy examination was performed, however, mitral valve fibrosis and dilated congestive cardiomyopathy cannot be excluded as possible causes for mitral regurgitation.

Peripheral Vascular Disease

A number of cases of peripheral vascular damage have been reported since 1899, when Gassmann found arterial changes in the skin of irradiated fields leading to intractable ulcers.[1] Fibrosis, inflammation, focal atherosclerosis, narrowing, occlusion, thrombosis, necrosis, and rupture of large vessels (such as the aorta, carotid, subclavian, and femoral arteries) have been attributed to radiation therapy.[61-66] The latent period between radiation and clinical presentation may vary from several months to more than 35 years. Rotman reported a 38-year-old woman who died after an attempted surgical repair of occlusions of the ascending aorta, arch, and brachiocephalic arteries occurring 36 years after radiation for tonsillitis.[67] Atheromatous changes and plaque formation occurred in the aorta and calcification of the branches of the aortic arch. Atherosclerotic changes occurred only within the field of irradiation. Heidenburg and associates reported a 21-year-old woman with Hodgkin's disease who developed "pulseless disease" 10 years after mediastinal radiation.[64] Histologic examination of both subclavian arteries revealed dense subintimal and intraluminal fibrosis. Hyalinization of the musculature of the vessel walls and thickening and fragmentation of the elastic membrane occurred. Conomy and Kellermeyer have reported the autopsy findings in a 27-year-old woman who presented with a devastating stroke 8 months after receiving 7200 cGy to the cervical area (over a 19 month period) for Hodgkin's disease.[63] Postmortem examination revealed unilateral thrombotic occlusion of the internal carotid artery with medial thickening, fibroblastic proliferation, and focal elastic membrane degeneration.

Experimental radiation in animal models has produced arteriosclerotic changes similar to the reported clinical findings in man. Lindsay et al. produced arteriosclerotic changes in irradiated segments of canine aortas after single doses up to 5500 cGy.[68] Fragmentation and reduplication of the internal elastic membrane and intimal thickening with deposition of collagen, mucopolysaccharide, and elastic tissue were noted in the irradiated segments.

SUMMARY

Recent evidence indicates that any part of the cardiovascular system can be subject to radiation injury. The relatively long cell-cycle time of the constituents of the cardiovascular system apparently is the primary reason why cardiac and vascular complications of radiation often do not manifest until years after therapy. Bloomer and Hellman have emphasized cell-cycle time, as well as the radiotherapy techniques, as important factors in determining the toxic effects of radiation on normal tissues.[69] Acute radiation reactions are produced by the reduction of actively proliferating cells, a function of dose rate and time-dose fractionation features rather than the total dose applied. Because of the long cell-cycle time of cardiac tissues, acute radiation effects are generally not observed in the cardiovascular system. Intermediate radiation reactions are caused by injury to cells of a slowly proliferating cell renewal system, such as endothelium or connective tissue. These intermediate effects are a function of both time-dose fractionation and the total dose applied and occur shortly after radiation. Radiation-induced pericarditis is the most common cardiac manifestation of this reaction. Late radiation reactions are postulated to be the result of injury to the endothelial cell system or alteration of the structural integrity of cellular macromolecules. These late effects are a function of the total dose administered to the cardiovascular system and may occur months to years after radiation. The manifestation of late sequellae are tissue fibrosis and necrosis. Myocardial fibrosis, constrictive pericarditis, and possibly accelerated atherosclerosis are the cardiovascular effects of late radiation reactions. This delay has become increasingly important as treatment for Hodgkin's disease has led to long disease-free intervals. The clinician must be aware of the consequences of radiation in distinguishing between recurrent disease and radiation injury.

The relationship of radiation dose to the occurrence of cardiovascular complications is not yet clearly defined. Investigators at Stanford[28] and at Massachusetts General Hospital[69] have reported evidence that cardiac complications increase with increasing total radiation dose and fractionation size. They suggest that administration of a total dose of 3500 to 4000 cGy to a large portion of the heart results in a dramatic increase in the incidence of pericardial disease. In addition, these authors believe that delivery of daily increments of more than 200 cGy results in important cardiac injury. On the other hand, researchers from the Baltimore Cancer Research Center did not demonstrate a significant increase in the incidence of cardiac complications with increasing applied radiation doses. Ruckdeschel[16] and Byhardt and associates[30] found that more frequent cardiac injury was associated with clinical factors unrelated to the quantitative aspects of radiation: elevated erythrocyte sedimentation rate, normal or increased lymphocyte count, extent of mediastinal tumor mass, and subsequent chemotherapy. They suggested that an autoimmune response to altered normal tissue antigens, sclerosis of cardiac lymphatic channels, or intercurrent viral infections may be important contributing factors. Clearly, numerous variables may determine the response of the cardiovascular system to radiation. The total administered dose, dose rate, amount of heart volume included in the irradiated field, and concomitant chemotherapy,[135] as well as extent of mediastinal tumor and immune status, are likely to be significant contributing factors to the development of radiation-induced cardiac disease.

The best management for radiation-induced cardiac damage is prevention. Recent modifications in the techniques of therapeutic irradiation, including shielding of the heart after 3500 cGy, shrinking fields, multiple portals, and irradiation through both anterior and posterior fields, may be expected to decrease the incidence and severity of cardiac injury after radiotherapy. Other approaches have aimed to reduce the response of normal tissues to the effects of radiation. Reeves et al. demonstrated that the early administration of methylprednisolone or ibuprofen in the experimental rabbit model improves survival, decreases the incidence of pericarditis and pericardial effusions, and reduces myocardial fibrosis after irradiation.[70] The administration of anti-inflammatory agents, as well as decreasing blood lipid levels, has not yet been examined in the clinical setting.

The current availability of powerful noninvasive cardiac diagnostic modalities, including echocardiography and radionuclide ventriculography, makes it possible to characterize cardiac anatomy and function before radiation therapy and to monitor changes that may occur during and after treatment. This allows careful study of the effects of radiation, the course of radiation-induced injury, and the prevention of complications to the cardiovascular system.

ADVERSE CARDIOVASCULAR EFFECTS OF CHEMOTHERAPY

DOXORUBICIN (ADRIAMYCIN)

Cardiotoxicity is a unique effect of the anthracycline chemotherapeutic agents. This toxic effect has clearly limited the total dose that can be safely administered in the treatment of Hodgkin's disease. The clinical success in treating Hodgkin's lymphoma with doxorubicin in conjunction with other chemotherapeutic agents and physical modalities has made the cardiac toxic effects an important problem, both in the limitation of doxorubicin administration and the late development of congestive cardiomyopathy in patients who have received curative or palliative chemotherapy. The underlying mechanism by which doxorubicin produces cardiac injury, as well as the interventions required to limit the cardiac effects, have not been sufficiently elucidated to provide clinical benefit. Recent investigations have identified a threshold dose below which the development of clinically detectable cardiac toxicity is rare. The search continues for reliable techniques to identify those individuals at risk for the development of particularly significant cardiotoxicity and to permit recognition of the earliest preclinical manifestations of cardiac disease. Identification of these characteristics allows individualization of doxorubicin treatment protocols so that potential curative chemotherapy may be continued in those patients not immediately at risk for the development of doxorubicin cardiotoxicity.

A number of cytotoxic mechanisms have been suggested as accountable for the antitumor and cardiotoxic effects of doxorubicin. Doxorubicin is known to bind DNA and may stimulate free-radical formation, affect cell membranes, and promote the release of vasoactive substances. Intercalation of anthracycline chemotherapeutic agents into DNA blocks the synthesis of DNA, RNA, and protein, causes fragmentation of DNA, and inhibits DNA repair. Clearly, intercalation into DNA may result in significant antitumor effects. However, it is unlikely to result in damage to the nondividing cell population found in myocardial tissue.

It has been demonstrated that doxorubicin binds to cell membranes and alters membrane function at or below the concentrations that affect DNA function. Although all membrane binding sites have not been identified, doxorubicin has been shown to bind to spectrin and cardiolipin. The binding to cardiolipin is of particular interest, since cardiolipin content is relatively high in membranes of both malignant cells and cardiac mitochondria, prompting Tritton to propose that this common membrane characteristic is responsible for both antineoplastic and cardiotoxic effects.[71] In addition, increased sodium permeability[72] and altered calcium metabolism in guinea-pig atria[73] and chick hearts[74] have been reported; these may provide an explanation for the altered sodium and calcium concentrations observed in cardiac tissue with the development of chronic cardiomyopathy.[75]

Bristow and colleagues have speculated that a cascade of vasoactive-substance release is responsible for the cardiac effects of doxorubicin.[76] In animal models of the acute effects of the drug, doxorubicin causes release of cardiac histamine, which subsequently causes catecholamine release and then increased prostaglandin synthesis; all these agents are vasoactive. In addition, doxorubicin-induced myocarditis is identical to histamine-induced myocarditis in other animal models; when these animals were pretreated with antihistamines and adrenergic blockade, doxorubicin caused no detectable acute cardiac effects. There was also a significant amelioration of chronic doxorubicin cardiomyopathy in rabbits treated with antihistamines and adrenergic blockers, suggesting that an association between the acute and chronic effects exists. Cromolyn sodium also limited the subacute cardiotoxic effects when given to rabbits before the administration of doxorubicin. Therefore, Bristow has postulated that the acute, subacute, and chronic cardiotoxic effects of doxorubicin are related to cardiac histamine release, resulting in cardiac effects similar to those produced by adrenergic substances.

Finally, Sato and co-workers first noted the ability of anthracyclines to trigger formation of oxygen radicals.[77–79] He and his associates demonstrated that the microsomal enzyme P450 reductase was able to catalyze the reduction of doxorubicin to a semiquinone free radical, which rapidly reduced molecular oxygen to the superoxide ion. Myers demonstrated that a free radical scavenger, alpha-tocopherol, ameliorated the cardiac injury from the administration of doxorubicin, providing the first evidence that free radical reactions might be the mechanism of action of the anthracyclines.[80] Since then, the ability of free radical scavengers to limit the acute myocardial damage has been confirmed in a number of animal models.[81–83] However, the utility of these agents in limiting the more chronic effects leading to cardiomyopathy has not been well established.[84] Further support for the cardiotoxic mechanism of superoxide-radical generation is provided by the identification of two processes accounting for the cardioselective nature of free-radical generation. First, mitochondria, which are known to be sites of doxorubicin-induced free radical generation, are present in large numbers in myocardial tissue. In addition, cardiac mitochondria have an unusually active electron-transport chain. Therefore, cardiac mitochondria may provide a particularly fertile source of doxorubicin-induced free radical stimulation. Second, cardiac tissue defends itself from oxygen radical damage by enzymatic mechanisms, which are different from other mammalian cells. Myers and associates have compared the detoxification process of free radicals in the cardiac tissue and in the liver of the mouse model.[85,86] Cardiac defense against free radicals depends primarily on superoxide dismutase and cytosolic glutathione peroxidase. Doxorubicin administration results in a rapid decrease in cardiac glutathione peroxidase, followed by a gradual restoration over 3 to 4 days. The administration of reduced glutathione to mice treated with doxorubicin protects against the characteristic early histologic changes associated with doxorubicin cardiotoxicity.[87] Thus, doxorubicin not only stimulates free-radical production in cardiac tissue, but also limits the ability of myocardial cells to metabolize the toxic-free radicals. A similar decrease in liver glutathione peroxidase levels was not observed.

The pathologic examination of cardiac tissue from both animal models and patients has identified characteristic changes.[76,88,89] The only morphologic change observed shortly after the administration of doxorubicin is the development of nucleolar segregation. The clinical significance of this nuclear change is unclear because it is reversed within 14 hours. Chronic morphologic changes consist of cardiac dilatation and mural thrombosis, degeneration and atrophy of cardiac muscle cells, and interstitial edema and fibrosis. The degeneration of cardiac myocytes appears to be the result of two forms of injury. The first type is characterized by myofibrillar loss apparent on light microscopy. The second type is characterized by cytoplasmic vacuolization usually associated with myofibrillar loss. The variable response of cardiac muscle cells to the same toxic stimulus remains unexplained. These pathologic changes appear to be related to the total cumulative dose and to the time interval between doses. Thus, in the mouse model, these lesions occur within 24 hours after the administration of a single large dose of doxorubicin;[89] however, these lesions are observed only after weeks or months following the administration of smaller repeated doses. Early morphologic changes are focal, becoming more diffuse as the toxic effects progress. Electron microscopic evidence has revealed that the degeneration of cardiac myocytes in chronic doxorubicin cardiomyopathy is a complex process involving the myofibrils, the nuclei, the membrane systems of the T-tubules, the sarcoplasmic reticulum and intercellular junctions, and the mitochondria. To allow quantitative estimates and thus more meaningful clinical and pathologic investigations, Billingham has developed a grading system based on the percentage of cells in a specimen exhibiting myofibrillar loss.[88]

With the aid of noninvasive and invasive assessments of cardiac structure and function, the natural history of the development of cardiac toxicity from doxorubicin has been elucidated. The clinical manifestations of cardiotoxicity may be divided into acute and chronic presentations. The acute toxicity appears to have two aspects. Disturbances in rhythm or conduction are relatively common after the administration of anthracyclines and are usually limited to sinus and supraventricular tachycardias or ventricular premature complexes.[90,91] Generally, these arrhythmias are not clinically important. However, complete heart block, ventricular tachycardia, and sudden death have been reported.[90] Neither the occurrence nor the severity of these arrhythmias has any relationship to the subsequent development of chronic cardiomyopathy.[91] The other acute toxic effect, the myocarditis-pericarditis presentation, is relatively rare.[92] The most severe expression of this form is characterized by the sudden onset of congestive heart failure, which is associated with pericardial effusions and diffuse myocardial injury. These cardiac effects may result in death, progress to chronic cardiac dysfunction, or completely resolve. Singer[93] has reported an acute toxicity manifested by a reduction in left ventricular ejection fraction observable between 24 and 72 hours after administration of greater than 60 mg/M^2. The drop in left ventricular function was at least partially reversed by 72 to 96 hours. Necropsy evaluation of several cases has revealed active myocardial inflammation as well as the characteristic anthracycline-induced myocyte degeneration.[92,94,95] The relation between this transient drop in left ventricular function or acute myopericardial inflammation and the subsequent development of chronic cardiac dysfunction remains unclear.

The chronic toxic effects of anthracyclines result in the most important adverse clinical syndrome associated with these agents. Patients may present with rapidly progressive biventricular congestive heart failure following the insidious onset of symptoms weeks to months after administration of the last dose of doxorubicin. The occurrence of symptomatic congestive heart failure secondary to anthracycline cardiomyopathy is associated with a 50 to 60% early mortality. The incidence of clinically apparent congestive heart failure in patients treated with anthracyclines clearly depend on the total cumulative dose administered. In 1973, Lefrak[90] suggested limitation of the total dose of doxorubicin to less than 550 mg/M^2 based on the incidence of ventricular failure of 0.27% in patients receiving less than 550 mg/M^2 and 30% in patients receiving greater than 550 mg/M^2. Recent evidence using invasive and noninvasive assessments of cardiac function and structure suggest that chronic cardiac toxicity occurs more frequently and at lower doses than had been appreciated earlier. Whereas only 1 to 2% of patients have overt evidence of congestive heart failure at a dose of 550 mg/M^2, more than 50% of asymptomatic patients have physiologic or pathologic evidence of cardiac damage.[96,97]

The detection of cardiac injury by doxorubicin may be accomplished by a number of noninvasive and invasive techniques. Some methods are relatively insensitive and nonspecific but are readily available. Others are more sensitive, but require special equipment. Others are reported to be sensitive and specific, but are available only in a few centers.

Electrocardiography, a universally obtainable modality, revealed a 30% decrease in limb lead QRS voltage associated with the development of congestive cardiomyopathy in one study.[98] Many investigators believe, however, that the identification of decreased voltage occurs too late to be used as an indicator of the need to stop therapy to prevent irreversible damage. Serial assessment of left ventricular function by noninvasively determined systolic time intervals (as from external pulse recording) permits detection of transient and permanent time interval abnormalities that correlate with increasing doses of administered doxorubicin. In assessments employing this approach, however, predictive value in identifying patients at risk of developing congestive heart failure was limited.[99,100]

More direct serial assessment of left ventricular function by echocardiography or by rest and exercise radionuclide cineangiography provides a more useful and accurate noninvasive estimate of myocardial damage with doxorubicin therapy. However, echocardiographic evaluation of left ventricular systolic function, obtainable in only 60% of the patients studied in one investigation, has also been associated with some limitation in predictability of clinical deterioration.[101] Left ventricular ejection fraction measurement by radionuclide cineangiography has provided more encouraging data, and appears to permit reliable identification of patients with toxic effects of doxorubicin therapy prior to the clinical development of congestive heart failure.

In a study of 55 patients receiving doxorubicin therapy, Alexander[102] retrospectively documented dramatic decreases in left ventricular ejection fraction at rest, to clearly subnormal values in studies that immediately preceded the administration of the doxorubicin dose, which appeared to be directly associated with clinical decompensation in all five patients who subsequently developed congestive heart failure. A therapy administration scheme based on this finding was then applied prospectively to the remainder of the study group: doxorubicin therapy was terminated when a patient manifested moderate reduction in left ventricular function (defined as a decrease in ejection fraction of greater than or equal to 15% from baseline to a final level of less than or equal to 45%, the pre-failure indicator in the observational study). When his algorithm was applied, none of the patients in whom moderate dysfunction occurred progressed to develop severe cardiotoxicity with congestive heart failure. In addition, no further deterioration in ejection fraction was observed in these patients over the next 1 to 4 months; the persistent mild decrease in left ventricular function was not predictive of later cardiac decompensation. These investigators concluded that serial assessment of left ventricular function by radionuclide ventriculography permitted noninvasive identification of those individuals at risk for the development of congestive heart failure so that appropriate timing of doxorubicin termination could be accomplished. Furthermore, this method allowed the identification (and continued monitoring) of patients who were not particularly sensitive to doxorubicin, and who could tolerate cumulative doses far in excess of 550 mg/m^2; thus, they could receive high-dose chemotherapy if clinically indicated. The clinical utility of monitoring left ventricular systolic function as an aid in the decision to continue or terminate doxorubicin therapy has recently been confirmed by the retrospective study of 282 high-risk patients by Schwartz.[103] In a study of 32 patients, Gottdiener[97] and associates, using rest and exercise radionuclide cineangiography, similarly demonstrated that clinically evident cardiomyopathy did not occur after the development of only moderate left ventricular dysfunction at the termination of therapy with 550 mg/M^2. Among 32 patients (Fig. 12–4) followed for as long as 43 months after completion of the doxorubicin regimen, left ventricular ejection fractions at rest were subnormal (less than 45%) in eight patients. An additional 12 patients with decreased left ventricular functional reserve were identified by exercise ventriculography. Sequential studies were performed in 13 patients 6 to 15 months after the initial evaluation (Fig. 12–5). Persistent depression of left ventricular ejection fraction at rest and with exercise was observed, and of note, findings suggestive of modest continued deterioration were present in six patients. However, none of these patients developed clinically evident congestive heart failure.

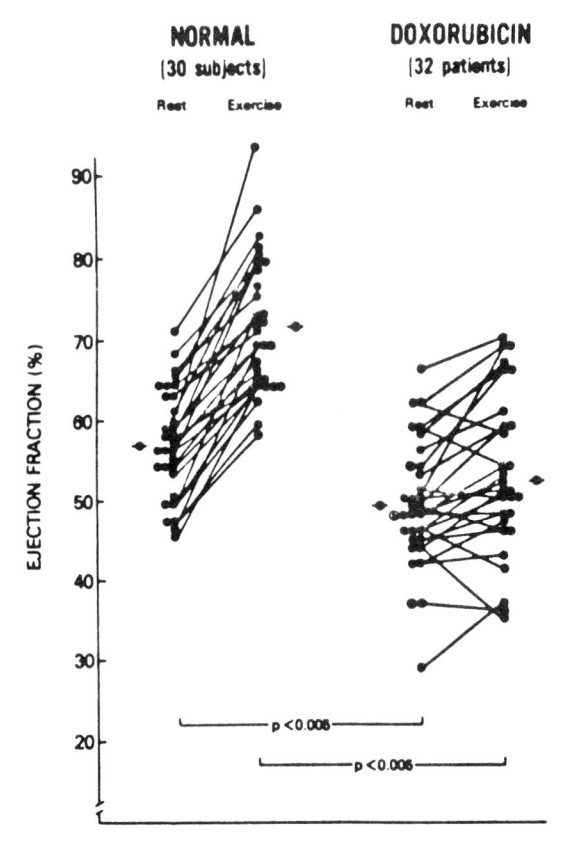

Fig. 12-4. Ejection fractions at rest and during maximal, symptom-limited supine bicycle exercise in 30 normal subjects compared with 32 doxorubicin-treated patients. ● = Average ejection fraction. ☉ = Rest study only. (From Gottdiener, J.S., Mathisen, D.J., Borer, J.S., Bonow, R.O. Myers, C.F., Barr L.H., Schwartz, D.B., Bacharach, S.L., Green, M.V., and Rosenberg, S.A. Doxorubicin cardiotoxicity: assessment of late left ventricular dysfunction by radionuclide cineangiography. Ann. Intern. Med. 94:430, 1981.)

Palmeri[104] also using rest and exercise radionuclide cineangiography, has shown that some degree of left ventricular dysfunction relative to pretreatment baseline values is common, occurring in 92% of the patient population after completing doxorubicin therapy (522 ± 22 mg/m^2). This study suggests that radionuclide cineangiography is a sensitive method of monitoring the cardiotoxic effects of doxorubicin. However, it is also important to recognize that 62% of the patients still had a normal ejection fraction (EF) at rest and 35% had a normal exercise response. Only 4 of the 48 patients studied developed clinical evidence of congestive heart failure after completing the course of doxorubicin therapy.

Endomyocardial biopsy and cardiac catheterization may provide the most accurate assessment of the risk status of an individual receiving doxorubicin chemotherapy.[105] Studies from several centers have suggested that the characteristic pathologic findings of myofibrillar loss and cytoplasmic vacuolization on biopsy precedes the development of left ventricular dysfunction.[106-108] This invasive, relatively costly procedure, however, is not universally available. To evaluate the relative predictive efficacy of competing modalities, McKillop compared radionuclide-determined rest and exercise left ventricular ejection fractions with echocardiographic and systolic time interval assessments of left ventricular function, regarding the capacity of each modality to identify patients with endomyocardial biopsy and right heart catheterization abnormalities previously found to be highly accurate in predicting the risk of congestive heart failure after doxorubicin.[109] An abnormal left ventricular ejection fraction at rest had a sensitivity of 53% and a specificity of 75% for identifying patients thus defined as being at moderate or high risk. The addition of exercise left ventricular ejection fraction (LVEF) increased the sensitivity to 89%, but reduced the specificity to 41% in identifying patients at moderate or high risk. Exercise LVEF improved the sensitivity of detection of high risk patients from 58 to 100%. Echocardiography and systolic time interval assessments proved less sensitive. McKillop concluded that determination of exercise left ventricular ejection fraction provides sufficient sensitivity for screening for anthracycline cardiotoxicity, but the lack of specificity does not allow its use as a definitive test. According to these authors, determination of left ventricular ejection fraction at rest did not provide sensitivity or the specificity sufficient for use as either a screening tool or a definitive test. Of course, this result must be evaluated in light of the fact that the authors defined the efficacy of the noninvasive tests only in terms of invasive descriptors, rather than clinical end points. The possible inadequacy of this approach is indicated by the work of Isner,[110] who identified seven of 20 (35%) pa-

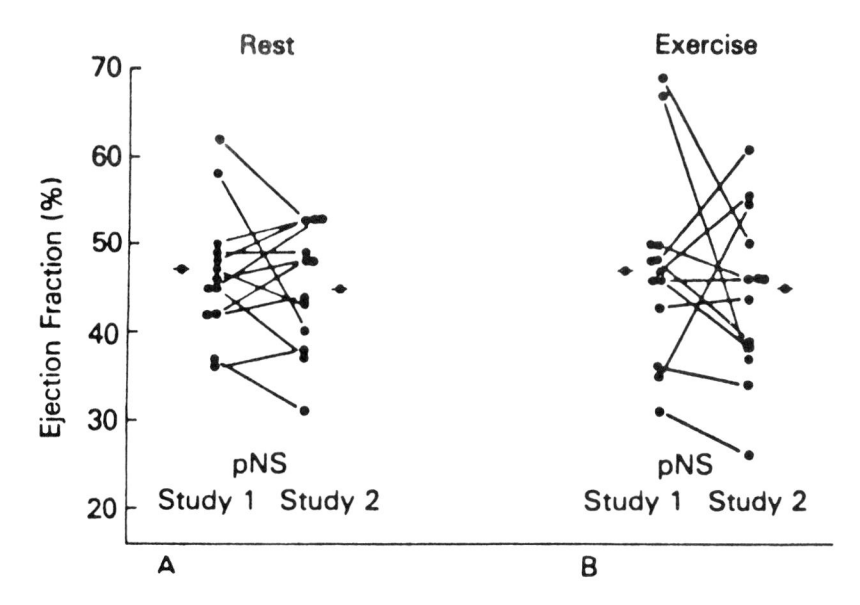

Fig. 12-5. Sequential determination of ejection fraction in 13 patients at rest (panel A) and during exercise (panel B). They were restudied an average of 9.2 months after initial postdoxorubicin evaluation which was performed an average of 21.4 months after completing the drug treatment. (From Gottdiener, J.S., Mathisen, D.J., Borer, J.S., Bonow, R.O., Myers, C.E., Barr, L.H., Schwartz, D.B., Bacharach, S.L., Green, M.V., and Rosenberg, S.A. Doxorubicin cardiotoxicity: assessment of late left ventricular dysfunction by radionuclide cineangiography. Ann. Intern. Med. 94:430, 1981.)

tients who had unequivocal clinical signs of congestive cardiomyopathy (jugular venous distention, rales and/or S3 gallop) on examination and did not manifest histologic signs of cardiotoxicity on multiple sections of myocardium. The investigators asserted that this finding limits the clinical utility of histologic prediction of significant anthracycline cardiotoxicity: in these seven patients, an endomyocardial biopsy would have predicted that doxorubicin chemotherapy could have been continued safely, and could not have been attributed merely to sampling errors associated with biopsy. Moreover, the findings of these investigators suggested that myofibrillar dropout and cytoplasmic vacuolization, histologic hallmarks of doxorubicin toxicity, are not the only factors predictive of doxorubicin-induced cardiac failure. Consequently, they argued that functional assessment of the left ventricle, including determination of exercise left ventricular ejection fraction, might be an important adjunct to any efforts at monitoring patients for latent cardiotoxicity. Long-term followup of patients who have received doxorubicin will be necessary to determine whether "latent toxicity," detected by either morphologic or functional parameters, ultimately will progress to overt congestive heart failure.

A number of clinical parameters may aid in the recognition of patients at risk for doxorubicin-induced cardiomyopathy. Clearly, the most significant risk factor contributing to the development of anthracycline cardiomyopathy is the total dose of doxorubicin administered. In a retrospective study of 3941 patients, Von Hoff and associates demonstrated a continuum of increasing risk related to increasing total dose of the drug (Fig. 12-6).[111] Palmeri[104] has identified a pattern of initial functional tolerance to doxorubicin. Although resting left ventricular function, as measured by radionuclide cineangiographic ejection fraction, progressively declined during the course of therapy, there was a greater decrease in ejection fraction per mg of doxorubicin after the administration of approximately 340 mg/M² total dose. In fact, patients with baseline resting left ventricular dysfunction may tolerate at least low doses of doxorubicin.[104,112] These studies strongly suggest that the dosage of doxorubicin should be tailored to the individual patient based on the evaluation of cardiac function by noninvasive and invasive methods, rather than by arbitrary limitation of 550 mg/M². Several studies have indicated that the schedule of doxorubicin administration also has significant impact on the risk of developing congestive heart failure (Fig. 12–6). Data from Weiss,[113] Chlebowski,[114,136] Von Hoff,[111] Torti,[115] and Legha[116] suggest that patients treated with smaller doses on a weekly schedule or by continuous infusion have a lower incidence of congestive heart failure than patients receiving larger doses every 3 weeks. The decrease in cardiotoxic complications with the more frequent dosing schedule is attributed to lower peak doxorubicin concentrations. It is important to note that this regimen does not seem to compromise antitumor efficacy. Increasing age, pre-existing cardiac disease, hypertension, radiotherapy to the mediastinum, and concomitant cyclophosphamide, actinomycin D, mitomycin C, and decarbazine administration have been reported to be associated with increased risk of doxorubicin-induced cardiomyopathy.[111,117–124]

Current treatment of anthracycline-induced congestive heart failure is limited to withdrawal of the drug and institution of conventional treatment for heart failure. Controversy exists concerning the efficacy of standard treatment with digoxin, diuretics, and vasodilators because some investigators have described good results and others have reported progressive deterioration. Recent investigations have examined pharmacologic interventions aimed at limiting or preventing congestive heart failure. Some, though not all, investigators have reported that the cardiac glycosides, digoxin and acetylstrophanthidin, decrease the cardiac toxic effects of doxorubicin, a process attributed to competition between the glycosides and doxorubicin for a common membrane carrier.[73,125,137] Coenzyme Q10, a component of the mitochondrial electron-transport chain that is reportedly decreased in anthracycline-induced cardiomyopathies, has also been reported to limit cardiac toxicity when administered to patients receiving doxorubicin.[126] Free radical

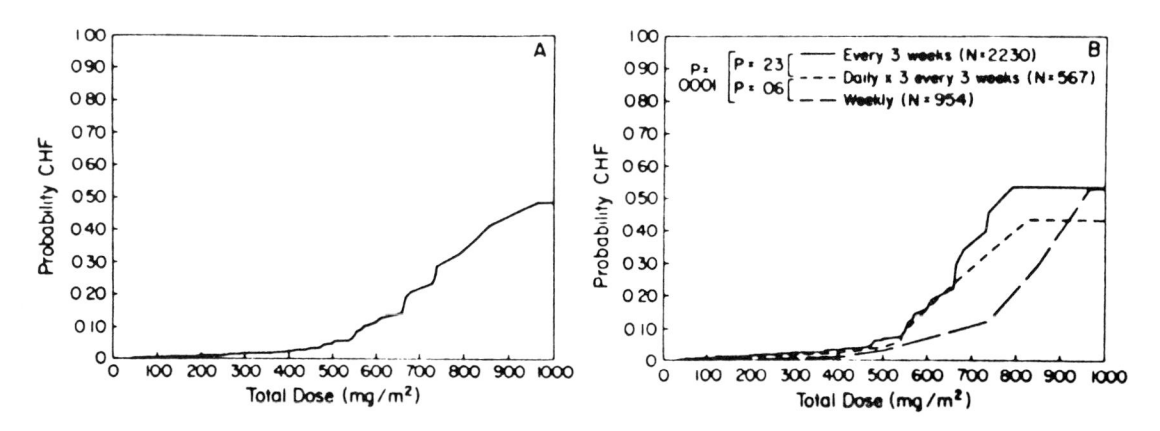

Fig. 12–6. (a) Cumulative probability of developing doxorubicin-induced congestive heart failure (CHF) versus total cumulative dose of doxorubicin in all patients receiving the drug (3941 patients—88 cases of congestive heart failure). To estimate the probability of developing congestive heart failure with a further dose (y) of doxorubicin in a patient who has already received a total dose (x) without drug-induced congestive heart failure, calculate

$$\frac{Q_{x+y} - Q_x}{1 - Q_x}$$

where Q is the probability of suffering congestive heart failure at a particular dose. (b) Cumulative probability of developing doxorubicin-induced congestive heart failure (CHF) versus total cumulative dose of doxorubicin in patients on three different dose schedules of the drug. (From Von Hoff, D.D., Layard, M.V., Basa, P., Davis, H.L., von Hoff, A.L. Rozencwieg, M. and Muggia, F.M. Risks factors for doxorubicin-induced congestive heart failure. Ann. Intern. Med. 9:710, 1979.)

scavengers, such as alpha tocopherol (Vitamin E) and N-acetylcysteine, appear to lessen the acute myocardial damage in animal models.[81,82] The efficacy of these agents in preventing chronic cardiac damage in clinical practice has not been established.[127,128] Cromolyn sodium may also provide cardioprotective effects by preventing the release of histamine.[76] In addition, the development of new anthracycline derivatives and analogs continues to be a major investigative focus in the effort to limit anthracycline-induced cardiomyopathy.

CYCLOPHOSPHAMIDE

Cyclophosphamide, an alkylating agent frequently used in combination with other chemotherapeutic drugs in treating patients with Hodgkin's disease, has been commonly used in modest doses without adverse cardiovascular effects. However, higher doses, particularly in preparation for bone marrow transplantation, have been associated with electrocardiographic changes and acute myopericarditis. A number of centers have reported cases of myopericarditis, some fatal, occurring after administration of 120 to 270 mg/M^2 of cyclophosphamide over 4 to 10 days.[129-134] Gottdiener and associates reported the occurrence of congestive heart failure in 9 of 32 patients (28%) treated with high dose cyclophosphamide for hematologic neoplasms.[132] Of these 9 patients, 6 (66%) died of myocardial failure. Of the 32 patients, 6 (19%) developed pericardial tamponade. In those patients surviving more than 3 weeks after cyclophosphamide therapy, none manifested late cardiotoxic reactions. A decrease in the summated electrocardiographic QRS voltage was noted in 91% (29/32) of these patients 5 to 14 days after beginning cyclophosphamide therapy. Echocardiographic evaluation before and after therapy in 13 of these patients revealed a significant decrease in left ventricular systolic function in eight (61%) patients, 5 to 16 days after initiation of therapy, and pericardial effusions in 5 of 15 (32%) patients. Left ventricular function returned to baseline in all of the six patients evaluated one month after therapy. There were no significant changes in left atrial dimension, aortic dimension, or left ventricular wall thickness. Pathologic examination of the heart in those patients who died of myocardial failure revealed thickening of the left ventricular wall with increased heart weight. All had serosanguinous pericardial effusions and fibrinous pericarditis of varying severity. Myocardial hemorrhage has occasionally been described. Histologic examination has revealed extravasation of blood, interstitial edema, and multifocal myocardial necrosis associated with fibrin microthrombi. Fibrin strands and red-blood cells were present in the interstitium adjacent to areas of capillary endothelial damage.

Cyclophosphamide cardiotoxicity has been attributed to direct myocardial endothelial damage resulting in the extravasation of blood containing high levels of the drug. High myocardial tissue levels and microvascular injury subsequently led to direct and ischemic myocardial cell damage, fibrin precipitation, interstitial edema, and focal hemorrhage.

As discussed previously, cyclophosphamide has been reported to potentiate the cardiotoxic effects of doxorubicin. It is not clear whether previous therapy with doxorubicin increases the risk of cyclophosphamide-induced cardiac injury.

SUMMARY

Historically, cardiovascular complications of chemotherapy for neoplastic diseases were initially limited to rare occurrences of orthostatic hypotension or myocardial infarctions related to chemotherapy with vincristine, a vinca alkaloid, and mild pulmonary hypertension resulting from pulmonary fibrosis during treatment with bleomycin or busulfan. The incidence of cardiovascular toxicity has become more significant not only with the advent of the anthracycline class of chemotherapeutic agents, but also with the increasingly successful treatment of neoplastic disease, allowing prolonged survival of patients with doxorubicin. The current invasive and noninvasive diagnostic modalities available to the investigator and clinician provide the capability for close monitoring of cardiovascular status with serial evaluations of cardiac anatomy and function. Through continued refinement of the therapeutic regimen based on the evaluation of cardiovascular status, limitation of cardiovascular toxicity without compromise of antineoplastic activity may be realized.

REFERENCES

1. Warren, S. Effects of radiation on normal tissues. Arch. Pathol. 34:1070, 1942.
2. Emery, E.S., Jr. and Gordon, B. The effect of roentgenotherapy on the human heart. Am. J. Med. Sci. 170:884, 1925.
3. Desjardins, A.N. Action of roentgen rays and radium on the heart and lungs. Experimental data and clinical radiotherapy. Am. J. Roentgen. 27:149, 303, 477, 1932.
4. Levy, R.L. and Golden, R. Roentgen therapy of active rheumatic heart disease. Am. J. Med. Sci. 194:597, 1937.
5. Hartman, F.W., Bolliger, A., Daub, H.P. et al. Heart lesions produced by the deep X-ray. Bull. Johns Hopkins Hospital, 41:36, 1927.
6. Applefeld, M.M., Slawson, R.G., Hall-Craigs, M. et al. Delayed pericardial disease after radiotherapy. Am. J. Cardiol. 47:210, 1981b.
7. Ross, J.M. A case illustrating the effects of prolonged action of radium. J. Pathol. Bact. 352:899, 1932.
8. Gottesman, J. and Bendick, A.J. Pneumopericardium from radium necrosis. Am. J. Med. Sci. 171:715, 1926.
9. Warren, S.L. and Whipple, G.H. Roentgen ray intoxication. J. Exper. Med. 35:187, 1922.
10. Warthin, A.S. and Pohle, E.A. The effect of roentgen rays on the heart. Arch. Intern. Med. 43:15, 1929.
11. Hellman, S. Principles of radiation therapy. In Cancer: Principles and Practice of Oncology. Edited by V.T. DeVita, S. Hellman, and S.A. Rosenberg. Philadelphia, J.B. Lippincott, 1982.
12. Phillips, T.L. Acute and late effects of multimodal therapy on normal tissues. Cancer 40:489, 1977.
13. Castellino, R.A., Glatstein, E., Turbow, M.M. et al. Latent radiation injury of lungs or heart activated by steroid withdrawal. Ann. Intern. Med. 80:593, 1974.
14. Fajardo, L.F. and Stewart, J.R. Pathogenesis of radiation-induced myocardial fibrosis. Lab. Invest. 29:244, 1973.
15. Wolf, G.L. and Kuman, P.P. Radiation-induced pericarditis. Pract. Cardiol. 6:41, 1980.
16. Ruckdeschel, J.C., Chang, P., Martin, R.G. et al. Radiation-related pericardial effusions in patients with Hodgkin's disease. Medicine 54:245, 1975.
17. Sjogren, H.O., Hellstrom, I., and Klein, G. Resistance of polyoma versus immunized mice to transplantation of established polyoma tumors. Exp. Cell Res. 23:204, 1961.
18. McKhann, C.F. The effect of X-ray on the antigenicity of donor cells in transplantation immunity. J. Immunol. 92:811, 1964.
19. Alexander, P. and Bacq, Z.M. The nature of the initial radiation damage at the subcellular level. In The Initial Effects of Ionizing Radiation on Cells. Edited by R.J.C. Harris. New York, Academic Press, 1961.
20. Allen, J.B., Sagerman, R.H., and Stuart, M.J. Irradiation decreases vascular prostacyclin formation with no concomitant effect on platelet thromboxane production. Lancet 2:1193, 1981.
21. Dollinger, M.R., Lavine, D.M., Foye, L.V., Jr. Myocardial infarction following radiation. Lancet 1:246, 1965.
22. Dollinger, M.R., Lavine, D.M., Foye, L.V. Myocardial infarction due to post-irradiation fibrosis of the coronary arteries. JAMA 195:316, 1966.
23. McReynolds, R.A., Gold, G.L., and Roberts, W.C. Coronary heart disease after mediastinal irradiation for Hodgkin's disease. Am. J. Med. 60:39, 1976.
24. Iqbal, S.M., Hanson, E.L., and Gensini, G.G. Bypass graft for coronary arterial stenosis following radiation therapy. Chest 71:664, 1977.
25. Tracy, G.P., Brown, D.E., Johnson, L.W. et al. Radiation-induced coronary artery disease. JAMA 228:1660, 1974.
26. Huff, H. and Sanders, E.M. Coronary artery occlusion after radiation. N. Engl. J. Med. 286:780, 1972.
27. Prentice, R.T.W. Myocardial infarction following radiation. Lancet 1:388, 1965.
28. Stewart, J.R. and Fajardo, L.F. Radiation-induced heart disease. Clinical and experimental agents. Radiol. Clin. North Am. 9:511, 1971.
29. Cohn, K.E., Stewart, J.R., Fajardo, L.F., Hancock, E.W. Heart disease following radiation. Medicine 46:281, 1967.
30. Byhardt, R., Brace, K., Ruckdeschel, J. et al. Dose and treatment factors in radiation relation pericardial effusion associated with the mantle technique for Hodgkin's disease. Cancer 35:795, 1975.
31. White, D.C. An atlas of radiation histopathology. Technical information center. Office of Public Affairs. U.S. Energy Research and Development Administration, 1975.
32. Posner, M.R., Cohen, G.I., and Skaris, A.T. Pericardial disease in patients with cancer. The differentiation of malignant from idiopathic and radiation-induced pericarditis. Am. J. Med. 71:407, 1981.
33. Gottdiener, J.S., Katin, M.J., Borer, J.S. et al. Late cardiac effects of therapeutic mediastinal irradiation. N. Engl. J. Med. 308:569, 1983.
34. Applefeld, M.M., Cole, J.F., Pollock, S.H. et al. The late appearance of chronic pericardial disease in patients treated by radiotherapy for Hodgkin's disease. Ann. Intern. Med. 94:338, 1981a.
35. Applefeld, M.M. and Wiernik, P.H. Cardiac disease after radiation therapy for Hodgkin's disease: analysis of 48 patients. Am. J. Cardiol. 51:1679, 1983.
36. Morton D.L., Glancy, D.L., Joseph, W.L., et al. Management of patients with radiation-induced pericarditis with effusion: a note on the development of aortic regurgitation. Chest 64:291, 1973.
37. Morton, D.L., Kagan, A.R., Roberts, W.C. et al.

Pericardiectomy for radiation-induced pericarditis with effusion. Ann. Thorac. Surg. 8:195, 1969.
38. Fajardo, L.F., Stewart, J.R., and Cohn, K.E. Morphology of radiation-induced heart disease. Arch. Pathol. 86:512, 1968.
39. Brosius, F.C., Waller, B.F., and Roberts, W.C. Radiation heart diseases. Am. J. Med. 70:519, 1981.
40. Burns, R.J., Bar-Shlomo, B.Z., Druck, M.N. et al. Detection of radiation cardiomyopathy by gated radionuclide angiography. Am. J. Med. 74:297, 1983.
41. Gomez, G.A., Park, J.I., Panahon, A.M. et al. Heart size and function after radiation therapy to the mediastinum in patients with Hodgkin's disease. Cancer Treat. Rep. 67:1099, 1983.
42. Kopelson, G. and Herwig, K.J. The etiologies of coronary artery disease in cancer patients. Int. J. Rad Oncol. Biol. Phys. 4:895, 1978.
43. Carmel, R.J. and Kaplan, H.S. Mantle irradiation in Hodgkin's disease. Cancer 37:2813, 1976.
44. Couch, R.D., Loh, K.K., Sugino, J. Sudden cardiac death following adriamycin therapy. Cancer 48:38, 1981.
45. Boivin, J.F. and Hutchison, G.B. Coronary heart disease mortality after irradiation for Hodgkin's disease. Cancer 49:2470, 1982.
46. Muggia, F.M., Ghosein, N.A., and Hanok, A. Creative phosphokinase and other serum enzymes during radiotherapy. JAMA 211:1345, 1970.
47. Pearson, H.E.S. Coronary occlusion following thoracic radiotherapy: two cases. Proc. R. Soc. Med. 50:516, 1957.
48. Prentice, R.T.W. Myocardial infarction following radiation. Lancet 1:388, 1965.
49. Andrews, J.T. and Etheridge, M.I. Electrocardiographic abnormalities following post-operation radiotherapy for carcinoma of the breast. Br. J. Radiol. 41:453, 1968.
50. Dunsmore, L.D., LoPonte, M.A., and Dunsmore, R.A. Radiation induced coronary artery disease. J. Am. Col. Cardiol. 8:239, 1986.
51. Radwaner, B.A., Geringer, R., Goldman, A.M. et al. Left main coronary artery stenosis following mediastinal irradiation. Am. J. Med. 82:1017, 1987.
52. Gold, H. Production of arteriosclerosis in the rat: effect of X-ray and a high fat diet. Arch. Pathol. 71:268, 1961.
53. Gold, H. Arteriosclerosis in the rats. Effect of X-ray and a high fat diet. Proc. Soc. Exptl. Biol. Med. 111:593, 1962.
54. Amromin, G.D., Gildenhorn, H.L., Solomon, R.D. et al. The synergism of x-irradiation and cholesterol-fat feeding on the development of coronary artery lesions. J. Atheroscler. Res. 4:325, 1964.
55. Ali, M.K., Kahlil, K.G., Fuller, L.M. et al. Radiation-related myocardial injury. Cancer 38:1941, 1976.
56. Cohen, S.I., Bharati, S., Glass, J., Lev, M. Radiotherapy as a cause of complete atrioventricular block in Hodgkin's disease. Arch. Intern. Med. 141:676, 1981.
57. Rubin, E., Camara, J., Grayzel, D.M. et al. Radiation-induced cardiac fibrosis. Am. J. Med. 34:71, 1963.

58. Tzivoni, D., Ratzkowski, E., Brian, S. et al. Complete heart block following therapeutic irradiation of the left side of the chest. Chest 71:231, 1977.
59. Walz, B.J., Rider, R.E., Pastove, J.O. et al. Cardiac pacemakers. Does radiation therapy affect performance? JAMA 234:72, 1975.
60. Lee, R.W., Huang, S.K., Mechling, E. et al. Runaway atrioventricular sequential pacemaker after radiation therapy. Am. J. Med. 81:883, 1986.
61. Cade, S. Malignant disease and its treatment by radium. Baltimore, Williams & Wilkins, 1940.
62. Thomas, F. and Forbus, W.D. Irradiation injury to the aorta and the lung. Arch. Pathol. 67:256, 1959.
63. Conomy, J.P., Kellermeyer, R.W. Delayed cerebrovascular consequences of therapeutic radiation. Cancer 36:1702, 1975.
64. Heidenberg, W.J., Lupovitch, A., and Tarr, N. "Pulseless disease" complicating Hodgkin's disease. JAMA 195:488, 1966.
65. Fajardo, L.F. and Lee, A. Rupture of major vessels after radiation. Cancer 36:904, 1975.
66. Silverberg, G.D., Britt, R.H., and Goffinet, D.R. Radiation-induced carotid artery disease. Cancer 41:130, 1978.
67. Rotman, M., Seidenbert, B., Rubin, I. et al. Aortic arch syndrome secondary to radiation in childhood. Arch. Intern. Med. 124:87, 1969.
68. Lindsay, S., Kohn, H.I., Daker, R.L. et al. Aortic arteriosclerosis in the dog after localized aortic X-irradiation. Circ. Res. 10:51, 1962.
69. Bloomer, W.D. and Hellman, S. Normal tissue responses to radiation therapy. N. Engl. J. Med. 293:80, 1975.
70. Reeves, W.C., Cunningham, D., Schwiter, E.J. et al. Myocardial hydroxyproline reduced by early administration of methylprednisolone or ibuprofen to rabbits with radiation-induced heart disease. Circulation 65:924, 1982.
71. Tritton, T.R., Murphree, S.A., and Sartorelli, A.C. Adriamycin: a proposal on the specificity of drug action. Biochem. Biophys. Res. Commun. 89:802, 1978.
72. Solie, T.N. and Yuncker, C. Adriamycin-induced changes in translocation of sodium ions in transporting epithelial cells. Life Science 22:1907, 1978.
73. Villani, F., Peccinini, F., Merelli, P. et al. Influence of adriamycin on calcium exchangeability in cardiac muscle and its modification by ouabain. Biochem. Pharmacol. 27:985, 1978.
74. Azuma, J., Sperelakis, N., Hasegawa, H. et al. Adriamycin cardiotoxicity: possible pathogenic mechanisms. J. Mol. Cell Cardiol. 13:381, 1981.
75. Olson, H.M., Young, D.M., Prieus, D.L. et al. Electrolyte and morphologic alterations of myocardium in adriamycin treated rabbits. Am. J. Pathol. 77:439, 1974.
76. Bristow, M.R. Toxic cardiomyopathy due to doxorubicin. Hosp. Pract. 17:101, 1982a.
77. Handa, K. and Sato, S. Generation of free radicals of quinone group-containing anti-cancer chemicals in NADPH-microsome systems as evidenced by initiation of sulfide oxidation. Gann 66:43, 1975.

78. Handa, K. and Sato, S. Stimulation of microsomal NADPH oxidation by quinone group containing anti-cancer chemicals. Gann 67:523, 1976.
79. Sato, S., Iwaizumi, M., Handa, K. et al. Electron spin resonance study on the mode of generation of free radicals of daunomycin, adriamycin, and carboquone in NADPH-microsome system. Gann 68:603, 1977.
80. Myers, C.E., McGuire, W.P., Liss, R.H. et al. Adriamycin: the role of lipid peroxidation in cardiac toxicity and tumor response. Science 197:165, 1977.
81. Doroshow, J.H., Locker, G.Y., Myers, C.E. The prevention of doxorubicin cardiac toxicity by N-acetyl-L-cysteine. Proc. Am. Assoc. Cancer Res. Am. Soc. Clin. Oncol. 20:253, 1979.
82. Olson, R.D., MacDonald, J.S., Harbison, R.D. et al. Altered myocardial glutathione levels: a possible mechanism of adriamycin toxicity. Fed. Proc. 36:303, 1977.
83. Sonneveld, P. Effect of α-tocopherol on the cardiotoxicity of adriamycin in the rat. Cancer Treat. Rep. 62:1033, 1978.
84. Herman, E.H. and Ferrans, V.J. Effects of vitamin E on the chronic doxorubicin toxicity in immature swine. Fed. Proc. 39:859, 1980.
85. Doroshow, J.H., Locher, G.Y., Myers, C.E. Enzymatic defenses of the mouse heart against reactive oxygen metabolites: alternations produced by doxorubicin. J. Clin. Invest. 65:128, 1980.
86. Katki, A.G. and Myers, C.E. Membrane-based glutathione peroxidase-like activity in mitochondria. Biochem. Biophys. Res. Commun. 96:85, 1980.
87. Yoda, Y., Nakazawa, M., Abe, T. et al. Prevention of doxorubicin myocardial toxicity in mice by reduced glutathione. Cancer Res. 46:2551, 1986.
88. Billingham, M.E., Mason, J.W., Bristow, M.R. et al. Anthracycline cardiomyopathy monitored by morphologic changes. Cancer Treat. Rep. 62:865, 1978.
89. Ferrans, V.J. Overview of cardiac pathology in relation to anthracycline cardiotoxicity. Cancer Treat. Rep. 62:955, 1978.
90. Lefrak, E.A., Pitha, J., Rosenheim, S. et al. A clinicopathologic analysis of adriamycin cardiotoxicity. Cancer 32:302, 1973.
91. Steinberg, J.S., Cohen, A.J., Wasserman, A.G. et al Acute arrhythmogenicity of doxorubicin administration. Cancer 60:1213, 1987.
92. Bristow, M.R., Thompson, P.D., Martin, R.P. et al. Early anthracycline cardiotoxicity. Am. J. Med. 65:823, 1978.
93. Singer, J.W., Narahara, K.A., Ritchie, J.L. et al. Time- and dose-dependent changes in ejection fraction determined by radionuclide angiography after anthracycline therapy. Cancer Treat. Rep. 62:945, 1978.
94. Starkebaum, G.A. and Durack, D.T. Early onset of daunorubicin (Daunomycin) cardiotoxicity. Lancet 2:711, 1975.
95. Harrison, P.T. and Sanders, L.A. Pericarditis in a case of early daunorubicin cardiomyopathy. Ann. Intern. Med. 85:339, 1976.
96. Mason, J.W., Bristow, M.R., Billingham, M.E. et al. Invasive and noninvasive methods of assessing adriamycin cardiotoxic effects in man: superiority of histopathologic assessment using endomyocardial biopsy. Cancer Treat. Rep. 62:857, 1978.
97. Gottdiener, J.S., Mathisen, D.J., Borer, J.S. et al. Doxorubicin cardiotoxicity: assessment of late left ventricular dysfunction by radionuclide cineangiography. Ann. Intern. Med. 94:430, 1981.
98. Minow, R.A., Benjamin, R.S., Lee, E.T. et al. QRS voltage change with adriamycin administration. Cancer Treat. Rep. 62:931, 1978.
99. Balcerzak, S.P., Christakis, J., Lewis, R.P. et al. Systolic time intervals in monitoring adriamycin-induced cardiotoxicity. Cancer Treat. Rep. 62:893, 1978.
100. Henderson, I.C., Sloss, L.I., Jaffe, N. et al. Serial studies of cardiac function in patients receiving adriamycin. Cancer Treat. Rep. 62:923, 1978.
101. Ewy, G.A., Jones, S.E., Friedman, M.J. et al. Noninvasive cardiac evaluation of patients receiving adriamycin. Cancer Treat. Rep. 62:915, 1978.
102. Alexander, J., Dainiak, N., Berger, H.J. et al. Serial assessment of doxorubicin cardiotoxicity with quantitative radionuclide angiocardiography. N. Engl. J. Med. 300:278, 1979.
103. Bristow, M.R., Ginsberg, R., Harrison, D.C. Histamine and the human heart: The other receptor system. Am. J. Cardiol. 49:249, 1982.
104. Palmeri, S.T., Bonow, R.O., Meyers, C.E. et al. Prospective evaluation of doxorubicin cardiotoxicity by rest and exercise angiography. Am. J. Cardiol. 58:607, 1986.
105. Bristow, M.R., Lopez, M.B., Mason, J.W., et al. Efficacy and cost of cardiac monitoring in patients receiving doxorubicin. Cancer 50:32, 1982.
106. Bristow, M.R., Mason, J.W., Billingham, M.E. et al. Dose-effect and structure-function relationships in doxorubicin cardiomyopathy. Am. Heart J. 102:709, 1981.
107. Druck, M.N., Gulenchyn, K.Y., Evans, W.K., et al. Radionuclide angiography and endomyocardial biopsy in the assessment of doxorubicin cardiotoxicity. Cancer 53:1667, 1984.
108. Ewer, M.S., Ali, M.K., Mackay, B. et al. A comparison of cardiac biopsy grades and ejection fraction estimations in patients receiving adriamycin. J. Clin. Oncol. 2:112, 1984.
109. McKillop, J.H., Bristow, M.R., Goris, M.L. et al. Sensitivity and specificity of radionuclide ejection fractions in doxorubicin cardiotoxicity. Am. Heart J. 106:1048, 1983.
110. Isner, J.M., Ferrans, V.J., Cohen, S.R. et al. Clinical and morphologic cardiac findings after anthracycline chemotherapy: analysis of 64 patients studied at necropsy. Am. J. Cardiol. 51:1167, 1983.
111. Von Hoff, D.D., Layard, M.W., Basa P. et al. Risk factors for doxorubicin-induced congestive heart failure. Ann. Intern. Med. 9:710, 1979.
112. Choi, B.W., Berger, H.J., Schwartz, P.E., Alexander, J., et al. Serial radionuclide assessment of doxorubicin cardiotoxicity in cancer patients with ab-

normal baseline resting left ventricular performance. Am. Heart J. *106*:638, 1983.
113. Weiss, A.J., Metter, G.E., Fletcher, W.S. et al. Studies on adriamycin using a weekly regimen demonstrating its clinical effectiveness and lack of cardiac toxicity. Cancer Treat. Rep. *60*:813, 1976.
114. Chlebowski, R.T., Pugh, R., Paroly, W. et al. Adriamycin on a weekly schedule: clinically effective with low incidence of cardiotoxicity. Clin. Res. *27*:53A, 1979.
115. Torti, F.M., Bristow, M.R., Howes, A.E. et al. Reduced cardiotoxicity of doxorubicin delivered on a weekly schedule. Assessment by endomyocardial biopsy. Ann. Intern. Med. *99*:745, 1983.
116. Legha, S.S., Benjamin, R.S., Mackay, B. et al. Reduction of doxorubicin cardiotoxicity by prolonged continuous intravenous infusion. Ann. Intern. Med. *96*:133, 1982.
117. Minow, R.A., Benjamin, R.S., and Gottlieb, J.A. Adriamycin (NSC-123127) cardiomyopathy—a overview with determinants of risk factors. Cancer Chemother. Rep. *6*:195, 1975.
118. Minow, R.A., Benjamin, R.S., Lee, E.T. et al. Adriamycin cardiomyopathy—risk factors. Cancer *39*:1397, 1977.
119. Cortes, E.P., Lutman, G., Wanka, J., et al. Adriamycin (NSC-123127) cardiotoxicity: A clinicopathologic correlation. Cancer Chemother. Rep. *6*:215, 1975.
120. Merrill, J., Greco, F.A., Zimbler, H. et al. Adriamycin and radiation: synergistic cardiotoxicity. Ann. Intern. Med. *82*:122, 1975.
121. Billingham, M.E., Bristow, M.R., Glatstein, E. et al. Adriamycin cardiotoxicity: endomyocardial biopsy evidence of enhancement by irradiation. Am. J. Surg. Pathol. *1*:17, 1977.
122. Kushner, J.P., Hansen, V.L., and Hamman, S.P. Cardiomyopathy after widely separated courses of adriamycin exacerbated by actinomycin-D and Mithramycin. Cancer *36*:1577, 1975.
123. Buzdar, A.V., Legha, S.S., Tashima, C.K. et al. Adriamycin and mitomycin C: possible synergistic cardiotoxicity. Cancer Treat. Rep. *62*:1005, 1978.
124. Smith, P.T., Ekert, H., Waters, K.D. et al. High incidence of cardiomyopathy in children treated with adriamycin and DTIC in combination chemotherapy. Cancer Treat. Rep. *61*:1736, 1977.
125. Somberg, J., Cagin, N., Levitt, B. et al. Blockade of tissue uptake of the antineoplastic agent, doxorubicin. J. Pharmacol. Exp. Ther. *204*:226, 1978.
126. Cortes, E.P., Gupta, M., Chow, C., Amin, V.C., Volker, K. Adriamycin cardiotoxicity: Early detection by systolic time interval and possible prevention by coenzyme Q. Cancer Treat. Rep. *62*:887, 1978.
127. Myers, C., Bonow, R., Palmeri, S. et al. A randomized controlled trial assessing the prevention of doxorubicin cardiomyopathy by N acetylcysteine. Semin. Oncol. *10*:(Suppl. I) 53, 1983.
128. Unverferth, D.V., Mehegan, J.P., Nelson, R.W., et al. The efficacy of N-acetylcysteine in preventing doxorubicin-induced cardiomyopathy in dogs. Semin. Oncol. *10*:2, 1983.
129. Santos, G.W., Sensenbrenner, L.L., Burke, P.J. et al. The use of cylophosphamide for clinical marrow transplantation. Transplant Proc. *4*:559, 1972.
130. Santos, G.W., Sensenbrenner, L.L., Burke, P.J. et al. Marrow transplantation in man following cyclophosphamide. Transplant Proc. *3*:400, 1971.
131. Bulkner, C.P., Rudolph, R.H., Fefer, A. et al. High dose cyclophosphamide therapy for malignant disease. Cancer *29*:357, 1972.
132. Gottdiener, J.S., Appelbaum, E.R., Ferrans, V.J. et al. Cardiotoxicity associated with high-dose cyclophosphamide therapy. Arch. Intern. Med. *141*:758, 1981.
133. Appelbaum, F.R., Stranchen, J.P., Graw, R.G. et al. Acute lethal carditis caused by high-dose combination chemotherapy. Lancet *1*:58, 1976.
134. Mills, B.A. and Roberts, R.W. Cyclophosphamide-induced cardiomyopathy. Cancer *43*:2223, 1979.
135. Greco, F.A., Brereton, H.D., Kent, H. et al. Adriamycin and enhanced radiation reaction in normal esophagus and skin. Ann. Intern. Med. *85*:294, 1976.
136. Chlebowski, R.T., Paroly, W.S., Pugh, R.P., et al. Adriamycin given as a weekly schedule without a loading course: clinically effective with reduced incidence of cardiotoxicity. Cancer Treat. Rep. *64*:47 1980.
137. Guthrie, D. and Gibson, A.L. Doxorubicin cardiotoxicity: possible role of digoxin in its prevention. Brit. Med. J. *2*:1447, 1977.
138. Martin, R.G., Ruckdeschel, J.C., Chang, P. et al. Radiation-related pericarditis. Am. J. Cardiol. *35*:216, 1975.
139. Minow, R.A., Benjamin, R.S., and Gottlieb, J.A. A clinicopathologic analysis of adriamycin cardiotoxicity. Cancer *32*:302, 1973.

CHAPTER 13

Pulmonary Complications of Hodgkin's Disease Treatment: Radiation Pneumonitis, Fibrosis, and the Effect of Cytotoxic Drugs

NANCY J. TARBELL
PETER MAUCH
SAMUEL HELLMAN

Treatment with mantle irradiation for lymph node involvement in Hodgkin's disease requires irradiation of the surrounding lung tissue. When there is extensive nodal involvement, more lung is initially treated. Some chemotherapeutic agents used in conjunction with irradiation affect the lung, requiring that the interactions between these modalities be understood. A number of acute and chronic lung complications can occur following either radiation therapy alone or combined modality therapy for Hodgkin's disease. These include the development of radiation pneumonitis, pneumothorax, pulmonary fibrosis, pulmonary insufficiency, and superimposed parenchymal or bronchial infections. The risk of pulmonary complications is related to radiation technique, fraction size, total dose, and the volume of lung irradiated. Although radiation pneumonitis is considered an acute complication, it characteristically occurs 1 to 6 months after completion of radiation therapy. This is the most common pulmonary complication seen after mantle irradiation.

RADIATION PNEUMONITIS

The clinical course of radiation pneumonitis has been well described.[1-4] It typically appears about 1 to 3 months after completion of the mantle field, although it may be delayed as long as 6 months.[4] Dyspnea on mild exertion, a nonproductive cough, and a low-grade fever are the common clinical symptoms. Less frequent symptoms include dull or pleuritic chest pain. Table 13–1 lists the frequency of presenting signs and symptoms from a review of pneumonitis in Hodgkin's patients

Table 13-1. Signs and Symptoms of Radiation Pneumonitis in 75 Patients

Signs and Symptoms	Patients
Shortness of breath or dyspnea on exertion	57
Cough	50
Pleurisy	6
Fever	1
Hemoptysis	1
Pleural rub	1
Decreased breath sounds	2
Rales	2
Radiographic signs of pneumonitis	67

Modified from Carmel and Kaplan[2]

treated at Stanford University Medical Center.[1] Physical findings depend on the severity of the pneumonitis and range from no signs to tachypnea, tachycardia, nasal flaring, and increased breath sounds. On chest roentgenogram, the mediastinal silhouette usually becomes less well defined. Irregular densities appear in the paramediastinal lung parenchyma that frequently outline the mantle field. These roentgenographic changes are usually confined to the high-dose regions; however, they may extend outside the radiation field in severe cases.[5] Infections, recurrent Hodgkin's disease, and drug toxicity are the major components in the differential diagnoses. Serial chest films are frequently of value in demonstrating progressive interstitial changes.

Figure 13-1 illustrates acute radiation pneumonitis with the infiltrates confined to the original radiation field. There is no clear-cut relationship between acute pneumonitis and the later development of fibrosis. Acute pneumonitis is thought to result from the temporary loss of alveolar lung cells with eventual repopulation, while fibrosis is the result of permanent destruction of this cell renewal compartment with resultant fibrosis. The overall incidence of secondary pneumonia or bronchitis following mantle irradiation does not appear to be increased. When pneumonitis is present in immunocompromised patients receiving both chemotherapy and irradiation, however, superimposed infections such as *Pneumocystis carinii* need to be ruled out.

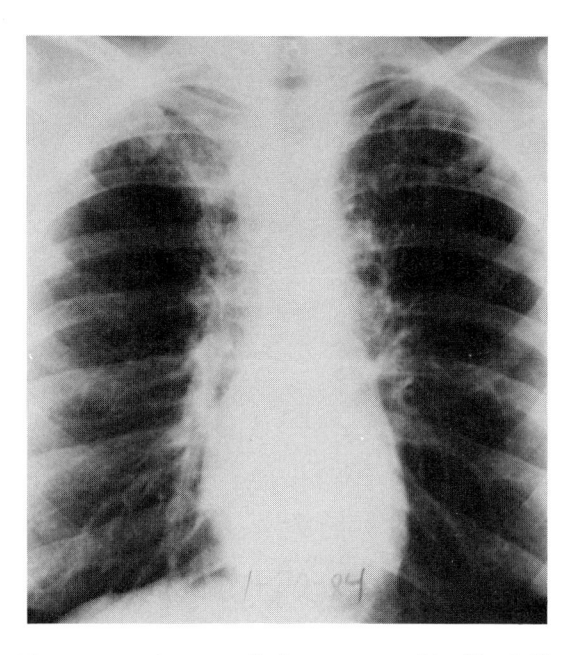

Fig. 13-1. Acute radiation pneumonitis. The infiltrates outline the mantle field and are confined to the paramediastinal and bilateral upper-lung fields.

TREATMENT

Most cases of pneumonitis should be managed conservatively. Rest, cough suppressants, and nonsteroidal anti-inflammatory agents are usually adequate for relief of mild symptoms.

With more severe symptoms, treatment with high-dose corticosteroids may be indicated. Clinical reports on the role of steroids in pneumonitis have been controversial.[4,6] However, high-dose steroids (prednisone 60 mg/day) administered at the time of progressive symptoms often have a beneficial effect.[3,4,6] Objective pulmonary studies may be of value. Associated findings include impairment of alveolar-capillary oxygen diffusion, which is characterized by hyperventilation, low arterial P_{CO_2}, and reduced oxygen consumption with exercise.[4]

Corticosteroids appear to reduce the severity of acute radiation-induced lung damage as measured by chest compliance studies.[6] Chronic changes, however, do not appear to be influenced by the use of steroids. This is not surprising because other chronic progressive lung disorders are similarly unaffected by the use of steroids. Thus, steroids are of benefit only in those patients with a severe acute course that might otherwise be fatal, but in whom the radiation damage is acute and reversible. Extreme care must be taken to taper steroids gradually, as abrupt steroid withdrawal may cause a recrudescence of the disease. Because such tapering requires an extended period of steroid administration, we are reluctant to use these agents unless the symptoms are severe.

HISTOPATHOLOGY

The pathology of radiation injury to the lung is well described by Rubin and Casarett.[4] The early histopathologic changes seen in the lung after irradiation include hyperemia and vascular congestion, as well as edema of the alveolar walls and an increase in phagocytic cells. The acute reaction is distinguished by the significant edema, the deposition of fibrin-like material in the alveoli, and the degeneration of the alveolar lining cells. Inflammatory cell infiltration is minimal in contrast to that occurring in other inflammatory conditions of the lung. This reaction may resolve or may progress to a late fibrotic stage.

Histologically, there is no clear separation, but rather a continuum from the acute exudative phase to the chronic fibrotic phase. Jennings and Arden[7] reported on the pathology of radiation pneumonitis in a human autopsy series. They felt that the accumulation of a fibrin-rich exudate within the alveoli and the thickening of alveolar septa by cellular proliferation of fibrous tissue were characteristic of radiation changes in the lung.

These acute changes may resolve, or when severe, may progress to a fibrotic stage. The fibrotic stage is characterized by excessive proliferation of connective tissue in the alveolar walls and hyalinization of the blood-vessel walls with reduction of the fine vasculature. Rare foci of collagen necrosis may be seen. Slight bronchial epithelial proliferation may also be seen. There is a resulting loss of cilia and an increase in secretions. Thus, the late fibrotic stage is associated with prominent vascular changes and fibrosis of the alveolar walls.[4,7]

CLINICAL PICTURE

The incidence of clinically significant radiation pneumonitis is related to the total radiation dose, the volume of lung irradiated, the daily dose, the number of fractions used, as well as the technique and equipment used for giving mantle irradiation.[7-10]

As noted by Kaplan,[1] the frequency of radiation pneumonitis depends strongly on the criteria that define the condition. Carmel and Kaplan[2] defined the syndrome of symptomatic pulmonary radiation reaction (SPRR) as unexplained cough, shortness of breath, dyspnea on exertion, and/or pleurisy on at least two follow-up clinic visits.

The importance of technique and method of treating the mantle field in Hodgkin's disease, and its relationship to radiation pneumonitis, is illustrated by the reports from Stanford.[2,10] Initially, patients were treated with large daily fractions (about 275 cGy per day). Patients received a dose of 4000 to 4400 cGy to the mediastinum in approximately 4 weeks. Sixteen of the 248 patients (6.4%) developed radiation pneumonitis. Nine were mild to moderate and seven were considered severe. One of the severe cases was fatal. The risk of pneumonitis was much greater when one or both whole lungs were treated either therapeutically for pulmonary involvement due to Hodgkin's disease or prophylactically in patients with significant hilar lymphadenopathy. Sixty-nine patients received treatment to one or both lungs, usually to a total of 1500 cGy in 10 to 12 days. Twenty-three patients (33%) developed radiation pneumonitis and four cases were fatal (5.8%).

As a result of this relatively high incidence, a method of treatment called the "thin block" technique was adopted at Stanford in 1970. The thin lung block technique uses partial thickness lung blocks so the midplane lung dose is approximately 37% of the midplane mediastinal dose.[11] Thus, the whole lung dose is approximately 75 cGy per day. With this technique, the total whole lung dose was limited to 1650 cGy and the incidence of pneumonitis dropped dramatically.[2] The incidence was still volume-related, with 4 of 27 (15%) of patients treated to one or both lungs with the new technique developing radiation pneumonitis. These findings are summarized in Table 13–2.

In a review of 307 patients wth supradiaphragmatic Hodgkin's disease seen and treated at the Joint Center for Radiation Therapy, clinically significant pneumonitis was seen in 10 patients (3.8%) treated with radiation alone. Four required treatment with prednisone. There was one fatality and this occurred in a patient who received bilateral whole lung irradiation using 200 cGy fractions to 2000 cGy.[12] The risk of pneumonitis was increased with the use of whole lung irradiation. This was comparable to the incidence of pneumonitis in patients receiving combined-modality therapy. There were 40 patients in this group and three of the 40 (7.3%) developed pneumonitis. All three of these patients required treatment with prednisone. We currently recommend that the fraction size not exceed 150 cGy when the whole lung is irradiated.

Patients with large mediastinal adenopathy necessitate irradiation of large volumes of lung and thus are at increased risk of radiation penumonitis. These patients may require a modification of the standard mantle technique.[11] Patients may be treated in the sitting position, which reduces the transverse diameter of the mediastinal mass compared to the standard prone or supine position. However, this is a more difficult technical set up and may be less reproducible. In addition, the details of matching the para-aortic field are more difficult. Alternatively, patients may have a large volume treated to 1500 cGy and then the blocks may be enlarged as significant shrinkage of the mediastinal mass occurs. This may require a treatment interruption to allow tumor reduction. This should not exceed a week to 10 days. Care must be taken when reducing the irradiated volume to be sure that all the tumor is included in the field. Another treatment option is to use combined-modality therapy in patients with large mediastinal adenopathy.[14] Initial treatment with MOPP chemotherapy may allow tumor shrinkage with the subsequent use of smaller fields of irradiation. This combined approach is generally used when the disease extent is such that large volumes of heart and lung would otherwise be irradiated.

DRUG EFFECT

Steroids

The most frequently seen drug-radiation reaction in patients with Hodgkin's disease involves the use of corticosteroids. The onset of pneumonitis may be related to the rapid withdrawal of steroid therapy, which has been described with the use of MOPP chemotherapy.[3] The recognition of this syndrome, which responds to high doses of steroids, is important and may be lifesaving. Progressive pneumonitis can improve dramatically after institution of corticosteroids. Figures 13–2a,

Table 13–2. The Influence of Dose Rate on the Incidence of Radiation Pneumonitis

Area Treated	Number of Patients	Radiation Pneumonitis		Fatal Pneumonitis	
		Number	%	Number	%
Program A					
Mediastinum	248	16	6	1	0.25
Mediastinum plus one or both lungs	69	23	33	4	6
Total	317	39	12	5	1.6
Program B					
Mediastinum	99	1	1	0	0
Mediastinum plus one or both lungs	27	4	15	0	0
Total	126	5	4	0	0

Program A—Dose rate of 1100 cGy/week (4 times a week) 1964–69
Program B—Dose rate of 375 cGy/week to the lung via "thin block" technique 1970–72
Modified from Kaplan[9]

b, and c illustrate the dramatic results that can be seen after initiation of steroids for pneumonitis. This patient had received combined-modality therapy with MOPP and irradiation. She developed severe progressive pneumonitis, which initially outlined the mantle field (Figure 13–2a). Her symptoms progressed, however, and Figure 13–2b demonstrates the fulminant bilateral interstitial process that developed in both lung fields. The patient was febrile, dyspneic, tachycardic. Her PO_2 was 50 with a P_{CO_2} of 36 on a 30% oxygen mark. High-dose corticosteroids were initiated and the patient was afebrile and resting comfortable in less than 12 hours. Figure 13–2c shows the improvement in her chest roentgenogram just 2 days after initiation of steroids. This patient had complete resolution of her symptoms and her steroids were tapered slowly over the following 3 months. One year later she was without evidence of any pulmonary problems.

Radiation pneumonitis related to steroid withdrawal should be considered a cause of clinical and radiographic abnormalities in irradiated patients who have received corticosteroids. The association of abrupt steroid withdrawal and prior irradiation should alert the clinician to the diagnosis of radiation pneumonitis rather than recurrent tumor or opportunistic infection. Once corticosteroids have been started for the treatment of pneu-

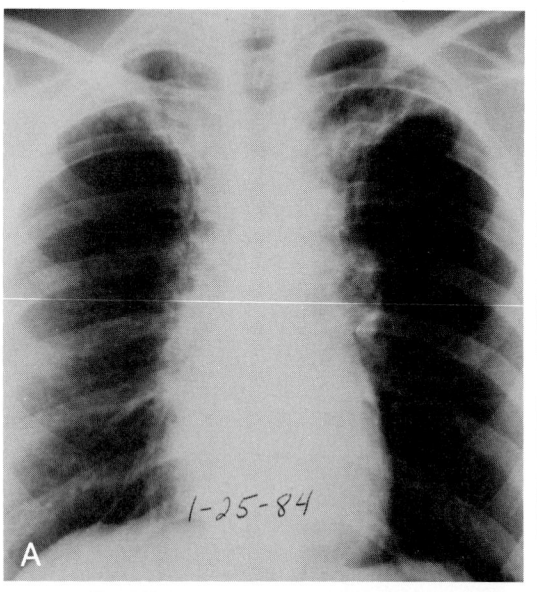

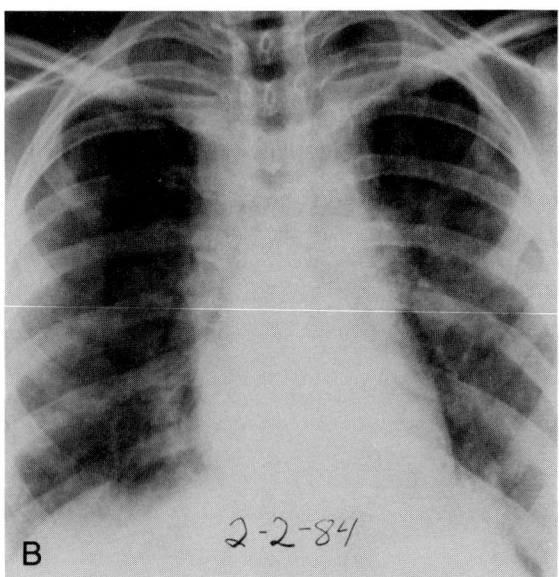

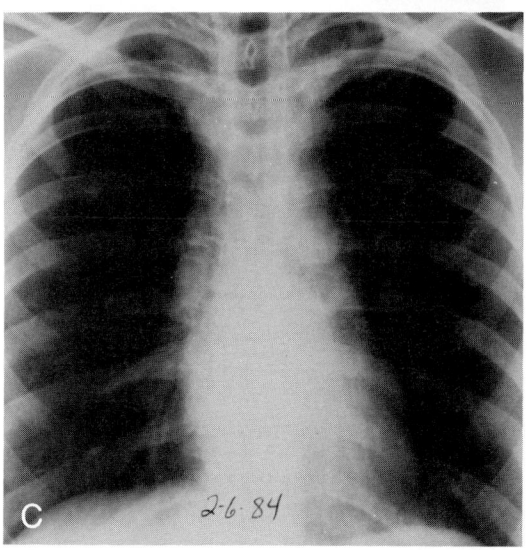

Fig. 13–2. (A) Acute pneumonitis after MOPP chemotherapy and mantle irradiation. (B) Progressive, fulminant, bilateral interstitial process encompassing both lung fields. (C) Chest x ray two days after initiation of high dose steroids. The patient improved symptomatically within 12 hours of treatment with steroids.

monitis, they must be gradually tapered.[3] Kaplan has recommended a dose of about 40 mg of prednisone daily with tapering over 3 months. Tapering doses should not be in excess of 2.5 mg per week.[2] We have generally started with 60 to 100 mg prednisone daily and gradually tapered the dose once symptoms improved.

Cytotoxic Drugs

Many chemotherapeutic agents have been reported to be associated with pulmonary damage.[15-21] These include the alkylating agents busulfan, chlorambucil, cyclophosphamide, BCNU, and melphalan; the antibiotics bleomycin and actinomycin-D; and the nitrosoureas. The most commonly reported drugs associated with pulmonary injury are bleomycin and BCNU.[15] Of the drugs used in MOPP, procarbazine has been reported to cause hypersensitivity pneumonitis[17,18] and nitrogen mustard may be implicated in some cases of drug-induced pulmonary disease.[19]

Since the reports of Bonadonna et al.,[22,23] ABVD has become common salvage therapy after MOPP failure in Hodgkin's disease. In addition, it is sometimes first-line therapy in alternating programs for advanced stage Hodgkin's disease.[24-25] Thus, the pulmonary toxicity of bleomycin has taken on more clinical importance and has been well described.[20,26,27] The clinical symptoms of toxicity may be abrupt and include cough, dyspnea, and pleuritic pain. On examination, rales are frequently present at the lung bases. Pulmonary function studies show a decrease in diffusion capacity. Chest roentgenograms of early pulmonary damage show a fine reticular pattern, usually located at the lower-lung zones and at the level of the costophrenic angle. Figure 13-3a shows the interstitial infiltrate characteristic of the early toxicity. A CT scan may demonstrate the full extent of the abnormality (Figure 13-3b).

The infiltrate may resolve with the discontinuation of bleomycin. In more advanced cases, the infiltrate may become more widespread and patchy and progress to alveolar consolidation. Ultimately, chronic pulmonary insufficiency may result. Figure 13-4 shows the peripheral nature of the infiltrate with sparing of the perihilar region. Significant clinical pulmonary abnormalities are noted in less than 15% of patients undergoing treatment with bleomycin. Less than 5% of reactions are fatal. Two forms of toxicity have been described. The more common toxicity is thought to be dose-dependent, increasing at cumulative doses exceeding 200 units per square meter.[27] However, an idiosyncratic toxicity, with fatal bleomycin-induced pulmonary reactions, has been reported at doses as low as 50 to 165 units.[20,26,27] Some of these cases have received prior lung irradiation.

The histopathology reveals interstitial edema, intra-alveolar hyaline membrane formation, increased numbers of alveolar macrophages, and the deposition of collagen in the alveolar walls.[20] The mechanism of pulmonary damage is not completely understood, but appears to be related to the preferential distribution of the drug in the lung tissue. Thus, pulmonary toxicity is increased by administering high single and total doses of bleomycin.

Because of the potential for severe pulmonary toxicity, patients must be assessed carefully with chest roentgenograms and pulmonary function tests at regular intervals. Early detection is extremely important because initial lesions may regress with prompt discontinuation of bleomycin.[26] Administration of bleomycin is contraindicated in the face of any evidence of pulmonary disease.

Chemotherapeutic agents may add to the effects of irradiation or may actually act synergistically to cause an enhanced irradiation effect. Such interactions in the lung have been described with the use of actinomycin-D, adriamycin, bleomycin, and cyclophosphamide.[20,28,29] The interaction of bleomycin and radiation is not well documented, but both clinically[27,29,30,31] and experimentally,[32,33] bleomycin appears to enhance radiation lung damage. When bleomycin is given with thoracic irradiation, lung damage occurs earlier and at lower radiation doses than with radiation alone.[29,30,33,34] It seems prudent to avoid concurrent bleomycin and irradiation.

FIBROSIS

Radiation-induced pulmonary fibrosis begins to appear at about 6 months after radi-

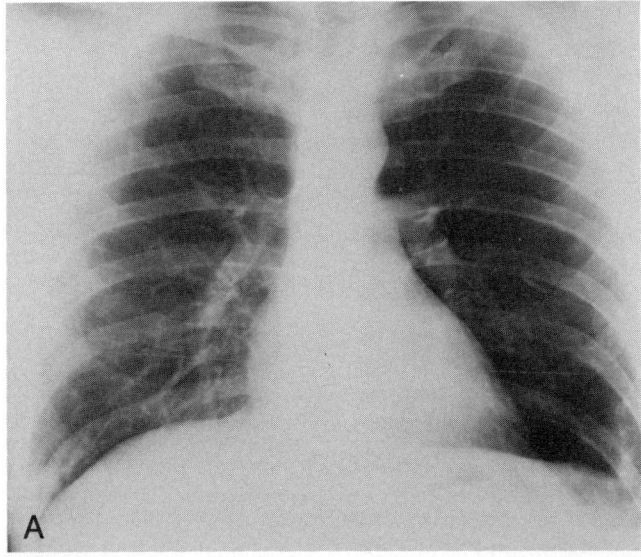

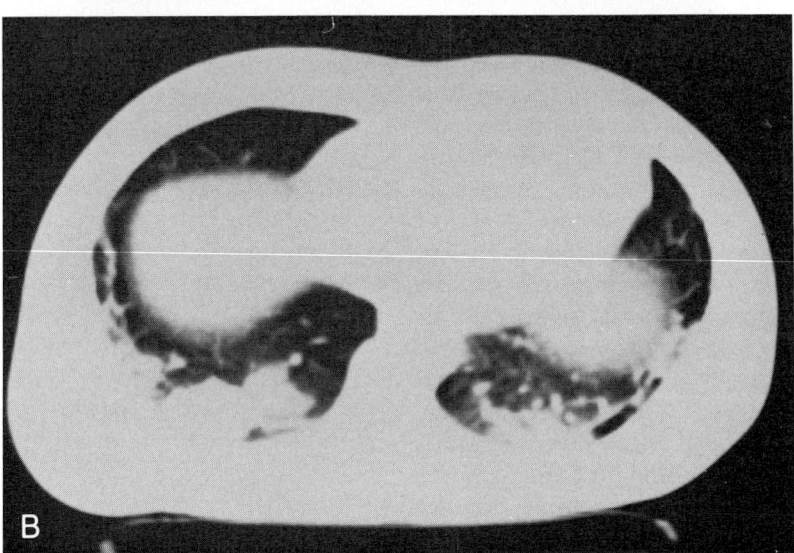

Fig. 13–3. (A) CXR showing the interstitial infiltrate at the lung bases, particularly at the costophrenic angle. This is characteristic of early bleomycin pulmonary toxicity. (B) CT scan dramatically demonstrates the changes noted on the chest x ray at the costophrenic angle.

ation treatment and usually stabilizes at 12 to 18 months. The pathology of the chronic phase reveals excessive proliferation of connective tissue, mainly in the alveolar walls, hyalinization and thickening of blood vessel walls, and reduction of fine vasculature.[4] The late fibrotic reaction is characterized by prominent vascular change with reduction of lumens associated with fibrosis of alveolar walls. These changes are nonspecific and are similar to other disorders causing chronic pulmonary fibrosis.[4] The volume irradiated appears to be the most important factor in determining the clinical significance of the irradiation. Even half-lung irradiation at high doses (5000 cGy), which produces severe pathologic changes, results in little clinical dysfunction if the remaining lung is normal. This may be comparable to pneumonectomized patients.[4] Although extensively fibrotic lung often retains significant pulmonary blood flow, this can result in shunting pulmonary artery blood through unaerated lung, thus decreasing arterial oxygen and causing

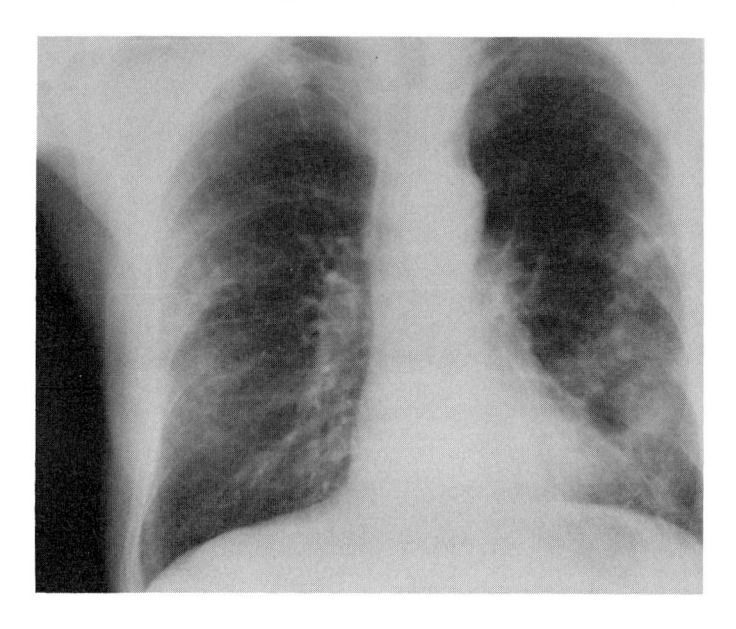

Fig. 13–4. Progressive bleomycin toxicity. Note peripheral nature of the infiltrate with relative sparing of the perihilar region.

symptoms. When bilateral irradiation is given at doses of 3000 cGy or greater, the result is usually fatal.[4] In contrast to acute pneumonitis, fraction size appears less important than the volume and the total dose in predicting long-term fibrosis. The former seems to depend on the balance of cell depopulation and repopulation while the latter depends on total cell kill. This is described in more detail elsewhere.[35]

After mantle irradiation, the fibrosis usually occurs at the apex of both lungs and in the paramediastinal region, sharply outlining the radiation portals. There may be elevation of the hila along with paramediastinal fibrosis. The mediastinum may appear wider as a result of the blending of the mediastinal pulmonary fibrosis with the true mediastinum.

Chest roentgenogram findings after mediastinal irradiation for Hodgkin's disease were evaluated by Slanina[36] and are shown in Table 13–3. The overall percentage of long-term pulmonary side effects is high in this study. This is probably related to the fact that the study included patients treated from 1948 to 1974 and, until 1964, kilovoltage therapy was in use.

Lung function has been studied in patients undergoing mantle irradiation.[28,37–40] Host and Vale[37] studied 17 patients in whom there was no mediastinal, hilar, or lung involvement by Hodgkin's disease. They found the vital capacity was reduced by about 10% shortly after the end of treatment. They did not see any further deterioration in ventilatory function beyond 3 months after treatment. Although on average, lung volume decreased by about 10%, there was no effect seen on pulmonary gas exchange at rest or during moderate exercise. Lassvik et al.[40] also found no evidence of impairment of pulmonary gas exchange or spirometric function in any of the eight patients with Hodgkin's disease. More significant pulmonary fibrosis is possible in those patients who require larger volumes of irradiation due to involvement of the mediastinum, hilum, or lung with Hodgkin's.

Morgan et al.[39] recently reported pulmonary function testing in 18 patients after mantle irradiation. They found a reduced mean diffusion capacity in 13 of the 18 (72%) patients analyzed. DLCO was significantly lowered in those patients who received both chemotherapy and irradiation (64% of pre-

Table 13–3. Roentgenogram Findings After Mediastinal Irradiation for Hodgkin's Disease

Paramediastinal Fibrosis	Dose of Irradiation	
	<4000 cGy	>4000 cGy
	n = 10	n = 55
None	10%	11%
Slight	60%	44%
Distinct	30%	36%
Severe	—	9%

*Modified from Slanina[36]

dicted) when compared to those who received irradiation alone (78% of predicted) (p<0.05).

PNEUMOTHORAX

Spontaneous pneumothoraces have been reported after treatment for Hodgkin's disease.[12,41,42] Radiation fibrosis may be instrumental in the development of pneumothorax.[41] It has been proposed that radiation-induced fibrosis promotes subpleural bleb formation; rupture of the bleb leads to a pneumothorax.[40] In our early-stage Hodgkin's patients, we have seen three cases of spontaneous pneumothoraces in 307 patients who underwent mantle irradiation.[12] In two patients, the pneumothoraces were small, about 10%, and resolved without treatment. The third patient had received whole-lung irradiation at 1950 cGy and had bilateral pneumothoraces that required thoracotomy. She is currently alive without evidence of Hodgkin's disease 10 years after treatment, but has severe restrictive lung disease.

This risk of pneumothorax appears to be increased by chemotherapeutic agents as well, but this occurrence is rare, with only isolated case reports.[42-45]

SUMMARY

Acute pneumonitis is primarily related to the volume irradiated and the fraction size used; the total dose appears to be less important. The occurrence of acute pneumonitis does not necessarily lead to eventual pulmonary fibrosis.

Chemotherapeutic agents may also cause pulmonary damage. In particular, agents such as bleomycin have significant pulmonary toxicity, which is enhanced by combined use with irradiation.

Corticosteroids have a special role in acute pneumonitis. Abrupt withdrawal from steroids may cause the acute onset of pneumonitis in the irradiated patient. This effect is important to appreciate when treating patients with MOPP chemotherapy and mantle irradiation. Corticosteroids appear to be effective in treating severe acute pneumonitis.

Fibrosis appears to be related primarily to the volume irradiated and the total dose of irradiation used. Typically, the fibrosis occurs at the apices of the lung and around the mediastinum. This pattern of fibrosis is directly related to the volume irradiated, unlike bleomycin, which usually causes fibrosis at the costophrenic angles. Spontaneous pneumothoraces occasionally occur in areas of previous fibrosis.

REFERENCES

1. Kaplan, H.S. Hodgkin's Disease. 2nd Ed. Cambridge, Harvard University Press, 1980.
2. Carmel, R.J. and Kaplan, H.S. Mantle irradiation in Hodgkin's disease: an analysis of technique, tumor eradication, and complications. Cancer 37:2813–2825, 1976.
3. Castellino, R.A., Glatstein, E., Turbow, M.M. et al. Latent radiation injury of lungs or heart activated by steroid withdrawal. Ann. Intern. Int. Med. 80:593–599, 1974.
4. Rubin, P. and Casarett, G.W. Clinical radiation pathology. Vol. 3. Philadelphia, W.B. Saunders, 1968.
5. Smith, J.C. Radiation pneumonitis. A review. Am. Rev. Respir. Dis. 87:647–655, 1963.
6. Moss, W.T., Haddy, F.J., and Sweeny, S.K. Some factors altering the severity of acute radiation pneumonitis: variations with cortisone, heparin, and antibiotics. Radiology 75:50–55, 1960.
7. Jennings, F.L. and Arden, A. Development of radiation pneumonitis. Time and dose factors. Arch. Pathol. 74:351–360, 1962.
8. Phillips, T.L. and Margolis, L. Radiation pathology and the clinical response of lung and esophagus. Front. Radiat. Ther. Oncol. 6:254–273, 1972.
9. Kaplan, H.S., Stewart, J.R., and Bissinger, P.A. Complications of intensive megavoltage radiotherapy for Hodgkin's disease. Natl. Cancer Inst. Monogr. 36:439–444, 1973.
10. Wara, W.M., Phillips, T.L., Margolis, L. et al. Radiation pneumonitis: A new approach to the derivation of time-dose factors. Cancer 32:547–552, 1973.
11. Palos, B., Kaplan, H.S., and Karzmark, C.J. The use of thin lung shields to deliver limited whole lung irradiation during mantle-field treatment of Hodgkin's disease. Radiology 101:441–442, 1971.
12. Leslie, N.T., Mauch, P., and Hellman, S. Evaluation of long term survival and treatment complications in patients with stage IA-IIB Hodgkin's disease. Int. J. Radiat. Oncol. Biol. Phys. 9 (Suppl.):127–128, 1983.
13. Hoppe, R.T. Radiation therapy in the treatment of Hodgkin's disease. Semin. Oncol. 7:144–154, 1980.
14. Leslie, N.T., Mauch, P.M., and Hellman, S. Stage IA–IIB supradiaphragmatic Hodgkin's disease. Long term survival and relapse frequency. Cancer 55 (9):2072–2078, 1985.
15. Rosenow, E.C. The spectrum of drug-induced pulmonary disease. Ann. Intern. Med. 77:977–991, 1972.

16. Phillips, T. Pulmonary section cardiorespiratory workshop. Cancer Clin. Trials 4 (Suppl):45–52, 1981.
17. Jones, S.E., Moore, M., Blank, N. et al. Hypersensitivity to procarbazine (matulane) manifested by fever and pleuro-pulmonary reaction. Cancer 29:498–500, 1972.
18. Ecker, M.D., Jay, B., and Keohane, M.F. Procarbazine lung. Am. J. Roentgenol. 131:527–528, 1978.
19. Farney, R.J., Morris, A.H., Armstrong, J.D. Jr. et al. Diffuse pulmonary disease after therapy with nitrogen mustard, vincristin, procarbazine and predisone. Am. Rev. Respir. Dis. 115:135–145, 1977.
20. DeLena, M., Guzzon, A., Monfardini, S. et al. Clinical, radiologic, and histopathologic studies on pulmonary toxicity induced by treatment with bleomycin. Cancer Chemother. Rep. 56:343–356, 1972.
21. Balikian, J.P., Jochelson, M.S., Bauer, K.A. et al. Pulmonary complications of chemotherapy regimens containing bleomycin. Am. J. Roentgenol. 139:455–461, 1982.
22. Bonadonna, G. and Santoro, A. ABVD chemotherapy in the treatment of Hodgkin's disease. Cancer Treat. Rev. 9:21–35, 1982.
23. Santoro, A. Bonfante, V., and Bonadonna, G. Salvage chemotherapy with ABVD in MOPP-resistant Hodgkin's disease. Ann. Intern. Med. 96:139–143, 1982.
24. Bonadonna, G., Santoro, A., Bonfante, V. et al. Cyclic delivery of MOPP and ABVD combinations in Stage IV Hodgkin's disease: rationale, background studies, and recent results. Cancer Treat. Rep. 66:881–887, 1982.
25. Santoro, A., Bonadonna, G., Bonfante, V. et al. Alternating drug combinations in the treatment of advanced Hodgkin's disease. N. Engl. J. Med. 306:770–775, 1982.
26. Bonadonna, G., DeLena, M., Monfardini, S. et al. Clinical trials with bleomycin in lymphomas and in solid tumors. Eur. J. Cancer 8:205–215, 1972.
27. Iacovino, J.R., Leitner, J., Abbas, A.K. et al. Fatal pulmonary reaction from low doses of bleomycin. An idiosyncratic tissue response. JAMA 235:1253–1255, 1976.
28. Phillips, T.L. and Fu, K.K. Quantification of combined radiation therapy and chemotherapy effects on critical normal tissues. Cancer 37:1186–1200, 1976.
29. Lamoureux, K.B. Increased clinically symptomatic pulmonary radiation reactions with adjuvant chemotherapy. Cancer Chemother. Rep. (part 1) 58:705–708, 1974.
30. Santoro, A., Vivian, S., Pagnon et al. Long-term therapeutic and toxicologic results of MOPP-RT-MOPP vs ABVD-RT-ABVD in PS B-III Hodgkin's disease. ASCO C-777, 1985.
31. Catane, R., Schwade, J.G., Turrisi, A.T. et al. Pulmonary toxicity after radiation and bleomycin: A review. Int. J. Radiat. Oncol. Biol. Phys. 5:1513–1518, 1979.
32. Mansfield, C.M., Kimler, B.F., Henderson, S.D. et al. Development of normal tissue damage in the rat subsequent to thoracic irradiation and prior treatment with cancer chemotherapeutic agents. Am. J. Clin. Oncol. (CCT) 7:425–430, 1984.
33. Collis, C.H., Down, J.D., Pearson, A.E. et al. Bleomycin and radiation induced lung damage in mice. Br. J. Radiol. 56:21–26, 1983.
34. Einhorn, L., Krause, M., Hornback, N. et al. Enhanced pulmonary toxicity with bleomycin and radiotherapy in oat cell lung cancer. Cancer 37:2414–2416, 1976.
35. Hellman, S. and Botnick, L.E. Stem cell depletion: An explanation of the late effects of cytotoxins. Int. J. Radiat. Oncol. Biol. Phys. 2:181–184, 1977.
36. Slanina, J., Musshoff, K., Rahner, T. et al. Long term side effects in irradiated patients with Hodgkin's disease. Int. J. Radiat. Oncol. Biol. Phys. 2:1–19, 1977.
37. Host, H. and Vale, J.R. Lung function after mantle field irradiation in Hodgkin's disease. Cancer 32:328–332, 1973.
38. Evans, R.F., Sagerman, R.H., Ringrose, T.L. et al. Pulmonary function following mantle-field irradiation for Hodgkin's disease. Radiology 111:729–731, 1974.
39. Morgan, G.W., Freeman, A.P., McLean, R.G. et al. Late cardiac, thyroid and pulmonary sequelae of mantle radiotherapy for Hodgkin's disease. Int. J. Radiat. Oncol. Biol. Phys. 11:1925–1931, 1985.
40. Lassvik, C., Rosengren, B., and Wranne, B. Pulmonary gas exchange following irradiation of cervical, mediastinal, hilar and axillary nodes. Acta Radiol. 16:27–31, 1977.
41. Libshitz, H.I. and Banner, M.P. Spontaneous pneumothorax as a complication of radiation therapy to the thorax. Radiology 112:199–201, 1974.
42. Jochelson, M., Tarbell, N.J. and Weinstein, H.J. Unusual thoracic radiographic findings in children treated for Hodgkin's disease. J. Clin. Oncol. 4(6):874–882, 1986.
43. Lote, K., Dahl, O., and Vigander, T. Pneumothorax during combination chemotherapy. Cancer 47:1743–1745, 1981.
44. Tucker, A.S., Newman, A.J., and Alvorado, C. Pulmonary, pleural, and thoracic changes complicating chemotherapy. Radiology 125:805–809, 1977.
45. D'Angio, G.T. and Iannacoccone, G. Spontaneous pneumothorax as a complication of pulmonary metastases in malignant tumors of childhood. Am. J. Roentgenol. 86:1092–1102, 1961.

CHAPTER 14

Renal and Genitourinary Complications from the Treatment of Hodgkin's Disease

SUSAN M. DIAMOND
MOSHE LEVI

HODGKIN'S DISEASE AND THE KIDNEY

A rare clinical problem for physicians practicing in the 1980s, renal and genitourinary function impairment has been an important cause of morbidity and mortality in patients with Hodgkin's disease.[1,2] Although Hodgkin's disease infrequently affects the kidney and genitourinary system directly, in earlier years, radiation and chemotherapy were associated with a high incidence of radiation nephritis, acute tubular necrosis, and hemorrhagic cystitis. Today, with a better knowledge of the adverse affects of radiation and chemotherapy, and better means of preventing most of the side effects, the kidney and the genitourinary tract are better protected, and most of the earlier mentioned complications are usually avoided. This chapter reviews some of the more common renal and genitourinary complications of Hodgkin's disease.

PRIMARY RENAL COMPLICATIONS OF HODGKIN'S DISEASE

The primary renal complications of Hodgkin's disease include: (1) infiltrative disease; (2) glomerulonephritis; (3) amyloidosis; and (4) renal vein thrombosis.

Infiltrative Disease. The incidence of renal involvement has been estimated from the various autopsy studies at approximately 15%.[3,4,5] Bone marrow involvement has been correlated with a higher incidence of renal lesions, presumably because it indicates more widespread disease. Most often, renal involvement is bilateral and in the form of multiple nodules.[6] Solitary involvement of the kidney has not been reported and is extremely rare even in lymphoma, where the kidney may be the primary site of disease.[5] The infiltrative lesions in Hodgkin's disease do not usually result in a significant impairment of renal function,[7] although cases of renal failure associated with Hodgkin's disease,[8,9] with improvement in renal function following successful chemotherapy, have been reported.

Glomerulonephritis. Glomerulonephritis is considered a paraneoplastic syndrome associated with Hodgkin's disease.[10] The incidence of glomerulonephritis and the frequency of specific glomerular lesions are difficult to estimate because much of the literature consists of case reports in which no renal biopsies were performed. The association of renal involvement in Hodgkin's disease is, however, infrequent. Most patients with Hodgkin's disease and renal involvement have the nephrotic syndrome. The nephrotic syndrome usually occurs concomitantly with other manifestations of the disease, or within several months of the diagnosis of Hodgkin's disease. Almost uniformly, the nephrotic syndrome resolves when Hodgkin's disease regresses with chemotherapy or radiation therapy, but it may reappear with relapses.[11-16] As the nephrotic syndrome resolves with the treatment of Hodgkin's disease, hypertension, azotemia, and renal failure are rare sequelae.

Minimal change disease or lipoid nephrosis is the glomerular lesion most often confirmed by biopsy.[10,14,15,16] There are additional case reports of proliferative,[17,18] membranoproliferative,[15,19] focal sclerosing,[19,20] and membranous[21] glomerulonephritis. In a minority of cases, the renal lesions cannot be classified. The etiology of the glomerular lesions remains uncertain. In one case, proliferative glomerulonephritis has been associated with immunoglobulin deposition.[18] But in most instances, no immunologic mechanism causing renal damage is apparent. Because the renal pathology closely parallels the clinical course of Hodgkin's disease, some investigators have suggested that the tumor may elaborate a toxic factor. In this regard, lymphokines that damage the glomerular basement membrane and alter glomerular permeability have been thought to play a role in the development of glomerulonephritis. In view of the alterations in T-cell function in Hodgkin's disease, a role for lymphokinase and other immunoregulatory molecules in the pathogenesis of the glomerular lesions seems likely.

Amyloidosis. Amyloidosis was first reported to be associated with Hodgkin's disease in 1856 by Wilks based on autopsy findings that suggested the coexistance of these entities.[22] With increasing awareness of the association between amyloidosis and Hodgkin's disease, physicians began diagnosing amyloidosis in these patients with greater frequency.[23] One clue to the diagnosis of amyloidosis is the presence of significant proteinuria. The nephrotic syndrome is found in over one half of the cases.[24] The prognosis of amyloidosis complicating Hodgkin's disease is poor, with death generally occurring within one year of its documentation.

Prior to 1970, the occurrence of both amyloidosis and Hodgkin's disease was reported to be between 3 and 8% of the total cases of Hodgkin's disease.[7] Currently, amyloidosis is rarely seen and no longer presents a significant problem for the clinician. The significant decrease in the number of patients with Hodgkin's disease also having amyloidosis may have resulted from the successful use of chemotherapy, eliminating the chronic antigenic stimulus that is believed to initiate amyloid deposition.

The pathogenesis of amyloidosis in Hodgkin's disease remains unresolved. Several forms of amyloid protein have been described. In the variety of amyloid associated with multiple myeloma and also in primary amyloidosis, the amyloid protein is composed of immunoglobulins. A second kind of amyloid is seen in patients with persistent antigenic stimuli, as in rheumatoid arthritis, chronic familial Mediterranean fever, and malignancies other than multiple myeloma. The amyloid fibrils are composed of amyloid protein derived from serum amyloid protein, which behaves as an acute phase reactant. It is the secondary type of amyloidosis that is associated with Hodgkin's disease and typically involves the parenchymous organs—the liver, spleen, and kidney, as opposed to primary amyloid, which is associated with deposition in the heart, tongue, and skin. Other forms of amyloid proteins have been described in familial amyloid polyneuropathy and amyloid associated with certain endocrine disorders.[25] Early reports related the development of amyloid protein to the treatment of Hodgkin's disease with drug combinations, some of which included nitrogen mustard.[26,27] Experimental evidence in support of this observation has been provided.[28] Increased deposition of amyloid protein in mice treated with subcutaneous injections of nitrogen mustard and sodium caseinate, as compared to mice that received only the control vehicle sodium caseinate, has been demonstrated. The importance of chemotherapy in initiating the development of amyloidosis remains unclear, however, as amylodosis developed rapidly in this animal model following treatment. Furthermore, amyloidosis can also develop in patients with untreated Hodgkin's disease.

Renal Vein Thrombosis. Renal-vein thrombosis may be a complication of Hodgkin's disease in patients with the nephrotic syndrome, usually associated with either membranous nephropathy, lipoid nephrosis, or amyloidosis.[29] The nephrotic syndrome is a hypercoagulable state. The urinary loss of proteins stimulate the liver to synthesize fibrinogen and various other clotting factors that predispose the patient to thrombosis. In addition, the urinary loss of antithrombin III, a heparin cofactor, as well as protein C and S may also play an important role in the pathogenesis of renal-vein thrombosis.[30,31]

RENAL COMPLICATIONS FOLLOWING THERAPY

The renal complications following therapy of Hodgkin's disease include: (1) renal dysfunction secondary to cardiac and thyroid disease; and (2) deleterious effects of radiation or chemotherapy leading to the impairment of renal and/or genitourinary function.[32]

CARDIAC AND THYROID INVOLVEMENT AFFECTING THE KIDNEY

Kidney function may be indirectly impaired by complications of Hodgkin's disease and its treatment, thereby affecting the heart and thyroid gland. Acute pericarditis resulting from radiotherapy to the chest, or cardiomyopathy caused by doxorubicin, may lead to decreased cardiac output, resulting in decreased renal blood flow and prerenal azotemia. In addition, hyponatremia may also be observed. The decrease in serum sodium may result from a decrease in the "effective" arterial blood volume, which results in (1) stimulation of the nonosmotic release of antidiuretic hormone; and (2) an increase in sympathetic tone causing a decrease in glomerular filtration rate and an increase in the proximal reabsorption of sodium, which all impair the ability of the kidney to dilute the urine.[33]

Additionally, hypothyroidism caused by radiation injury can result in peripheral edema. This may occur secondary to hypothyroid cardiomyopathy or myxedema. Myxedema has been associated with increased capillary permeability and sodium binding to the anionic mucopolysaccharides in the subcutaneous tissue, leading to excess salt and water retention with edema formation. Hyponatremia and an impaired diluting capacity may also occur; however, the mechanism underlying this disturbance is unsettled. The syndrome of inappropriate antidiuretic hormone (SIADH), impaired renal hemodynamics (specifically decreased glomerular filtration rate and renal blood flow), and chronic hypercapnia may all contribute to the decreased excretion of free water.[34]

RADIATION THERAPY

Nephropathy. Although earlier descriptions exist, Domagk in 1927 was the first to diagnose and report a case of radiation nephropathy that occurred in a 9-year-old girl who received radiation for tuberculous mesenteric lymph nodes.[35] This, and subsequent clinical observations, were ignored for a number of years because studies of the acute effects of sublethal doses of radiation on renal function in dogs led physicians to believe that the kidneys were radioresistant.[36] It was not until the 1950s that these conclusions came into doubt. Luxton is credited with the first comprehensive description of a series of 27 patients.[37] Based on a number of problematic cases using high-dose radiation with subsequent renal complications, Luxton and coworkers proposed that 2300 cGy given over 5 weeks was the maximal tolerable dose.[38] Doses higher than 2300 cGy have been associated with unilateral renal destruction[39] and hence are avoided in present-day practice.[40]

Improved techniques of radiation therapy and proper shielding of the kidney have significantly decreased the incidence of radiation nephritis or, more properly designated, radiation nephropathy because there is rarely evidence of an inflammatory process.[41,42] In one series of over 1200 patients with Hodgkin's disease treated with radiation therapy since 1961, no cases of radiation nephritis were reported.[2] In another series, a smaller group consisting of 23 patients with stage IA to IIIB Hodgkin's disease were followed for 3 to 6 years.[43] These patients were treated with extended-field radiation that included the spleen, which unavoidably irradiates the upper pole of the left kidney. These investigators found that the patients had good tumor control with little evidence of renal complications. In this study, of the 17 patients who underwent evaluation of renal function, all maintained a normal serum blood-urea nitrogen and creatinine level. One patient developed hypertension associated with a 30-pound weight gain, while only one of the four patients who were hypertensive prior to radiation therapy remained hypertensive. Renal scan done with ^{99m}Tc-DPTA did, however, show decreased activity in the upper pole of the left kidney in 10 of 16 cases, while excretory studies obtained using ^{131}I hippurate indicated that the anatomic lesion was not associated with any constant functional impairment. Similar findings have been reported in 74 patients who were also treated with irradiation of the spleen for Hodgkin's disease and nonHodgkin's lymphoma.[44] In this study, creatinine clearances were normal in all patients studied 3 to 5 years following radiation treatment, in spite of some abnormalities detected in the superior pole of the left kidney by ^{131}I hippuran and ^{99m}Tc-DTPA renal scan as well as the latent appearance of cortical atrophy in the same location evident on renal tomograms 18 months after therapy. These clinical studies document that while modern techniques of radiation therapy may cause some damage to the renal tissue, overall function is well preserved, and radiation nephropathy is no longer a routine consequence of treatment with carefully planned and executed radiotherapy. Cases of radiation nephropathy, however, are still occasionally reported following treatment of Wilms' tumors, seminomas of the testes, ovarian carcinoma, and retroperitoneal nonHodgkin's lymphoma.[42] In these cases, the kidneys are in the way of the radiation beams and therefore are at great risk to develop radiation nephropathy.

Pathology. Current knowledge of the pathogenesis of radiation nephritis is derived from human renal biopsy and autopsy studies and from animal experiments.[45-49] Still debate continues about which structures are most sensitive to radiation and where the initial damage occurs. The course and severity of the lesions also depend on the volume of tissue irradiated, the total dosage delivered, the dose per fraction, and the time over which radiation is given.[42] No clear pattern of injury and response by the kidney has been outlined as of the writing of this chapter.

Glomeruli. The response of glomeruli to radiation injury may vary from focal areas of fibrinoid necrosis to complete hyalinization.[50] Experimental studies in rats and mice confirm that the glomeruli are sensitive to damaging effects of radiation.[47,51,52] In mice, Glastein demonstrated that either a single large dose of radiation (1100 to 1900 cGy) or a larger dose of radiation (3500 to 5000 cGy) given sequentially over 10 treaments in 9 days caused striking alterations in the glomerular histology well before the development of tubular atrophy. Blood vessels larger than the capillaries were only minimally involved.[47] Employing a rat model of radiation injury, Madriazo and coworkers demonstrated significant glomerular lesions by electron microscopy 4 to 6 days after a single dose of radiation (4800 or 9600 cGy); these were the first signs of renal injury.[51,52] In fact, in mice and rats, the glomeruli appear to be the most sensitive element of the kidney to radiation injury, in contrast to dogs and rabbits where glomerular lesions represent secondary changes.[53] The pathologic changes in response to radiation injury in mice and rats, as well as humans, are similar. There is glomerular endothelial cell swelling with separation of these cells from the basement membrane. Electron micoscopy reveals subendothelial expansion and deposition of electron lucent material on the endothelial side of the basement membrane with splitting of the basement membrane.[42,53-55] Depending on the extent of the vascular damage and the severity of the accompanying hypertension, total glomerular hyalinization may replace the more benign lesions just described.

Tubulointerstitial Cells. Tubular damage may be part of the early lesions in radiation nephropathy. This involves mostly the cells of the proximal convoluted tubule.[55] Initially, the renal interstitium may be edematous with congestion. As the injury progresses (chronic radiation nephritis), the interstitial edema is replaced by fibrosis.[55]

Blood Vessels. Fibrinoid necrosis and minimal thickening of the arterioles are prominent features of radiation nephropathy. The relationship between these vascular lesions and radiation therapy, however, has been difficult to clarify because not all patients who have radiation therapy initially have significant vascular lesions.[50] Furthermore, these vascular changes in other circumstances are attributed to elevated blood pressure irrespective of the etiology of the renal insufficiency. These conflicting observations have prompted several investigators to conduct animal studies to sort out the cause-and-effect relationship of these vascular lesions, hypertension, and radiation nephritis. Early studies in animals demonstrated that radiation therapy can cause vascular lesions. Fisher and Hellstrom showed that this effect of radiation could be disassociated from that of hypertension.[46] In their experiment in the rat, these investigators placed a clip on one renal artery causing hypertension and this maneuver was followed by bilateral irradiation. With this protocol, vascular changes were noted in both kidneys. Since the clipped kidney should have been protected from the effect of hypertension, these lesions were proposed to have been caused by radiation treatment. In another study, Asscher et al. subjected a group of rats to irradiation followed by the induction of hypertension in a subset of rats via unilateral nephrectomy and renal artery clipping of the remaining kidney.[47] They showed that no vascular lesions developed in the rats that failed to become hypertensive. Thus, irradiation alone did not produce vascular changes, but rather sensitized the vessels to the damaging effects of hypertension. The experimental evidence is thus confusing, and the contribution of hypertension to human vascular pathology remains unresolved.

Clinical Manifestations and Treatment. Radiation injury to the kidney presents in two distinct clinical forms, which was first described in a large series of patients by Luxton.[37,57] Acute radiation nephropathy, which comprised 13 of the original 27 cases described by Luxton, derives its name from the rapid and severe course that usually appears 6 to 12 months following therapy. Patients with acute radiation nephropathy traditionally present with severe hypertension and symptoms of renal insufficiency, including lassitude, vomiting, headache, dyspnea on exertion, and peripheral edema. Their laboratory tests reveal a deterioration of renal function, a normocytic normochromic anemia, proteinuria, hematuria, and granular casts. Proteinuria ranges from 0.5 to 4 g per day, but is usually less than 2 g per day. Serial radioisotope renograms may be useful in distinguishing acute radiation nephritis from Hodgkin's disease.[58,59]

At the present time, no effective therapy is available for prevention or treatment of acute radiation nephritis. One study showed that dogs and patients were protected against the development of radiation therapy nephropathy by the infusion of epinephrine into the renal artery during radiotherapy.[60] The number of patients involved was small and this experimental treatment cannot be recommended. In a case report, where radiation nephritis was complicated with disseminated intravascular coagulation, heparin ameliorated while prednisone aggravated the clinical course of acute radiation nephritis.[61] Currently, therapy is aimed at controlling complications. Hypertension is usually treated medically, while advanced renal failure may necessitate the institution of dialytic therapy.

Prior renal disease and the use of certain chemotherapeutic agents in conjunction with radiation therapy have been shown to decrease the renal threshold to injury. Several drug regimens when used prior to or concomitently with radiation therapy, have been linked with increased incidence of radiation nephropathy. Synergy between radiation and chemotherapy has been reported with the use of the following drugs: (1) cyclophosphamide and doxorubicin in a child with neuroblastoma;[62] (2) actinomycin D and vincristine in two cases of nephroblastoma;[63] and (3) bleomycin and vinblastine in testicular cancer.[64] When using these drug regimens with radiation therapy, radiation nephropathy occurs much sooner than would be expected. Evidence of radiation nephropathy may appear in 4 to 6 weeks following treatment, instead of 6 to 12 months after therapy.

Chronic radiation nephropathy may evolve from the acute form or may have a smouldering course over several years.[57] In either case, the clinical presentation and pathology is similar to other patients with chronic interstitial nephritis, but they may have severe hypertension secondary to vascular damage produced by radiation injury. In addition, these patients present with evidence of renal interstitial damage, including proteinuria (usually less than 2 g/day), pyuria, hematuria, and hyporeninemic hypoaldosteronism, causing hyperkalemic, hyperchloremic metabolic acidosis.[42] Chronic radiation nephritis usually pursues a prolonged and indolent course and is usually not a cause of mortality.[57] In the initial description of radiation nephropathy, these other syndromes were felt to be associated with renal exposure to radiation: (1) asymptomatic proteinuria; (2) benign hypertension; and (3) malignant hypertension. These three syndromes probably represent part of the spectrum of chronic radiation nephropathy.

Obtaining an estimate of kidney size is most valuable in patients with chronic radiation nephropathy and hypertension. A significant discrepancy in renal size may indicate the presence of radiation-induced ischemic renal injury to one of the kidneys. The removal of the injured kidney has been reported to ameliorate the hypertension.[65–68]

In surviving patients treated with radiotherapy when they were children, another long-term effect is renal artery stenosis or occlusion.[69] The affected patients present with hypertension years after treatment, which is caused by injury to the large- and medium-size arteries. Larger doses of irradiation in smaller vessels result in occlusion, whereas smaller doses of radiation in larger vessels cause stenosis or hypoplasia.[69] These patients present with severe hypertension secondary to these renovascular lesions and can be differentiated from those with radiation nephropathy by their disproportionately elevated selective renal-vein renins, their lack of proteinuria, and their normal renal function. Their abnormal vasculature is easily delineated by angiography.[70,71] Potentially, these vascular malformations can be corrected by revascularization procedures[69] or by nephrectomy,[70] especially when an impaired blood supply has rendered the kidney nonfunctional. Similar to the situation in chronic radiation nephrectomy, removal of the unsalvageable kidney has cured the patients' hypertension.

Genitourinary Effects of Radiation. Ureteral injury secondary to radiation therapy rarely occurs. The ureters are considered radioresistant.

With supervoltage x-ray therapy and better means of shielding the bladder, radiation cystitis in the 1980s is an uncommon problem. Both acute and chronic forms of radiation cystitis, however, may complicate treatment when radiotherapy is begun within 3 weeks of surgery.[72]

Acute radiation cystitis develops when over 3000 cGy are delivered to the pelvic area in 3 to 4 weeks. The symptoms include dysuria, frequency, and nocturia; gross hematuria does not usually develop. Cystoscopy, when performed during an episode of acute radiation cystitis, reveals hyperemia, petechiae, occasional ulcers, and significant edema of the bladder mucosa. Acute radiation cystitis is self-limited, resolving without sequelae.

Chronic radiation cystitis has been reported in patients as early as 4 months after treatment and as late as 4 years after treatment. In chronic radiation cystitis, cystoscopy reveals tortuous blood vessels, bleeding ulcers, erythemia, and edema of the bladder mucosa. Interstitial fibrosis, obliterative endarteritis, and telangiectases are the most common microscopic findings.[73] Further problems occur when improper radiation tehniques are used. A small contracted bladder, fistulae (ureteralvesical, retrovesical, and vesicovaginal), and adhesions are additonal complications.

CHEMOTHERAPY

Nephrotoxicity. Combination chemotherapy is currently the treatment modality of choice in disseminated Hodgkin's disease (Stage IIIB and IV). Probably the most commonly used regimen is MOPP (nitrogen mustard, vincristine, procarbazine, and prednisone). Those who fail MOPP are frequently given ABVD (doxorubicin, bleomycin, vinblastine, and DTIC). Other regimens including BVPP (BCNU, cyclophosphamide, vinblastine, procarbazine, and prednisone) and single agents have been used in providing palliation.

Despite the large number of drugs used in the treatment of Hodgkin's disease, nephrotoxicity is not a major complication of therapy. However, 17 of 18 patients given BCNU in excess of 1.5 g/M^2 over a year for brain tumors developed impaired renal function.[74,75] In these patients, renal insufficiency developed insidiously without any abnormalities in the urinary sediment, evidence of hypersensitivity, or documented episodes of acute renal failure. Kidney biopsies obtained in 7 of 17 cases revealed chronic interstitial nephritis without immunoglobulin deposition in the kidney. In some patients, renal function continued to deteriorate despite the cessation of chemotherapy.[74,76] Most likely, the renal insufficiency is the result of a direct toxic effect of the BCNU, but the pathogenesis of the continuing renal damage is unknown. The renal toxicity of BCNU has not been reported in patients receiving this therapy for Hodgkin's disease.

Therapy with cyclophosphamide and vincristine may cause hyponatremia. Cyclophosphamide administration has been associated with impaired water excretion, weight gain, inappropriately concentrated urine, and dilutional hyponatremia when given in doses of more than 50 mg/kg intravenously.[77,78] Several studies have documented no consistent change in the glomerular filtration rate or solute excretion after intravenous cyclophosphamide, suggesting either a hemodynamic or tubular effect as the cause of this syndrome.[79–81] The onset of the electrolyte derangements occur within 4 to 8 hours of administration of cyclophosphamide and resolves within 24 hours, a time course related to the excretion of the active metabolites of cyclophosphamide. Further consideration has been given to whether the metabolites stimulate the release of antidiuretic hormone or vasopressin. Defronzo et al.[81] measured vasopressin levels in three patients given high-dose intravenous cyclophosphamide and in only one patient could the increase in urine osmolality be accounted for by the concomitant rise of vasopressin. Direct tumor release of vasopressin seems unlikely as the cause of these derangements because the patients studied have included those with leukemia and asplastic anemia. Whether this effect of cyclophosphamide is the direct result of toxicity directed at the distal tubules or represents an increased sensitivity of the tubules to vasopressin remains unresolved.

With vincristine therapy, on the other hand, the syndrome of inappropriate antidiuretic hormone (SIADH) has clearly been documented as the cause of the hyponatremia. These cases are characterized by a significant decrease in serum osmolarity, an inappropriately concentrated urine, and an elevated vasopressin level.[82] This syndrome coincides with the appearance of other signs of vincristine toxicity, including peripheral neuropathy and adynamic ileus in both adults and children.[83–86]

Genitourinary Complications. Cyclophosphamide is the chemotherapeutic agent most often associated with bladder toxicity, an association recognized since 1961. Animal studies have shown that the metabolites of cyclophosphamide are directly toxic to the bladder mucosa. Two major complications of cyclophosphamide therapy have been reported. Bladder fibrosis occurs when dosages of cyclophosphamide exceed 6 g/M^2 of body-surface area.[87] The second and far more common complication of cyclophosphamide therapy is hemorrhagic cystitis. The incidence of hemorrhagic cystitis varies in different series, ranging from 2 to 40% of patients treated depending on the dosage used, dose schedule, and duration of treatment. Radiation therapy to the pelvis in conjunction with cyclophosphamide therapy significantly raises the incidence of bladder complication.[88] Cystitis usually resolves 2 to 6 weeks after the cyclophosphamide is discontinued.[89] There is at least one report of this complication in patients treated with cyclophosphamide for Hodgkin's disease.[90] Similarly, a case of hemorrhagic cystitis in a young black male patient receiving MOPP therapy for Hodgkin's disease, which was clinically and histologically similar to that induced by cyclophosphamide, was reported.[91] Additionally, one case of hematuria seen after treatment with procarbazine was reported.[92]

A retrospective study of de novo bladder cancer, involving patients treated with cyclophosphamide for nonuroepithelial neoplasm showed a ninefold increase in the incidence of bladder cancer.[93] Specifically in Hodgkin's disease, cyclophosphamide, most often used in conjunction with radiation therapy, has been associated with the following bladder tumors: (1) squamous cell cancer;[94] (2) transitional cell carcinoma;[93] (3) fibrosarcoma;[95] (4) fibroblastic tumor;[96] and (5) leiomyosarcoma.[97] In all of these case reports, the patients received cyclophosphamide for several years as a part of maintenance therapy.[93,98-100]

Patients who have received oral cyclophosphamide therapy for a long period of time should, therefore, have regular follow-up visits. If hematuria is noted, then a comprehensive work-up, including cystoscopy and retrograde urography, is indicated to rule out a neoplastic process.

ACKNOWLEDGEMENTS

The authors would like to thank Ms. Ginny Mitchell for expert secretarial assistance, and Dr. Mortimer J. Lacher and Dr. John R. Redman for inviting us to be part of this courageous undertaking.

REFERENCES

1. Fer, M.J. et al. Cancer and the kidney: renal complications of neoplasm. Am. J. Med. 71:704, 1981.
2. Kaplan, H.S. Hodgkin's Disease. Cambridge, Harvard University Press, 1980.
3. Lalli, A.F. Lymphoma and the urinary tract. Radiology 93:1051, 1969.
4. Wentzell, R.A., Berheigher, S.W. Malignant lymphomatosis of the kidneys. J. Urol. 74:177, 1955.
5. Richmond, J. et al. Renal lesions associated with malignant lymphomas. Am. J. Med. 32:184, 1962.
6. Martinez-Maldonado, M., Ramirez de Arellando, G.A. Renal involvement in malignant lymphomas: A survey of 49 cases. J. Urol. 95:485, 1966.
7. Kiely, J.M., Wagoner, R.D., and Holley, K.E. Renal complications of lymphoma. Ann. Intern. Med. 71:1159, 1969.
8. Champion, A.D., Coup, A.J., and Hancock, B.W. Hodgkin's disease and chronic renal failure. Cancer 38:1867, 1976.
9. McNeal, R.M. et al. Hodgkin's disease presenting as renal failure: improvement in renal lesion and renal function with chemotherapy. J. Pediatr. Nephrol. 2:99, 1981.
10. Eagan, J.W. and Edmund, J. Glomerulopathies of neoplasia. Kidney Int. 11:297, 1977.
11. Kramer, P., Sizoo, W., and Twiss, E.E. Nephrotic syndrome in Hodgkin's disease. Neth. J. Med. 24:114, 1981.
12. Sherman, R.L., Sartiano, G.P., Vinciguerra, V.P. et al. Nephrotic syndrome in Hodgkin's disease. Ann. Int. Med. 72:805, 1970.
13. Shitara, T. et al. Hodgkin's disease complicated by nephrotic syndrome. New clinical observations on the response of both diseases to radiotherapy to the neck. Am. J. Pediatr. Hematol. Oncol. 3:177, 1981.
14. Walker, F., O'Neill, S., Carmody M. et al. Nephrotic syndrome in Hodgkin's disease. Int. J. Pediatr. Nephrol. 4:39, 1983.
15. Dabbs, D.J., Morel-Maroger, L., Mignon, F. et al. Glomerular lesions in lymphomas and leukemias. Am. J. Med. 80:63–70, 1986.
16. Alpers, C.E. and Cotran, R.S. Neoplasia and glomerular injury. Kidney Int. 30:465, 1986.
17. Moortney, A.V., Zimmerman, S.W., and Burkholder, P.M. Nephrotic syndrome in Hodgkin's disease: evidence for pathogenesis alternative to immune complex deposition. Am. J. Med. 61:471, 1976.
18. Froom, D.W. et al. Immune deposits in Hodgkin's disease with nephrotic syndrome. Arch. Pathol. 94:547, 1972.
19. Powderly, W.G., Cantwell, B.M.J., Fennelly, J.J. et al. Renal glomerulopathies associated with Hodgkin's disease. Cancer 56:874, 1985.
20. Watson, A., Stachura, I., Fragola, J. et al. Focal segmental glomerulosclerosis in Hodgkin's disease. Am. J. Nephrol. 3:228–232, 1983.
21. Hardin, J.G., Jr., Cooke, A.S., and Blinton, J.H. Medicine Grand Rounds. South. Med. J. 62:1111, 1969.
22. Wilks, S. Cases of lardaceous disease and some allied affections. Guys Hosp. Res. 52:103, 1856.
23. Wallace, S.L. et al. Amyloidosis in Hodgkin's Disease. Am. J. Med. 8:552, 1950.
24. Brandt, K., Cathart, E.S., and Cohen, A.S. A clinical analysis of the course and prognosis of 42 patients with amyloidosis. Am. J. Med 44:955, 1968.

25. Glenner, G.G. Amyloid deposits and amyloidosis. N. Engl. J. Med. 302:1333, 1980.
26. Cardell, B.S. The role of cytotoxic agents in the production of amyloidosis in Hodgkin's disease. Br. Med. J. 1:1145, 1961.
27. Spain, D.M. Rapid and extensive development of amyloidosis in association with nitrogen mustard therapy. Am. J. Clin. Pathol. 26:52, 1956.
28. Teilum, G. Studies on the pathogenesis of amyloidosis: II. Effect of nitrogen mustard in inducing amyloidosis. J. Lab. Clin. Med. 43:367, 1954.
29. Llach, F. Acute renal vein thrombosis. In Diseases of the Kidney. Edited by R.W. Schrier and C.W. Gottschalk. Boston, Little Brown and Co., 1988.
30. Kauffman, R.H. et al. Acquired antithrombin III deficiency and thrombosis in the nephrotic syndrome. Am. J. Med. 65:607, 1978.
31. Vigano-D'Angelo, S. et al. Protein S deficiency occurs in the nephrotic syndrome. Ann. Intern. Med. 107:42–47, 1987.
32. Martinez-Maldonado, M. et al. Nonrenal neoplasma and the kidney. In Diseases of the Kidney. Edited by R.W. Schrier and C.W. Gottschalk. Boston, Little Brown and Co., 1988.
33. Bichet, D. and Schrier, R.W. Water metabolism in edematous disorders. Semin. Nephrol. 4:325, 1984.
34. Weiss, N.M. and Robertson, G.L. Water metabolism in endocrine disorders. Semin. Nephrol. 4:303, 1984.
35. Domagk, G. Die Runtgenstrahlenwirkurg auf das Gewebe, im besonderen betrachtet an den Nieren: Morphologische and functionelle veranerungen. Beitraeye zue Pathologoschen Anatomie und zur Allgemenein Pathologie 77:525, 1927.
36. McQuarrier, I. and Whipple, G.H. Study of renal function in roentgen ray intoxication; resistance of renal epithelium to direct radiation. J. Exp. Med. 35:225, 1922.
37. Luxton, R.W. Radiation nephritis. Q. J. Med. 22:25, 1953.
38. Kunkler, P.B., Farr, R.F., and Luxton, R.W. The limit of renal tolerance to x-rays. Br. J. Radiol. 25:190, 1952.
39. Danforth, D.N. and Javadpous, N. Total unilateral renal destruction caused by irradiation for Hodgkin's disease. Urology 5:790, 1975.
40. Castleman, B., Scully, R.E., and McNeely, B.U. Case records of the Massachusetts General Hospital. Weekly clinicopathological exercises. Presentation of a case.
41. Greenberger, J.S., Weichselbaum R.R., and Cassady, J.R.: Radiation nephropathy. In Cancer and the Kidney. Edited by R.E. Rieselbach and M.B. Garnick. Philadelphia, Lea & Febiger, 1982, 814.
42. Arruda, J. Radiation nephritis. In Tubulo-interstitial Nephropathies. Edited by R.S. Cotran. New York, Churchill Livingston Inc., 1983, 275–285.
43. Birkhead, B.M. et al. Assessment of renal function following irradiation of the intact spleen for Hodgkin's Disease. Radiology 130:473, 1979.
44. Le Bourgeois, J.P. et al. Renal consequences of irradiation of the spleen in lymphoma patients. Br. J. Radiol. 52:56, 1979.
45. Antopol, W. and Glaubach, S. Renal Lesions in mice receiving 600 whole body radiation. Fed. Proc. 15:505, 1956.
46. Fischer, E.R. and Hellstrom, H.R. Pathogenesis of hypertension and pathological changes in experimental irradiation. Lab. Invest. 19:530, 1968.
47. Glastein, E., Fagardo, L.F., and Brown, J.M. Radiation injury in the mouse kidney. Int. J. Radiol. Oncol. Biol. Phys. 2:933, 1977.
48. Jordan, S.W., Tuhas, J.M., and Key, C.R. Late effects of unilateral radiation on the mouse kidney. Radiat. Res. 76:429, 1978.
49. Williams, M.V. and Denekamp, J. Sequential functional testing of radiation-induced renal damage in the mouse. Radiat. Res. 94:305, 1983.
50. Hepinstall, R.H. Radiation Injury. In Pathology of the Kidney. Boston, Little, Brown and Co., 1983.
51. Madrazo, A., Suzuki, Y., and Churg, J. Radiation nephritis: acute change following high dose radiation. Am. J. Pathol. 54:507, 1969.
52. Madrazo, A., Suzuki, Y., and Churg, J. Radiation nephritis II: Chronic changes after high doses of radiation. Am. J. Pathol. 61:37, 1970.
53. Rosen, S., Swerdlow, M.A., Mehhrlee, R.C. et al. Radiation nephritis: Light and electron microscopic observations. Am. J. Pathol. 41:487, 1967.
54. Keane, W.F. et al. Radiation induced renal disease: A clinicopathologic study. Am. J. Med. 60:127, 1976.
55. Madrazo, A., Schwarz, G., and Churg, J. Radiation Nephritis: A review. J. Urol. 114:822, 1975.
56. Asscher, A.W., Wilson, C., and Ansson, S.G. Sensation of blood vessels to hypertensive damage by irradiation. Lancet 1:580, 1961.
57. Luxton, R.W. Radiation nephritis: A long-term study of 54 patients. Lancet 2:1221, 1961.
58. Cohen, Y. and Robinson, E. The role of the radioisotope renogram in the diagnosis and evaluation of radiation nephritis. J. Urol. 112:268, 1974.
59. Koholin, V.V. et al. Kidney function study by radioisotope renography in lymphogranulomatosis patients subjected to radiation treatment. Vopr. Onkol. 27:13, 1981.
60. Johnson, R.E. et al. Prevention of radiation nephritis with renal artery infusion of vasoconstrictors. Radiology 91:103, 1968.
61. Cogan, M.G. and Arieff, A.I. Radiation nephritis and intravascular coagulation. Clin. Nephrol. 10:74, 1978.
62. Dhalval R.S. et al. Radiation nephritis with hypertension and hyperreninemia following chemotherapy: cure by nephrectomy. J. Pediatr. 96:68, 1980.
63. Arneil, G.C. et al. Nephritis in two children after irradiation and chemotherapy for nephroblastoma. Lancet 1:960, 1974.
64. Churchill, D.N., Hong, K., and Gault, M.H. Radiation nephritis following combined abdominal radiation and chemotherapy (bleomycin-vinblastine). Cancer 41:2162, 1978.
65. Shapiro, A.P. et al. Hypertension in radiation nephritis. Arch. Int. Med. 137:848, 1977.

66. Crummy, A.B., Hellman, S., Stansel, H.C. et al. Renal hypertension secondary to unilateral radiation damage relieved by nephrectomy. Radiology 84:108, 1965.
67. Kim, T.H., Sommervill, P., Genest, P. et al. Unilateral radiation nephropathy—long-term significance. Int. J. Radiat. Oncol. Biol. Phys. 9:108, 1983, (abstract).
68. Stabb, G.E., Tegtmeyer, C.J., and Constable, W.C. Radiation-induced renovascular hypertension. Am. J. Roentgenol. 126:634, 1976.
69. McGill, C.W., Holder, T.M., Smith, T.H. et al. Post radiation renovascular hypertension. J. Pediatr. Surg. 14:831, 1979.
70. Salvi, S. et al. Renal artery stenosis and hypertension after abdominal irradiation for Hodgkin's disease. Urology 21:611, 1983.
71. Gerlock, A.J. and Goncharenko, V.A. Radiation induced stenosis of the renal artery causing hypertension. J. Urol. 118:1064, 1977.
72. Aron, B.S. and Schlesinger, A. Complications of radiation therapy: The genitourinary tract. Semin. Roentgenol. 9:65, 1974.
73. Goldberg, I.D., Garnick, M.B., and Bloomer, W.D. Urinary tract toxic effects of cancer therapy. J. Urol. 132:1, 1984.
74. Schacht, R.G. et al. Nephrotoxicity of nitrosoureas. Cancer 48:1328, 1981.
75. Schacht, R.G. and Baldwin, D.S. Chronic interstitial nephritis and renal failure due to nitrosourea (NU) therapy. Kidney Int. 14:66, 1978.
76. Schilsky, R.S. Renal and metabolic toxicities of cancer chemotherapy. Semin. Oncol. 9:75, 1982.
77. Healy, H.G. and Clarkson, A.R. Renal complications of cytotoxic therapy. Aust. N.Z. J. Med. 13:531, 1983.
78. Harlow, P.J. et al. Fatal cases of inappropriate ADH secretion induced by cyclophosphamide therapy. Cancer 44:896, 1979.
79. Steele, T.H., Serpick, A.A., and Block, J.B. Antidiuretic response to cyclophosphamide in man. J. Pharmacol. Exp. Ther. 185:245, 1973.
80. DeFronzo, R.A., Braive, H., Calvin, O.M. et al. Water intoxication in man after cyclophosphamide therapy. Ann. Int. Med. 78:86, 1973.
81. DeFronzo, R.A. et al. Cyclophosphamide and the kidney. Cancer 33:483, 1974.
82. Robertson, G.L., Bhoopalam, N., and Zelkowitz, L.J. Vincristine neurotoxicity and abnormal secretion of antidiuretic hormone. Arch. Intern. Med. 132:717, 1973.
83. Cutting, H.O. Inappropriate secretion of antidiuretic hormone secondary to vincristine therapy. Am. J. Med. 51:269, 1971.
84. Fine, R.N., Clarke, R.R., and Shore, N.A. Hyponatremia and vincristine therapy syndrome possibly resulting from inappropriate antidiuretic hormone secretion. Am. J. Dis. Child. 112:256, 1966.
85. Slater, L.M., Wainer, R.A., and Serpick, A.A. Vincristine neurotoxicity with hyponatremia. Cancer 23:122, 1969.
86. Suskind, R.M. and Brusilow, S.W. Syndome of inappropriate secretion of antidiuretic hormone produced by vincristine toxicity (with bioassay of ADH level). J. Pediatr. 81:90, 1972.
87. Johnson, W.W. and Meadows, D.C. Urinary-bladder fibrosis and telangiectasia associated with long term cyclophosphamide therapy. N. Engl. J. Med. 284:290, 1977.
88. Jayalkshamma, B. and Pinkel, D. Urinary bladder toxicity following pelvic irradiation and simultaneous cyclophosphamide therapy. Cancer 28:701, 1976.
89. Watson, N.A. and Notely, R.G. Urologic complications of cyclophosphamide. J. Urol. 45:606, 1973.
90. Reynolds, R.D. et al. Hemorrhagic cystitis due to cyclophosphamide. J. Urol. 101:45, 1969.
91. Royal, J.E. and Suler, R.A. Hemorrhagic cystitis with MOPP therapy. Cancer 41:1261, 1978.
92. Schmidt, J.D. et al. Comparison of procarbazine imidazole-carboxamide and cyclophosphamide in relapsing patients with advanced carcinoma of the phosphate. J. Urol 121:185, 1974.
93. Fairchild, W.V. et al. The incidence of bladder cancer after cyclophosphamide therapy. J. Urol. 122:163, 1979.
94. Wall, R.L. and Caulsen, K.P. Carcinoma of the urinary bladder in patients receiving cyclophosphamide. N. Engl. J. Med. 243:271, 1975.
95. Rupprecht, L. and Blessing, M.H. Fibrosarkom der Harnblase nach siebenjähriger Chemotherapie einer Lymphogranulomatose in Kidesalter. Dtsch. Med. Wochenschr. 98:1663, 1973.
96. Carney, L.N., Stevens, P.S., Fried, F.A. et al. Fibroblastic tumor of the urinary bladder after cyclophosphamide therapy. Arch. Pathol. Lab. Med. 106:247, 1982.
97. Rowland, R.G. and Eble, J.N. Bladder leiomyosarcoma and pelvic fibroblastic tumor following cyclophosphamide therapy. Br. J. Urol. 130:344, 1983.
98. Ansell, J.D. and Castro, J.E. Carcinoma of the bladder complicating cyclophosphamide therapy. Br. J. Urol. 47:413, 1975.
99. Chivalier, R.L. et al. Bladder polyp and heavy proteinuria in a patient with Hodgkin's disease in remission. Cancer 54:777, 1984.
100. Fuchs, E.F. et al. Uroepithelial carcinoma in association with cyclophosphamide ingestion. J. Urol. 126:544, 1981.

CHAPTER 15

Gastrointestinal Complications of Staging and Treatment of Hodgkin's Disease

ELIOT ZIMBALIST
MOSHE SHIKE

Recent advances in the diagnosis and treatment of Hodgkin's disease have resulted in a dramatic improvement in survival.[1,2] The success we are now witnessing in the treatment of this disease has shifted some of the attention from cure to the complications of the diagnostic procedures and treatment. In the current setting of long-term survival and a potential cure rate of 80%,[3] several previously unrecognized complications arising from therapy have emerged. This chapter reviews the gastrointestinal complications that stem from the diagnosis, staging, and treatment of Hodgkin's disease.

THE STAGING LAPAROTOMY

Glatstein and coworkers introduced the staging laparotomy and splenectomy for Hodgkin's disease in 1969.[4] In the subsequent years, numerous reports about the morbidity and mortality from this procedure emerged.[5-10] The overall incidence of complications ranged from 5 to 35%. The wide range of reported complications is the result of differences in patient populations, surgical experience, and the protocol for the staging procedure used in the different institutions. Rutherford[6] compiled the results in nearly 2000 patients from these various reports and found a 6.4% incidence of major complications, such as pulmonary embolus, subphrenic abscess, and intestinal obstruction requiring operations. There were 10 deaths resulting from the staging laparotomy, amounting to a mortality rate of 0.5%, which is comparable to that reported for other groups of patients undergoing elective abdominal exploration.[6] Age-specific mortality rates were not available, but there were generally lower rates in younger patients.

Mechanical small-bowel obstruction secondary to adhesions, volvulus or intussusception, and prolonged paralytic ileus are well-known complications of any abdominal surgery and have been reported in patients with Hodgkin's disease who have undergone a staging laparotomy. Among the first 400 consecutive patients undergoing staging laparotomies at Stanford University Hospital, four cases (1%) of small-bowel obstruction secondary to adhesions occurred.[7] All these patients required surgery for lysis of adhesions and recovered. In a series of 316 patients reported from the Mayo Clinic, major complications due to staging laparotomy occurred in 25 patients (7.9%) and required operation in 6 (1.9%).[8] Included in this group of complications were small-bowel obstruction in one, peritonitis caused by a lymphatic leak in one, and left subphrenic fluid collection in three (of which one was a subphrenic abscess and two were hematomas). All these patients recovered following surgery.

Post-traumatic pancreatic injury during surgery, resulting in both an asymptomatic rise in serum amylase as well as symptomatic pancreatitis, has also been reported.[9] In the previously mentioned Mayo Clinic study,[8] two patients experienced mild pancreatitis. Liver biopsy performed during laparotomy was reported to cause hemobilia and death in one patient.[10] Isolated cases of injury to the colon with resultant fecal fistula have also been reported.[11,12]

In addition to complications arising directly from the operative procedure, the staging laparotomy, as well as any intra-abdominal surgery, has been found to be a predisposing factor for radiation-induced damage to the gastrointestinal tract.[13,14] The staging laparotomy can result in adhesions and an immobility of the bowel, exposing some of its segments to high doses of irradiation. Thus, the staging laparotomy may contribute to the development of radiation enteropathy. In a report on patients with Hodgkin's disease undergoing subdiaphragmatic radiation, the incidence of radiation enteritis was 23% among patients who had exploratory laparotomy, significantly higher than the 7% in patients without previous laparotomy.[13] In this report, age, sex, disease stage, and histology did not seem to affect the rate of radiation-induced gastrointestinal damage.

The potential complications of the staging laparotomy may be avoided by the use of laparoscopic examinations. Laparoscopy has been found to be useful for the staging of Hodgkin's disease[15-18] and may be used with a high degree of accuracy in selected patients; however, it does not provide information as complete as the staging laparotomy. Laparoscopic examination can visualize up to 75% of the liver surface and a portion of the splenic and peritoneal surfaces. Small Hodgkin's disease nodules, undetected by prior abdominal CT scans, may be seen and a biopsy may be performed with direct visualization. By obtaining histologic and visual evidence of Hodgkin's disease in the liver, spleen, or abdominal cavity by laparoscopic examination, surgery may be avoided.

Laparoscopy is not a substitute for a formal staging laparotomy because only a portion of the liver and spleen are evaluated and the retroperitoneal lymph nodes cannot be examined. Another advantage of laparotomy is the ability to do an oophoropexy in young women who will be receiving pelvic irradiation.

The indications for a staging laparoscopy or laparotomy in Hodgkin's disease remain controversial and depend on the approach of the physician or institution.

INTESTINAL COMPLICATIONS OF RADIOTHERAPY

Radiation therapy plays a major role in the treatment of Hodgkin's disease. The gastrointestinal tract is frequently the major normal tissue limiting the dosage of abdominal and pelvic radiation. The incidence and severity of radiation-induced gastrointestinal damage depends primarily on the total radiation dose and its fractionation. However, a number of additional factors have been identified as predisposing an individual to gastrointestinal damage from radiation. These include: the part of the intestine irradiated, previous abdominal surgery, vascular disease from diabetes or hypertension, and concomitant chemotherapy with actinomycin D, doxorubicin, bleomycin, and 5-fluorouracil.

The extent of radiation injury of the gastrointestinal tract depends on the dose of radiation and the radiation sensitivity of the segment to which it is directed. The incidence of serious radiation-induced injury to the intestine increases sharply when the dose exceeds 5000 cGy.[19] Rubin and Casarette have defined the "minimum" and "maximum" doses of radiation tolerated by the intestine.[20] The minimum tolerance dose is defined as the dose at which 1 to 5% of the patients are expected to manifest chronic radiation damage within 5 years of therapy, and the maximum tolerance dose is the dose at which 25 to 50% would develop damage in 5 years. The minimum and maximum dosages vary according to the part of the gastrointestinal tract evaluated. For instance, the stomach has a minimum tolerance dose of 4500 cGy and a maximum tolerance dose of 5000 cGy, while the rectum has a minimum tolerance dose of 5500 cGy and a maximum dose of 8000 cGy.[20]

ACUTE INTESTINAL COMPLICATIONS

The acute effects of radiation on the gastrointestinal tract reflect a disruption of the mucosal cell-renewal system, decreased enzymatic activities, and disturbances of motility and absorption.[21–24] Trier and Browning[23] described the morphology of the small intestinal mucosa following exposure to therapeutic abdominal radiation in nine patients, four of whom had Hodgkin's disease. They noted that within 12 hours following radiotherapy, the number of mitoses in the crypts decreased. The height of the crypt epithelial cells decreased while their width increased, so they assumed a cuboidal appearance. As exposure to radiation continued, cell loss from the villous tips exceeded cell replacement from the crypts. This resulted in shortening of the villi and a decrease in the total absorptive epithelial surface. In contrast to celiac disease in which the villi are also shortened or absent but the crypts are deep, the radiation-induced lesion was shown to be characterized by shortened villi and shallow crypts. There is an infiltration of the lamina propria and submucosa with plasma cells, eosinophils, and polymorphonuclear leukocytes, with occasional crypt-abscess formation. The radiation-induced mucosal lesion was found to be limited to the small bowel directly exposed.

The endoscopic appearance of the intestinal mucosa following radiotherapy is similar to what has been described in the nonspecific inflammatory bowel diseases. Mucosal and submucosal erythema and edema, superficial ulcerations, mucosal friability, and necrosis have all been observed.[24,25] More extensive injury can result in intestinal perforation and formation of fistulas. Adhesions and intestinal stenosis may develop both acutely from edema and chronically from fibrosis. While emphasizing the rarity of perforation during radiation of patients with gastric lymphoma, Elliot and Jenkinson[26] reported a gastric perforation in a patient receiving 2180 cGy because of generalized Hodgkin's disease involving the stomach. They found that the ulcer had occurred in an area not involved with tumor and assumed it was caused by radiation.

Transient symptoms of anorexia, abdominal pain, nausea, vomiting, diarrhea, ulcerations, and bleeding may occur secondary to the acute radiation-induced changes in the gastrointestinal tract. Disrupted mucosal surface, a decreased absorptive surface area, decreased enzyme activity, and disturbances in motility all contribute to these symptoms. More commonly, however, these symptoms are minimal or absent, even when a significant mucosal lesion is present. Since the morphologic changes are limited to segments of the bowel exposed to radiation, the remaining bowel is unaffected and able to compensate for the dysfunction of the radiated segments.[25] The acute effects of radiation on the gastrointestinal tract usually subside within days to weeks after discontinuation of radiotherapy. With the rapid rate of epithelial regeneration, ulcerations heal, inflammation subsides, and symptoms gradually decrease and disappear.

Acute damage to the ileum wih resultant bile salt malabsorption and diarrhea or vitamin B_{12} malabsorption has been reported in patients receiving pelvic radiation for gynecologic malignancies.[24] Although there are no specific reports of this occurring after extended-field radiotherapy in Hodgkin's disease patients, it is a potential problem when the terminal ileum is in the radiation field. Absorptive defects of D-xylose, trioctanoin, and cholylglycin due to losses of mucosal absorptive surface and enzymes have been reported in radiation-induced enteropathy in patients treated for cervical cancer.[25] Whether this occurs after radiotherapy for Hodgkin's patients has not been studied. It must be noted that usually the dose of radiotherapy to patients with gynecologic malignancies (5000 to 6000 cGy) exceeds the usual dose given to patients with Hodgkin's disease (2000 to 4500 cGy).

Acute radiation-induced colitis can occur after abdominal and pelvic radiotherapy. As in the upper intestinal tract, disruption of the mucosal cell-renewal systems results in mucosal erythema, edema, and ulceration. The resultant inflammatory colitis can induce a loss of colonic fluid and electrolyte absorption with severe diarrhea, lower gastrointestinal bleeding, and crampy lower abdominal pain. With time, these acute symptoms usually subside.

CHRONIC INTESTINAL COMPLICATIONS

The true incidence of chronic gastrointestinal damage following abdominal irradiation is unknown. It has been estimated to occur in about 1 to 2% of patients with gynecologic malignancies[27,28] and in up to 10% of patients receiving radiotherapy for various other abdominal neoplasms.[20,29,30] The interval from time of radiation exposure to presentation with symptoms of chronic radiation enteritis may vary from 2 months to over 30 years.[29-32]

The mechanisms of the late effects of radiation on the intestinal tract involve progressive damage to the supportive stroma and vasculature. This results in an endarteritis of the submucosal vessels with subsequent fibrous and thrombotic obliteration of the small intestinal arterioles. The vascular damage leads to progressive ischemia with various clinical manifestations.

Most commonly, patients with chronic radiation enteritis present with recurrent abdominal pain. The pain is due to intestinal obstruction or a motility disorder secondary to progressive fibrosis of the intestinal wall. Other clinical presentations include diarrhea and malabsorption, chronic gastrointestinal blood loss and anemia, bloody mucoid discharge due to proctitis, abdominal fistulas,[33] and intestinal perforation. Diarrhea and malabsorption occur secondary to extensive damage to the surface epithelium, lymphatic obstruction, bacterial overgrowth, or bile salt deficiency from damage to the terminal ileum.

Chronic radiation damage has also been reported in the stomach and esophagus of patients with Hodgkin's disease who have had radiation to these organs. Kellum et al.[31] described gastric ulcers, hemorrhagic gastritis, radiation-induced pseudotumor, and pyloric stricture in six patients treated with a cumulative dose of at least 4500 cGy for Hodgkin's disease and other lymphomas. These complications occurred from 2 months to 11½ years after irradiation.

During the course of mantle radiotherapy, acute esophagitis can occur. Several years later this can develop into fibrous stenosis of the esophagus or a bronchioesophageal fistula.[34-36] In a collaborative study of Hodgkin's disease, there was one case of esophageal stenosis and stricture requiring bypass surgery, with death ensuing as a complication of this surgery.[37] Radiation damage to the esophagus may also result in the development of inflammatory pseudopolyps and dysphagia.[38]

We have treated patients who developed dysphagia due to benign esophageal strictures after mantle radiotherapy. These patients were successfully managed with esophageal dilatation. Initial dilatation may at times require the use of the more sophisticated dilators (such as Eder-Peustow or pneumatic dilators) but subsequently patients can be dilated with bougies such as Maloney or Savory dilators.

MANAGEMENT OF INTESTINAL RADIATION INJURY

The management of radiation injury to the intestinal tract can be divided into preventive measures and therapeutic measures. The therapy for radiation enteritis can be further subdivided into medical and surgical.

The incidence of radiation enteritis is minimized by careful attention to the time, dose, and fractionation of radiation, use of multiple fields, and calculation of dose to be administered.[39] If the patient had either prior abdominal surgery or a previous inflammatory abdominal process, a preradiation barium study to exclude fixed loops of bowel in the radiation field can be helpful in adjusting the dose and radiation field. Results of recent experiments have demonstrated a cytoprotective effect of prostaglandin E2 in irradiated rat ileum.[40] Whether this form of pretreatment will be useful in the prevention of human radiation enteropathy remains to be seen.

In evaluating current forms of therapy for radiation enteritis, Haddad et al.[41] identified three clinical groups: Group I. Patients with minimal to moderate symptoms of acute enteritis may be managed with symptomatic medical treatment. This group includes patients with acute symptoms of anorexia, nausea, vomiting, diarrhea, and crampy abdominal pain; Group II. Patients who present with an acute surgical problem, namely intestinal obstruction, perforation, or severe proctitis, requiring emergency surgery; Group III. Patients with chronic radiation enteropathy who have had a long history of intermittent partial obstruction, fistulas, intractable abdominal pain, diarrhea, or blood loss.

The symptoms of Group I patients are caused by direct toxic effects of radiation on the rapidly dividing cells of the intestinal mucosa and usually are self-limited.[42] They can be treated with antiemetic, antispasmotic, or antidiarrhea medications and low-residue lactose-restricted diets.[39] In a report by Donaldson et al.,[43] five children with delayed radiation enteritis secondary to abdominal radiation for lymphomas, Wilms' tumor, rhabdomyosarcoma, or teratoma were treated with a diet free of lactose and gluten and low in fat and fiber. All five patients had symptomatic improvement with the modified diet and their previously abnormal small-bowel roentgenographs and small-bowel biopsies returned to normal. This form of therapy, however, has not been evaluated in a prospective randomized trial. Clinical observations at the Institute Gustave Roussy in France suggest that dietary therapy in the form of a low-residue, low-fat, gluten-free, lactose-free regimen during abdominal radiation can prevent significant bowel injury.[39] Prospective randomized studies substantiating this observation are also required. We have used similar dietary manipulations, mainly after therapy for cervical cancers, and have been impressed with the symptomatic improvement. In patients with radiation-induced diarrhea, we also limit the quantity of food and water per meal and increase the frequency of feedings to six per day.

Anti-inflammatory drugs such as corticosteroids, acetylsalicylates, and salicylazosulfapyridines have been used in the management of acute and chronic radiation enteritis,[44-46] but the benefit of such therapy is controversial. Goldstein et al.[45] found improvement in four patients treated with salicylazosulfapyridines for chronic radiation enteritis. In a report by Rauch and Weiland, 48 of 50 patients with varying degrees of diarrhea during cobalt therapy showed prompt improvement with salicylazosulfapyridines.[46] However, other case reports have found these drugs to be ineffective.[49]

A prospective randomized trial comparing four treatment regimens for chronic radiation enteropathy was reported by Louidice and Lange.[47] Twenty-four patients were randomized to one of four treatment groups: (1) Methylprednisolone, 80 mg intravenously, plus Vivonex-HN (a chemically defined nutrient solution), 2 L/day orally; (2) Methylprednisolone, 80 mg intravenously, plus total parenteral nutrition (TPN), 2.5 L/day; (3) Total parenteral nutrition, 2.5 L/day; and (4) Vivonex-HN, 2 L/day orally. Improvement was gauged by overall nutritional assessment measurements, nitrogen balance data, and by radiologic and clinical parameters. After the patients were treated for an 8-week period, it was found that the treatment regimen of TPN and bowel rest resulted in improvement in the patients' nitrogen balance data and nutritional status. Steroids were found to enhance this effect of TPN; however, when steroids were combined with enteral feedings they were not effective. All patients had varying symptoms of obstruction, diarrhea, and malabsorption; however, there was no comment on how the different forms of therapy affected these symptoms.

Miller et al.[48] reported their experience with 10 patients with chronic radiation enteritis unresponsive to conventional medical and surgical therapy who were placed on long-term home TPN. The indications for radiotherapy included carcinoma of the colon, ovary, cervix, or bladder. The average duration of home TPN was 15.7 months (range 1 to 52 months). These patients had improvement in their nutritional status manifested by weight gain and an increase in serum albumin. Six of the patients were alive and at home; at the time of this report four patients died, two from recurrent cancer, the third from a cerebrovascular accident, and the fourth from ischemic bowel necrosis. In a similar fashion, Lavery et al.[49] treated five patients with functional and/or anatomic short bowel resulting from radiation enteritis with home TPN.[53] He was also able to maintain or improve the nutritional status of the patients. However, it remains doubtful whether the nutritional manipulations truly modify the primary damage to the bowel.[50]

In our experience in 24 patients with gynecologic malignancies and chronic radiation enteritis who were referred for nutritional management, the onset of symptoms occurred between 5 months and 6 years following radiation therapy. The most common manifestation was that of weight loss (83%), followed by diarrhea (63%) and nausea and vomiting (46%). Investigations revealed various degrees of malabsorption. Successful management of the nutritional problems of these patients has been accomplished by dietary modifications (low-fat, low-fiber diets with mineral and vitamin supplementation), home enteral feeding, or home TPN in cases of severe malabsorption.

When evaluating a patient with chronic radiation enteropathy who develops diarrhea, treatable causes should not be overlooked. Bile salt malabsorption secondary to radiation-induced ileal damage can produce diarrhea, which responds to cholestryramine and a low-fat diet.[51] Bacterial overgrowth secondary to impaired motility, strictures, or fistulas may be treated with antibiotics; however, some form of surgery is usually necessary to correct the primary lesion that predisposed to bacterial overgrowth.

Surgical management of radiation enteritis can be extremely difficult. Patients who require emergency surgery should be treated preoperatively by controlling sepsis and correction of fluid and electrolyte imbalance. In addition, if the patient is malnourished or a prolonged course of inadequate oral intake is anticipated, supporting these patients with parenteral nutrition is advisable. The choice of a surgical procedure in patients who present with chronic symptoms of obstruction due to strictures, fistulas, intractable abdominal pain, diarrhea, and severe bleeding unresponsive to medical therapy is controversial. Swan and his colleagues,[52] in a review of the literature, noted a lower operative mortality (10% versus 21%) and a lower incidence of anastomotic dehiscence (6% versus 36%) in patients having intestinal bypass in comparison to those treated with resection. They therefore suggested that simple bypass of the involved segment of intestine provides adequate palliation with the least morbidity and mortality. Other authors advocate wide resection of all involved intestine with either primary anastomosis or initial proximal diversion.[53,54]

RADIATION-INDUCED LIVER DAMAGE

The liver was initially thought to be extremely resistant to radiotherapy damage. With the use of megavoltage radiotherapy, however, this has been shown to be a misconception. Until 1963, there were only scattered reports of damage to the liver following radiation.[55-60]

Subsequently, numerous authors[56,57,61,62] found that injury to the small hepatic veins was the earliest lesion in radiation hepatitis. A fine network of reticulum fibers and secondary thrombosis occluded the small hepatic veins. This then resulted in sinusoidal and hepatic congestion, centrilobular necrosis, and subsequent fibrosis. The histologic appearance of chronic radiation hepatitis is characterized by a shrunken liver showing severe vascular damage, liver cell atrophy, lobular collapse, and fibrosis centered around the portal vein and bile ducts.[58,62,63]

Potential predisposing factors to radiation damage to the liver include the dose and fractionation of radiation, concomitant use of cytotoxic agents, tumor infiltration of the liver, and previous chronic liver disease or resection.[63-65]

In 1965, Ingold et al.[55] described the clinical features as well as the pathologic findings of radiation hepatitis. This series included 40 patients who received varying doses of radiation to the entire liver either for ovarian cancer or lymphoma. In order to define the effect of radiation on the liver, the authors chose patients who were free of clinically significant hepatic metastases and who after irradiation of the entire liver had: (1) significant alteration in liver function tests; (2) hepatomegaly not present prior to radiation; (3) ascites; or (4) a needle biopsy of the liver showing the previously described radiation-induced liver damage. In this series, 13 of the 40 patients met the above criteria. No case of liver damage was seen when the radiation dose to the liver was less than 3000 cGy. In 3 of 14 patients who received 3000 to 3800 cGy, evidence of hepatic damage was present, and the rate increased to 7 of 17 (42%) patients who received 3800 to 4000 cGy. Above 4000 cGy, three of four patients treated had evidence of liver dysfunction. The authors concluded that the development of radiation hepatitis is dose dependent, and the clinical presentation is similar to that seen in veno-occlusive disease reported from Jamaica, as well as the Budd-Chiari syndrome (hepatomegaly, predominance of ascites, and mild to moderate abnormalities of the liver function tests).

Liver damage resulting from radiation may be asymptomatic and manifests only in liver function tests and imaging abnormalities. In 23 patients with stage III Hodgkin's disease treated by Poussin-Rosillo,[67] 2000 cGy were delivered to the entire liver, and an additional 2000 cGy to the left lobe were given. Seventy-eight percent of the patients developed elevated serum alkaline phosphatase, and 35% had elevated glutamic oxaloacetic transaminase. These abnormalities appeared 3 to 12 months (median 5 months) after radiotherapy and persisted for 2 to 23 months (median 10 months). None of these patients had symptoms.

Tefft[63] found clinical evidence of chronic liver damage in 66 of 116 irradiated children, as judged by radioisotope liver scan and glutamic oxaloacetic transaminase values. His study population consisted of children irradiated for Wilms' tumor or neuroblastoma with various doses. Although Ingold[55] did not see any evidence of radiation hepatitis in patients who received less than 3000 cGy, Tefft found hepatic toxicity in patients receiving as low as 1200 cGy.

The manifestations of acute hepatitis of the veno-occlusive or Budd-Chiari type described by Ingold and Poussin-Rosillo usually appear 2 to 6 weeks following completion of radiation therapy, are sustained for several weeks or months, and then gradually disappear. Although the majority of patients recover, severe cases of chronic hepatic dysfunction have been reported. Supporting evidence for radiation-induced chronic liver damage in Hodgkin's patients is found in a paper by Reed and Cox.[57] Seventeen liver biopsies from twelve patients were examined after variable doses of radiation to the liver. Five of these specimens were from Hodgkin's disease patients and in one of them, histologic findings of hepatic cell loss, hepatic vein occlusion, parenchymal fibrosis, and irregular hyperplasia were found. The other four liver specimens from Hodgkin's patients revealed only acute changes of hyperemia in three, hepatic cell loss in one, and hepatic vein lesions in two.

A morphologic study emphasizing the late changes of radiation hepatitis was reported by Lewis and Millis.[68] A total of 19 patients received radiation to the liver, seven of whom had Hodgkin's disease. Three of these seven patients developed histologic changes compatible with chronic radiation hepatitis. The main changes were fibrosis, primarily of the portal tracts, central and sublobular hepatic vein narrowing and perivenous sclerosis, moderate cellular atrophy, and lobular collapse and distortion.

To circumvent the hepatic toxicity of radiation, the group at Stanford University tried the approach of radioactive gold combined with external radiation.[69,70] Other groups have persisted in attempts to radiate the liver.[71] These authors compared total-nodal irradiation (TNI) alone to TNI plus low-dose irradiation to the liver in patients with stage IIIA Hodgkin's disease. Serial liver function studies were performed in 14 patients. Fifty percent showed mild and 21% showed significant elevation of alkaline phosphatase. They found that recurrence-free survival improved significantly when the liver was irradiated and recommended total-nodal irradiation plus low-dose irradiation to the liver as the primary modality of treatment for stage IIIA patients.

The current view is that direct radiation therapy to the liver is to be avoided as much as possible. It is now well documented that the liver is very sensitive to radiotherapy. Radionuclide scans have shown decreased function after doses as low as 1200 to 1500 cGy.[63] Although the central portion of the liver is included in axial radiotherapy portals used in the treatment of Hodgkin's disease, late liver failure or portal hypertension from such radiation is rarely encountered.[55] Since the realization that the liver is radiosensitive, recommendations have been made to either limit the total dose to the liver to a maximum of 2500 cGy or to limit the total hepatic volume to be irradiated.[72]

The treatment of radiation hepatitis is symptomatic and centered on the control of ascites, encephalopathy, and coagulopathy, which can develop secondary to hepatic insufficiency. An adequate diet with salt and fluid restriction is helpful in the treatment of ascites. Bedrest and careful use of diuretics may be good additional measures. When the prothrombin time is prolonged, vitamin K supplementation should be tried initially, and if indicated, the coagulopathy may require fresh frozen plasma. In the presence of hepatic encephalopathy, restriction of dietary proteins and either lactulose or neomycin may be useful.

LIVER AND PANCREATIC DAMAGE FROM CHEMOTHERAPY

The chemotherapeutic agents used in the management of patients with Hodgkin's disease include representatives of virtually all classes of antineoplastic drugs. A detailed listing of the acute and chronic hepatic complications of some of these agents is beyond the scope of this chapter and can be found in comprehensive reviews of the subject.[73-76]

Devita et al.[76] reported on liver dysfunction in patients with Hodgkin's disease treated with nitrogen mustard, vincristine sulfate, procarbazine hydrochloride, and prednisone. Seven of 43 patients treated with these drugs developed evidence of hepatic dysfunction. Five patients had mild transient elevations of serum alkaline phosphatase, and three patients had minor transient increases in serum glutamic oxaloacetic transaminase. Two of the patients developed a clinical picture similar to that of viral hepatitis. Needle biopsy of the liver in these two patients was compatible with viral hepatitis, subsequently one patient recovered, the other developed chronic hepatitis. Although the two biopsies showed hepatic lesions compatible with viral hepatitis, it is possible to assume they had drug-induced hepatitis because they received chemotherapy prior to developing liver dysfunction. It was unlikely that they had hepatitis B or non-A non-B hepatitis because the hepatitis B surface antigen was negative and they did not receive blood transfusions. Care must be taken when evaluating reports of liver function abnormalities in Hodgkin's disease patients. In evaluating liver function test abnormalities in patients with Hodgkin's disease, it must be remembered that, in addition to a potential toxicity or hypersensitivity from chemotherapy, Hodgkin's disease by itself can cause a variety of liver-function abnormalities.[77]

Liver damage caused by methotrexate has been well documented,[78-82] and ranges from fatty changes[81] to fibrosis of the portal tracts, and the eventual development of cirrhosis.[82] However, methotrexate is not commonly used in present-day protocols for Hodgkin's disease. Of the more commonly used agents, nitrogen mustard and the vinca alkaloids have not been shown to cause hepatic damage. Dimethyltriazeneimidazole carboxamide (DTIC) commonly causes mild hepatic dysfunction, reflected by an elevated serum glutamic oxaloacetic transaminase (SGOT). In a series of 200 patients treated with DTIC for melanoma, at a dose of 6.0 mg/kg, SGOT elevation occurred in 50.5% of the patients and diarrhea occurred in 0.5%.[83] Minow et al.[84] reported 11 patients treated with a combination of 6-mercaptopurine (6MP) and doxorubicin for refractory leukemia who developed elevations of serum bilirubin, alkaline phosphatase, and SGOT. Liver tissue obtained at necropsy showed intrahepatic cholestasis in eight, hepatocellular necrosis in 10, and fatty changes in nine cases. Although doxorubicin has not been found to be hepatotoxic as a single agent, it has been shown to potentiate the hepatotoxicity of both 6MP and radiation.[85-88] Bleomycin has been reported to cause hyperbilirubinemia as an acute toxicity. However, a review of more than 1000 patients treated with bleomycin concluded that hepatic toxicity was not consistently reported and could not be specifically ascribed to bleomycin in many cases.[89] Procarbazine was reported to cause granulomatous hepatitis in a single case in a selected series of 74 patients.[90] Corticosteroids have long been recognized to be associated with acute pancreatitis. One 1977 review[91] counted 51 cases up to 1975.

Abt et al.[92] compared the liver biopsy results from 25 patients with Hodgkin's disease who received multiple chemotherapeutic regimens with those of 103 untreated patients. It was found that there was some increase, although not statistically significant, in fatty infiltration and hemosiderosis in the treated patients. The etiology of the hemosiderosis was felt to be the result of hypersplenism and hemolysis, and there is some suggestion that the steatosis may be caused by one of the chemotherapeutic agents.

In reviewing available data on the complications from chemotherapy for Hodgkin's disease, it was notable to find relatively few reports of hepatotoxicity, although the major site of metabolism of many of these agents is the liver. Since there is a limited number of reported cases of chemotherapy-induced hepatic abnormalities in Hodgkin's patients, the prognosis of such liver abnormalities is not clearly defined. Suggested modifications of chemotherapy dosage in the presence of liver dysfunction have been made in reviews of this subject.[93,94]

INTESTINAL DAMAGE FROM CHEMOTHERAPY

The rapid turnover of the intestinal epithelium makes it particularly susceptible to the effects of cytotoxic drugs.[95] Cytotoxic drugs block cell mitosis in the crypts; however, the migration of preexisting differentiated cells from the crypt floor to the villous apex is not affected. Trier studied the acute morphologic alterations induced by methotrexate in the mucosa of the small intestines.[96] Mitosis in the crypts decreased within 3 hours of the drug administration, became negligible in 6 to 48 hours, and returned to normal 96 hours after methotrexate was stopped. Although changes varied from cytoplasmic inclusion bodies to villous shortening, gastrointestinal symptoms were absent or mild. Most treatment regimens for Hodgkin's disease use cyclical combination drug programs. Since cell migration from the crypt floor to the villous apex takes 5 to 7 days,[97] recovery of the regenerating zone of the crypt epithelium usually occurs between cycles, limiting the intestinal toxicity of these drugs.

Parrilli et al.[98] determined the intestinal permeability to lactulose, D-xylose absorption, and the intestinal mucosal histologic pattern in five Hodgkin's patients treated with MOPP. They found that D-xylose absorption and the intestinal mucosal pattern were the same before and 10 days after the beginning of treatment. However, there was an early occurrence and prompt resolution of an increased permeability to lactulose. They theorized that this was the result of a transient increase in the size of the junctional complexes between adjacent enterocytes. Despite these early and rapidly reversible increases in passive lactulose permeability, there were no changes in active absorption of D-xylose or in intestinal biopsy specimens. However, with the institution of newer multidrug regimens and radiotherapy combinations,[99] the additive crypt cell kill or prolonged periods of low proliferative activity could result in significant gastrointestinal damage.

Chemotherapy-induced nausea and vomiting are mediated by the vomiting center in the medullary reticular formations.[100,101] Emesis results when the vomiting center is stimulated by the chemoreceptor trigger zone in the area posterior to the fourth ventricle. Of the previously used drugs for Hodgkin's disease, nausea and vomiting occur commonly in patients given nitrogen mustard and nausea and vomiting may also occur in 75 to 95% of patients given procarbazine,[90] while the vinca alkaloids usually produce only minimal symptoms. The management of nausea and vomiting associated with chemotherapy can be accomplished by the use of antiemetics, intravenous hydration and dietary adjustments. These symptoms resolve with termination of therapy.

Autonomic nerve dysfunction manifesting as colicky abdominal pain, constipation, and adynamic ileus has been reported in patients receiving vincristine.[102] In one report,[103] vincristine-induced constipation was found in one-third of patients, with higher frequency, greater severity, and earlier onset in those treated with large doses. Vincristine-induced adynamic ileus usually resolved with conservative therapy; however, deaths resulting from this complication have been reported.[103] Mucositis is seen with methotrexate, 5-fluorouracil, actinomycin D, doxorubicin, and bleomycin, drugs commonly used for Hodgkin's disease.

Perforation of the bowel, either secondary to tumor or to various cytotoxic agents, has been reported in patients with lymphoma.[104,105] When the lymphoma has diffusely infiltrated the bowel wall, treatment with chemotherapy may result in tumor-cell necrosis, sloughing, and subsequent perforation. Two of 613 patients treated with MOPP died after the initial cycle of chemotherapy as a result of rapid necrosis of tumor masses and small-bowel perforation.

Adrenal corticosteroids have been implicated in the genesis of gastric and duodenal ulcers, as well as predisposing the patient to the development of gastrointestinal moniliasis. In a retrospective study from Memorial Sloan-Kettering Cancer Center, 310 patients were evaluated for upper gastrointestinal bleeding.[106] Forty-nine patients had massive bleeding defined by a fall in blood pressure, a 5% drop in hematocrit, or hematemesis. Acute stress ulcers were found to be the most common cause of the massive gastrointestinal hemorrhage, occurring in 16 of the 49 patients. Hodgkin's disease patients were most commonly found to have this type of bleeding, although this did not represent the most common neoplasm seen at the institution. These patients were all receiving steroids or other chemotherapy at the time of their bleeding episode, and it has been suggested that the therapy played a contributing role in the development of ulcers and bleeding.

Esophageal or gastric moniliasis is a frequent complication in patients with Hodgkin's disease receiving steroids, radiation, or chemotherapy. In an autopsy series, 11% of patients with Hodgkin's disease had candidal infection of the gastrointestinal tract.[107] Acute symptoms of gastrointestinal bleeding, dysphagia, and odynophagia, as well as fatal complications secondary to bleeding, perforation, and disseminated moniliasis have been reported.[107] When identified, institution of treatment should begin with either nystatin (Mycostatin), ketoconazole, or amphotericin, depending on the severity of the infection.

A case of terminal diarrhea during chemotherapy for Hodgkin's lymphoma secondary to herpes simplex colitis has been described.[108] It is well recognized that herpes simplex and cytomegalovirus can cause infection of the upper gastrointestinal tract in immunosuppressed patients.[109–111] Hodgkin's disease patients undergoing chemotherapy belong in this category and are therefore at risk of developing this infection too.

SECONDARY MALIGNANCIES IN THE GASTROINTESTINAL TRACT

Second malignancies in patients previously treated for Hodgkin's disease have been extensively reported.[112-117] Such malignancies may involve the gastrointestinal tract. In a report from Stanford University Medical Center[112] on 598 patients treated for Hodgkin's disease and followed prospectively, six patients developed widely disseminated nonHodgkin's lymphoma at a time when none had evidence of the presence of Hodgkin's disease. The actuarial risk of development of nonHodgkin's lymphoma at 10 years was 4.4% in this group. In five of the six cases there was abdominal or gastrointestinal involvement. This pattern of involvement is unusual in Hodgkin's disease and occurs more commonly in lymphomas of B-cell origin. Therefore, apparent late recurrences in the abdomen or gastrointestinal tract in patients treated successfully for Hodgkin's disease with radiation and chemotherapy should raise the possibility of secondary malignancy and should not be accepted as being due to Hodgkin's disease without biopsy.

It has also been noted that there may be an increased occurrence of nonhemopoietic malignancies in patients with Hodgkin's disease. A report from Memorial Sloan-Kettering Cancer Center identified 41 patients from a group of 1028 Hodgkin's disease patients who had a second malignancy.[115] A total of 44 antecedent, synchronous, and metachronous cancers were identified. Of the 23 reported metachronous cancers, two were adenocarcinomas of the colon, two were adenocarcinomas of the stomach and one was a leiomyosarcoma of the duodenum. In another report from the National Cancer Institute,[113] six among 62 patients treated with combined radiotherapy and chemotherapy developed multiple cancers in addition to Hodgkin's disease. This represented a higher incidence of second tumors than expected. In a series of 630 Hodgkin's disease patients reported by the Southeast Oncology Group,[114] 11 metachronous cancers were identified, seven were acute leukemia, and four were solid tumors (two lung and two colon). The development of secondary malignancies in patients treated successfully for Hodgkin's disease with radiation therapy or chemotherapy underscores the importance of continual medical care and follow-up in these patients.

Therapy has become more aggressive and successful in the management of Hodgkin's disease. Long-term survival can now be expected in 80% of the patients. Long-term gastrointestinal complications are uncommon; when they do occur occasionally, they can be serious. Regular observations and study of these complications have resulted in modifications of the diagnostic evaluation and treatment of the disease. In general, the indication for a staging laparotomy has been limited to the situation in which a change in stage would change the treatment plan. Radiation damage to the liver and gastrointestinal tract has been decreased by the identification of "minimum" and "maximum" tolerance doses of these organs. Predisposing factors that increase the risk of gastrointestinal damage from radiation damage have also been identified. It is unusual for chronic radiation enteritis to occur after radiotherapy for Hodgkin's disease. When it is present, however, it is a difficult management problem that often requires some form of surgery. Unlike bone-marrow toxicity, liver and intestinal-tract toxicity from chemotherapy is not dose limiting. The cycle combination drug programs used in Hodgkin's disease rarely cause significant complications. As our understanding of the complications that arise from the therapy for Hodgkin's disease grows, new modalities of treatment for the complications will be evaluated. These advances will undoubtedly add to the excellent long-term survival presently enjoyed by these patients.

REFERENCES

1. DeVita, V.T. The consequences of the chemotherapy of Hodgkin's disease. The 10th David A. Karnofsky Memorial Lecture. Cancer 47:1–13, 1981.
2. DeVita, V.T. Hodgkin's disease: Conference sum-

mary and future directions. Cancer Treat. Rep. 66:1045–1055, 1982.
3. Longo, D.L., Young, R.C., and DeVita, V.T. Chemotherapy for Hodgkin's disease: The remaining challenges. Cancer Treat. Rep. 66:925–936, 1982.
4. Glatstein, E., Guernsey, J.M., Rosenberg, S.A., et al. The value of laparotomy and splenectomy in the staging of Hodgkin's disease. Cancer 24:709–718, 1969.
5. Rosenstock, J.G., D'Angio, G.J., and Kiesewetter W.B. Proceedings: The incidence of complications following staging laparotomy for Hodgkin's disease disease in children. Am. J. Roentgenol. Radium Ther. Nucl. Med. 120:531–535, 1974.
6. Rutherford, C.J., DesForges, J.G., Davies, B. et al. The decision to perform staging laparotomy in symptomatic Hodgkin's disease. Br. J. Haematol. 4:347–358, 1980.
7. Cannon, W.B., Kaplan, H.S., Dorfman, R.F. et al. Staging laparotomy with splenectomy in Hodgkin's disease. Surg. Ann. 7:103–114, 1975.
8. Martin, J.K., Clark, S.C., Beart, R.W. et al. Staging laparotomy in Hodgkin's disease. Mayo Clinic Experience. Arch. Surg. 117:586–591, 1982.
9. Kaiser, C.W. Complications from staging laparotomy for Hodgkin's disease. J. Surg. Oncol. 16:319–325, 1981.
10. Lanzkowsky, P., Shende, A., Karayalcin, G. et al. Staging laparotomy and splenectomy: Treatment and complications of Hodgkin's disease in children. Am. J. Hematol. 1:393–404, 1976.
11. Slavin, R.S. and Nelsen, T.S. Complications from staging laparotomy for Hodgkin's disease. Natl. Cancer Inst. Monogr. 36:457–459, 1976.
12. Baretta, G., Spinelli, P., Rilke, F. et al. Sequential laparoscopy and laparotomy combined with bone marrow biopsy in staging Hodgkin's disease. Cancer Treat. Rep. 60:1231–1237, 1976.
13. Gallez-Marchal, D., Henry-Amar, M. Radiation injuries of the gastrointestinal tract in Hodgkin's disease: the role of exploratory laparotomy and fractionation. Radiother. Oncol. 2:93–99, 1984.
14. Loiudice, T., Baxter, D., and Balint, J. Effects of abdominal surgery on the development of radiation enteropathy. Gastroenterology 73:1093–1097, 1977.
15. Casirola, G., Ippoliti, G., and Marini, G. Laparoscopy in Hodgkin's disease. Acta. Haematol. 49:1, 1973.
16. DeVita, V.T., Jr., Bagley, C.M. Jr., Goodell, B. et al. Peritoneoscopy in the staging of Hodgkin's disease. Cancer Res. 31:1746–1750, 1971.
17. Bagley, C.M. Jr., Thomas, L.B., Johnson, R.F. et al. Diagnosis of liver involvement by lymphoma: Results of 96 consecutive peritoneoscopies. Cancer 31:840–847, 1973.
18. Coleman, M., Lightdale, C.J., Vinciguerra, V.P. et al. Peritoneoscopy in Hodgkin's disease. Confirmation of results by laparotomy. JAMA 236:2634–2636, 1976.
19. Strockbine, M.F., Hancock, J.E., and Fletcher, G.H. Complications in 831 patients with squamous cell carcinoma of the intact uterine cervix treated with 3,000 rads or more whole pelvis radiation. Am. J. Roentgenol. 108:293–304, 1970.
20. Rubin, P. and Casarette, G. A direction for clinical radiation pathology. In Frontiers of Radiation Therapy and Oncology. Edited by J.N. Vaeth. Vol. 6. Baltimore, University Park Press, 1972, pp. 1–16.
21. Tarpila, S. Morphologic and functional response of human small intestine to ionizing irradiation. Scan. J. Gastroenterol. 6 (suppl.):9–48, 1971.
22. Tarpila, S. and Jussila, J. The effect of radiation on the disaccharidase activities of human small intestinal mucosa. Scan. J. Clin. Lab. Invest. 23 (suppl.):44, (abstract), 1969.
23. Trier, J.S. and Browning, T.H. Morphologic response of the mucosa of human small intestine to x-ray exposure. J. Clin. Invest. 45:194–204, 1966.
24. Greenberger, N.J. and Isselbacher, K.J. Malabsorption following radiation injury to the gastrointestinal tract. Am. J. Med. 36:450–456, 1964.
25. Roswit, B. Complications of radiotherapy: The alimentary tract. Semin. Roentgenol. 1:51–63, 1974.
26. Elliott, A.R. and Jenkinson, E.L. Ulceration of the stomach and small intestine following roentgen therapy. Radiology 23:149–156, 1934.
27. Graham, J.B. and Vallalba, R.J. Damage to the small intestine by radiotherapy. Surg. Gynecol. Obstet. 116:665–668, 1963.
28. Palmer, J.A. and Bush, R.S. Radiation injuries to the bowel associated with the treatment of carcinoma of the cervix. Surgery 80:458–464, 1976.
29. DeCosse, J.J., Rhodes, R.S., Wantz, W.B. et al. The natural history and management of radiation-induced injury of the gastrointestinal tract. Ann. Surg. 170:369–384, 1969.
30. Wellwood, J.M. and Jackson, B.T. The intestinal complications of radiotherapy. Br. J. Surg. 60:814–818, 1973.
31. Kellum, J.M., Jaffe, B.M., Calhoun, T.R. et al. Gastric complications after radiotherapy for Hodgkin's disease and other lymphomas. Am. J. Surg. 134:314–317, 1977.
32. Novak, J.M., Collins, J.T., and Domowitz, M. Effects of radiation on the human gastrointestinal tract. J. Clin. Gastroenterol. 1:9–14, 1979.
33. Kinsella, T.J., Fraciss, B.A., and Glatstein, E. Late effects of radiotherapy in the treatment of Hodgkin's disease. Cancer Treat. Rep. 66:991–1001, 1982.
34. Katin, M.J. et al. Surgical repair of esophagobronchial fistula following successful treatment of Hodgkin's disease. Cancer 44:121, 1979.
35. Marks, J.E., Moran, E.M., Gbriem, M.L. et al. Extended mantle radiotherapy in Hodgkin's disease and malignant lymphoma. Am. J. Roentgenol. Radium Ther. Nucl. Med. 121:772–788, 1974.
36. Morichau-Beauchant, M., Briaud, M., and Maire, P. Oesophagites postradiques chroniques apres irradiation pour cancer oropharyngo-larynge: une entite meconnue. Gastroenterol. Clin. Biol. 6:87A, 1982.
37. Nickenson, J.J., Fuller, L.M., Hutchison, G.B. et al. Survival and complications of radiotherapy following involved and extended field therapy of Hodg-

kin's disease, stages I and II: A collaborative study. Cancer 38:288–305, 1976.
38. Papazian, A., Capron, J.P., Ducroix, J.P. et al. Mucosal bridges of the upper esophagus after radiotherapy for Hodgkin's disease. Gastroenterology 84:1028–1031, 1983.
39. Donaldson, S.S. Nutritional consequences of radiotherapy. Cancer Res. 38:2407–2414, 1977.
40. Thomas-de-la-Vega, J.E., Banner, B.F., Hubbard, M. et al. Cytoprotective effect of prostaglandin E2 in irradiated rat ileum. Surg. Gynecol. Obstet. 158:39–45, 1984.
41. Haddad, G.K., Grodsinsky, C., and Allen, H. The spectrum of radiation enteritis: Surgical considerations. Dis. Colon Rectum 26:590–594, 1983.
42. Rubin, P. and Casarette, G.W. Alimentary tract: Small and large intestine and rectum. In Clinical Radiation Pathology. Vol. 1. Philadelphia, WB Saunders, 1968, pp. 193–240.
43. Donaldson, S.S., Jundt, S., Ricour, C. et al. Radiation enteritis in children—A retrospective review, clinicopathologic correlation and dietary management. Cancer 35:1167–1178, 1975.
44. Mennie, A.T., Dalley, V.M., and Dineen, L.C. Treatment of radiation-induced gastrointestinal distress with acetylsalicylate. Lancet 2:942–943, 1975.
45. Goldstein, F., Khouy, J., and Thornton, J. Treatment of chronic radiation enteritis and colitis with salicylazosulfapyridine and systemic corticosteroids. Am. J. Gastroenterol. 65:201–208, 1976.
46. Rauch, K. and Weiland, H. Behandlung des radiogenen kolitis mit salicylazosulfapyridine (Azulfidine). Strahlentherapie 143:660–663, 1972.
47. Louidice, T.A. and Lange, J.A. Treatment of radiation-induced injuries of the intestine. Surg. Gynecol. Oncol. 153:896–900, 1981.
48. Miller, D.G., Ivey, M., and Young, J. Home parenteral nutrition in treatment of severe radiation enteritis. Ann. Intern. Med. 91:858–860, 1979.
49. Lavey, I.C., Steinger, Z., and Fazio, V.W. Home parenteral nutrition in management of patients with severe radiation enteritis. Dis. Colon Rectum 23:91–93, 1980.
50. Brown, M.S., Buchanan, R.B., and Kanan, S.J. Clinical observations on the effects of elemental diet supplementation during irradiation. Clin. Radiol. 31:19–20, 1980.
51. Heusinkveld, R.S., Manning, M.R., and Aristizabal, S.A. Control of radiation-induced diarrhea with cholestryramine. Radiat. Oncol. Biol. Phys. 4:687–690, 1978.
52. Swan, R.W., Fowler, W.C., and Boronow, R.C. Surgical management of radiation injury to the small intestine. Surg. Gynecol. Obstet. 42:325–327, 1976.
53. Russell, J.C. and Welch, J.P. Operative management in radiation injuries to the intestinal tract. Am. J. Surg. 137:433–442, 1979.
54. Schmidt, E.H. and Symmondo, I. Surgical treatment of radiation-induced injuries of the intestine. Surg. Gynecol. Oncol. 153:896–900, 1981.
55. Ingold, J.A., Reede, G.B., Kaplan, H.S. et al. Radiation hepatitis. Am. J. Roentgenol. Radium Ther. Nucl. Med. 93:200–208, 1965.
56. Ogata, K., Hyawa K., Yoshida, M. et al. Hepatic injury following irradiation: A morphologic study. Tukushima J. Exp. Med. 9:240–251, 1963.
57. Reed, G.B. and Cox, A.J. The human liver after radiation injury. A form of veno-occlusive disease. Am. J. Pathol. 48:597–612, 1966.
58. Brick, I.B. Effects of million volt irradiation on gastrointestinal tract. AMA Arch. Intern. Med. 96:26–31, 1955.
59. Case, J.T. and Warthin, A.S. Occurrence of hepatic lesions in patients treated by intensive deep roentgen irradiation. Am. J. Roentgenol. Rad. Therapy 12:27–46, 1924.
60. Phillips, R., Karnofsky, D.A., Hamilton, L.D. et al. Roentgen therapy of hepatic metastases. Am. J. Roentgenol. Rad. Ther. Nucl. Med. 71:826–834, 1954.
61. Hahn, P.F., Jackson, M.A., and Goldie, H. Liver cirrhosis and ascites, induced in dogs by chronic massive hepatic irradiation with radioactive colloid gold. Science 114:303–305, 1951.
62. Fellows, K.E., Vawter, G.F., and Tefft, M. Hepatic effects following abdominal irradiation in children: Detection by Au-198 scan and confirmation by histologic examination. Am. J. Roentgenol. Rad. Ther. Nucl. Med. 103:422–431, 1968.
63. Tefft, M., Mitus, A., and Das, L. Irradiation of the liver in children: review of experience in the acute and chronic phases, and in the intact normal and partially resected. Am. J. Roentgenol. Radium Ther. Nucl. Med. 108:365–385, 1970.
64. Bernard, A. Study of hepatic damage resulting from irradiation of nephroblastomas in children. Thesis, University of Paris, 1974.
65. Tefft, M., Traggis, D., and Filler, R.M. Liver irradiation in children: Acute changes with transient leukopenia and thrombocytopenia. Am. J. Roentgenol. 106:750–765, 1969.
66. Tefft, M., Mitus, A., and Jaffree, N. Irradiation of the liver in children: Are the effects enhanced by chemotherapeutic administration? Am. J. Roentgenol. 111:165–173, 1971.
67. Poussin-Rosillo, H., Nisee, L.Z., D'Angio, G.J. Hepatic radiation tolerance in Hodgkin's disease patients. Radiology 121:461–464, 1976.
68. Lewis, K. and Millis, R. Human radiation hepatitis: A morphologic study with emphasis on the late changes. Arch. Pathol. 96:21–26, 1973.
69. Kaplan, H.S. and Bagshaw, M.A. Radiation hepatitis: possible prevention by combined isotopic and external radiation therapy. Radiology 91:1214–1220, 1968.
70. Krant, J.W., Kaplan, H.S., and Bagshaw, M.A. Combined fractionated isotopic and external irradiation of the liver in Hodgkin's disease. A study of 21 patients. Cancer 30:39–46, 1972.
71. Lee, C.K.K., Bloomfield, C., and Levitt, S.H. Liver irradiation in stage IIIA Hodgkin's disease with splenic involvement. Am. J. Clin. Oncol. 7:149–157, 1984.

72. Kaplan, H.S. Radiotherapy. *In* Hodgkin's Disease, 2nd Ed. Cambridge, Harvard University Press, 1980, pp. 366–444.
73. Carter, S.K. and Slavik, M. Chemotherapy of cancer. Am. Rev. Pharmacol. 14:157–179, 1974.
74. Ludwig, J. Drug effects on the liver. A tabular compilation of drugs and drug-related hepatic diseases. Dig. Dis. Sci. 24:785–796, 1979.
75. DeVita, V.T., Lewis, B.J., Rosenzweitg, M. et al. The chemotherapy of Hodgkin's disease. Past experiences and future directions. Cancer 42:979–990, 1978.
76. DeVita, V.T., Serpick, A.A., and Cerbone, P.P. Combination chemotherapy in the treatment of advanced Hodgkin's disease. Ann. Intern. Med. 73:881–895, 1970.
77. Levitan, R., Diamond, H.D., and Craver, L.F. The liver in Hodgkin's disease. Gut 2:60–71, 1961.
78. Nesbit, M., Krivit, W., Heyn, R. et al. Acute and chronic effects of methotrexate on hepatic, pulmonary, and skeletal systems. Cancer 37:1048–1054, 1976.
79. Dahl, M.G.C., Gregory, M.M., and Scheuer, P.J. Liver damage due to methotrexate in patients with psoriasis. Br. Med. J. 1:625–630, 1971.
80. Hersh, E.M., Wong, V.G., Henderson, E.S. et al. Hepatoxic effects of methotrexate. Cancer 19:600–606, 1966.
81. Klatskin, G. Toxic and drug-induced hepatitis. *In* Diseases of the Liver. Edited by L. Schiff. 4th Ed. Philadelphia, J.B. Lippincott Co., 1975, pp. 604–710.
82. Podurgiel, B.J., McGill, D.B., Ludwig, J. et al. Liver injury associated with methotrexate therapy for psoriasis. Mayo Clin. Proc. 48:787–792, 1973.
83. Johnson, R.O., Metter, G., Wilson, W. et al. Phase I evaluation of DTIC (NSC-45388) and other studies in malignant melanoma in the central oncology group. Cancer Treat. Rep. 60:183–187, 1976.
84. Minow, R.A., Stern M.N., Casey, J.H. et al. Clinicopathologic correlation of the liver damage in patients treated with 6-mercaptopurine and adriamycin. Cancer 38:1524–1528, 1976.
85. Kun, L.E. and Bruce, M.C. Hepatopathy following irradiation and adriamycin. Cancer 42:81–84, 1978.
86. Cassady, J.R., Richter, M.P., Piro, A.J. et al. Radiation-adriamycin interactions: Preliminary clinical observations. Cancer 36:946–949, 1975.
87. Mayer, E.G., Poulter, C.A., and Aristizabal, S.A. Complications of irradiation related to apparent drug potentiation by adriamycin. Int. J. Radiat. Oncol. Biol. Phys. 1:1179–1188, 1976.
88. Wang, J.J., Corets, E., Sinks, L.F. et al. Therapeutic effect and toxicity of adriamycin in patients with neoplastic disease. Cancer 28:837–843, 1971.
89. Baum, R.H., Carter, S.K., and Agre, K. A clinical review of bleomycin: A new antineoplastic agent. Cancer 31:903–914, 1973.
90. Stolinsky, D.C., Solomon, J., Pugh, R.P. et al. Clinical experience with procarbazine in Hodgkin's disease, reticulum cell sarcoma, and lymphosarcoma. Cancer 26:984–990, 1979.
91. Nakashima, Y. and Howard, J.M. Drug induced acute pancreatitis. Surg. Obstet. Gynecol. 145:105–109, 1977.
92. Abt, A.B., Kirschner, R.H., Belliveau, R.E. et al. Hepatic pathology associated with Hodgkin's disease. Cancer 33:1564–1571, 1974.
93. Perry, M.C. Hepatotoxicity of chemotherapeutic agents. Semin. Oncol. 9:65–74, 1982.
94. Woolley, P.Y. Hepatic and pancreatic damage produced by cytotoxic drugs. Cancer Treat. Rev. 10:117–137, 1983.
95. Trier, J.S. Morphology of the epithelium of the small intestine. *In* Handbook of Physiology. Section 6: Alimentary Canal. Vol III, Intestinal Absorption. Edited by C.F. Code and W. Heidel. Washington, Am. Physiol. Soc., 1968, pp. 1125–1175.
96. Trier, J.S. Morphologic alterations induced by methotrexate in the mucosa of human proximal intestine. Gastroenterology 2:295–305, 1968.
97. Hartwich, G. Side effects of a cytostatic treatment on the gastrointestinal tract. Acta Hepatogastroentero. 121:89–92, 1974.
98. Parrilli, G., Iaffaioli, R.V., Capuano, G. et al. Changes in intestinal permeability to lactulose induced by cytotoxic chemotherapy. Cancer Treat. Rep. 66:1435–1436, 1982.
99. Young, C.W., Straus, D.J., Myers, J. et al. Multidisciplinary treatment of advanced Hodgkin's disease by an alternating chemotherapeutic regimen of MOPP/ABDV and low-dose radiation therapy restricted to originally bulky disease. Cancer Treat. Rep. 66:907–914, 1982.
100. Borison, H.L. and Wang, W.C. Physiology and pharmacology of vomiting. Phamacol. Rev. 5:193–230, 1953.
101. Scogna, D. and Smalley, R. Chemotherapy induced nausea and vomiting. Am. J. Nurs. 79:1562–1564, 1979.
102. Rosenthal, S. and Kaufman, S. Vincristine neurotoxicity. Ann. Int. Med. 80:733–737, 1979.
103. Holland, J.F., Schanlan, C. and Gailani, C. Vincristine treatment of advanced cancer: A cooperation study of 392 cases. Coma Res. 33:1258–1264, 1973.
104. Irvine, W.T. and Johnstone, J.M. Lymphosarcoma of the small intestine with special reference to perforating tumours. Brit. J. Surg. 42:611–621, 1955.
105. Sherlock, P. and Oropeza, R. Jejunal perforation in lymphoma after chemotherapy. Arch. Intern. Med. 110:102–107, 1962.
106. Klein, M.S., Ennis, F., Sherlock, P. et al. Stress erosions: A major cause of gastrointestinal hemorrhage in patients with malignant disease. Am. J. Dig. Dis 18:167–171, 1973.
107. Eras, P., Goldstein, M.J., and Sherlock P. Candida infection of the gastrointestinal tract. Medicine 51:367–379, 1972.
108. Boulton, A.J.M., Slater, D.N., and Hancock, B.W. Herpes virus colitis: A new cause of diarrhea in a patient with Hodgkin's disease. Gut 23:247–249, 1982.
109. Casazza, A.R., Duvall, C.P., and Carone, P.P. Infection in lymphoma. JAMA 197:710–716, 1966.
110. Howiler, W. and Goldberg, H.I. Gastroesophageal

involvement with herpes simplex. Gastroenterology 70:775–778, 1976.
111. Rosen, P. and Hajdu, S.I. Visceral herpes virus infection in patients with cancer. Am. J. Clin. Pathol. 56:459–465, 1971.
112. Krikorian, J.G., Burke, J.S., and Rosenberg, S.A. Occurrence of non-Hodgkin's lymphoma after therapy for Hodgkin's disease. N. Engl. J. Med. 300:452–458, 1979.
113. Canellos, G.P., DeVita, V.T., Arseneau, J.C. et al. Second malignancies complicating Hodgkin's disease in remission. Lancet 1:947–949, 1975.
114. Toland, D.M. and Coltman, C.A. Jr. Second malignancies complicating Hodgkin's disease. Blood 46:1013, 1975. Casazza A.R., Duvall, C.P., Carbone, P.P. Infection in lymphoma. JAMA 197:710–716, 1966.
115. Brody, R.S., Schottenfeld, D., and Reid, A. Multiple primary cancer risk after therapy for Hodgkin's disease. Cancer 40:1917–1926, 1977.
116. Boivin, J.F. and Hutchinson, G.B. Second cancers after treatment for Hodgkin's disease: a new review. In Radiation Carcinogenesis: Epidemiology and Biological Significance. Edited by J.D. Boice and J.F. Fraumeni. New York, Raum Press, 1984, p. 181.
117. Arseneau, J.C., Canellos, G.P, Johnson, R. et al. Risk of new cancer in patients with Hodgkin's disease. Cancer 40:1912–1916, 1977.

CHAPTER 16

Cutaneous Sequelae of Hodgkin's Disease

BIJAN SAFAI
GRETCHEN ANDERSON
PATRICIA L. MYSKOWSKI

With the advent of radiation and chemotherapy for the treatment of Hodgkin's disease, the prognosis has greatly improved. Radiation and chemotherapy, however, may have later consequences on many organs, including the skin. In addition, there are a number of specific and nonspecific cutaneous findings that are associated with Hodgkin's disease itself.

Since most of the treatments of Hodgkin's disease are aimed at rapidly dividing cells, it is not surprising that the skin and mucous membranes are frequently affected by the complications of antitumor therapy. Indeed, it has been estimated that 15 to 30% of all patients with Hodgkin's disease will develop some sort of cutaneous disorder during the course of their illness.[1-2] Although many of these problems are the direct results of therapy, several complications appear to be related to the underlying Hodgkin's disease itself or are representative of paraneoplastic syndromes.

PRURITUS

Pruritus, or itching, is the irritating sensation in the skin that results in an impulse to scratch. While pruritus may be related to a number of diseases, it appears to have a special significance in Hodgkin's disease. Generalized pruritus occurs as a presenting symptom in a significant portion of patients with Hodgkin's disease.[3] It has also been noted in other lymphoproliferative disorders, such as mycosis fungoides and leukemia.[3] There is some debate, however, concerning the importance of generalized pruritus and its relationship to prognosis in Hodgkin's disease.[3-4] In the past, severe generalized pruritus had been included as a symptom in the B category, for the staging of disease. In 1971, however, pruritus was dropped from this category. Recently Feiner et al. have argued that pruritus in its most severe generalized forms is indeed a significant prognostic sign and should be re-evaluated as staging criteria.[4] Gobbi et al. reviewed the records of 360 patients with Hodgkin's disease in a retrospective study and reached similar conclusions.[4] They defined severe pruritus as being generalized, accompanied by multiple excoriations, and persisting despite multiple forms of antipruritic therapy. The authors observed that 5.8% of patients with Hodgkin's disease presented with severe generalized pruritus. They noted that this group of patients had shorter survival times when compared with individuals who had only mild pruritus prior to the onset of their disease.[4] Since numerous medical conditions may also result in itching, other possible causes for pruritus must always be sought in patients with Hodgkin's disease. Frequently, drug reactions, with or without cutaneous findings, may be associated with pruritus and may be a result of the chemotherapeutic agents used in the treatment of disease. Other medications, including multiple antibiotics, may be used in the treatment of infectious complications in patients and again may result in pruritic reactions. Endocrine disorders, anemia, renal dysfunction, and even severe anxiety may result in itching in the predisposed patient. Thus, the evaluation of pruritus in patients with Hodgkin's disease must be thorough and include a complete search for medical conditions both related and unrelated to the primary disorder.

PARANEOPLASTIC SYNDROMES

A number of cutaneous manifestations may be found with Hodgkin's disease. These findings typically precede the diagnosis of Hodgkin's disease, and often will be eliminated when the disease responds to therapy. However, the development of any of the cutaneous signs associated with malignancy in a patient in remission may signal the reactivation of disease and should be evaluated appropriately.

Acquired ichthyosis is the cutaneous syndrome most typically associated with Hodgkin's disease.[5,6] The term "ichthyosis" is used to describe a number of disorders characterized by large fish-like scales and generalized xerosis. A number of the ichthyosiform dermatoses are inherited. The most common of these is ichthyosis vulgaris, a relatively common genodermatosis that is inherited in autosomal dominant pattern. In this disorder, there is a strong family history of severe dry skin, which becomes much worse in the winter, with a significant exacerbation in the xerosis developing at puberty. Scaling is present primarily on the extensor surfaces of the extremities. Several other forms of ichthyosis are also recognized and may be inherited in different genetic patterns. However, the hereditary forms of ichthyosis do not have any increased association with malignancy. In contrast, when ichthyosis develops in adult life, the patient must be throughly evaluated for the possibility of internal neoplasms.[5-8] Hodgkin's disease is the most common malignancy associated wih the onset of acquired ichthyosis, occurring in approximately 70% of patients with this symptom and cancer.[7] Other malignancies have also been reported, however, including lymphosarcoma, aplastic anemia, mycosis fungoides, multiple myeloma, and carcinomas of breast and lung.[8] While the onset of acquired ichthyosis usually parallels the diagnosis of Hodgkin's disease, it may occasionally precede the onset of symptoms by several years.[8] Less frequently, other medical problems may account for the onset of ichthyosis in adult life.[9] Pharmacologic agents that interfere with lipid metabolism, such as triparanol or nicotinic acid,[9] also result in an ichthyotic dermatosis. Acquired ichthyosis may also be seen in the setting of chronic renal dialysis.[9]

Other paraneoplastic syndromes may also be associated with Hodgkin's disease, particularly those that have features of autoimmune dysfunction.[10,11] Dermatomyositis is a syndrome of proximal muscle weakness and characteristic skin findings; it is frequently associated with malignancy when it begins in adult life. In individuals over 50 years of age, the incidence of associated malignancy has been reported to be 25 to 40%.[12] Dermatomyositis associated with malignancies is characterized by a polymyositis, accompanied by the typical skin lesions of periorbital erythema and edema, periungual erythema and telangiectasias, and erythematous patches and plaques overlying bony prominences. Hodgkin's disease is one of the malignancies that is associated with dermatomyositis.[12] It has also been estimated that nearly 2% of patients with lymphoma will have other accompanying collagen vascular diseases, of which polymyositis is the most common.[10] Other autoimmune disorders, including scleroderma and systemic lupus erythematosis, have also been occasionally reported with Hodgkin's disease.[11]

CUTANEOUS INVOLVEMENT BY HODGKIN'S DISEASE

It is well known that a variety of lymphoproliferative disorders may involve the skin. For example, leukemic infiltrations of the skin are found frequently in acute myelogenous leukemia and often occur late in the course of disease. Lymphomas may also involve the skin in a number of different patterns. Cutaneous T-cell lymphoma, or mycosis fungoides, often remains localized to the skin for many years, before progressing to nodal and visceral disease. Primary cutaneous lymphomas of other cell types, including B-cell disorders, are less common, but may also present in the skin. The typical appearance of lymphoma in the skin ranges from erythematous papules to more indurated plaque-like lesions or tumors (Fig. 16–1). These lesions reflect the dermal infiltration by neoplastic cells. A number of benign lymphocytic infiltrations of the skin (e.g., lymphocytoma cutis, lymphomatoid papulosis, and lymphocytic infiltrate of Jessner-Kanof) may mimic cutaneous lymphomas both clinically and histologically.[1,8]

Primary cutaneous Hodgkin's disease, without evidence of visceral involvement, has been reported rarely in the skin.[1,8] However, some controversy in the current literature surrounds the reportedly benign course of primary cutaneous Hodgkin's disease.[1,8] Hodgkin's disease has also been reported to secondarily involve the skin with an incidence of 0.5 to 7.5%.[8,9] The types of lesions described in secondary Hodgkin's disease include papules, nodules, plaques, infiltrated lesions, and erythroderma. The most frequently reported site of involvement is the trunk.[8] There have been a number of etiologies proposed for the development of secondary cutaneous involvement by the lymphoma, including direct invasion from underlying lymph nodes,[8] hematogenous spread,[1] and retrograde lymphatic spread from involved lymph nodes.[8] However, the relatively high frequency of cutaneous Hodgkin's disease has been questioned for a number of factors. First of all, a spuriously high incidence may have been attributable to the small amount of tissue used for diagnosis from skin lesions and to the difficulty in distinguishing cutaneous Hodgkin's disease from other benign and malignant lymphoproliferative disorders of the skin.

CONSEQUENCES OF TREATMENT: RADIATION THERAPY

Radiation therapy is widely used in the treatment of Hodgkin's disease, especially stage I and II disease.[13] While the treatment may be curative, radiation therapy often has significant acute and chronic effects. The skin is a common site for both early and late reactions to radiation therapy; indeed, early efforts at successful radiation therapy of internal disease were often limited by the acute cutaneous side effects.[13]

Radiation therapy exerts it tumoricidal effect through its absorption by nuclear DNA, resulting in inhibition of cell division. In addition, mutations may also be induced, with the resulting potential for malignant transformation of cells. The adverse reactions to radiation therapy are determined by the duration of radiation treatment, total dose, distribution of radiation, and the location and sensitivity of the radiated tissues.[14] The skin is a

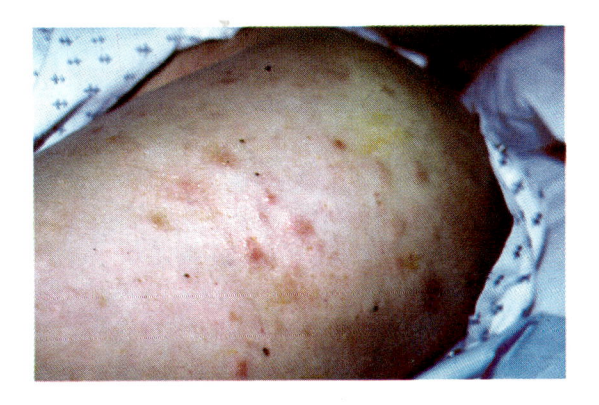

Fig. 16–1. Cutaneous infiltration by Hodgkin's disease. Infiltrated, ill-defined erythematous plaques and papules.

relatively radiosensitive organ, with the relative sensitivity of the individual components being inversely proportional to the cellular differentiation. Thus, the most sensitive components of the skin are the rapidly dividing basal epidermal cells, as well as the endothelial cells of the blood vessels, and to a lesser degree, melanocytes. Hair follicles, sebaceous glands, arrector pili muscles, and sweat glands are less sensitive (in that order) to the effects of radiation.[15] A number of factors may influence the sensitivity of the skin to the early and late effects of radiation.[13,16] Thin vascular areas of skin are relatively more radiosensitive, while hyperpigmented areas are more resistant to the effects of radiation. Obesity also predisposes an individual to increased cutaneous sensitivity to radiation. Certain anatomic sites also have differences in their sensitivity to radiation. The scalp, neck, and chest are relatively radioresistant, while the perineal area and intertriginous areas, such as the axillae, are more susceptible to radiation reactions.[13]

ACUTE RADIATION INJURY

Acute radiation damage is seen days to weeks after irradiation, with a peak period at days 10 to 14.[17] The earliest sign of inflammation is transient erythema. This erythema occurs as a result of increased blood flow, secondary to the release of various chemical mediators. Although diphasic erythema may occur, this is usually not seen with Hodgkin's disease because of the fractionation of radiation doses.[14] The threshold dose for skin erythema has been reported to be 800 cGy for 300 to 200-KV radiation.[14] It has also been suggested that the threshold of the erythema increases with increasing fractionation of the radiation, thereby allowing intracellular repair of the sublethally injured nonmalignant cells. Thus, with the fractionation of radiation, acute cutaneous reactions can be minimized. Another early consequence of radiation is dermal edema, caused by the increase in permeability of the capillaries and venules. This appears to be a direct result of endothelial damage.[14] Radiation injury to melanocytes is manifested by hyperpigmentation, which may develop in the early days and weeks following the radiation, but which may last for months to years. Although the incidence of postradiation hyperpigmentation has been significantly reduced with increased fractionation, it does not necessarily correlate with clinically apparent erythema.[14] Epilation, or loss of hair, is often seen after radiation. The threshold dose for epilation of scalp and facial hair is approximately 300 cGy.[16] Epilation is apparently achieved by the effect of radiation on the anagen, or growing hair follicle; this appears to be reversible in most situations. Slanina and his colleagues have reported that 26% of patients with Hodgkin's disease treated only with radiation experienced hair loss, thus making it a relatively common occurrence.[16]

The histology of acute radiation injury supports the clinically evident findings. In the early erythematous stage, there is congestion of the dermal blood cells and a perivascular infiltrate is present. On days 2 to 7 following radiation, epidermal changes develop, including pyknotic nuclei and abnormal mitotic figures in the epidermis. This is followed by epidermal atrophy, with subsequent regeneration. In severe radiation injury, significant tissue edema with collapse of small blood vessels occurs. Blisters may develop in a subepidermal pattern, followed by epidermal necrosis. Skin appendages may also be destroyed in such reactions.[14]

Acute skin reactions may also occur outside the irradiated area, but these are an indirect consequence of radiation therapy. It has been suggested that these reactions are the result of an autosensitization through tissue breakdown following irradiation. These eruptions included generalized maculopapular eruptions as well as urticaria and erythema multiforme.[14]

CHRONIC RADIATION INJURY

Chronic radiation injury is more insidious in its onset than the acute reactions, and is seen months to years after radiation therapy. It may occur as a consequence of acute radiation injury or may develop de novo in patients without any clinical evidence of radiation damage. Clinically, the features of chronic radiodermatitis include atrophic, dry skin with areas of hyperpigmentation, hypopigmentation, and telangiectasia (poikiloderma) (Fig. 16–2). Hyperkeratotic papules may develop as well as ulcerations. In a series of patients with Hodgkin's disease who were treated with 3000–5000 cGy,[16] Slanina et al. reported a 25% incidence of telangiectasia, a 1.8% incidence of erosions and ulcerations, and an 8% incidence of chronic symptoms of discomfort in the irradiated field. Lymphedema may also occur as a consequence of radiation therapy to regional lymph nodes and is usually seen 2 to 6 months after treatment.[14]

The histologic findings of chronic radiodermatitis include a thin epidermis, with variable absence of appendageal structures, including sebaceous glands, hair follicles and, less frequently, eccrine glands. Within the dermis, there are dilated capillaries and collagen hyalinization.[14,16]

The course of radiation-damaged skin can be variable. The changes of radiodermatitis may remain stable or may degenerate into malignant and premalignant lesions. Ulcer formation, with delayed healing, is a common problem in secondarily damaged sites. The factors that may contribute to the development of chronic radiation ulcers include trauma, mechanical pressure, ultraviolet light, and intense cold exposure.[15,18] These areas of radiodermatitis may be symptomatic, with chronic pain occurring in some patients. Radiation keratoses are not infrequent. The most serious consequence of radiation therapy, however, is the development of cutaneous malignancies, as will be discussed later.

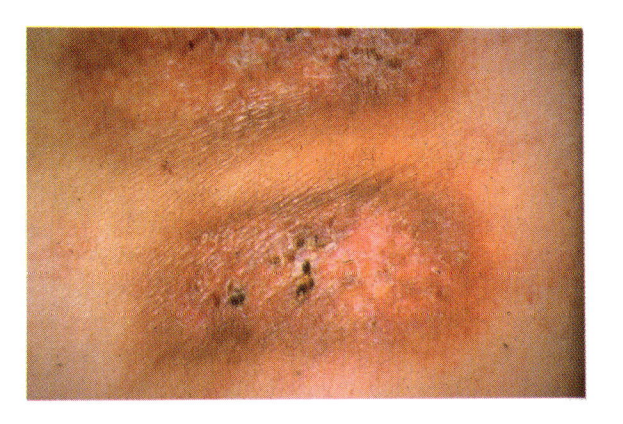

Fig. 16–2. Chronic radiodermatitis. Hyperpigmentation, hypopigmentation, and atrophy are present.

CUTANEOUS COMPLICATIONS OF CHEMOTHERAPY

The survival of patients with advanced or relapsed Hodgkin's disease has been dramatically improved by the use of combination chemotherapy.[13] However, although the survival rate has increased, the incidence of both early and late cutaneous complications from chemotherapy has also increased.[19,20] These complications may be caused from a number of mechanisms, including direct toxic effects of chemotherapy, hypersensitivity reactions, and indirect effects of chemotherapy that result in altered inflammatory reactions.

The most common chemotherapeutic agents used in the treatment of Hodgkin's disease include MOPP (nitrogen mustard, vincristine, procarbazine and prednisone) and ABVD (doxorubicin, bleomycin, vinblastine and dacarbazine). It may be difficult to determine the etiology of acute skin eruptions in patients on chemotherapy because they are often immunocompromised and may additionally be taking a number of medications, such as antibiotics, for concomitant medical illnesses. However, a number of cutaneous complications may be anticipated with the current chemotherapeutic regimens. The most common of these are alopecia, stomatitis, and hyperpigmentation, with local chemical injury, onychodystrophy, hypersensitivity reactions, and photosensitivity also occurring in patients undergoing treatment for Hodgkin's disease (Table 16–1).

ALOPECIA

Alopecia is the most common cutaneous side effect of chemotherapy. The scalp hair is most frequently involved, although pubic, axillary, and facial hair may also be affected. Chemotherapeutic agents act primarily on the anagen, or growing hair follicles, resulting in a thin, malformed, and weakened hair shaft. The loss of anagen hairs results in diffuse, although not complete, alopecia. Complete alopecia occurs when telogen (resting) hairs as well as catagen hairs are affected.[20] This is usually dose-dependent and occurs most commonly with a combination of doxorubicin

Table 16–1. Mucocutaneous Reactions Related to Chemotherapy

Reaction	Drug
Alopecia	Doxorubicin,* cyclophosphamide,* bleomycin, mechlorethamine, vincristine, vinblastine
Stomatitis	Doxorubicin,* bleomycin,* cyclophosphamide, procarbazine, vincristine
Hyperpigmentation	Bleomycin, doxorubicin
Nail changes	Bleomycin, doxorubicin
Delayed hypersensitivity reactions	Doxorubicin,* mechlorethamine
Photosensitivity	Dacarbazine, vinblastine
Chemical phlebitis	Dacarbazine, doxorubicin, mechlorethamine, vinblastine
Chemical cellulitis	Doxorubicin,* mechlorethamine, vincristine, vinblastine
Transient facial erythema	Procarbazine
Increased radiosensitivity	Doxorubicin, bleomycin
Radiation recall	Doxorubicin

*Relatively more common

and cyclophosphamide.[21] Other agents that often result in hair loss include bleomycin, mechlorethamine (nitrogen mustard), vincristine, and occasionally vinblastine.[21] Hair loss caused by chemotherapy usually begins approximately 2 weeks after the administration of the drug. It is most severe 1 to 2 months following therapy, and regrowth is usually seen within 2 to 3 months.[20,22] Alopecia is almost always reversible, although the hair may occasionally regrow to a different color or texture.[23,24] The use of scalp tourniquets and local hypothermia (cold packs) has been shown to reduce the hair loss associated with chemotherapy.[20]

STOMATITIS

The agents that most commonly result in ulceration of the oral mucosa include doxorubicin[21] and bleomycin,[21,22] occurring in 20 to 40% of patients. Less frequently, cyclophosphamide, procarbazine, and vincristine have also been implicated.[21] Stomatitis appears to be dose-dependent, and its incidence has been shown to increase significantly with combination chemotherapy.[25] In most cases, stomatitis is first manifested shortly after drug administration, with mucosal erythema and a burning sensation being reported by the patient. Erosions and painful ulcers follow within a few days. Most ulcerations heal within 2 weeks following discontinuation of the drug.[20] However, secondary bacterial and fungal infections may retard the healing process. In addition to the oral mucosa being a target for the direct effect of chemotherapeutic agents, there are indirect causes of oral ulcerations, including thrombocytopenia and delayed hypersensitivity reactions such as the Stevens-Johnson syndrome.[20]

HYPERPIGMENTATION

Hyperpigmentation is a relatively common consequence of chemotherapy. The etiology generally appears to be attributed to direct stimulation of melanocytes. The hyperpigmentation may be generalized or localized to one area of skin, mucous membrane, or nail bed.

Bleomycin is the most commonly implicated agent in hyperpigmentation of the skin. Approximately 30% of patients treated with this drug will develop hyperpigmentation.[24] Although a normal number of melanocytes appear to be present in the skin, individual melanocytes are enlarged with an increased amount of endoplasmic reticulum[26] and dopa-oxidase activity.[27] A unique pattern of reaction seen with bleomycin is the presence of hyperpigmented areas at sites of trauma, often resulting in linear streaks on the trunk and proximal extremities. Minimal trauma, such as excoriation, pressure or even the application of an adhesive dressing, may result in this postinflammatory hyperpigmentation.[28] Nail changes are also frequently reported with bleomycin.[29] Darkening of the nail cuticles and palm creases have also been described,[20] as well as hyperpigmented banding of the nails.[22,29]

Doxorubicin is another common cause of chemotherapy-induced hyperpigmentation. The skin is usually affected at the skin creases, nail beds, the palms and dorsa of the hand, the soles, the face, and the oral mucosa and tongue.[30,31] Hyperpigmentation of the nail plate has also been described and may appear diffuse, or longitudinal or horizontal banding occurs.[31] The histologic changes that correlate with this hyperpigmentation from doxorubicin include increased melanin deposits within the epidermis and an increased number of melanocytes.[32]

NAIL CHANGES

Nail changes other than hyperpigmentation have also been described with a number of chemotherapeutic agents. These include Beau's lines (transverse depressions in the nail plate), which are nonspecific and may be seen with any severe illness as well as following chemotherapy.[19] Muehrke's lines (paired transverse lines on the nail plate) have also been seen.[17,22,23] Muehrke first described these diseases in 1956 as a sign of chronic hyperalbuminemia, but they have often been reported following chemotherapy. Onycholysis, loss of nails, and dystrophic nail changes have all been reported with bleomycin therapy.[27]

LOCAL INJURY

Direct toxic effects of chemotherapeutic agents may follow the intravenous administration of drugs, including phlebitis of the infused blood vessel or a local chemical cellulitis. The first signs of an adverse local reaction include an erythematous flare of the skin over the involved vein, which usually lasts less than one hour. Persistent erythema often indicates the beginning of a chemically induced phlebitis. Dacarbazine, doxorubicin, mechlorethamine, and vinblastine are most commonly implicated in the development of chemical phlebitis.

Chemical cellulitis follows the accidental extravasation of a chemotherapeutic drug into the subcutaneous tissue and may result in considerable morbidity.[34,35] The first sign is a painful erythema, which occurs immediately following extravasation, with edema resulting over the next few hours. This may resolve spontaneously, leaving an indurated or hyperpigmented area. If the reaction is severe, progressive dusky erythema, necrosis, and ulceration may occur (Fig. 16–3), occasionally causing damage to underlying nerves, muscles, and tendons. Surgical debridement may be necessary.[35] Doxorubicin has the highest incidence of cellulitis following extravasation, although this is seen in less than 1% of patients.[20] Chemical cellulitis has also been seen following extravasation of mechlorethamine, vinblastine, and vincristine.[19]

Another local injury phenomenon is that of the "recall" phenomenon. This has been described in areas of local injury, in which the previously inflamed tissue is reactivated by a subsequent administration of the offending drug. This has been seen in cases of phlebitis as well as chemical cellulitis.[36]

DELAYED HYPERSENSITIVITY REACTIONS

In the first minutes following administration of chemotherapy, delayed hypersensitivity reactions may be manifested by urticaria and angioedema, with or without anaphylaxis. This has rarely been reported with intravenous doxorubicin.[19] In addition, localized reactions have been seen in 3% of patients receiving this drug.[37] These reactions are usually manifested by erythematous

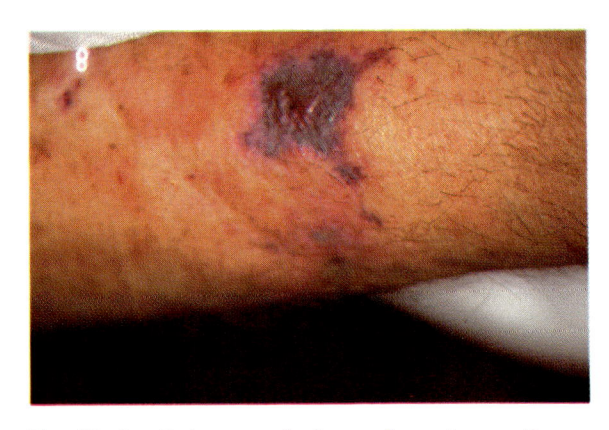

Fig. 16–3. Cutaneous findings after extravasation of chemotherapy into subcutaneous tissue. A central area of necrosis has developed.

streaks or urticarial lesions along the infused vein. This reaction occurs shortly after the drug is infused, is usually pruritic, and subsides within 30 minutes. This appears to be a histamine-mediated reaction, either as a result of direct stimulation of mass cells or basophils, or perhaps a complement-mediated mechanism.[37] There has been an additional report of nonfatal anaphylaxis following localized urticaria from doxorubicin.[38] Procarbazine has also been reported to cause urticaria.[39] Another immediate cutaneous reaction is a transient flushing of the face and neck due to a vasomotor reaction, which may also follow the administration of intravenous procarbazine.[39] Mechlorethamine has been reported to cause hypersensitivity reactions when used intravenously. In two cases, angioedema and pruritis have been recorded.[40] In another instance, an erythema multiform-like reaction has been reported.[41] Delayed hypersensitivity reactions may also occur with different chemotherapeutic regimens. Bleomycin has been shown to cause a delayed hypersensitivity reaction of a morbilliform eruption in 11% of one group of patients.[24] This drug has also been responsible for cutaneous reactions such as vesiculation[25] and edema and erythema of the extremities.[22] Some later effects of bleomycin therapy may reflect the actions of bleomycin on collagen formation. Bleomycin has been shown to stimulate the production of dermal collagen,[27] possibly through increasing the production of type I procollagen.[28,42] The late cutaneous sequelae of bleomycin therapy may resemble scleroderma.[27] Other autoimmune phenomena, specifically those related to sclerosing disorders, have also been seen following bleomycin administration. Some of these include thickening of the nail beds,[22] diffuse sclerosis of the hands and feet, and infiltrated nodules and plaques in a generalized distribution.[27] In one instance, aggressive sclerosis was so severe that gangrenous changes occurred in the finger tips.[27] Raynaud's syndrome has also been described both with and without ischemic ulcerations of the digits following bleomycin therapy.[64]

PHOTOSENSITIVITY REACTIONS

A number of chemotherapeutic agents may result in increased sensitivity to ultraviolet light. Dacarbazine and vinblastine are most frequently implicated as sources of increased sun sensitivity.[44,45] Erythematous and edematous eruptions in sun-exposed areas have been well documented following the administration of dacarbazine.[44] These areas have been described as being accompanied by a stinging sensation. Photopatch testing has shown that this reaction is associated with a lowered minimal erythema dose to ultraviolet light rays of 280 to 320 lambda (UV-B).[20] Vinblastine lowers the minimal erythema dose to ultraviolet light in a similar fashion.[45] These changes are often manifested by pruritis, followed by a vesicular eruption in sun-exposed areas. Similar lesions have also been evoked in volunteers by intradermal injections of vinblastine, followed by exposure of the skin to a suberythema dose of ultraviolet light.[45]

CORTICOSTEROIDS

The use of corticosteroids, most commonly prednisone, as part of chemotherapeutic regimens may have many consequences in the skin.[20] The typical Cushingoid features of truncal obesity, moon facies, striae, and easy bruisability are well known. Steroid acne is another common finding in patients receiving prednisone. Steroidal acne is manifested by the presence of erythematous papules and pustules, without comedones, on the chest and back. The face is often less frequently involved in steroid-related acne than it is in typical acne vulgaris.

INTERACTION OF CHEMOTHERAPEUTIC AGENTS WITH RADIATION

While a number of drug-radiation interactions are possible in Hodgkin's disease, radiation enhancement by chemotherapy is most important clinically.[46] For this reason, the doses of radiation used with combination chemotherapy are significantly lower (1500 to 3000 cGy) than those in treatment regimens of radiation alone (3500 to 4500 cGy).[13] The enhancement effect of radiation by chemotherapy may be subadditive, additive, or superadditive.[46] Enhanced radiation responses occur more frequently in the skin than in the other tissues and may result in significant morbidity.

The enhancement of radiation response by a drug has a similar appearance to that caused by radiation alone. Erythema is first seen, followed by scaling and desquamation. Vesiculation may occur in the most severe cases and may be followed by necrosis, ulceration, and postinflammatory hyperpigmentation.[20,47] Doxorubicin has been reported to cause significantly enhanced radiation effects.[48] It is felt that doxorubicin inhibits the repair of sublethal radiation damage, thereby enhancing the effects of radiation.[20] Other authors have questioned this proposed mechanism of action.[49] The greatest amount of enhancement is seen when doxorubicin is given concomitantly with radiation. In addition to the prolonged enhancement of radiosensitivity, there is significant suppression of cellular proliferation following the administration of this drug. Animal studies have shown that the gastrointestinal mucosa of mice has a 50% decrease in its expected proliferative response to radiation up to 7 weeks after the administration of doxorubicin.[46] Thus the radiation-enhancing effect may endure. Bleomycin is another agent that has been reported to produce radiation enhancement with its concomitant administration.[50] Mucous membranes may also be the targets of enhanced drug-radiation responses, including mucositis, necrosis, and ulceration. This has been seen with the concurrent administration of radiation with bleomycin,[51] as well as with various combination chemotherapy regimens.[52]

Radiation recall is another drug-radiation reaction that involves an inflammatory response in previously irradiated tissues with the administration of the drug. This phenomenon has been frequently reported with doxorubicin.[20,52] Clinical evidence of radiation damage is not a prerequisite for the development of a radiation recall reaction. The radiation recall reaction clinically resembles acute radiation injury. Recall reactions may recur with each subsequent course of chemotherapy.[20] In one instance, three separate episodes of erythema occurred in a previously irradiated site following three courses of doxorubicin. The erythema occurred 4 to 7 days after the drug was injected, with each episode lasting approximately 7 days.[20]

INFECTIOUS COMPLICATIONS

Infections involving the skin may occur in a number of settings in patients with Hodgkin's disease. The patient's predisposition to infection is most pronounced during chemotherapy-induced immunosuppression, but their increased susceptibility may remain a life-long problem even after treatment is stopped. This predisposition to infection may be associated with Hodgkin's disease itself, perhaps related to a primary T-lymphocyte defect, the late immunosuppressive effects of chemotherapy, or even the susceptibility to bacterial infections that is the result of splenectomy done for staging.[53] Patients with Hodgkin's disease, even in remission, are more prone to develop a number of viral, fungal, and bacterial infections.

Viral infections present a threat to the patient in remission as well as patients undergoing therapy for Hodgkin's disease. Perhaps the best known of these viruses is the varicella-zoster virus, resulting in either primary infection (chickenpox) or herpes zoster (shingles).[54] Infection with the varicella-zoster virus has been reported relatively frequently; in one series of patients with Hodgkin's disease followed for an average period of 5.7 years, 35% of patients experienced varicella-zoster infections, with cutaneous dissemination being seen in 42%.[53] This most frequently took the form of the re-exacerbation of the herpes zoster virus in a dermatomal distribution. Disseminated herpes zoster, with systemic manifestations, may also affect the Hodgkin's patient, whether he is under treatment or in remission (Fig. 16-4). This is manifested by the presence of disseminated umbilicated vesicles on an erythematous base, both in a dermatomal distribution as well as in a generalized fashion, with occasional involvement of the mucous membranes. With the advent of effective antiviral agents, such as acyclovir, this infection presents much less of a risk to the Hodgkin's disease patient. Other herpes

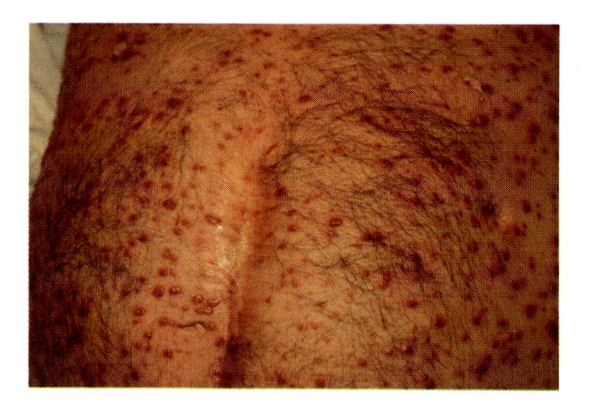

Fig. 16–4. Umbilical vesicles of disseminated herpes zoster in a patient with Hodgkin's disease.

viruses may also pose a problem.[55] Cytomegalovirus infections, as well as severe herpes simplex infections, may occur in this group of patients.[55] Another common cutaneous viral infection is the presence of common warts (verruca vulgaris), as a result of infection with a papova virus. These verrucae may prove relatively resistant to the usual therapeutic modalities. Treatments are often prolonged, with new lesions occurring frequently.

Fungal infections also pose a problem for patients with Hodgkin's disease.[56] Common dermatophyte infections, including tinea cruris and tinea pedis, are found frequently in individuals both undergoing and following treatment. More pathogenic fungi may also produce cutaneous infections in patients with Hodgkin's disease. *Coccidioides imitis* and *Cryptococcus neoformans* may affect the skin both primarily and secondarily, resulting in small erythematous papules, plaques, or occasionally abscesses.[56,57] Histoplasmosis may also be seen in these patients, with mucosal ulcerations being present in 25% of cases and other cutaneous manifestations such as erythema nodosum and erythema multiforme being reported.[56]

Bacterial infections may also occur in Hodgkin's disease, especially as a consequence of splenectomy. The increased susceptibility to *Streptococcus pneumoniae* after splenectomy is well known.[58,59] Infections with *Haemophilus influenzae* are also seen more commonly following splenectomy[53,59] and may both result in haemophilus cellulitis, which is typically reddish-purple with an irregular and rapidly advancing border, as well as the more common sinopulmonary infections.

SECOND MALIGNANCIES

The increased risk of second primary neoplasms in Hodgkin's disease patients is widely known.[60–62] It is not clear whether patients are predisposed to second malignancies by the Hodgkin's disease itself, or whether this predisposition is the result of radiation and chemotherapy used in the treatment. These data are especially difficult to obtain because of the lack of information comparing treated with untreated patients.

Chemotherapeutic agents are well recognized to be carcinogenic in animal models.[51] Procarbazine, in particular, has been shown to induce carcinomas and myelogenous leukemias in nonhuman primates.[63] However, some studies in humans have questioned the incidence of second malignancies in patients treated with chemotherapy alone for Hodgkin's disease.[61] It is clear, however, that combined-modality therapy carries with it a greater risk for the induction of second malignancies than either radiation or chemotherapy alone.[62]

The late effects of radiation therapy on the induction of cutaneous and internal malignancies are well known.[14,47,61,64] A statistically significant increased incidence of second malignancies, other than and including acute leukemias, has been reported in patients with Hodgkin's disease treated with radiation therapy alone.[61] Malignancies may occur through a number of possible mechanisms including radiation-induced nonlethal mutations of somatic cells.[47,64] The latency period after radiation therapy for the induction of skin cancers may be variable, ranging from 4 to 40 years, with an average of 7 to 12 years.[14] Cutaneous malignancies may arise in areas of chronic radiation damage or in areas that appear clinically normal.[60] The type of malignancy that develops may depend on a number of factors, including the type of radiation given, the amount of injury, and the anatomic location of the radiation.[15,65] Multiple skin cancers, including squamous cell carcinomas, basal cell carcinomas, and melanomas, may all arise in areas of radiation damage.[15]

Another factor that may contribute to the development of second cutaneous malignancies is the presence of immunodeficiency, whether primary[66] or iatrogenic.[67,68] One may consider that patients with Hodgkin's disease are not immunologically intact, perhaps as a result of the disease itself, but more likely as a result of the immunosuppressive therapy of treatment. Patients who are immunologically suppressed by drugs, especially renal transplant recipients, are well known to have an increased incidence of neoplasms.[67] Some examples of cutaneous neoplasms that have been seen in both Hodgkin's disease and in immunosuppressed patients include mycosis fungoides, Kaposi's sarcoma, basal cell carcinoma, squamous cell carcinoma, and malignant melanoma (Table 16–2).[68]

Squamous cell carcinoma is the cutaneous malignancy that is most commonly associated with immunosuppression and radiation injury. Squamous cell carcinomas frequently arise on sun-damaged skin; they occasionally arise de novo, but frequently evolve from premalignant lesions (actinic keratoses). Squamous cell carcinoma is typically an erythematous, ill-defined nodule that often grows relatively rapidly. Nodal and distant metastases are not common in healthy individuals but appear to be more frequent in immunosuppressed patients. In healthy individuals, squamous cell carcinomas occur one-third as often as basal cell carcinomas and are primarily limited to areas of sun-damaged skin. In immunosuppressed patients, however, this ratio is reversed; squamous cell carcinomas are three times as common as basal cell carcinomas. Squamous cell carcinomas also arise more commonly de novo in immunosuppressed patients, such as renal transplant recipients.[67] However, patients with lymphoproliferative malignancies have a sevenfold increase in all types of skin cancers, including basal cell carcinoma, squamous cell carcinoma, and melanoma.[68] In addition, chemotherapy such as cyclophosphamide and immunosuppressant drugs such as azathioprine are associated with an increased development of cancers. While the overall incidence of skin cancers is not known in Hodgkin's disease patients, some data may be extrapolated from the experience in renal transplant recipients. Marshall noted that 17% of patients who had received renal transplants developed skin cancers, with 28% developing premalignant lesions such as actinic keratoses or Bowen's disease.[67] There is also evidence that squamous cell carcinoma may behave more aggressively in patients with lymphoproliferative diseases, with rapid growth, local recurrence, and metastatic spread being more common in these individuals than in healthy patients.[69]

Basal cell carcinoma is another form of skin cancer that is found in immunosuppressed cancer patients. In the United States, basal cell carcinoma is the most common form of skin cancer in (healthy) Caucasians, and is usually found on the sun-exposed skin of fair-skinned individuals. Clinical features of this tumor typically include a slowly enlarging, pearly, pink, or flesh-colored nodule (Fig. 16–5). The lesion is often surrounded by telangiectasia and may have a central ulceration. Radiation exposure greatly increases the risk of basal cell carcinoma and indeed these are the most common malignancies found at irradiated sites.[14,18,70] Immunosuppression may also contribute to both the incidence and more aggressive behavior of basal cell carcinoma.[69] While basal cell carcinoma is easily controlled by locally destructive means, its early detection is especially important in patients with Hodgkin's disease because of its potentially aggressive behavior.

Malignant melanoma is the most common life-threatening form of skin cancer. Clinically, melanoma is characterized by a flat or slightly elevated lesion, with irregular pigmentation (i.e., black, white, pink, shades of

Table 16–2. Cutaneous Neoplasms in Hodgkin's Disease

Squamous cell carcinoma[68]
Basal cell carcinoma[14,18,70]
Malignant melanoma[68,71]
Kaposi's sarcoma[72,73]
Spindle cell squamous cell carcinoma[65]
Mycosis fungoides[74,75]
Sebaceous carcinoma[15]
Sweat-gland carcinoma[15]

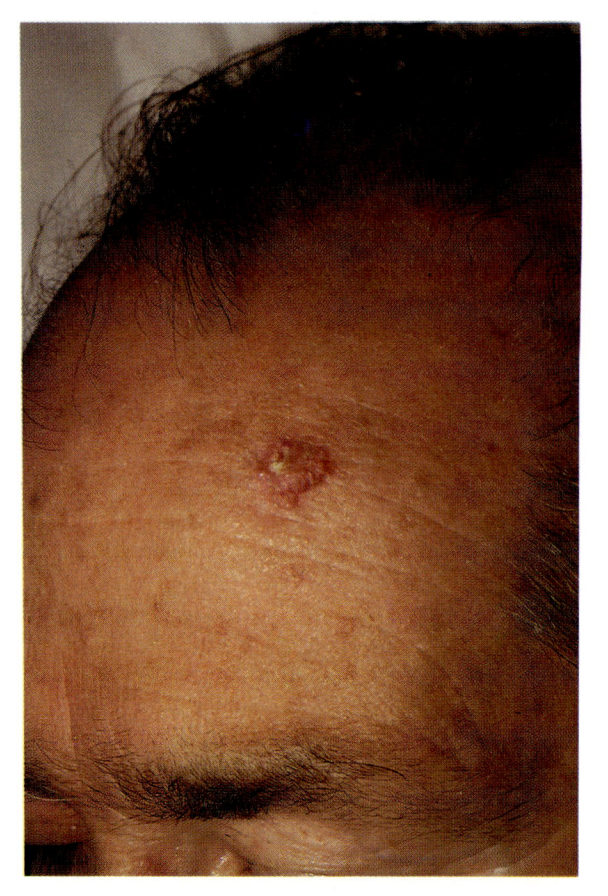

Fig. 16–5. Pearly, flesh-colored nodule of basal cell carcinoma.

brown) (Fig. 16–6). Melanomas also occur with greater frequency in patients with lymphoma,[68] and specifically in Hodgkin's disease,[71] than in the general population. Since malignant melanoma is a potentially curable lesion, early detection in predisposed individuals is crucial.

Other cutaneous malignancies may also arise with greater frequency in areas of radiation injury. Spindle cell squamous cell carcinomas are aggressive tumors that may occur in radiation-damaged sites.[65] Other malignant tumors, such as sebaceous carcinomas and sweat-gland carcinomas, have also been reported in this setting.[15]

Kaposi's sarcoma is another neoplasm that has been closely linked to lymphoproliferative disorders and immunodeficiency states.[72,73] Kaposi's sarcoma is characterized by reddish-purple nodules in the skin and is often multifocal in its presentation (Fig. 16–7). In its classic form, Kaposi's sarcoma typically involves the lower extremities of elderly men. However, when Kaposi's sarcoma occurs in immunodeficient patients, such as in the variant associated with the acquired immune deficiency syndrome, the tumors may be widespread, even involving lymph nodes and internal organs. The incidence of Kaposi's sarcoma is significantly increased in patients with Hodgkin's disease;[73] conversely, patients presenting with classic Kaposi's sarcoma have a twentyfold increase in the incidence of lymphoid malignancies.[72]

Finally, the patient with a history of Hodgkin's disease may also be predisposed to the development of other lymphomas in the skin.[74–76] Mycosis fungoides, or cutaneous T-

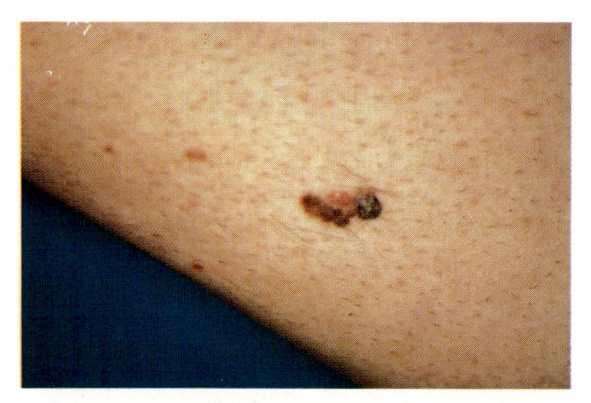

Fig. 16–6. Malignant melanoma. Irregularity of pigmentation with peripheral nodular component.

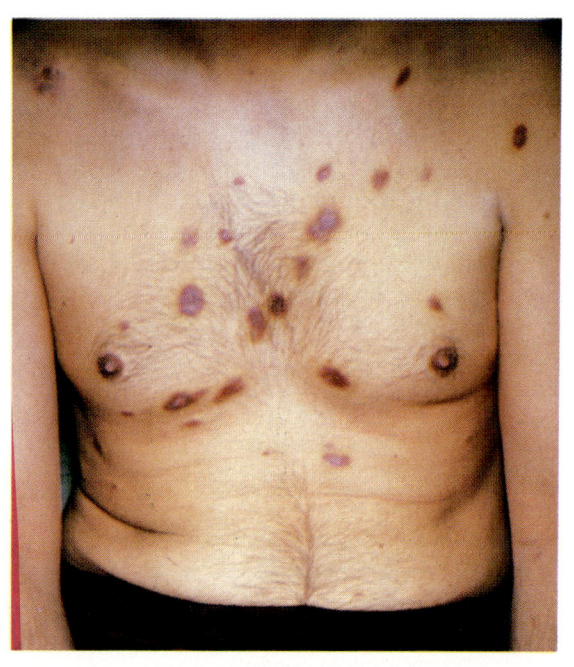

Fig. 16–7. Reddish-purple nodules of Kaposi's sarcoma.

cell lymphoma, has been reported both preceding and following the diagnosis of Hodgkin's disease.[74,75] Sézary syndrome, in which a T-cell leukemia accompanies the cutaneous T-cell lymphoma, has also been reported in this setting.[76]

The patient with Hodgkin's disease faces a number of cutaneous complications as a result of both therapy and the disease itself. In the earliest stages of treatment, the skin is often the site of various reactions to chemotherapy and/or radiotherapy. An increased susceptibility to infections involving the skin, especially fungi and viruses, may persist indefinitely following treatment and may in fact be related to Hodgkin's disease itself. The late sequelae of Hodgkin's disease primarily involve the increased risk of skin cancers. With the early recognition of these cutaneous sequelae, the patient with Hodgkin's disease can avoid further morbidity from these problems.

REFERENCES

1. Rubins, J. Cutaneous Hodgkin's disease: Indolent course and control with chemotherapy. Cancer 42:1218, 1978.
2. Kaplan, H.S. Hodgkin's disease: Unfolding concepts concerning its nature, management and prognosis. Cancer 45:239–2474, 1980.
3. Gobbi, P.G., Attardo-Parinello, G., Laltizaio, G. et al. Severe pruritus should be a B-symptom in Hodgkin's disease. Cancer 51:1934–1936, 1983.
4. Feiner, A., Mahmood, T., and Wallner, S. Prognostic importance of pruritus in Hodgkin's disease. JAMA 240:2738–2740, 1978.
5. Cooper, M.F. et al. Acquired ichthyosis and impaired lipogenesis in Hodgkin's disease. Br. J. Dermatol. 102:689, 1980.
6. Stevanovic, D.V. Hodgkin's disease of the skin: Acquired ichthyosis preceding tumor and ulcerating lesions for seven years. Arch. Dermatol. 82:96, 1960.
7. Belisario, J.C. Cutaneous manifestations associated with internal cancer. Cutis 1:513–522, 1965.
8. Smith, J.L. and Butler, J.L. Skin involvement in Hodgkin's disease. Cancer 45:354–361, 1980.
9. Winkelman, R.K. et al. Cutaneous syndromes produced as side effects of triparanol therapy. Arch. Dermatol. 87:372–377, 1963.
10. Kedor, A. et al. Autoimmune disorders complicating adolescent Hodgkin's disease. Cancer 44:112, 1979.
11. Efremidis, A., Eiser, A.R., Grishman, E. et al. Hodgkin's lymphoma in an adolescent with systemic lupus erythematosus. Cancer 53:142, 1984.
12. Callen, J.P. The value of malignancy evaluation in patients with dermatomyositis. J. Am. Acad. Dermatol. 6:253–259, 1982.
13. Sanders, C. and Kathren, R. Lymphoid tissue. In Ionizing Radiation Tumorigenic and Tumorifidal Effects. Columbus, Battelle Press, 1983.
14. Wiskemann, A. Effects of ionizing radiation of the skin. In Dermatology in General Medicine. Edited by J.B. Fitzpatrick et al. New York, McGraw Hill, 2nd Edition, 1979.
15. Tranenkle, H.L. Late radiation injury and cutaneous neoplasms. In Cancer Dermatology. Edited by F. Helm. Philadelphia, Lea & Febiger, 1979.
16. Slanina, T. et al. Long-term side effects in irradiated patients with Hodgkin's disease. Int. J. Radiat. Oncol. Biol. Phys. 2:1, 1977.
17. McMeekin, T.V. and Moshella, S.L. Iatrogenic complications of dermatologic therapy. Primum non nocere. Med. Clin. North Am. 63:441, 1979.
18. Martin, H., Strong, F., and Spiro, R.H. Radiation-induced skin cancer of the head and neck. Cancer 25:61–71, 1970.
19. Dunogin, W.G. Clinical toxicity of chemotherapeutic agents: dermatologic toxicity. Semin. Oncol. 9:14, 1982.
20. Brunner, A.K. and Hood, A.F. Cutaneous complications of chemotherapeutic agents. J. Am. Acad. Dermatol. 9:645, 1983
21. Levine, N. and Greenwald, F.S. Mucocutaneous side effects of cancer chemotherapy. Cancer Treat. Rev. 5:67–84, 1978.
22. Blum, R.H., Carter, S.K., and Agre, K. A clinical review of bleomycin a new antineoplastic agent. Cancer 31:903–914, 1973.
23. Falksun, G. and Schulz, E.J. Changes in hair pigmentation associated with cancer chemotherapy. Cancer Treat. Rep. 65:529, 1981.
24. Yagoda, A. et al. Bleomycin, an antitumor antibiotic. Clinical experience in 274 patients. Ann. Intern. Med. 77:861–870, 1972.
25. Bennett, J.M. et al. Bleomycin. Ann. Intern. Med. 90:945–948, 1979.
26. Perrot, H. and Ortonne, J.P. Hyperpigmentation after bleomycin therapy: Ultrastructural study. Arch. Derm. Res. 261:245–252, 1978.
27. Coeh, I.S. et al. Cutaneous toxicity of bleomycin therapy. Arch. Dermatol. 107:553, 1973.
28. Lowitz, B.B. Streaking with bleomycin. (letter) N. Engl. J. Med. 242:1300, 1975.
29. Shetty, M.R. Case of pigmented banding of the nail caused by bleomycin. Cancer Treat. Rep. 61:501–502, 1977.
30. Moris, D., Aisner, J., and Wiernik, P.H. Horizontal pigmented banding of the nails in association with adriamycin chemotherapy. Cancer Treat. Rep. 61:499–501, 1977.
31. Pratt, C.B. Hyperpigmentation of the nails from doxorubicin. JAMA 228:460, 1974.
32. Orr, L.F. and Mckernan, J.F. Pigmentation with doxorubicin therapy. Arch. Dermatol. 116:273, 1980.
33. Schwartz, R.A. and Vickerman, C.E. Muehrke lines of the fingernails. Arch. Intern. Med. 134:242, 1979.

34. Reilly, J.J., Weifeld, J.P., and Rosenberg, S.A. Clinical course and management of accidental adriamycin extravasation. Cancer 40:2053–2056, 1977.
35. Ruldolph, R., Suzuki, M., and Luce, J.K. Experimental skin necrosis produced by adriamycin. Cancer Treat. Rep. 63:529–537, 1979.
36. Buer, D. and Wilkinson, L.S. Daunorubicin, adriamycin and recall effect. Ann. Intern. Med. 85:259–260, 1976.
37. Weiss, R.B. and Bruna, S. Hypersensitivity reactions to cancer chemotherapeutic agents. Ann. Intern. Med. 94:66–72, 1981.
38. Etcunbonus, E. and Wilbur, J.R. Uncommon side effects of adriamycin. Cancer Chemother. Rep. 58:757–758, 1974.
39. Brunner, K.W. and Young, C.W. Amethyhydrozine derivative in Hodgkin's disease and other malignant neoplasms: therapeutic and toxic effect studies in 51 patients. Ann. Intern. Med. 63:69–86, 1965.
40. Wilsop, K.S. and Alexander, S. Hypersensitivity to mechlorethamine. Ann. Intern. Med. 94:823, 1981.
41. Brauer, M.J., McEvoy, B.F., and Mitus, W.J. Hypersensitivity to nitrogen mustards in the form of erythema multiforme: a unique reaction. Intern. Med. 120:499, 1967.
42. Clark, J.G., Starcher, B.C., and Vitts, J. Bleomycin-induced synthesis of type I pro-collagen by human lung and skin fibroblasts in culture. Biochem. Biophys. Acta. 631:359–370, 1980.
43. Chernicoff, D.R., Bukowski, R.M., and Young, J.R. Raynaud's syndrome phenomenon after bleomycin treatment. Cancer Treat. Rep. 62:570–571, 1978.
44. Yung, C.W., Winston, E.M., and Lorinez, A.L. Dacarbazine-induced photosensitivity reaction. J. Am. Acad. Dermatol. 4:541–543, 1981.
45. Breza, T.S., Halprin, K.M., and Taylor, J.R. Photosensitivity reaction to vinblastine. Arch. Dermatol. 111:1168–1170, 1975.
46. Schenken, L.L., Burholt, D.R., and Kovacs, C.J. Adriamycin radiation combinations: drug-induced delayed gastrointestinal sensitivity. Int. J. Radiat. Oncol. Biol. Phys. 5:1265–1269, 1979.
47. Carmel, R.J. and Kaplan, J.S. Mantle irradiation in Hodgkin's disease. Cancer 37:2813, 1976.
48. Philips, J.L. Chemical modification of radiation effects. Cancer 39:987–999, 1977.
49. Field, S.B. and Michalowski, A. Endpoints for damage to normal tissues. Int. J. Radiat. Oncol. Biol. Phys. 5:1185–1196, 1974.
50. Philip, T.L. and Fu, K.K. Quantification of combined radiation therapy and chemotherapy effects on critical normal tissues. Cancer 37:1186–1200, 1976.
51. Arseneau, J.C., et al. Risk of new concerns in patients with Hodgkin's disease. Cancer 40:1912–1916, 1977.
52. Phillips, J.L. Tissue Toxicity of Radiation Drug Interactions in the Treatment of Cancer. New York, John Wiley, 1975, 1980.
53. Notter, D.T. et al. Infections in patients with Hodgkin's disease: A clinical study of 300 consecutive adult patients. Rev. Int. Dis. 2:761–800, 1980.
54. Reboul, F., Donaldson, S.S., and Kaplan, H.S. Herpes zoster and varicella infections in children with Hodgkin's disease: analysis of contributing factors. Cancer 41:95–99, 1978.
55. Luna, M.A. and Lichtiger, B. Disseminated toxoplasmosis and cytomegalovirus infection complicating Hodgkin's disease. Am. J. Clin. Pathol. 55:499–505, 1971.
56. Rosen, R.P. Opportunistic fungal infections in patients with neoplastic disease. Pathol. Annu. 11:255–315, 1976.
57. Zimmerman, L.F. and Rappaport, H. Occurrence of cryptococcosis in patients with malignant disease of the reticuloendothelial system. Am. J. Clin. Pathol. 24:1050–1072, 1954.
58. Weitzman, S.A. et al. Impaired humoral immunity in treated Hodgkin's disease. N. Engl. J. Med. 297:245–248, 1977.
59. Weitzman, S. and Aisenberg, A.C. Fulminant sepsis after the successful treatment of Hodgkin's disease. Am. J. Med. 62:47–50, 1977.
60. Schomberg, P.J. et al. Second malignant lesions after therapy for Hodgkin's disease. Mayo Clin. Prol. 59:493–497, 1984.
61. Arsenea, J.C. et al. Non-lymphomatous malignant tumors complicating Hodgkin's disease—Possible associations with intensive therapy. N. Engl. J. Med. 287:1119–1122, 1972.
62. Canellos, G.P., DeVita, V.J., Arsenear, J.L. et al. Carcinogenesis by cancer chemotherapeutic agents. Second malignancies complicating Hodgkin's disease in remission. Recent Results. Cancer Res. 49:108–114, 1974.
63. O'Gara, R.W. et al. Neoplasms of the hematopoietic system in non-human primates—Report of one spontaneous tumor and two leukemias induced by procarbazine. J. Natl. Cancer Inst. 46:1121–1130, 1971.
64. Pack, G.T. and Dovis, J. Radiation cancer of the skin. Radiology 84:436–442, 1965.
65. Hanke, C.N. et al. Chemosurgical reports: basal cell carcinoma resulting from radiation therapy for hypertrophic tonsils. J. Dermat. Surg. Oncol. 11:108–110, 1985.
66. Gatti, R.A. and Good, R.A. Occurrence of malignancy in immuno-deficiency states. Cancer 28:84–98, 1971.
67. Walder, B.K., Robertson, M.R., and Jeremy, D. Skin cancer and immunosuppression. Lancet 2:1282–1283, 1971.
68. Berg, J.W. The incidence of multiple primary cancers. I. Development of further cancers in patients with lymphomas, leukemias and myeloma. J. Natl. Cancer Inst. 38:741–752, 1967.
69. Weimar, V.M., Ceilley, R.I., and Goeke, J.A. Aggressive biologic behavior of basal and squamous cell cancers in patients with chronic lymphocytic leukemia or chronic lymphocytic lymphoma. J. Dermatol. Surg. Oncol. 5:609–614, 1979.
70. Allison, J.R. Radiation-induced basal-cell carcinoma. J. Dermatol. Surg. Oncol. 10:200, 1984.
71. Tucker, M.A. et al. Cutaneous malignant melanoma after Hodgkin's disease. Ann. Intern. Med. 102:37–412, 1985.
72. Safai, B. et al. Association of Kaposi's sarcoma with

second primary malignancies. Possible etiopathologic implications. Cancer 45:1472–1479, 1980.
73. Ulbright, T.M. and Santa Cruz, D.J. Kaposi's sarcoma: Relationship with hematologic, lymphoid and thymic neoplasia. Cancer 47:963–973, 1981.
74. Chan, W.C. et al. Mycosis fungoides and Hodgkin's disease occurring in the same patient: report of three cases. Cancer 44:1408, 1979.
75. Caya, J.G. et al. Hodgkin's disease followed by mycosis fungoides in the same patient. Cancer 53:463–467, 1984.
76. Buchner, S.A. Sezary syndrome after successful treatment of Hodgkin's disease. Arch. Dermatol. 117:50, 1981.

CHAPTER 17

Dental Complications After Treatment for Hodgkin's Disease

PHILIP TERMAN
MORTIMER J. LACHER

The treatment of Hodgkin's disease with primary radiation therapy, polychemotherapy, or both has resulted in an extraordinary percentage of 5-year survivals. These successes are now expected to extend patients lives beyond the 10-year mark. This will result, it is hoped, in "normal" life expectancies for the majority of patients. Because of this anticipation of a "normal" life for the majority of patients, it is now more important than ever to review the management of the patients' dentition as part of the overall initial treatment plan and with respect to the complications that might occur as a result of the Hodgkin's treatment itself.

Plans for dental management after radiation therapy have usually depended on data obtained from patients treated with radiation therapy for primary tumors of the head and neck region. These patients with head and neck tumors typically have a history of alcoholism and excessive cigarette smoking. They are usually past the age of 50. Their radiation treatment, usually employing intensive external radiation therapy, encompasses all of the salivary glands, with doses of radiation, commonly one-and-a-half to two times the doses applied to Hodgkin's patients. Patients with head and neck tumors typically receive 6000 to 8000 cGy and sometimes even higher doses using interstitial radiation sources.

Only in a general way do these extremely intense radiation factors apply to the Hodgkin's patient. Adult Hodgkin's patients, for instance, typically receive only 3600 to 4400 cGy to the neck areas and the lower jaw, with only limited radiation of the salivary glands;[1] in children with Hodgkin's disease, the effort now is to restrict the dose of radiation to 2000 to 3000 cGy (the lesser dose being more desirable) to prevent the suppression of bone growth, while adding combination chemotherapy[2,3] to insure long survival. Most of the adult Hodgkin's patients are between the ages of 20 to 40 years and have never been characterized as excessive smokers or alcoholics, characteristics that are common to patients who develop head and neck tumors involving the mouth and pharynx. Furthermore, radical surgery of the neck or the partial removal of the mandible or other important bony structures that play an important role in dentition (commonly part of the treatment of tumors arising in the head and neck region) is no longer even considered as part of the treatment of Hodgkin's patients.[4] These important differences in primary treatment must be considered when setting a treatment plan to conserve the dentition of the Hodgkin's patient.

Hodgkin's patients fall into two groups of concern when considering the effects of treatment on dentition. First, patients usually less than 13 years of age, in their formative years are now treated with less radiation and more chemotherapy in an attempt to avoid bone growth defects. The majority of Hodgkin's patients fall into the second category. They are treated between the ages of 20 and 40 and receive radiation therapy in doses that rarely exceed 4400 cGy, which affects only a limited area of the jawbone and salivary glands when the upper mantle-field radiation therapy is employed.

With appreciation of the differences between the treatment that head and neck patients receive compared to Hodgkin's patients, we try to extrapolate the data from the existing literature as it may apply to the Hodgkin's patient. In time, many more studies specifically about the Hodgkin's patient will be developed. Because specific data concerning Hodgkin's patients is limited, we also use data concerning other lymphoma patients to complete as comprehensive a review as possible.

The nature of objective complications of treatment, such as alterations in growth and development of the jaw and the teeth, radiation-induced osteonecrosis, and dental caries, are reviewed. Reasonable plans to prevent, control, and treat these problems are outlined.

GROWTH DEFECTS

THE EFFECT OF RADIATION ON BONE AND TOOTH DEVELOPMENT

Depending on the age of the patient, even when the treatment is not delivered directly to the jawbones, the effect of the scatter radiation on developing teeth can produce complete agenesis of some teeth. A case report by Weyman[5] demonstrated that in a patient 2 to 3 years of age in whom whole lung radiation took place, only nine permanent teeth developed.

The changes to the developing tooth structure depend on the point of development of the dentition at the time of initiating therapy. Guggenheimer, Fischer, and Pechersky[6] reported a case of a 7-year-old boy who received 5500 cGy to the palate, nasopharynx, and base of the skull, and an additional 4500 cGy to the cervical lymph nodes from an external ionizing radiation source (Cobalt 60). This was instituted after complete excision of the soft palate for an embryonal rhabdomyosarcoma. The field of radiation included the areas of dentition from the cuspids through the molars and the parotid glands. For the next 7 years, extensive dental care was necessary because of the development of radiation caries. By the age of 20, except for the incisors and first molars, all the teeth had arrested root development. Only rudimentary maxillary and mandibular molars were present.

Guggenheimer et al. noted the following: "Immature teeth are most sensitive to the teratogenic effects of large doses of radiation. Susceptibility is considerably prolonged for the permanent dentition, because it usually does not become permanently calcified until 15 or 16 years of age. At any time prior to this, therapeutic irradiation of the head or neck regions is likely to produce malformation and developmental arrest of the noncalcified components. The full impact of irradiation will not become apparent until the teeth erupt; unfortunately, even the most severely malformed teeth are capable of eruption. This factor contributes to the delayed morbidity of radiation therapy, because such teeth require extensive treatment and may be lost anyway due to insurmountable structural defects."[6]

The degree of calcification at the time of therapy is the critical line of demarcation for prognosticating malformation. When calcified, the direct effects of irradiation are negligible, and even with damage to the root structure the teeth will erupt.

Although it is anticipated that relatively large doses of radiation ordinarily employed to treat malignant tumors will result in significant and serious alterations in growth and development of bony structures and dentition in children, even limited low-dose radiation may alter the development of the developing teeth. Weyman[5] reported the instance of a 5-month-old child who had been treated for a congenital nevus of the left lower lip and the adjacent cheek with a single application of superficial x-radiation of 400 r; the underlying bone received an approximately 200 to 250 r. The growth and development of the child's teeth were observed for a period of 15 years, and it was concluded that ". . . the effect of low-dosage irradiation on developing teeth at the center of application is similar to that which occurs if the dental development area is at the periphery of a sphere of heavy dosage. There was earlier eruption at the affected site and slightly advanced root completion. That this effect was so slight presumably accounts for the fact that there was no observable shortening of the roots. The result not previously recorded was the defective enamel on the two deciduous and first permanent molars in the quadrant."[5]

Radiation to the head and neck of children with Hodgkin's disease can cause malformation and arrest development of the (prenatal) teeth as well as produce developmental abnormalities of the jaws. Facial bone growth retardation can result from indirect radiation (scatter radiation) as well as direct radiation during therapy for malignant disease.[7,8]

Lines et al.[7] reported using radiation dosages varying from 3600 to 4000 cGy to the mantle field for Hodgkin's disease with extreme efforts to assure against direct radiation of the jaw in three children aged 9, 9, and 12. Analysis in two of the cases showed that there was no direct irradiation to the mandibles and in one case the mantle field bordered on, but did not include, the entire mandible. Since the patients were carefully immobilized and special emphasis was placed on the reproducibility of patient position for daily treatment, it must be presumed that the mandibles received only indirect radiation. Even in this meticulously monitored situation, the carefully measured radiation to the mandible was found to be significant. From their data, it was suggested that an estimated 25% of children treated with extended-field irradiation using the upper mantle field (for Hodgkin's disease) "are at risk for altered development of the mandibular structures."[7]

In the cases of Lines et al.,[7] the following abnormalities were observed: Case I: roentgenograms revealed premature apical closure of roots of the bicuspids and the second and third molar teeth in the lower jaw with foreshortening of these teeth. Case II: premature apical closure of the roots and foreshortening of the lower cuspids and the first and second bicuspids occurred, with no root formation of the lower third molars. In addition, the patient developed a severe malocclusion. Case III: roentgenograms suggested early apical closure of roots and foreshortening of lower cuspids, bicuspids, and second molars.

Damage to the growth centers in the body and the condyle of the mandible and stimulus to the erupting teeth may occur from direct or scatter radiation from mantle field radiation therapy in the treatment of Hodgkin's disease. Radiation effects on the teeth are characterized by malformation of the crowns, dwarfing of the tooth structure as evidenced by shortness and tapering, and premature apical closure of the root.

At The University of Texas M. D. Anderson Hospital and Tumor Institute, long-term survivors of childhood cancer returning for follow-up in 1979 were referred to the Department of Dental Oncology for evaluation. This follow-up study by Jaffe et al.[8] is a comprehensive analysis of dental and maxillofacial abnormalities detected in long-term survivors of childhood cancer radiation and chemotherapy. Their study, published in 1984, concerned 45 long-term survivors of childhood cancer who had received radiation of the maxillofacial region; this included 14 patients who had been treated for Hodgkin's disease between the ages of 3 to 16 years (median 5 years). In Hodgkin's patients "The interval between treatment and examination was 3 to 16 years (median 6 years). The radiation dose varied from 2,000 to 4,900 rad (median 3,000 rad), and radiation was administered to a mantle or right or left neck port. The majority of the patients developed root and crown abnormalities without facial deformities. However, mild mandibular hypoplasia was noted on the side that received radiation."

A Memorial Hospital Case Report

A striking example of the disastrous effects of radiation therapy and chemotherapy that could affect the developing child treated for lymphoma is illustrated by the following case:

L.M. was initially referred to the Dental Department of the Memorial Sloan Kettering Cancer Center the first time on January 7, 1972, with the following history:

In October, 1971, at the age of five, she first noted rhinorrhea. In November, 1971, she had epistaxis occurring almost every day. In December, 1971, the mother noticed that her appetite had decreased and that she began to lose weight. Enlarged right anterior cervical nodes then appeared. On December 22, 1971, an adenoidectomy and tonsillectomy was performed at another hospital. A diagnosis of diffuse, undifferentiated, malignant lymphoma of the nasopharynx with cervical-node involvement was established. After an extensive work-up, which included a negative lymphangiogram and normal bone marrow and peripheral blood studies, it was concluded that disease was present only in the nasopharynx and cervical nodes. A diagnosis of American Burkitt's lymphoma was considered. On January 14, 1972, she started on an intense chemotherapy protocol and simultaneously began radiation therapy to the nasopharynx, receiving a total dosage of 5500 cGy. In addition, radiation therapy was delivered to both side of the neck, with each area receiving a total of 4500 cGy. This was the radiation dosage presumed to be necessary to be curative, the clinicians did not fully anticipate what the local toxicity and morbidity would be.

All visible tumor rapidly disappeared. She was continued on intermittent maintenance chemotherapy for 2 years and then all therapy was stopped. No further antitumor therapy has been given since 1974. It soon became obvious during the latter time of her treatment period that her growth development and her normal expected pattern of weight gain had stalled. In addition, she developed a significant degree of lymphedema of the head and neck area exacerbated with every recurring upper respiratory infection. Microphthalmia then became evident. Tooth development was delayed and hypothyroidism appeared. A decreased production of growth hormone was documented. Despite hormone replacement, the damage to growth and development has been severe.

The radiographic effects on the facial bones and the teeth are illustrated in Figures 17–1 and 17–2. The nature of the dental destruction is shown by the dwarfed roots, by the malformation of the last molar crowns, and by the continuing tooth decay. The roots, although dwarfed, did erupt normally, but there is crowding of the teeth. Furthermore, this patient has extreme trismus adding to the difficulties of interventive treatment. The size of the facial bones are all diminutive. Her dental prognosis is poor and it is anticipated that she will experience continued tooth decay and tooth loss.

Other Reported Cases

Carl and Wood[9] observed that if destructive doses of radiation therapy have to be used to control childhood cancer and normal tissues are in the path of the radiation beams, no current methods or radiation techniques are available to prevent these destructive byproducts of the therapy. They reported two cases of children treated at ages 4 and 9 for embryonal rhabdomyosarcoma in the left submandibular and left cheek area respectively. Initial surgery and then radiation therapy were followed by chemotherapy (actinomycin D and vincristine). Six years after treatment, the child who was initially treated at 4-years-of-age had no root development of the permanent mandibular anterior teeth and premolars and only partial root development of the molars. The mandible was generally underdeveloped. The child initially treated at 9 years of age had more complications of her treatment, and 3 years after her initial treatment a panoramic radiograph showed underdevelopment of the left side of the mandible, indicating that growth had been arrested on the side of greatest concentration of radiation. Carl and Wood noted that, "Functionally, considerable trismus had de-

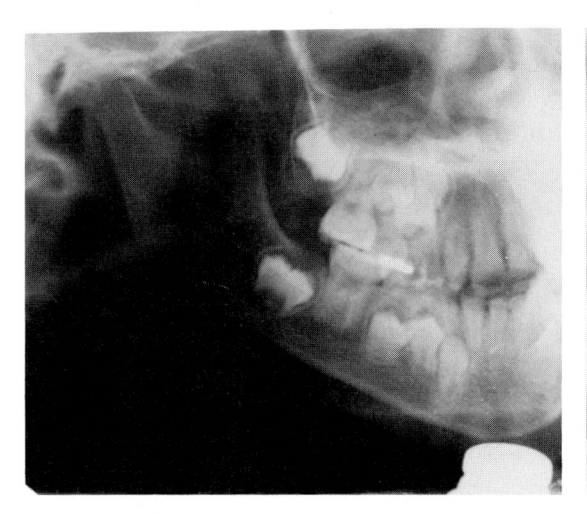

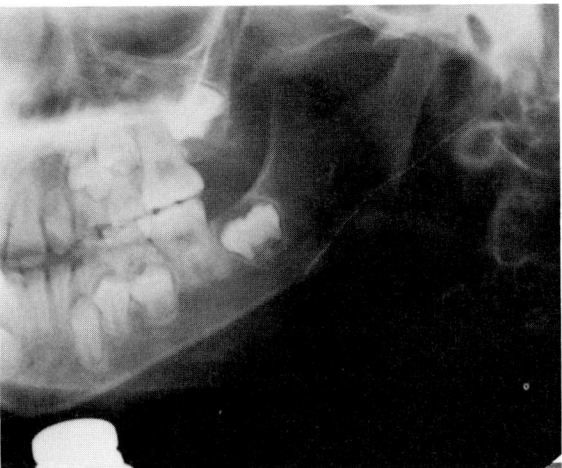

Fig. 17–1. The radiograph documents the developing dentition at the beginning of treatment (February 27, 1974). There is no evidence of the developing third molar on the radiograph and the patient is free of decay. The developing roots are straight up and down and do not appear to be crowded. The apices of the roots are open and the anatomy appears to be normal.

veloped as a result of the surgery and the radiotherapy. The oral condition had deteriorated to the point at which the teeth on the left side had to be extracted with use of general anesthesia."[9]

With a far greater appreciation of the late or long term effects of cancer therapy on the developing child when there are therapeutic choices, the risks versus the benefits to be derived should determine the therapeutic approach. These choices have been especially important in the management of children with Hodgkin's disease, and protocols of combined limited radiation therapy and

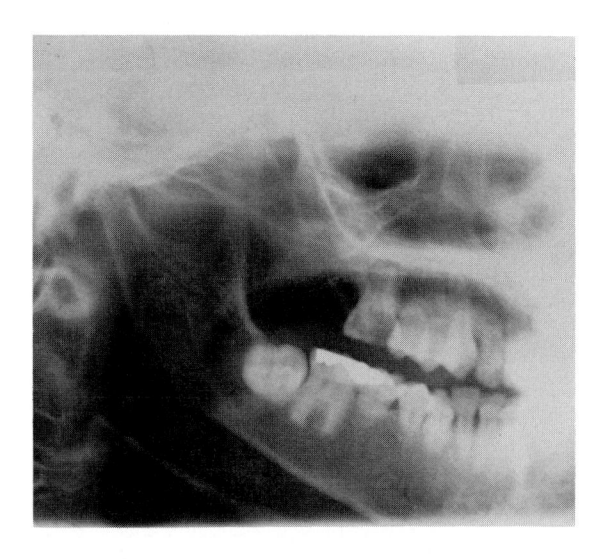

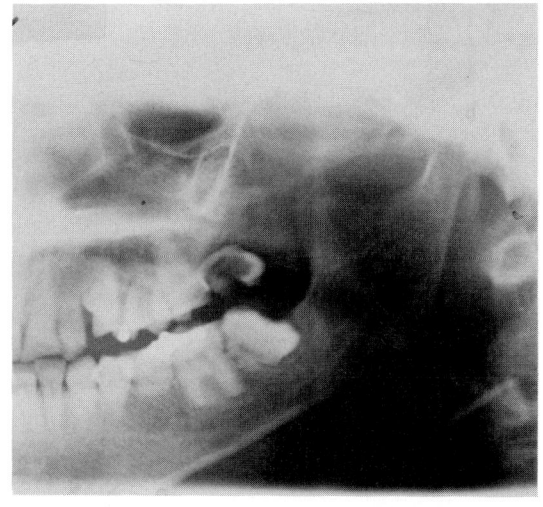

Fig. 17–2. Ten years after the radiograph in Figure 17–1, the roots have continued their upward movement and forced the deciduous teeth out, but they have not developed. The apices of the teeth have closed, but the length is attenuated at the exact same length as it was at the start of treatment. There is no evidence of the third molar bud and will not be. There is evidence of radiation caries in spite of a vigorous fluoride program.

chemotherapy are now being used to produce the greatest numbers of survivors with the least damage to the developing organs.[2,3]

THE EFFECT OF HERPES ZOSTER INFECTION ON TOOTH AND BONE GROWTH

Devitalization and exfoliation of teeth and necrosis of bone may occur following herpes zoster infection, and this may occur at any age. Smith and Rose[10] reported a case of abnormal tooth development following herpes zoster infection in a 7-year-old. Herpes zoster is of particular interest in the management of the Hodgkin's patient as it may occur in as many as 25% of the population after treatment at some time. The incidence of this viral disease in Hodgkin's patients is greater than the general population and the clinical course of the disease may be more severe. In some instances, the infection becomes life threatening as it generalizes into a full blown chickenpox syndrome with the viral infection affecting every organ system.

The etiology of the herpes zoster effect on dentition, which results in the eventual loss of teeth, occurs when it affects dermatomes serving the dental areas, probably as a result of neurovascular changes induced by the viral infection. Herpes zoster also causes distress because of the severe neuralgia accompanying the infection; when the trigeminal nerve is involved, it may simulate a toothache of extreme severity. Herpes zoster may also result in painful oral mucosal ulcers. Because the zoster infection is usually self-limited, these acute changes on the mucosa need only to be treated symptomatically. It is hoped that newly developed antiviral agents will eventually control herpes zoster in adults. Acyclovir is an antiviral agent that does appear to have limited effectiveness against herpes zoster.[11] Varicella-zoster immune-globulin (VZIG) is effective in modifying the course of chickenpox in children, provided it is administered in less than 96 hours after exposure and preferably within the first 24 to 48 hours of exposure. The use of VZIG in adults with Hodgkin's disease is still not clearly established. In general, if VZIG is not applied within 48 to 96 hours of exposure to herpes zoster, it will not be useful. In established cases of zoster or varicella, VZIG is not useful. "VZIG is not known to be useful in treating clinical varicella or zoster or in preventing disseminated zoster, and is not recommended for such use."[12] Despite the absence of scientific data, VZIG may be recommended for use in adults, making the presumption that VZIG has a very low incidence of known serious side effects and that it might be helpful. According to the recommendations of the Immunization Practices Advisory Committee, as outlined in the Morbidity and Mortality Report of the Centers for Disease Control (March 1984), however, "VZIG has not been evaluated as a prophylactic measure for prevention or attenuation of varicella in normal or immunocompromised adults. Therefore, data do not exist with which to calculate the appropriate dose in adults."[12] Because no specific treatment can be applied directly to the teeth or the underlying bone in cases of herpes zoster, it is hoped that effective, specific treatment of the herpes zoster infection will be developed soon, thus ending the complications associated with this infection.

Case History

The following case history relates an unusual series of multiple dental abscesses following infection by herpes zoster.

SC presented with Stage IIA nodular sclerosing Hodgkin's disease. She underwent a course of radiotherapy as her initial treatment. The radiotherapy was given to a mantle port, which included direct radiation to the lower jaw. Her Hodgkin's disease recurred in late 1978 and in 1979 she underwent a year of combination chemotherapy. In September, 1981, she developed a herpes-zoster infection involving the third division of the left trigeminal nerve. The skin rash resolved, but the infection resulted in permanent damage to the nerves innervating the left lower jaw teeth. The teeth abscessed following the viral attack (Fig. 17–3).

THE DEVELOPMENT OF CARIES IN RELATION TO CHANGES IN SALIVARY-GLAND SECRETIONS

Salivary-gland changes following radiation therapy for Hodgkin's disease are probably

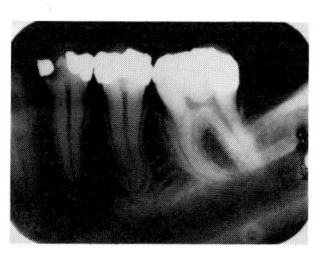

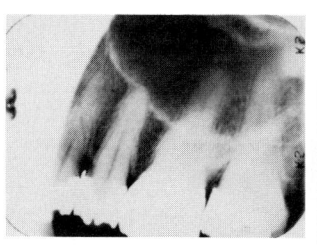

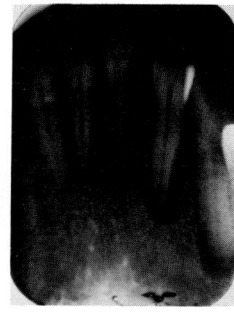

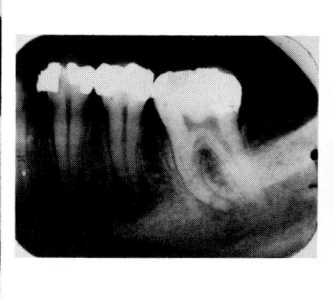

Fig. 17-3. Radiographs depicting teeth prior to the onset of herpes zoster and after the skin infection had subsided. The teeth abscessed following the viral attack.

not as severe as the changes accompanying cancericidal doses of radiation for other head and neck tumors because the dosages are lower and only a limited number of salivary glands are affected. However, when the radiation field includes Waldeyer's ring, both parotid glands, and the submaxillary glands, the effect may be just as severe. Even limited radiation therapy, affecting only the lower jaw and the salivary glands in that region and sparing the parotids, may result in significant acute and long-term changes in salivary secretions. This in turn may affect the development of caries in teeth of both the upper and lower jaw of Hodgkin's patients,[12,12a] even though the radiation dose is delivered only to the lower jaw and spares the upper jaw.

Typically, data regarding the effects of xerostomia on changes in salivary secretions and microbial content[13] were derived from patients treated for "midline cancers of the head and neck." The patients' mean age was 50 years, and they were scheduled to receive a minimum of 5000 cGy at the rate of 1000 cGy per week, including partial-to-total coverage of the major salivary glands. These studies, therefore, represent the maximum effect that can be anticipated secondary to radiation therapy of the head and neck region, with the Hodgkin's patients' reactions falling somewhere below this level of deprivation of saliva (and resulting alteration in the microbial changes of the oral flora and salivary electrolyte, protein, and mineral content). Until studies are forthcoming that specifically relate to the Hodgkin's patient (lower radiation doses in more youthful patients with only partial involvement of the major salivary glands), only estimates of the responses to treatment can be surmised.

HISTOLOGIC SALIVARY-GLAND CHANGES AFTER RADIATION THERAPY

Cellular changes observed in salivary glands after radiation treatment[14] are characterized by severe acute tissue damage with the serous glands and acini showing more susceptibility to injury. In the chronic stage of injury, the glands have few acini left and have a ductal framework with interlobular and periductal fibrosis and chronic inflammatory cells. Atrophy of the salivary glands reduces the volume of saliva and changes the composition of the saliva, which predisposes the patient to caries, periodontal disease, and the risk of severe infection. These changes in the volume, viscosity, pH, and the inorganic and organic constituents of the salivary secretions are the late sequelae that may be anticipated after irradiation of the major salivary glands.[14]

XEROSTOMIA

Atrophy of the salivary glands induced by radiation therapy results in the uncomfortable syndrome of xerostomia. The chronically dry mouth, without considering its far reaching effects on the patient's dentition, is extremely unpleasant. Patients affected with radiation-induced xerostomia need to constantly sip fluids; others with a minimal amount of residual salivary-gland tissue can maintain some moisture in the mouth by chewing gum.

On awakening from sleep, the mouth is especially dry and has been described by some patients as being filled with dry cotton balls. The xerostomia limits their ability to speak, even for ordinary periods of time, without artificially adding liquid to moisten the mucosal surfaces of the mouth. Usually, however, Hodgkin's patients do not have a severe persistent dry mouth syndrome similar to that seen in the head and neck cancer patient. This is undoubtedly because of the preservation of the parotid glands and the limited radiation dose delivered to the other salivary glands that permits at least partial, if not full, physiologic recovery.

ELECTROLYTE, MINERAL, AND BACTERIAL FLORA CHANGES AFTER SALIVARY GLAND RADIATION AND THE DEVELOPMENT OF CARIES

The danger of impaired production of saliva is not just its uncomfortable clinical effect, but rather that it "strips the teeth of an important natural defense against dental caries."[15] As del Regato[16] had suspected as far back as 1939, it is not the direct effect of radiation that leads to the rampant postradiation caries, but the absence of the salivary protection against caries that is lost. In 1965, Frank, Herdly, and Philippe[14] studied dental defects in 61 patients treated with "a cobalt 60 teletherapy unit for carcinomas of the oral cavity, oro- and nasopharynx, hypopharynx and larynx. Two patients with carcinomas of the floor of the mouth had radium implants combined with external roentgen-ray irradiation." The salivary glands on each side received at least "5000 to 6000 R." They concluded that "Acquired dental defects developed in only those patients in whom the salivary glands had been radiated during treatment . . ."

More importantly, as further proof that it was the effect of the deprivation of salivary gland secretions that led to the development of rampant caries, they also concluded: "The lesions developed in these patients whether the teeth had been outside or inside the field of irradiation. [Whereas] In patients in whom radiation doses had been administered directly to the jaws and teeth but not to the salivary glands, such dental defects did not develop" (even after three years of follow-up observation). This occurred independently of the direct damaging effect of radiation on the microstructure of the human mandible.[17]

The conclusion by Frank, Herdly, and Philippe that their study provided "evidence of the fundamental importance of the salivary system and saliva secretion in the maintenance of healthy tooth surfaces" is fully accepted today. The saliva affects the nature of the bacterial flora of the mouth, as well as acting as a cleansing, diluting, mineralizing, and buffering agent.[13,14]

Radiation-induced histologic changes in the salivary glands are accompanied by a physiologic alteration in the quantity and content of the saliva. This significant alteration in electrolyte content of the saliva, however, does not affect the general system in any readily detectable manner. Dreizen et al.[15] demonstrated that ". . . none of the serum electrolytes measured was significantly altered by the subtotal salivary shutdown." They determined that radiation-induced salivary deprivation may be accompanied by significant increases in saliva NA^+, Cl^-, CA^{++}, MG^{++}, and $Prot^-$ concentrations and a decrease in saliva HCO_3^- content. "The xerostomic saliva was more concentrated and had greater salinity than the pretreatment saliva. . ." This, however, had no measurable effect on serum electrolytes.

Xerostomia produces changes in the oral bacterial flora with a shift of the balance toward components characterized as highly cariogenic micro-organisms. Brown et al. demonstrated that while the total bacterial concentration remained the same, the changes toward a highly acidogenic microflora increased.[13] *Streptococcus mutans* is considered the predominant micro-organism associated with dental caries; the increase in numbers of this organism as well as significant increases in *Lactobacillus*, *Staphylococcus*, and *Candida* (primarily *C. albicans*) were noted after radiation-induced xerostomia. The significant shift in the proportional amount of *Streptococcus mutans* in the streptococcal population, either in the dental plaque or in the stimulated saliva samples, was at the expense of *S. sanguis*. Preradiation dental plaque *S. mutans* ranged from 0.6 to 2.4%, with *S. san*-

guis levels ranging from 37.6 to 41.2%. Three months after radiation, *S. mutans* constituted 25.9% of the cultivable streptococci, while *S. sanguis* levels dropped to a range of 3.9 to 11.9% Decreased levels of *S. sanguis, Neisseria,* and *Fusobacterium* were simultaneously noted. This study by Brown et al.[13] clearly demonstrated that microorganisms implicated in the production of caries ". . . quickly replaced many of the noncariogenic microorganisms before the onset of clinical caries" following radiation therapy and the change in salivary secretions.

Based on a short-term (3 month) follow-up, Brown et al.[13] concluded that these changes occurred whether or not fluoride applications were used to combat caries. A subsequent study and long-term follow-up of 1 to 13 years after radiotherapy from the same institution by Keene et al.[18] noted that "The inverse relationship between several of the S. mutans measurements employed . . . and the number of years post-radiotherapy is an intriguing finding which suggests that among cooperative patients, the caries-preventive regimen may actually limit the spread and/or reduce the degree of infection by S. mutans over a number of years."

Sites of Postradiation Caries

Dreizen et al.[19] stated that "irrespective of previous caries history no unprotected patient remains caries free after radiotherapy." There are naturally susceptible sites for caries and naturally resistant areas, but this distinction does not seem to operate following radiation, and all sites become vulnerable to caries attack. For example, the incisal edges of anterior teeth, cusps of molars and premolars, the facial surfaces of incisors, and canines at the cervical collar develop lesions that continue throughout the cementum and dentine and amputate the crowns. Lesions of all the crowns of the posterior teeth produce friable enamel and rapid breakdown. These carious lesions develop rapidly, and according to Dreizen et al.,[18] lesions can be seen within 3 months after radiation, and advanced destruction to the dentition, after one year.

Whether or not teeth decay faster following radiation as a direct result of changes in the structure of enamel, dentine, or cement is an unanswered question. There is no doubt that fibrosis and atrophy of the dental pulp occur early and the predisposition to pulpal infection and the response to dental procedures are unpredictable.

TOPICAL FLUORIDE PROGRAMS FOR THE PREVENTION OF DENTAL CARIES INDUCED BY RADIATION THERAPY

Prior to radiation therapy, a program of oral prophylaxis and thorough oral hygiene instruction should be instituted. During the period of radiation therapy, the accompanying mucositis and general malaise of the patient often precludes the possibility of effective self care and support. But this period of radiation treatment in the Hodgkin's patient rarely extends more than 2 months. The patient's vigor usually returns quickly and he or she is capable of continuing with appropriate topical applications of fluoride and any necessary urgent dental intervention.

The value of the recommended preventive regimen for caries, including daily topical fluoride applications, restriction of dietary sucrose, and good oral hygiene, greatly depends on the level of patient compliance.[18] "The extremely low caries increment observed in cooperative patients, despite the remarkable shift to a highly cariogenic oral microflora, provides good evidence for the effectiveness of these measures, especially the topical fluoride program."[18] This program of daily application of a 1% sodium fluoride gel containing a red, plaque-disclosing dye was developed by Day and Drane at the University of Texas Dental Branch and M.D. Anderson Hospital and Tumor Institute. Dreizen, Daly, Drane, and Brown[19] described the method as follows. "The gel is applied by means of flexible plastic carriers, which are custom fabricated on stone casts prepared from alginate impressions of the dental arches. Clenching the carriers pumps the gel onto and between the teeth. The gel must remain in contact with the teeth for at least five minutes. When the carriers are removed and the gel is rinsed off, the plaques are stained red and then can be removed by brushing and flossing."

Dreizen et al.[19] have emphasized that to be maximally effective, the application of fluoride must be instituted at the beginning of radiotherapy and continued every day in a diligent life-long program.

The efficacy of an aggressive fluoride program for the reduction of radiation-associated caries has been supported by various studies.[20-23] Brown et al.[21] demonstrated the effectiveness of daily topical application of 1% sodium fluoride (NaF) in a randomized study of three groups of patients: (1) those having daily application of 1% NaF; (2) those having daily topical NaF and restricted sucrose in the diet; and (3) those using a nonfluoride gel. Assessment was made prior to radiation therapy; weekly during radiation therapy, at 3-month intervals the following year, and at 6-month intervals thereafter. In the first posttreatment year, 81% of cases of caries appeared in the nonfluoride application group. All patients were then switched to the fluoride applications. No significant differences were detected between the fluoride group and the group randomized to fluoride plus a restricted sucrose diet.

Fleming reviewed the use of topical fluoride in patients receiving cancer therapy.[22] He noted that since the initial work of Daly and Drane using 1% sodium fluoride, further work showed the additional plaque-inhibition benefit of stannous fluoride (SnF_2). Outlining the current program (1983) at The University of Texas M.D. Anderson Hospital, Fleming indicated that the method now involved the daily topical application of a 0.4% SnF_2 gel to the teeth for a minimum of 5, but preferably 10, minutes by means of custom-fabricated polypropylene fluoride carriers. "After removing the fluoride carriers, the patients swish the accumulated saliva and residue gel for approximately 1 minute and then empty their mouths. The patients then do not disturb the applied fluoride film by further rinsing, drinking, or brushing for 30 minutes."[22] The 0.4% SnF_2 gel has a pH of 3.2 and is more acidic than the 1% NaF. Fleming states that the soft tissue irritations associated with the more acidic gel during radiation therapy and even into the postradiation period have been a problem in less than 2% of their patients.

From the viewpoint of Wescott, Starcke, and Shannon, "The ravaging form of dental caries associated with the postirradiation period can be essentially eliminated in cooperating patients."[20] That is, the patients had to cooperate in a program of oral hygiene that included the daily application of fluoride. Their method used topical applications of stannous fluoride (SnF_2) applied with a toothbrush. They emphasized that it was ". . . not necessary to use a tray with SnF_2 gel . . ." although they believe that some patients ". . . need paraphernalia to encourage them to use the gel on a daily basis."[20] More importantly, when using the SnF_2 gel and applying it to all tooth surfaces, either with a toothbrush or when using a tray, it is mandatory that the teeth be wet when the gel is applied. If they are not, the water-free stable SnF_2 gel does not release as many stannous and fluoride ions as needed to form stannous fluorophosphate, which is responsible for the protective effect.

The nature of caries prevention provided by fluoride application is most likely the result of surface phenomena uptake and remineralization of the tooth structure.[19] The preference for fluoride gels of higher pH rather than that of low pH acidulated gels, which enhance fluoride uptake, is predicated on several factors. Some patients report increased burning and pain upon use of the low pH gels, especially during radiation therapy when mucositis is likely to be at its greatest intensity. Furthermore, acidulated gels tend also to attack existing dental restorations, such as porcelain crowns, causing their disintegration.

The need to treat all patients with a preventative fluoride gel program, even when the parotids are spared during radiation therapy, is emphasized by Fleming.[22] This is based on the extraordinary variation in secretions of the individual salivary glands to total salivary secretion under circumstances of mechanical stimulation, during the resting state, during the waking hours, and during sleep. During mastication, for instance, the parotid supplies 58% of the total salivary secretion; submandibular, 33%; sublingual, 1.5%; and accessory salivary glands, 7.5%. During sleep, however, the parotid secretion is 0; the submandibular gland secretion, 72%; the sublingual glands, 14%; and the minor accessory glands, 14%. It is probable that fluoride treatments applied at only irregular intervals do not provide the appropriate protection, especially for cancer patients experiencing radiation-induced or drug-induced xerostomia, but long-term compliance with a complicated program of fluoride application is difficult to achieve.

Regezi et al.[24] proposed this oral hygiene program: (1) tooth brush instruction with soft brushes (patients were instructed to brush four times a day and to follow each brushing with oral lavage and fluoride rinse); (2) oral lavage instruction (1 l warm water with 1 tsp each of NaCl and $NaHCO_3$); (3) sodium fluoride rinse instruction (1 tsp 3% NaF held in mouth 1 minute, then expectorated). This rinse was discontinued during acute mucositis because of mucosal irritation.

During radiation therapy, the patient also had weekly prophylaxis with fluoridated polishing paste, and after radiation it was expected that the patient would continue the daily oral hygiene regimen as outlined above.

CHLORHEXIDINE AS AN ANTICARIES AGENT

Katz carried out a clinical study[23] that examined the caries-preventive ability of a combination of sodium fluoride and chlorhexidine applications, compared to the application of sodium fluoride solution alone. This study was carried out in Spain on 35 cancer patients treated for head and neck tumors with at least 5000 to 7000 cGy. None of the patients received any oral prophylaxis prior to radiotherapy, nor were any extractions performed because of the lack of adequate facilities and personnel to treat the patients before radiotherapy. Despite the absence of pretreatment oral prophylaxis, no post-treatment complications could be attributed to the poor oral health of the participants.

The purpose of adding chlorhexidine to the fluoride prophylaxis was to add an agent that has the effect of controlling the overgrowth of *Streptococcus mutans*, which as noted previously in this review, is particularly implicated in the production of dental caries. In addition the method allowed the patient to treat himself at home using simple mouth rinses, which it was hoped would result in a higher level of patient compliance. This study using chlorhexidine was carried out in Spain because, according to Katz, although "topical applications of chlorhexidine have been used for more than 20 years in the treatment of burns, for bladder irrigation, and other situations requiring antimicrobial action . . . as well as [being the active ingredient in] lozenges widely used or the treatment of throat infections and esophagitis . . . [It appeared that the toxicity of chlorhexidine was low] . . . at this time, the US Food and Drug Administration has not approved chlorhexidine for oral rinses and topical applications, although such uses of chlorhexidine are widespread in Europe."[23] Chlorhexidine alone had been used in England more than 20 years ago, in preference to fluoride, in the management of radiation caries.[25]

Dr. Katz, however, conluded that "a regime of four topical applications of 1.0% sodium fluoride—1.0% chlorhexidine digluconate plus daily rinses with an 0.05% sodium fluoride—0.2% chlorhexidine solution prevented radiation caries completely. It also resulted in remineralization of incipient existing lesions. Use of the chlorhexidine-fluoride rinses alone also stopped radiation caries but did not permit remineralization to occur." However, "use of four topical applications with a fluoride gel and daily rinses with an 0.05% sodium fluoride solution was not sufficient to prevent radiation caries," and finally, "no chlorhexidine staining was observed."[23] The chlorhexidine-fluoride combination appeared to be superior to fluoride alone.

Despite these favorable results, Katz recommended that in countries where the use of chlorhexidine was not permitted, the methods of Dreizen and his colleagues using topical fluoride were the treatment of choice.[23] The morbid nature of this problem is that as the teeth decay, there is an accompanying possibility of dental infection, bone infection, osteoradionecrosis, and major soft-tissue necrosis.

OSTEORADIONECROSIS

The pathologic process that develops following radiation of osseous tissue and characterized by a benign mucosal ulceration with exposure of the jawbone for more than 3 months duration is a reasonable definition of osteoradionecrosis for the purpose of this review. It is usually associated with pain, and suppuration is not evident in many patients. Pathologically, it is characterized by the presence of necrotic bone. Detailed histology of the microstructure of the human mandible after direct radiation of 6000 to 7200 cGy has been outlined by Savostin-Asling and Silverman.[17] Radiographically, some degree of decalcification is usually demonstrated.

Incidence and Causative Factors

The incidence of postradiation therapy osteonecrosis following treatment for head and neck cancer varies widely in different clinical reviews.[26-31] Many of the predisposing factors to the development of osteonecrosis of the jaw after head and neck radiation for oral, nasopharyngeal, and laryngeal cancers are not consistently agreed on by all observers. Factors such as the state of dentition prior to radiation treatment, post-treatment trauma, and infection seem to play variable roles.

Whether or not dental extractions prior to radiation treatment or following treatment lead to osteonecrosis is also not consistently reported. However, there is general agreement that the dose of radiation delivered to the dentition-bearing bones is the crucial factor. It has been stated that osteonecrosis of the jaw does not occur in patients who have received less than 6500 cGy.[30]

Morrish et al.[30] outlined various factors in the development of postradiation osteonecrosis:

1. Patients who were edentulous at the time of diagnosis of cancer had a relatively low risk for osteonecrosis.
2. Patients who were dentulous had a greater risk.
3. The increased risk in dentulous patients appeared to be associated with those who had tooth extractions following radiation therapy.
4. Dentulous patients with pretreatment extractions or no extractions appeared to have risks similar to the edentulous patients.
5. The most important risk factor for the development of osteonecrosis appeared to be the radiation dose to the bone, particularly in the less vascular mandible.

In their experience, "the risk of osteonecrosis is negligible when the bone dose was less than 6500 rads but great when the dose exceeded 7500 rads."[30]

Part of the confusion regarding the incidence of osteonecrosis in the radiated patient is characterized by the observation of Morrish et al.[30] that prior to 1971,[32] at the University of California, osteoradionecrosis developed in less than 4% of patients radiated for cancer of the oral cavity, oropharynx, and nasopharynx. When factors of selection entered into the analysis, such as availability of complete dental records, variable or inadequate follow-ups, the application of more modern, more aggressive radiation treatment plans, or early death of patients precluding a long follow-up, the incidence of osteonecrosis could be widely manipulated.

For instance, after 1971, at the University of California, 22% (or about one out of every five patients) selected for study developed osteonecrosis. In the period from January 1971 to July 1977, however, only 100 out of the 534 patients treated for head and neck tumors with radiation therapy qualified for review because there were complete dental records and a minimum follow-up of 6 months. Morrish et al. recognized that because of these factors, a true incidence of postradiation osteonecrosis was difficult for them to determine based on their data.[30] They concluded, however, that "the incidence of osteonecrosis appears to be directly related to the radiation dose to the bone. Osteonecrosis developed in 85% of the dentulous patients and in 50% of the edentulous patients who received more than 7500 rads to the bone. None of the patients who received less than 6500 rads developed osteonecrosis."[30]

An outline of the incidence of osteonecrosis in patients irradiated for head and neck cancer reported in the literature appears in Table 17–1.

Larson et al.[31] agreed that a major factor correlating with undesirable side effects after treatment of head and neck tumors was the dose of radiation: "When large doses were employed there was an increase in later major complications [osteonecrosis]."[31]

Because patients with Hodgkin's disease receive radiation dosage levels that reach only 3600 to 4400 cGy, the risk of osteoradionecrosis must be negligible. In fact, no case reports concerning the complications of postradiation osteonecrosis of the mandible in Hodgkin's patients have been noted.[12,33] This absence of risk must be taken into consideration when proposing a preradiation treatment dental plan for the Hodgkin's patient that includes recommendations for preradiation dental extractions, ostensibly to avoid the chance of post-treatment osteoradionecrosis.

At the M.D. Anderson Hospital, Bedwinek et al.[28] reviewed 381 patients with squamous-cell carcinoma of the oral cavity, nasopharynx, and oropharynx who were treated with radiotherapy between 1966 and 1971 with a minimum of 5-year follow-up. Osteoradionecrosis developed in 14% of the 381 patients. It was noted that in 65% of the patients (35 of 54), osteoradionecrosis was associated with dental extraction or dental irritation. In the remaining 35% (19 of 54), the onset of the disease was spontaneous (that is, unrelated to any previous dental extractions or known problems). Those who had undergone dental extraction before radiotherapy had a lower incidence of osteoradionecrosis (7.7%) compared to a 19.7% incidence of osteoradionecrosis occurring in patients who required dental extractions after their radiation treatment.

Pathogenesis of Osteoradionecrosis

The question of potentially greater danger of postradiation tooth extraction being associated with a higher probability of the development of osteoradionecrosis has been a subject of major concern and some controversy for years. It may be possible now to consider that the work of Marx[34,35] explains some of the confusion.

The classic sequence of radiation, trauma, and infection that once served to explain the initiating pathophysiologic factors in osteoradionecrosis has been questioned by Marx[34] and he has proposed a new concept of its pathophysiology. Based on 26 consecutive cases of osteoradionecrosis, from which 12 en-bloc resection specimens were cultured and stained for micro-organisms, it was indicated that micro-organisms play only a "contaminant role in osteoradionecrosis and that trauma is only one mechanism of tissue breakdown leading to the condition." The pathogenetic sequence suggested by Marx is "(1) radiation, (2) hypoxic-hypocellular hypovascular tissue, (3) tissue breakdown, and (4) chronic non-healing wound."[34]

The osteoradionecrosis that occurs after radiation treatment does not need any traumatic or infectious initiating factor. "Spontaneous osteoradionecrosis is a valid entity and is related to higher total irradiation doses and perhaps to implant sources."[34]

An outline of Marx's conclusions is as follows:

1. Osteoradionecrosis is not a primary in-

Table 17–1. Incidence of Osteonecrosis in Patients Irradiated for Head and Neck Cancer

Source (Year)	Location	Duration of Study	Radiation Dose (cGy)	Total No. Patients	No. (%) of Osteonecrosis Cases
Bedwinek (1976)	M.D. Anderson, TX	1966–1971	6000–7500	381	54 (14%)
Dodson (1962)	Geisenberger, VA	1948–1960	5000–9500	108	10 (9%)
Wildermuth (1958)	Swedish, D.C.	1939–1951	4000–8500	104	6 (6%)
Meyer (1958)	Westfield, MA	1940–1957	4000–18,000	491	26 (5%)
Beumer (1972)	Univ. Calif, CA	1961–1971	5000–7000	278	10 (4%)
Carl (1973)	Roswell Park, NY	1968–1972	3600–12,900	47	2 (4%)

Adapted from Morrish et al.[30]

fection of irradiated bone. It is a complex metabolic and tissue homeostatic deficiency created by radiation-induced cellular injury.
2. Micro-organisms play only a contaminant role in its pathophysiology.
3. Trauma may or may not be an initiating factor. When trauma is associated with osteoradionecrosis, it is usually caused by tooth removal (88%).
4. The occurrence of spontaneous osteoradionecrosis is related to the use of implant sources and higher total radiation doses.
5. The use of supervoltage irradiation has neither eliminated nor reduced the frequency of osteoradionecrosis of the jaws, despite claims as to its bone-sparing effects: 80% of cases of external beam-related osteoradionecrosis were associated with supervoltage sources. Perhaps this finding is related to the higher total radiation doses used when supervoltage sources were employed.

Does preradiation extraction promote osteonecrosis? It is possible that Marx's concepts can explain the confusing divergence between data from the University of Texas Dental Branch at Houston (and the M.D. Anderson Hospital and Tumor Institute) of Daly, Drane, and MacComb[27] versus the data from Roswell Park Memorial Institute reported by Carl, Schaaf, and Sako.[36] Carl et al.[36] indicated that over a period of 4 years they extracted 187 teeth from 47 previously irradiated patients without precipitating a case of osteoradionecrosis. Yet they observed two cases of osteoradionecrosis in two patients whose mandibular molars had been removed just prior to radiation therapy. On the other hand, Daly et al.[27] discovered 71 incidents of bone necrosis in 66 of 304 patients reviewed over a period from January 1966 to December 1971, and 20 of 71 (28%) instances of necrosis were associated with extractions before irradiation. Of 71 cases of bone necrosis, 3 (4%) occurred in association with extractions after irradiation; 10% occurred with trauma other than extractions; 17% were associated with jaw surgery for disease in the irradiated area; and 41% occurred "spontaneously" or were attributed to an "unknown cause."

Daly, Drane, and MacComb[27] concluded that "because of the high incidence of bone necrosis demonstrated in extraction sites prior to therapy . . . a more conservative approach has been taken in regard to extraction of teeth prior to treatment." This approach apparently resulted in a "considerable decrease" in the incidence and severity of bone necrosis as well as the necessity for fewer resections. Furthermore, "conservative thorough dental treatment utilizing fluoride, adequate patient education, and good cooperation have resulted in a reduced number of teeth being extracted in the post radiation period."[27]

Despite the observations and conclusions of Daly, Drane, and MacComb regarding postradiation osteonecrosis, some reviewers such as Main (University of Toronto) continue to recommend that the "majority of patients receiving radiotherapy should still be rendered edentulous before hand."[37] This certainly appears to be the most radical and unnecessary approach to the problem. Other reviews from the University of Texas by Murray et al.[29] showed that there was a high correlation between pre-existing dental disease and the incidence of postradiation osteonecrosis, but that it was impossible to predict reliably which patients with dental disease would devleop bone necrosis. On the other hand, when a patient was dentally healthy prior to treatment, he had a relatively low risk of osteoradionecrosis.

Despite previously contrary data from the same center (University of Texas[27]) and without any clear additional evidence, Murray et al.[29] concluded the following: "Once radiation has been given, diseased teeth cannot be extacted without a high risk of bone necrosis."[27] They therefore recommended that in irradiated patients dental disease must be treated conservatively. (That is, extractions should be avoided after radiation therapy). Taking all of these factors and varying data into account, extractions, before and after radiation therapy to the head and neck, should therefore probably be avoided as much as possible in both the pretreated patient and in the postirradiated patient.

If it is true that edentulous patients have a lower incidence of the development of osteoradionecrosis after radiation therapy, the decision to remove teeth might be based on the following criteria: (1) extensive caries; (2) moderate to advanced periodontal involvement; (3) lack of opposing teeth and consequent loss of function and self-cleaning action; (4) partial impaction or incomplete eruption and extensive periapical lesions.

Osteoradionecrosis occurs most frequently in the mandible and in the area of the molar teeth; therefore, this area requires careful evaluation with respect to preradiation extraction. The question also arises about whether or not to extract impacted molar teeth prior to treatment. The extraction of impacted molar teeth is generally not indicated due to the anticipated prolonged healing time and the necessity to remove much bone along with removal of the tooth.

A conservative approach that avoids pretreatment dental extractions appears to be most prudent. It is our opinion that teeth that are obviously at risk (gross dental caries, periapical pathosis with advanced periodontal disease) may be extracted, although a generally more conservative approach with the retention of teeth is advocated.

IS TOOTH EXTRACTION PRIOR TO TREATMENT FOR HODGKIN'S DISEASE NECESSARY?

In general, in the radiation technique for Hodgkin's disease only the mandible is at risk, and that risk limits the radiation dose to less than 4400 cGy or only scatter radiation. Any teeth that have periodontal deficiencies and bone loss may be considered for extraction, but because the incidence of bone necrosis may be nonexistent in patients treated with only a limited dose of radiation therapy (limited fields, sparing direct radiation to either the mandible or the maxilla, under 6500 cGy), tooth extraction in this setting may be considered a "radical" approach. Furthermore, the Hodgkin's patients salivary glands are also spared because they receive a limited dose and limited exposure (the parotids, for instance, are almost invariably spared in the radiation treatment planning); this added quantity of saliva helps protect even the careless patient who fails to consistently follow a recommended regime of life-long fluoride prophylaxis.

Every attempt must be made to assess the oral hygiene habits of the patient prior to therapy. An aware patient with adequate habits can usually be motivated to maintain and increase the regimen of oral self-care necessary to prevent complications. The effects of radiation therapy with respect to the patients' dental needs must be reiterated frequently. A patient who is not motivated sufficiently is at greater risk of complications. When extractions are performed, it is essential that they be performed with minimal trauma[36] and each extraction should be accompanied with prophylactic antibiotic coverage.

TASTE AND DIET

Alterations to taste have been studied by Henkin et al.[38] and Conger and Wells.[39] Taste is immediately affected by radiation therapy to the oral regions. Histologically, deterioration and atrophy of the taste buds occur at 1000 cGy,[39] and at cancericidal levels the architecture of the buds is almost completely eliminated. Return of taste to normal levels is associated with the presence of saliva; conversely, reduction of the salivary flow appears to decrease the number of taste buds and probably alters the function of the remaining buds.[38]

The effect on the patient's diet as a result of loss of taste and mucositis can be devastating. The nutritional impairment can lead to severe weight loss and the nature of the diet found to be acceptable and palatable to the patient (i.e., soft foods, cakes, starches, candy, and sugary foods) all add to the shift in microflora predisposing the patient to dental caries. These severe effects, which may be common in intensely treated patients with head and neck cancer, are not anticipated in the Hodgkin's patient.

TRISMUS

Trismus accompanies cancericidal doses of radiation in patients treated for head and neck tumors to a varying degree with no apparent

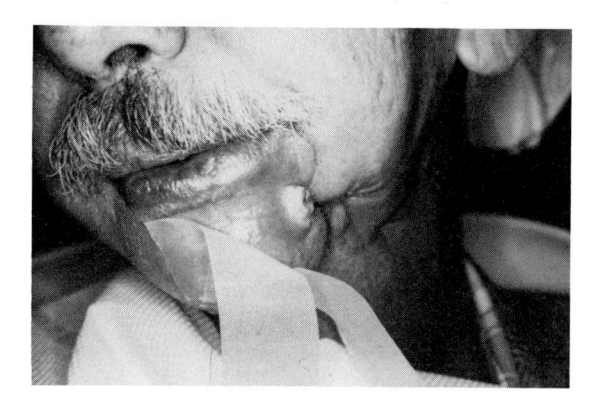

Fig. 17–4. Mr. W.C. following mandibulectomy for osteoradionecrosis still continues to show evidence of necrotic breakdown.

predictability in cases of nasopharyngeal nasal sinus and palatal tumors. It is rarely seen as a complication of the treatment of Hodgkin's disease.

If the radiation field includes the temporomandibular joints, the limitation of opening may be severe in the worst cases, even preventing the patient from placing a bolus of food or a toothbrush in the mouth. This impairment generally can be lessened by the use of exercises and bite openers immediately on cessation of therapy. If allowed to go untreated as a result of the discomfort precipitated during the required manipulations, the limitation of opening can last a lifetime, thereby increasing the risk of dental infection through poor oral hygiene and inadequate access for treatment of dental problems.

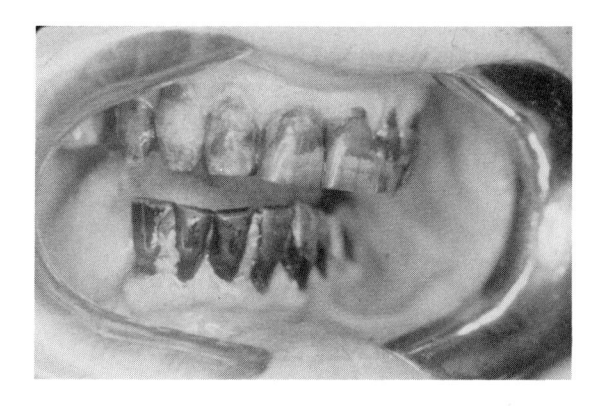

Fig. 17–5. Mr. C.C.'s failure to use the fluoride applications plus his initial poor oral hygiene led to severe dental breakdown within 2 years after radiation therapy.

ADDITIONAL CASE REPORTS

Mr. W.C. received 5500 cGy to the mandible following a marginal resection for cancer of the floor of the mouth. A spontaneous fracture of the mandible at the level of the second molar tooth occurred 3 months following the completion of therapy. Pain and disability necessitated hemimandibulectomy, which was followed 2 months later by soft-tissue necrosis exposing the underlying bone (Fig. 17–4). This had not healed with conservative therapy and further resection of the jaw was contemplated. Unfortunately, the patient developed lung metastases and expired 3 months later.

Mr. C.C. with Stage IIA Hodgkin's disease received 4500 cGy to the mantle field in 1976. His poor oral hygiene, coupled with his failure to follow a prescribed regimen of fluoride applications, led to dental breakdown associated with extensive caries within 2 years (Fig. 17–5).

REFERENCES

1. Nisce, L. and D'Angio, G.J. Radiation therapy for Hodgkin's disease: Memorial Hospital techniques. *In* Hodgkin's Disease. Edited by M.J. Lacher. John Wiley and Sons, 1976, pp 145–177.
2. Jenkin, D., Chan, H., Freedman, M. et al. Hodgkin's disease in children: Treatment results with MOPP and low-dose, extended-field irradiation. Cancer Treat. Rep. 66:949–959, 1982.
3. Donaldson, S.S. Pediatric Hodgkin's disease: Focus on the future. *In* Status of the Curability of Childhood Cancers. Edited by J. Van Eys, M.P. Sullivan. New York, Raven Press, 1980, pp. 235–249.
4. Lacher, M.J. The role of radical surgery in Hodgkin's disease. N. Engl. J. Med. 33:164–167, 1966.
5. Weyman, J. The effect of irradiation on developing teeth. Oral Surg. 25:623, 1968.
6. Guggenheimer, J., Fischer, W.G., and Pechersky, J.L. Anticipation of dental anomalies induced by radiation therapy. Radiology 117:405, 1975.
7. Lines, L.G., Hazra, T.A., Howells, R. et al. Altered growth and development of lower teeth in children receiving mantle therapy. Radiology 132:447, 1979.
8. Jaffe, N., Toth, B.B., Hoar, R.E. et al. Dental and maxillofacial abnormalities in long-term survivors of childhood cancer: effects of treatment with chemotherapy and radiation to the head and neck. Pediatrics 73:816, 1984.
9. Carl, W. and Wood, R. Effects of radiation on the

developing dentition and supporting bone. J Am. Dent. Assoc. *101*:646, 1980.
10. Smith, R. Herpes zoster effect on teeth, and bone growth.
11. Balfour, H.H. Jr., Bean, B., Laskin, O.L. et al. Acyclovir halts progression of herpes zoster. N. Engl. J. Med. *308*:1448–1453, 1983.
12. Morbidity and Mortality Weekly Report. Centers for Disease Control, Atlanta. JAMA *251*:1401–1413, 1984.
12a. Leslie, N.T., Mauch, P.M., and Hellman, S. Evaluation of long-term survival and treatment complications in patients with stage IA–IIB Hodgkin's Disease. Int. J. Radiat. Oncol. Biol. Phys. *9*(suppl. 1):127, 1983 (abstract 110).
13. Brown, L.R., Dreizen, S., Handler, S. et al. Effect of radiation-induced xerostomia on human oral flora. J. Dent. Res. *34*:740, 1975.
14. Frank, R.M., Herdly, J., and Phillipe, E. Acquired dental defects and salivary gland lesions after irradiation for carcinoma. J. Am. Dent. Assoc. *70*:868, 1965.
15. Dreizen, S.A., Brown, L.R., Handler, S. et al. Radiation-induced xerostomia in cancer patients. Cancer *38*:273, 1976.
16. Del Regato, J.A. Dental lesions observed after roentgen therapy in cancer of the buccal cavity, pharynx, and larynx. Am. J. Radiat. *42*:404, 1939.
17. Savostin-Asling, I. and Silverman, S. Effects of therapeutic radiation on microstructure of the human mandible. Am. J. Anat. *151*:295–306, 1978.
18. Keene, J.J. et al. Dental caries and Streptococcus mutans prevalence in cancer patients with irradiation induced xerostomia: 1–13 years after radiotherapy. Caries Res. *15*:416, 1981.
19. Dreizen, S.A., Daly, T.E., Drane, J.B. et al. Oral complications of cancer radiotherapy. Postgrad. Med. *61*:85, 1977.
20. Westcott, W.B., Starcke, E.N., and Shannon, I.L. Chemical protection against postirradiation dental caries. Oral Surg. *40*:709, 1975.
21. Brown, L.R. et al. Interrelations of oral microorganisms, immunoglobulins and dental caries following radiotherapy. J. Dent. Res. *57*:882, 1978.
22. Fleming, T.J. Use of topical fluoride by patients receiving cancer therapy. Curr. Probl. Cancer *7*:37, 1983.
23. Katz, S. The use of fluoride and chlorhexadine for the prevention of radiation caries. J. Am. Dent. Assoc. *104*:164–170, 1982.
24. Regezi, J.A., Courtney, R.M., and Kerr, D.A. Dental management of patients irradiated for oral cancer. Cancer *38*:994, 1976.
25. Coffin, F. The management of radiation caries. Br. J. Oral Surg. *11*:54–59, 1973.
26. Dodson, W.S. Irradiation osteomyelitis of the jaw. J. Oral Surg. *20*:467–474, 1962.
27. Daly, T.E., Drane, J.B., and MacComb, W.S. Management of problems of the teeth and jaws in patients undergoing irradiation. Am. J. Surg. *124*:539, 1972.
28. Bedwinek, J.M., Shukovsky, L.J., Fletcher, G.H. et al. Osteonecrosis in patients treated with definitive radiotherapy for squamous cell carcinoma of the oral cavity and naso and oropharynx. Radiology *119*:665–667, 1976.
29. Murray, C.G., Daly, T.E., and Zimmerman, S.O. The relationship between dental diseases and radiation necrosis of the mandible. Oral Surg. *49*:99, 1980.
30. Morrish, R.B., Chan, E., Silverman, S. et al. Osteonecrosis in patients irradiated for head and neck carcinoma. Cancer *47*:1980–1983, 1981.
31. Larson, D.L., Lindberg, R.D., Lane, E. et al. Major implications of radiotherapy in cancer of the oral cavity and oropharynx. Am. J. Surg. *146*:531, 1983.
32. Beumer, J., Silverman, Dcenak, et al. Of complications following preradiation dental extractions.
33. Sonis, S.T., Sonis, A.L., and Lieberman, A. Oral complications in patients receiving treatment for malignancies other than of the head and neck. J. Am. Dent. Assoc. *97*:468–472, 1978.
34. Marx, R.E. Osteoradionecrosis: A new concept of its pathophysiology. J. Oral Maxillofac. Surg. *41*:283–288, 1983.
35. Marx, R.E. A new concept in the treatment of osteoradionecrosis. J. Oral Maxillofac. Surg. *41*:351–357, 1983.
36. Carl, W., Schaaf, N.G., and Sako, K. Oral surgery and the patient who has had radiation therapy for head and neck cancer. Oral Surg. *36*:651, 1973.
37. Main, J.H.P. Dental care for cancer patients. Can. Med. Assoc. J. *128*:1062, 1983.
38. Henkin, R., Talal, N., Larson, A. et al. Abnormalities of taste and smell in Sjogren's syndrome. Ann. Intern. Med. *76*:375, 1972.
39. Conger, A.D. and Wells, M.A. Radiation and aging effect on taste structure and function. Radiation Res. *37*:31, 1969.

CHAPTER 18

Pediatric Hodgkin's Disease: The Uniqueness of the Pediatric Patient

SARAH S. DONALDSON

While the biology and natural history of Hodgkin's disease afflicting the child does not differ from Hodgkin's disease afflicting the adult, there are many aspects of the condition that have a particularly important impact on a child and therefore are unique to the pediatric population. These aspects present both a challenge and a dilemma when managing children with Hodgkin's disease and relate to the consequences of survival. The life span of a survivor of Hodgkin's disease when afflicted as a child will be appreciably longer than one who is afflicted as an adult. Thus, the quality of survival and the number of these survival-years become an important consideration. As well, the long-term complications related to the disease and its therapy have greatest impact on youngsters and children who are undergoing active growth and development at the time of treatment. This chapter discusses the consequences of long-term survival relative to children with Hodgkin's disease.

The single most important attribute of the long-term survivor is that he has overcome the disease itself; once it was considered a uniformly fatal malignancy. Proper prospective must be given to the fact that the disease is now curable; the majority of patients stricken with Hodgkin's disease today will be long-term survivors. This success is related to continual accomplishments in histopathology, imaging techniques, staging procedures, radiotherapy, chemotherapy, and a multidisciplinary approach. Every newly diagnosed child with Hodgkin's disease should be approached in a uniform and systematic manner, with curative intent. With such a goal we now can look at results of therapy that demonstrate curability and defend the need for carefully examining the quality of survival.

Although Hodgkin's disease in children was long thought to be associated with a poor prognosis, and children were once thought to fare less well than adults with the disease,[1] current data demonstrate that children fare as well, if not better, than adults. Figure 18–1 shows the influence of age on prognosis

---

Supported in part by research grant No. CA-34233 from the National Cancer Institute, National Institutes of Health.

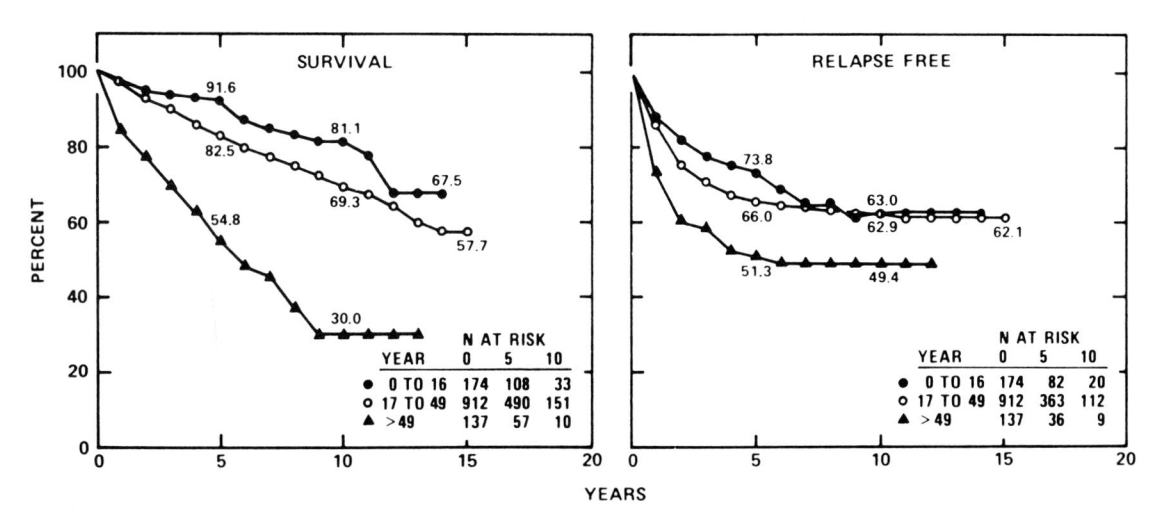

Fig. 18–1. Influence of age on prognosis. Actuarial analysis of survival and freedom from relapse of patients under 16 years of age as compared to those 17 to 49 years, and those older than 50 years of age seen between 1961 and 1977 at Stanford University Medical Center. (Reprinted by permission of Harvard University Press from Kaplan, H.S. Hodgkin's Disease, 2nd Ed. Fig. 12–20, p. 569, 1980.)

when looking at actuarial analysis of survival and freedom from relapse of 1223 consecutive patients seen at Stanford between 1961 and 1977. Children 16 years of age and less are compared against the cohort of patients between ages 17 and 49 years and against those greater than 49 years. The 5- and 10-year survival of 91.6% and 81.1%, respectively, for the pediatric age group compare favorably against the corresponding figures for the middle and older age groups. The actuarial relapse-free survival also demonstrates the favorability of the pediatric and young adult age group when compared against those who are over 49 years. The prognostic influence of age is clearly stage-dependent.[1] The pediatric age group fares slightly better than the young adult age group and much better than the older adult for every stage, both among symptomatic and asymptomatic subsets. Thus, there is no longer any justification for the outdated view that prognosis among children is unfavorable. On the contrary, current data demonstrate that survival in the pediatric age group is slightly superior to that of young adults. When age has been further examined among the subset of children 15 years of age and less, those 10 years of age or less were found to have a 5-year relapse-free survival of 83%, as compared to 61% for adolescents 11 years of age or more.[2] This influence of age correlates with improved 5-year survival among pathologically staged children of 82%, as compared to 55% among those clinically staged only. Furthermore, among the pediatric population, the prognostic influence of histopathology emerges with 5-year survival of 100% among children with lymphocyte predominant histology, 88% among those with nodular sclerosis, and 81% at 5 years among those with mixed cellularity disease.

The impact of improved staging as well as improvement in treatment techniques have been demonstrated among the pediatric population showing an improvement in cure rates following radiation alone,[3–5] chemotherapy alone,[6–8] stage-related therapeutic programs,[2,9–12] planned combined-modality programs using reduced radiotherapy volumes plus chemotherapy,[13] and/or reduced radiotherapy doses plus chemotherapy.[14–18] The gradual and progressive trend with each of these reports is toward improved survival so that now several groups reporting large numbers of consistently managed children referred to regional centers report greater than 90% survival and cure rates for all children.[12,13,15,18] These various reports represent differing philosophies regarding the importance of clinical versus pathologic staging and initial aggressive therapy versus aggressive salvage therapy. Each, however, concludes that attention to late effects is absolutely essential when treating children. We must look at the complication rates from treatment when devising therapeutic approaches for children. Appropriately, the therapeutic focus has now become one of minimizing complications of treatment. In general, this requires maximizing initial staging to select those children with localized disease from those with more extensive, unfavorable, or widespread disease. Evolving therapeutic programs now are directed towards minimizing therapy for those with earlier stage disease and least tumor burden, while reserving more aggressive therapy for those with unfavorable prognostic factors, large tumor burden, or advanced stage disease. With the goal of optimizing therapy for children with Hodgkin's disease, it is important to look at the recognized long-term complications among those who are long-term survivors.

EPIDEMIOLOGIC, GENETIC, AND FAMILIAL FACTORS

While the aspects of epidemiology and genetics of Hodgkin's disease are not unique to children, they do impact the pediatric population. There is a characteristic bimodal age-specific curve, with one peak occurring in young adults aged 15 to 40, and a second in the older age group, 45 to 70 years.[19] The epidemiologic patterns observed appear to reflect a variety of environmental and socioeconomic factors, suggesting that several environmental factors influence the incidence of Hodgkin's disease, as shown in studies of children.[20] The disease has been reported to occur more frequently in younger patients from developing countries as compared to those of advanced socioeconomic levels.[21] While there is a male to female predominance of approximately 1.5:1 among adults,[1] the male to female ratio among children greatly favors males with a 9:1 ratio in the 3 to 7 age range, dropping to 3:1 by age 7 to 9, and progressively falling toward adult proportions thereafter.[22]

A number of individual case reports of Hodgkin's disease occurring in more than one member of the family or in first-degree blood relatives have been reported,[23] as well as risk of Hodgkin's disease related to sibship size,[24] suggesting the incidence of Hodgkin's disease is low among persons from large families. Other childhood social environmental factors have been studied; they show decreased risk of Hodgkin's disease when living in multiple family homes rather than single family dwellings. An increased number of cases among children whose mothers were well educated and an increased number of cases among those who have had infectious mononucleosis as compared to control patients not having Hodgkin's disease, suggest the risk of Hodgkin's disease is associated with factors including protection from infectious exposure.[25] Cases of clustering of Hodgkin's disease have been reported, drawing attention to an outbreak of Hodgkin's disease occurring among students attending a particular school.[26,27] However, data regarding transmissibility of Hodgkin's disease are lacking. Whereas controversies exist regarding epidemiology, most observations favor environmental rather than genetic influences.

Children with congenital immunodeficiency states as well as patients receiving chronic immunosuppressive medications are highly susceptible to the development of malignant lymphomas, usually large-cell lymphoma. However, Hodgkin's disease has developed in children with Chédiak-Higashi syndrome[28] and ataxia-telangiectasia.[29] The latter poses difficulties in treatment with radiotherapy because of its known defect in the repair of radiation-induced cellular damage, which is manifested by extreme tissue reactions after therapeutic doses of ionizing radiation.[30] Coexistence of Hodgkin's disease and Down's syndrome has been reported, with chromosomal analysis of the involved lymph nodes containing Hodgkin's disease also demonstrating trisomy 21–22.[31]

HISTOPATHOLOGY

The histopathologic subtypes of Hodgkin's disease that affect children do not differ greatly from those occurring in adults, with the exception of a slightly higher percentage of lymphocyte predominant cases seen among children and fewer cases of lymphocyte depletion. Table 18–1 shows the histologic subtypes taken from three large pediatric series from America, West Germany, and France demonstrating rather uniform agreement. Whereas Strum and Rappaport[32] reported that 63% of their cases of Hodgkin's disease in the first decade of life represented the nodular sclerosis subtype, Poppema and Lennert were unable to show a significant difference in the West German series when contrasted with their adult experience.[33] The Stanford investigators[34] showed differing percentages of histologic subtypes among children less than 10 years of age as compared to those in the 11 to 15-year age subgroup. They noted a 70% incidence in the nodular sclerosing histologic subtype among the 11 to 15-year age group, while of those 10 and younger, equal numbers of children had mixed cellularity and nodular sclerosis subtypes. The lymphocyte predominant variant was also more frequently noted in the youngsters. Lymphocyte depletion was rare.

CLINICAL STAGING

The routine clinical staging of children with Hodgkin's disease involves a careful history and physical examination with special attention to the lymphoid system. In children, the evaluation of palpable or enlarged lymph nodes is often difficult because of the frequent finding of lymphadenopathy, reflecting a reactive benign process as opposed to involvement with lymphoma. Routinely, several physicians should exam every child. When differences of opinion arise regarding the presence or absence of palpable lymph nodes, suspicious nodes should be biopsied or treated as if involved with the disease. Commonly, the difficulty is not whether or not a gland is palpable, but whether the palpable node contains lymphoma. Knowledge of the recognized contiguity of spread of Hodgkin's disease, the location of the lymph nodes, and experience in the feeling of nodes is helpful in making this decision. Characteristically, involved lymph nodes are not painful or tender but have a "rubbery" firmness to the experienced examiner. They may become quite large before they are apparent (Fig. 18–2). The growth rate of involved lymph nodes may be variable. Frequently, the enlarged nodes have been present for several weeks or even months, often waxing and waning in size. While lymph nodes in the upper one half of the neck, in the anterior and posterior chains, and in the submandibular areas may often be associated with coexisting upper-respiratory-tract infections in children, firm lymph nodes presenting in the lower one half of the neck, including the supraclavicular fossa, are much more likely to be clinically significant. Approximately 80% of children present with disease in one or both sides of the neck, while only approximately one third have axillary adenopathy[15] (Fig. 18–3). Palpable "shotty" inguinal/femoral lymph nodes are common, but less than 5% are proven to show Hodgkin's disease by biopsy. Involvement of the lymphoid tissues of Waldeyer's ring is uncommon and unlikely to occur without associated high cervical lymphadenopathy. Epitrochlear, brachial, and popliteal involvement are rare in children. Whenever an enlarged lymph node is palpable in a site where involvement would significantly influence either staging or treatment, it is a wise policy to perform a biopsy on such a node to assess involvement.

Laboratory examinations routine in staging

Table 18–1. Distribution of Histologic Subtypes of Hodgkin's Disease in Children

Institution (ref)	Number of Patients	Subtype				
		Lymphocyte Predominance	Nodular Sclerosis	Mixed Cellularity	Lymphocyte Depletion	Unclassified
Stanford[34]	105	15%	58%	23%	1%	3%
Kiel[33]	278	23%	38.8%	33.5%	4.7%	
Villejuif/Paris[12]	178	16%	47%	30%	2%	6%

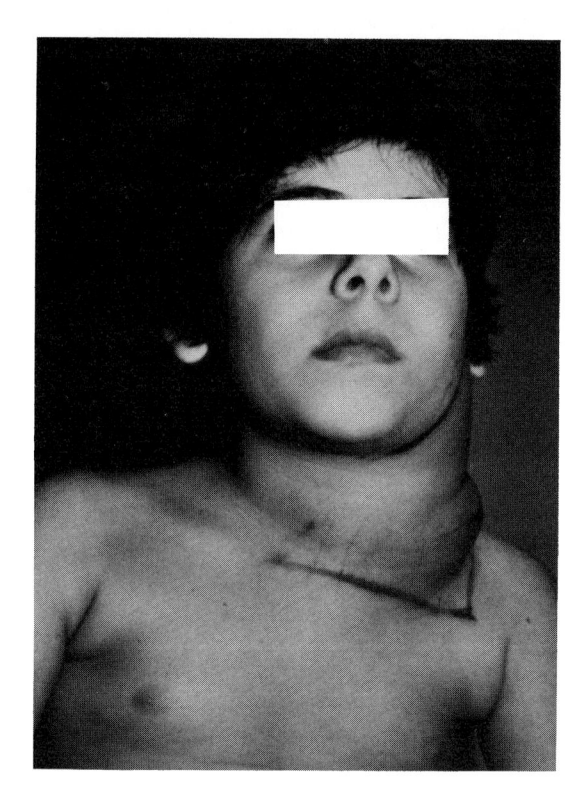

Fig. 18-2. Huge mass of confluent lymph nodes in the left cervical and supraclavicular region causing torticollis in a 7-year-old girl with Hodgkin's disease.

include a complete blood count, erythrocyte sedimentation test, liver function studies (including alkaline phosphatase) and serum copper. The alkaline phosphatase, a sensitive nonspecific indicator of disease activity, is less useful in children than in adults, since it characteristically is elevated as a function of active bone growth in addition to being a measure of disease activity. However, an unusually elevated alkaline phosphatase, with or without symptoms of bone pain, is a signal to evaluate the skeletal system by bone scan. Serum-copper examinations, a useful nonspecific marker of disease activity, often reflect normal hormonal activity in young patients. The elevated serum copper level is most useful as a means of following disease response in successfully treated patients and as a nonspecific indicator of detecting relapse.[35] However, false-positive elevations of serum copper have been observed in children with Hodgkin's disease secondary to infection and inflammatory disease,[36] as well as in pregnancy and in patients taking oral contraceptive medications.

Recommended radiographic staging procedures among the pediatric population do not differ from adults, although their interpretation may be more difficult in children. When assessing the chest, approximately 60% of children manifest intrathoracic Hodgkin's disease most commonly as disease in the anterosuperior mediastinum, paratracheal, and tracheobronchial lymph node groups. When using tomography for further delineation of the chest, 62% of children have been shown to have abnormal whole-lung tomograms.[34] Mediastinal adenopathy is present in 60%, hilar adenopathy in 30%, pulmonary involvement in 10%, and pleural infusions in 4% of children. Pulmonary involvement is rarely seen in the absence of hilar disease. Pleural effusions may be secondary to lymphatic obstruction from large central disease and do not necessarily represent advanced disease. Children aged 1 to 10 have a significantly lower incidence (33%) of mediastinal involvement as compared with children age 11 to 15 (76%).[34] This may relate to the higher incidence of nodular sclerosis subtype in adolescence, as it is a common form of intrathoracic Hodgkin's disease. Pericardial effusion is often associated with large mediastinal disease and is best delineated by echocardiography. Computed tomography (CT) has been shown in adults to be a sensitive method of evaluating the chest in adults, but has not been systematically studied in children. Children present the additional problem when evaluating the mediastinum of differentiating thymic infiltration by Hodgkin's disease from a normal thymus gland. Cases of thymic involution, secondary to immunosuppressive chemotherapy, have been observed in children receiving MOPP chemotherapy for Hodgkin's disease, with subsequent thymic enlargement with the cessation of chemotherapy. This observation has been made in several children at Stanford who presented with inguinal/femoral disease, but without supradiaphragmatic Hodgkin's disease. Following involved field pelvic radiotherapy and six cycles of MOPP, transient enlargement of the mediastinum has been observed, which initially was mistaken for disease extension,

ANATOMIC DISTRIBUTION OF 490 SITES OF INVOLVEMENT IN 129 SURGICALLY STAGED CHILDREN WITH HODGKIN'S DISEASE

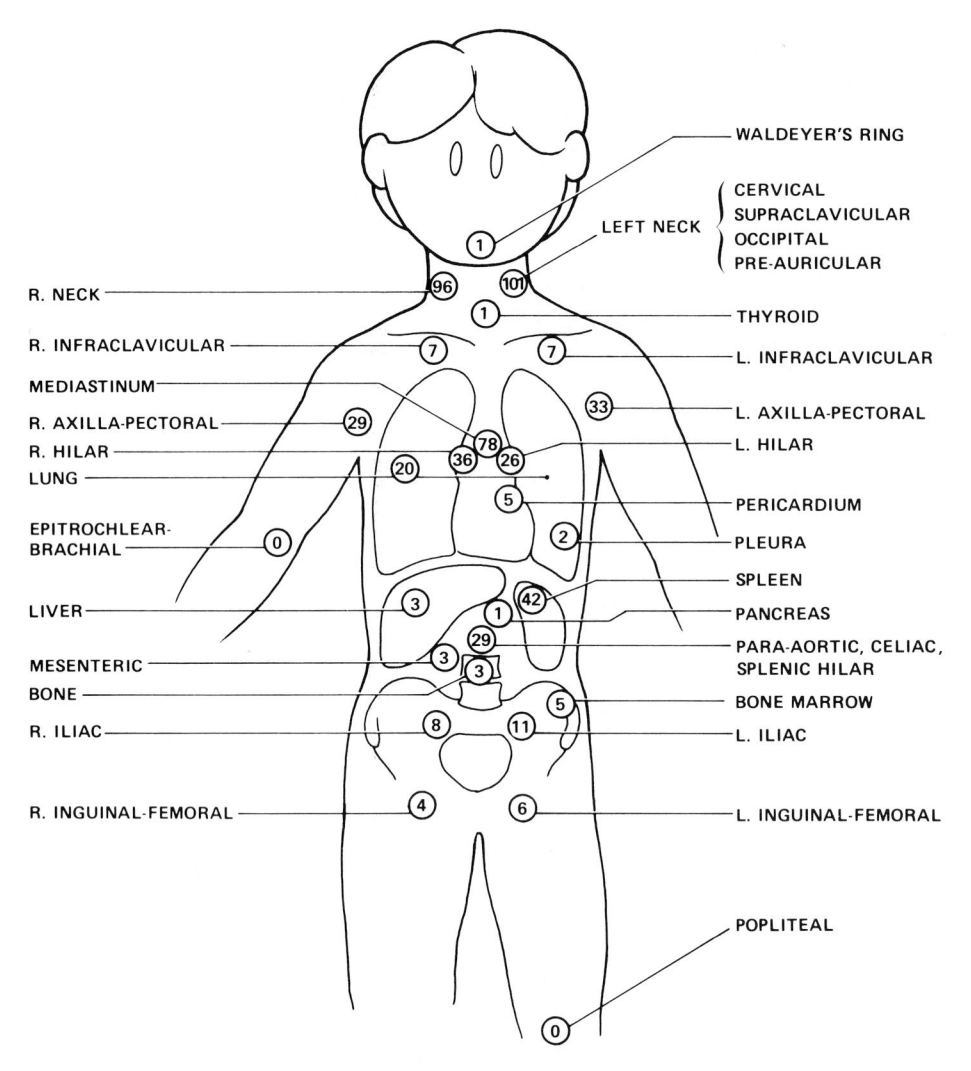

Fig. 18–3. Anatomic distribution of 490 lymphatic and extralymphatic sites of documented involvement occurring in 129 consecutive children with Hodgkin's disease. (From Donaldson, S.S. and Kaplan, H.S.: A survey of pediatric Hodgkin's disease at Stanford University: Results of therapy and quality of survival. In Malignant Lymphomas. Etiology, Immunology, Pathology, Treatment. Edited by S.A. Rosenberg and H.S. Kaplan. New York, Academic Press, 1982.)

but subsequently shown to subside spontaneously without treatment; this is consistent with normal thymic involution. This observation underscores the importance of histologically confirming possible recurrences before making therapeutic decisions.

Maximal assessment of the retroperitoneal lymph nodes in children requires lymphography as well as CT scanning. A bipedal lymphogram is the most direct method of visualizing the retroperitoneal node chains most frequently involved in Hodgkin's disease, the paralumbar and parailiac lymph nodes. In experienced hands and in those in whom histopathologic correlation has been possible, the lymphographic accuracy among children with Hodgkin's disease is 95%.[37] Whereas 70% of lymphograms at Stanford are interpreted as normal, the remaining 30% reveal abnormalities of Hodgkin's disease in 19% and abnormalities of reactive hyperplasia in 12%.[34] Reactive hyperplasia is seen most commonly in youngsters 1 to 10 years of age (19%) as compared to those 11 to 15 years of age (8%).[34] The incidence of reactive hyperplasia is highest in children and less a problem among the adult population. With expertise in performing and reading lymphograms, Castellino et al. have demonstrated success in repeat lymphography in children with Hodgkin's disease, with the same lymphatic cannulation success rate on repeat studies as upon initial lymphograms.[38] Furthermore, they have shown that a negative initial lymphogram was found to be positive on a repeat study in 39% of children studied.[38] The Stanford investigators have demonstrated the value of lymphography in children in accuracy of staging, guiding the surgeon to the appropriate lymph nodes for biopsy, aiding the radiotherapist in treatment planning, and usefulness in following patient response to therapy.

More recently, CT has become widely used as a noninvasive means to evaluate the retroperitoneum in patients with Hodgkin's disease. Among a small number of children with Hodgkin's disease studied by both CT and lymphography, an 82% correlation between the two studies was observed; however, the majority of patients had negative studies by both examinations.[39] Lymphography has been particularly useful in children less than 10 years of age and among those with a clearly negative CT scan.[39] Although a histopathologic correlation of CT and staging laparotomy among children is not available, studies in adults have shown significantly increased accuracy of lymphography, as compared with CT, in assessing the retroperitoneal lymph nodes.[40] Whereas CT does allow assessment of the upper abdomen and celiac axis lymph nodes, which are not opacified by a lymphogram, the CT criterion of abnormal adenopathy is based solely on size, usually considering that greater than 1.0 to 1.5 cm as positive; its theoretical advantage in detecting lymphomatous deposits in lymph nodes about the celiac axis has not been confirmed.[40] Computed tomography accuracy is impeded because nodal involvement of Hodgkin's disease is characteristically focal with small architectural filling defects, rather than one of uniform enlargement and replacement with disease. Furthermore, children frequently have enlarged nodes (>1.5 cm) because of reactive hyperplasia rather than replacement with Hodgkin's disease. In addition, optimal imaging with CT depends on an interface of nodal tissue against retroperitoneal fat to differentiate tissue planes. Children characteristically have a paucity of retroperitoneal adipose tissue and often are not able to tolerate adequate amounts of oral contrast material, which makes accurate visualization of normal structures even more difficult in a child than in an adult. Optimal radiographs by means of lymphography or CT scanning often require sedation or even anesthesia of young children. At present, the lymphogram and the abdominal-pelvic CT must be considered complementary studies for children. If only one study is available, the lymphogram is most useful in defining involvement with Hodgkin's disease.[40]

Involvement of the spleen represents a diagnostic challenge. Unfortunately, routine use of radionuclide liver/spleen scans have not proven useful in the detection of Hodgkin's disease.[41] Likewise, CT scanning of the abdomen is accurate in confirming splenic involvement in Hodgkin's disease in only one third of patients. Tumor nodules are often less than 1 cm in maximal dimension, which is smaller than the resolving power of modern-day scanners.[40] Furthermore, splenic size and weight do not correlate well with involvement. Gallium scanning is used by some in assessing lymph node involvement, but is most useful in evaluating sites above the diaphragm that are easily defined by chest roentgenogram and physical examination; gallium scanning has an accuracy of approximately 60%.[42] For infradiaphragmatic sites, however, gallium scanning provides true positive data in only 40%, with 60% of studies yielding false-negative interpretations, thus rendering it of little help in assessing the area most difficult to image in children.

Complete clinical staging that affords little to no long-term toxicity is known to be accurate only in approximately two thirds of children.[43] At least one third of children have their stage altered by the findings of surgical staging at laparotomy with splenectomy, most frequently by the finding of occult splenic disease in the setting of a normal lymphogram, normal CT scan, and normal physical exam. It is therefore appropriate to discuss the risk versus benefits to the child to undergo surgical staging including splenectomy.

SURGICAL STAGING

The issue of surgical staging including splenectomy represents one of the controversies regarding management of children with Hodgkin's disease, largely because of concerns of morbidity or mortality related to elective operating staging. When treatment policies depend on accurate staging and extent of disease, surgical staging is easily defended. General approaches regarding management of children have been to tailor treatment to the extent of disease, thus most investigators continue to rely upon operative staging.[44] Others, however, have opted for uniform therapy for all children irrespective of stage or extent, thus negating the value of surgical staging.[17]

Clinical staging using physical examination, chest radiographs, CT and whole lung tomograms, lymphography, and bone-marrow biopsy is accurate in only approximately 70% of children, with approximately one third found to have occult splenic disease in children otherwise thought to have only supradiaphragmatic disease. Approximately 8% of those with splenic disease are shown to have liver involvement at staging laparotomy.[15] Other areas of occult abdominal disease include nodal disease in the splenic pedicle, celiac axis, and porta hepatis—areas not opacified by the lymphogram. Staging laparotomy therefore provides data in an appreciable portion of children regarding the anatomic extent of disease at diagnosis that otherwise would not be obtainable. The technique of ovarian transposition (oophoropexy) at the time of staging laparotomy, with appropriate gonadal shielding prior to pelvic radiotherapy, allows preservation of ovarian function in young women with Hodgkin's disease.[45]

The acute complications of elective operative staging among children, including wound infection, wound dehiscence, retroperitoneal hematoma, subphrenic abscess, pancreatitis, hemobilia, and acute pulmonary complications of atelectasis and/or pneumonia have occurred in less than 1% of the pediatric series.[46] The routine administration of localized mediastinal irradiation prior to general anesthesia for those patients with extensive intrathoracic disease or airway compromise has been successful in avoiding airway problems following extubation. Late complications including bowel obstruction have ranged between 3 and 4% in pediatric series,[44,46] related to adhesions following the surgical procedure rather than recurrent disease. In the more recent era, however, even a lower incidence of acute and delayed surgical complications has ben observed, presumably because these patients are young, in good general health, and have been operated on and cared for by a team of surgeons with expertise in performing diagnostic staging laparotomies. There has not been morbidity related to surgical staging in the large pediatric series.

Among the long-term adult male survivors following splenectomy for trauma, concern about increased mortality due to ischemic heart disease related to postsplenectomy thrombocytosis and hypercoagulability has arisen.[47,48] Data supporting such problems following splenectomy for staging of Hodgkin's disease are not available.

INFECTIONS

Because of the concern of overwhelming septicemia in asplenic children, controversy exists over the risk/benefit of splenectomy as part of surgical staging in children. A partial or hemisplenectomy has been proposed as an alternative procedure to total splenectomy for children as a means of providing biopsy material for staging, while leaving some intact splenic tissue to protect against overwhelming sepsis.[49] However, it has been shown that partial splenectomy results in greater than an 11% false-negative rate, which underscores the risk of failing to diagnose occult splenic involvement.[50] Adequate assessment of splenic involvement cannot be made by inspection, palpation, or by currently available imaging techniques; it requires removal of the entire spleen with serial sectioning at millimeter intervals. The likelihood of splenic involvement cannot be accurately predicted on the basis of the circulation of the spleen or by the presence or absence of splenic hilar lymph-node involvement. Whereas a partially intact spleen can protect against sepsis in animal models,[51] comparable data in humans do no exist. It is now recognized that splenic irradiation can produce splenic atrophy and dysfunction capable of resulting in fatal overwhelming sepsis.[52,53] It is not known if this risk is related to dose of radiation or to chemotherapy. Splenic dysfunction, however, has been observed many years post-treatment, suggesting that postirradiation recovery of function is unlikely.

The incidence of serious bacterial infections with Hodgkin's disease has been reported in 10 to 13% of children,[54,55] whereas for older patients the risk is substantially less.[56] The most common offending organisms observed are the encapsulated bacteria including *Streptococcus pneumoniae, Haemophilus influenzae,* and group A streptococcus. The risk of developing a serious bacterial infection coincides with the timing of treatment in approximately one half of cases, with infections occurring during the time of active treatment for Hodgkin's disease when children are immunosuppressed from their disease and/or treatment and when periods of neutropenia are common.[54] Yet in the Stanford series, 52% of the episodes of serious bacterial infection in children occurred months or years following completion of treatment among a population presumed to be cured of Hodgkin's disease. Infection in this setting has been observed as an initial event at 13 years following therapy, with 4 of 12 off-treatment episodes being fatal.[54]

In the Stanford series, the risk of serious bacterial infection among children is related to the intensity of the treatment given rather than to whether or not a splenectomy was performed (Table 18–2). The serious infections were defined as bacteremia, meningitis, pneumonia, or pyelonephritis, requiring hospitalization and treatment with parenteral antibiotics. The risk of serious bacterial infection among irradiated children was 1 of 71 (1.4%) among splenectomized children and 2 of 71 (2.8%) among nonsplenectomized children. When chemotherapy was added to the treatment program, however, the risk rose to 13 of 71 (18.3%) for splenectomized children and 6 of 26 (23.1%) for nonsplenectomized children ($p<0.05$).

As the predominant organisms for these serious bacterial infections are penicillin-sensitive, many investigators now recommend routine use of prophylactic antibiotics for children with previous splenic irradiation or splenectomy. Whereas the optimal dose and duration of antibiotic administration is not known, the routine use of antibiotics has coincided with a drop in infection rate at Stanford from a previous incidence of 13% to less than 1%. The one asplenic youngster in the recent Stanford series who has developed pneumococcal bacteremia did so despite antibiotic prophylaxis and pneumococcal vaccine immunization one year after splenectomy; he was immunosuppressed and undergoing treatment with six cycles of chemotherapy and irradiation for stage IV Hodgkin's disease involving the bone marrow. Thus, although the liberal use of antibiotics has greatly reduced the incidence of infection, the risk of bacteremia and/or meningitis secondary to encapsulated organisms is not zero, thereby requiring patient/family education that emphasizes the importance of prompt physician evaluation with appropriate cultures during febrile episodes.

Although it was hoped that use of the pneumocccal vaccine would provide protection against the pneumococcus, studies of children with Hodgkin's disease demonstrate that its effect is not adequate to provide long-term protection.[57] Adequate antibody response is not observed when the vaccine is given postsplenectomy or postimmunosuppressive therapy. When administered prior to staging or treatment, only two thirds of patients will respond to the vaccine. Antibody

Table 18–2. Serious Bacterial Infections in 179 Children with Hodgkin's Disease

Treatment	Splenectomy		No Splenectomy	
Radiotherapy alone	1/71 (1.4%)	p < 0.05	2/71 (2.8%)	p < 0.05
Chemotherapy ± Radiotherapy	13/71 (18.3%)		6/26 (23.1%)	

Adapted from Donaldson, S.S., Glatstein, E., and Vosti, K.L.: Bacterial infections in pediatric Hodgkin's disease: Relationship to radiotherapy, chemotherapy, and splenectomy. Cancer 41:1949, 1978.)

responses vary among the various components of the multivalent vaccine and are not predictable or consistent from patient to patient. Furthermore, the duration of response is short, with the majority of responses equal to or less than baseline values 5 to 9 months following initial immunization. As there is no readily available commercial method to evaluate pneumococcal antibody response, we cannot rely upon pneumococcal vaccine for sole protection in a child with Hodgkin's disease.

The most frequently recognized viral infection in children with Hodgkin's disease is herpes zoster-varicella, which occurs in approximately 35% of all cases; localized herpes zoster, 25%; disseminated herpes zoster, 8%; varicella, 1.5%.[58] The risk of herpes zoster-varicella is not increased by splenectomy and does not carry prognostic significance.[59] As with bacterial infections, the incidence of herpes zoster-varicella infections correlates with the degree of immunosuppression and intensity of treatment. When irradiation is the sole modality of therapy, the risk of infection is 21%. The risk increases to 37% among the cohort of children given low-dose involved-field radiation with MOPP chemotherapy, and rises to 53% when MOPP is added to high-dose extended-field radiation. An incidence of 44% is observed among children being treated for relapsed Hodgkin's disease. In the Stanford series, one child died from disseminated zoster with visceral involvement.

Opportunistic and fungal infections occurring in children with Hodgkin's disease are also most common during periods of maximal immunosuppression from aggressive therapy. Pneumocystis carinii pulmonary infections are most apt to occur in children with intrathoracic Hodgkin's disease undergoing chemotherapy and irradiation. The use of specific antimicrobial therapy with Bactrim/Septra appears to have reduced the number of observed cases, although risk values are not available.

Approximately 30% of children with Hodgkin's disease have repeated and persistent verruca vulgara, common warts usually occurring on the backs of hands and fingers unrelated to treatment.[10]

SOFT-TISSUE AND BONE-GROWTH ALTERATIONS

Attention has been given to the impairment of bone growth and development known to accompany high-dose large-volume radiation since the initial reports describing a disproportionate alteration in sitting height as compared with standing height among a group of children at Stanford who received total-nodal irradiation.[60,61] Table 18–3 shows sitting and standing height data for 72 children from Boston and Stanford who received radiation doses of 3500 cGy or greater to the axial skeleton.[10,44] They are compared to Table 18–4 showing data for 44 children from Stanford who were given 2500 cGy or less to the axial skeleton. The growth impairment is most significant in those who received doses of more than 3500 cGy to the axial skeleton and is particularly significant among those children who are youngsters or in early adolescence, under 13 years at the time of treatment.[9–12] Growth disturbance is not a significant complication of high-dose radiation for children whose bone age is 14 to 15 years or greater at the time of radiotherapy. Boys appear to be more severely affected than girls.[62]

The bone-growth impairment can be minimized by reducing the doses and volumes of irradiation to youngsters, particularly those whose epiphyses are open at the time of treatment and whose bone age is less than their chronologic age at the time of radiotherapy.

Table 18-3. Heights for 72 Children Receiving More Than 3500 cGy*

Standing Heights

	Age at Treatment (years)		
	3-8	9-12	13-16
+2SD			
+1SD	1	1	9
Mean	9	19	19
-1SD	1	8	3
-2SD		1	1
-3SD			

Sitting Heights

	Age at Treatment (years)		
	3-8	9-12	13-16
+2SD			
+1SD			1
Mean	2	13	4
-1SD	6	10	22
-2SD	3	5	4
-3SD		1	1

*Numbers of children listed are children irradiated at 3-8 years, 9-12 years, or 13-16 years of age whose standing and/or sitting heights are within plus or minus one, two, or three standard deviation(s) (SD) from the mean as indicated. (Adapted from Donaldson, S.S. and Kaplan, H.S.: Complications of treatment of Hodgkin's disease in children. Cancer Treat. Rep. 66:977, 1982, and Mauch, P.M. et al.: An evaluation of long-term survival and treatment complications in children with Hodgkin's disease. Cancer 51:925, 1983.)

Table 18-4. Heights for 44 Children Receiving Less Than 2500 cGy*

Standing Heights

	Age at Treatment (years)		
	3-8	9-12	13-16
+2SD		1	
+1SD	2	3	1
Mean	10	15	4
-1SD	6	2	
-2SD			

Sitting Heights

	Age at Treatment (years)		
	3-8	9-12	13-16
+2SD			
+1SD		1	3
Mean	6	12	1
-1SD	9	6	1
-2SD	3	2	
-3SD			

*Numbers of children listed are children irradiated at 3-8 years, 9-12 years, or 13-16 years of age whose standing and/or sitting heights are within plus or minus one, two, or three standard deviation(s) (SD) from the mean as indicated. (Adapted from Donaldson, S.S. and Kaplan, H.S.: Complications of treatment of Hodgkin's disease in children. Cancer Treat. Rep. 66:977, 1982.)

Data for irradiated children receiving doses less than 2500 cGy show no abnormalities in standing height greater than 1 standard deviation from the mean and minimal sitting height alterations. These children have received chemotherapy in addition to radiotherapy.

Shortening of the clavicles with a decrease in the intraclavicular separation is also characteristic of children given high-dose irradiation to a mantle field at a young age, although it is difficult to quantitate. Underdevelopment and fibrosis of the soft tissues of the neck have also been seen and are explained by a high dose of irradiation given to a preadolescent child. Less common bone sequelae such as slipped femoral capital epiphyses, which are hypothesized to be related to an irradiation effect on chondrogenesis as well as vascular injury[63] or possibly to excess stress on a previously weakened bone structure,[64] have been reported. Of a more serious nature is the observation of avascular necrosis of bone reported as high as 10% among long-term survivors who receive chemotherapy including prednisone in addition to irradiation.[65] The Stanford series reports only a 1% incidence of this complication, presumably because of the routine use of humeral head and femoral head blocks in all mantle and pelvic fields.[44]

Prior to the use of megavoltage irradiation, changes in the sternum, occasionally with necrosis, were observed.[66] This problem has been eliminated by the use of symmetric megavoltage irradiation. Combination chemotherapy commonly accounts for a temporary growth impairment during the period of actual chemotherapy, when height frequently remains stationary and weight often decreases. This cessation of growth is temporary and is alleviated when a course of chemotherapy is completed.

The observation of hydrocele formation among adolescents and young adults with Hodgkin's disease following inverted-Y irradiation to doses in the range of 3500 cGy has been observed, presumably related to lymphatic fibrosis.[67] The incidence of this problem is small and easily corrected by hydrocelectomy.

PULMONARY—CARDIAC SEQUELAE

Significant pulmonary injury from irradiation is related to total radiation dose, daily fraction size, and volume of lung included in the high-dose irradiated area. The risk of pulmonary injury among children is not significantly different from the adult experience, and represents an approximate 4% risk according to the Stanford pediatric Hodgkin's disease experience.[44] Symptomatic pulmonary injury occurred in 3.6% of children receiving high-dose mantle radiotherapy, but increased to approximately 6% when chemotherapy was added to high-dose irradiation, either as planned therapy or as treatment for relapse. To date, significant pulmonary reactions have not been observed among the 55 children receiving low-dose radiotherapy and six cycles of MOP chemotherapy. This lower incidence reflects both a reduction in radiation dose and volume, as well as shrinking radiation fields and shaped and "thin" lung blocks.[68] The use of chemotherapy prior to mantle radiotherapy for children with large mediastinal masses has enabled smaller volumes to be irradiated. Bilateral whole lung fractionated radiation to doses not in excess of 1600 cGy appears to be within tolerance for children and not associated with symptomatic pulmonary reaction.

Early experience demonstrated the exacerbation of acute radiation injury with a rapid tapering of prednisone following the I and IV cycles of the MOPP chemotherapy program,[69] so that prednisone is now routinely omitted whenever thoracic radiotherapy is given. Asymptomatic pleural effusion occurring 6 and 8 years following high-dose mantle therapy has been observed in two children irradiated at Stanford.[44] In both children, careful evaluation failed to disclose a source of infection or recurrent Hodgkin's disease as an etiology for the effusion. Both patients have had stability of the effusion without therapy for many years, suggesting the etiology may be related to aberrant lymphatic drainage following pulmonary irradiation with subsequent fibrosis.

The incidence of pulmonary injury may increase as more liberal use of chemotherapeutic agents, which carry some degree of pulmonary toxicity, are employed. Pulmonary fibrosis secondary to bleomycin appears to be dose related, and is hoped to be reversible, alhough data from large groups of children with Hodgkin's disease are not yet available.

Cardiac injury from radiation is related to dose, volume, and fraction size, manifesting as pericarditis or pancarditis including myocardial injury.[70,71] Its severity may range from asymptomatic and transient cardiac enlargement, recognized only radiographically, to delayed constrictive pericarditis requiring pericardiectomy. The approximately 13% incidence among children following high-dose mantle irradiation does not differ from that observed in adults.

Coronary artery disease with coronary fibrosis and accelerated atherogenesis has been observed in long-term survivors of Hodgkin's disease who underwent mantle irradiation.[72] Two cases of premature coronary artery disease have been observed among 120 children receiving mantle radiotherapy at Stanford.[44] The cause-and-effect connection between coronary artery disease and radiotherapy remains questionable and appears to have a low incidence.[73] It has been suggested that myocardial ischemia from atheromatous plaques in coronary vessels may be formed by platelet accumulation and aggregation following splenectomy and subsequent thrombocytosis and hypercoagulability.[48] Attention to the techniques of radiotherapy, using pericardial and subcarinal blocks, as well as multiple shrinking fields, has reduced the risks of radiation-related injury in patients with Hodgkin's disease.[68] Five of 120 children irradiated for intrathoracic Hodgkin's disease have been observed with valvular abnormalities and myocardial dysfunction. These children have been successfully managed medically and/or surgically. The pathogenesis and relationship of heart disease to Hodgkin's disease among these long-term survivors remains unclear, but is of particular concern in the pediatric population having a high likelihood of long-term survival. Yet unknown is the degree of short- or long-term toxicity related to combination chemotherapy regimens containing doxorubicin and daunorubicin, agents known to have dose-related cardiotoxicity. Caution regarding synergistic effects must be maintained with long-term monitoring of cardiac function, otherwise the true risk of these sequelae will not be known.

ENDOCRINE SEQUELAE

Thyroid dysfunction among patients with Hodgkin's disease has been reported to occur in between 4 and 79% of irradiated patients, provided one uses an elevated TSH level as an indicator of hypothyroidism.[2,74-80] Interestingly, the pediatric series have consistently reported a high incidence of TSH elevations among children,[77,81-83] suggesting a greater sensitivity of the thyroid among the rapidly growing preadolescent or adolescent age group as compared to adults. The iodine load of a preradiotherapy lymphogram has been implicated, although the exact relationship of the lymphogram to thyroid injury is unclear and controversial. The Stanford investigators showed that dose of radiation to the thyroid is important in the incidence of thyroid dysfunction among children with Hodgkin's disease.[84] Only 17% of children who received neck irradiation doses of 2600 cGy or less developed thyroid abnormalities as compared to 78% of the children who received doses of 2600 cGy or greater. Of interest in the Stanford series was the spontaneous reversal of thyroid dysfunction with return of the elevated TSH to within normal limits. Also of interest was the substantial improvement in 36% of the biochemically hypothyroid children.[84] Thyroid nodules, hyperthyroidism,[85] and thyroid cancer[86] have also been observed among patients with Hodgkin's disease. It is recommended that children with chemical hypothyroidism manifested by elevated TSH levels following neck irradiation be given thyroid replacement therapy to reduce thyroid stimulation from prolonged TSH elevation.

Thyroid dysfunction is an observed sequela in long-term survivors but is easily managed by replacement therapy and is not considered a long-term complication. Its potential does, however, require observation and evaluation in the follow-up period and management if abnormalities occur.

Pancreatic dysfunction with insulin-dependent juvenile diabetes mellitus has been present in children who subsequently developed Hodgkin's disease. In the Stanford series, such patients have been successfully treated by total-nodal irradiation, including an irradiation field covering the entire pancreas as well as the spleen and para-aortic lymph nodes, without discernible exacerbation of the diabetes.[1]

Sterility, alterations in fertility, and potential gonadal injury following staging and treatment are important issues that must be addressed at the time of diagnosis and prior to therapy. Pelvic lymph-node irradiation is known to carry with it the high likelihood of ablation of ovarian function, hence consideration of ovarian transposition prior to pelvic radiotherapy is required. The technique of oophoropexy, ovarian transposition from the normal lateral position to a central location and tacked either in front of or behind the uterus, has allowed the preservation of ovarian function in young women with Hodgkin's disease.[45] The likelihood of maintenance of ovarian function is directly related to gonadal exposure and age at treatment.[87] The younger the woman at the time of therapy, the higher the probability of maintenance of regular menses following therapy. In an assessment of menstrual status among girls with Hodgkin's disease 13 to 18 years of age at the time of treatment, it was shown that following oophoropexy 100% of the girls treated with radiation alone maintained normal menses.[44] For those girls in whom multiagent chemotherapy was added to the treatment program, 88% maintained normal menses. Thus, the impact of aggressive therapy on ovarian function in girls and young women is less than in adult women, as only 48% of adult women maintain normal menses following total lymphoid irradiation and chemotherapy.[87] However, one chemotherapy series revealed that only 43% of women 12 to 39 years of age with

Hodgkin's disease continue to menstruate following MOPP chemotherapy with no correlation to age or cumulative drug exposure.[88] In another series, 69% of women younger than 30 and still in the reproductive age group continued with menstrual function following combination chemotherapy.[89] It is probable that the younger the patient, the greater the complement of oocytes at the time of treatment and hence the greater the likelihood of maintenance of ovarian function after radiation, chemotherapy, or combined modality therapy.

Pregnancies have been observed among these girls with no increased risk of fetal wastage or spontaneous abortion.[44,87] Of the pregnancies that have been carried to term, no birth defects have been observed.

In contrast to females, the sterility issue in males is of much greater severity, and yet available data are more scant, requiring longer periods of follow-up observation. High-dose irradiation to the pelvis in a standard inverted-Y field, as is used in Hodgkin's disease, may be associated with a transient oligospermia or azoospermia; however, recovery of function is common.[90] Testicular shields are routinely recommended in adult males when pelvic irradiation is used,[91] however, these generally are anatomically difficult to use effectively in prepubertal males. The early reports of testicular injury following combination chemotherapy, specifically MOPP, reported a more complete and nonreversble injury than that observed following irradiation; recovery was rare.[92,93] Among the pediatric population, 9 of 13 Ugandan adolescent boys with Hodgkin's disease, 10 to 16 years of age at the time of MOPP treatment, developed gynecomastia, complete germinal aplasia, increased follicle stimulating hormone, and luteinizing hormone and decreased serum testosterone.[94] In contrast, the prepubertal boys studied showed no change in gonadotropin levels and no clinical gynecomastia. The definitive evaluation is by way of semen analysis rather than hormonal assay. It now appears that germ-cell depletion and Leydig-cell dysfunction are expected and likely to be irreversible in adolescent and adult males following six cycles of MOPP chemotherapy. The cytotoxic damage to the testicular germinal epithelium appears to be dose related. Some data are available to suggest that recovery of spermatogenesis may be seen in adult males receiving three or fewer cycles of MOPP, as compared to the standard six cycles.[95] Of the MOPP combination, it is probable that the mechlorethamine (mustard) and procarbazine are the most toxic to the testes. Data with definitive semen analysis, sperm counts, and motility studies among boys prepubertal at the time of MOPP chemotherapy are still too premature to know if this subset will be spared the sterility that accompanies chemotherapy given to the postpubertal patient. It is hoped that four-drug combination chemotherapy approaches such as the ABVD combination will be equally efficacious therapeutically but have a lower risk of sterility.[96] Long-term follow-ups are necessary before these important issues will be clarified. Sperm banking is advised among males requiring chemotherapy who are desirous of a family. However, the disease itself may have an adverse effect on fertility before any form of staging or treatment.[97] Many males are subfertile prior to initiation of therapy, thus sperm banking itself is not a guarantee for future reproduction among these patients who have a high likelihood to be long-term survivors.

SECOND MALIGNANT TUMORS

The problem of second malignancies among patients surviving their initial cancer is well recognized.[98] Over 300 cases of acute leukemia have been reported among patients treated for Hodgkin's disease. The actuarial risk of developing leukemia is a function of the treatment administered. With 7 to 10 year follow-up among several series with large numbers of patients, the risk following radiation alone is less than 1%; following initial irradiation and chemotherapy, salvage irradiation and chemotherapy, or chemotherapy alone, the risk is in the range of 6%.[99–103] Most leukemias have been acute myelogenous leukemia and most are fatal.[104] Most studies have shown age to be a prognostic indicator, with an especially high risk of leukemia among older patients (over 40 years of age).[99,101,102] Conversely, children less than 20 have fared most favorably.[99,101] The carcinogenic effect of the chemotherapy appears to be drug- and dose-related. Most leukemias have occurred following the MOPP combination among patients receiving six cycles of drugs. It is hoped that a fewer number of cycles or that other drug combinations such as ABVD will prove to be less carcinogenic.[100]

Also of concern is the increased risk of solid tumors among these survivors, which is not related to treatment modality. Among large series, the actuarial risk of a second solid tumor following radiotherapy is 6 to 9%;[99,100,103] initial radiotherapy and chemotherapy or salvage radiotherapy and chemotherapy, 6 to 9%;[99,103] or chemotherapy alone, 7%.[103] The solid tumors that have been observed do not necessarily occur in the irradiation field. There does appear to be an increased risk of developing a solid tumor with increasing age.[103] A variety of solid tumors have been reported, most of which are bone or soft tissue sarcomas.[105] Approximately one half of the patients with these secondary lymphomas or solid tumors will be cured of their second neoplasm.[99,101] Table 18–5 shows the Stanford pediatric experience of second malignant tumors. The one case of thyroid cancer among 63 children who received radiotherapy alone (1.6%) appeared 10 years following treatment and was successfully managed by subsequent surgical resection. Among the 115 children who received combined modality therapy, 49 received initial low-dose radiotherapy and MOPP, and 66 received high-dose radiotherapy and MOPP, 30 as initial therapy and 36 as salvage therapy. There have been three cases of acute myelocytic leukemia and one case of acute lymphoblastic leukemia. Three of 49 children who received low-dose involved-field radiotherapy and MOPP developed leukemia, a crude incidence of 4%, and one of 36 children who received combined modality salvage treatment developed it.

The one case of undifferentiated sarcoma occurred after a 5-year disease-free interval in an abdominal irradiation field in a child treated with total lymphoid irradiation and adjuvant MOP. The tumor was nonresponsive to further chemotherapy. The one case of chondrosarcoma occurred 9 years after initial diagnosis in a boy with multiple enchondroses (Ollier's disease) and was fatal. One child treated with low-dose irradiation (1500 cGy) to the left neck and MOPP chemotherapy developed thyroid cancer in the nonirradiated right lobe of the thyroid 9 years following initial treatment for Hodgkin's disease. He was treated with a subtotal thyroidectomy and ^{131}I. Three months later he was found to have acute lymphoblastic leukemia. Long-term follow-up is essential in assessing the true risk of these second malignant tumors as the risk increases with age and length of follow-up. The dose and volume of radiotherapy is not related to the develop-

Table 18–5. Second Malignant Tumors in Children with Hodgkin's Disease

Treatments (Number of Patients)	Leukemia	NonHodgkin's Lymphoma	Solid Tumors			Total
			Thyroid Cancer	Undifferentiated Sarcoma	Chondrosarcoma	
Radiotherapy (63)			1			1/63 (1.6%)
Initial radiotherapy and chemotherapy (79)	3*		1*	1		4/79 (5%)
Salvage radiotherapy and chemotherapy (36)	1	1			1	3/36 (8%)
Chemotherapy (1)						0/1 (0%)
Total (179)						8/179 (4.4%)

*One child developed thyroid cancer and subsequently acute lymphoblastic leukemia. (Adapted and updated from Donaldson, S.S. and Kaplan, H.S.: Complications of treatment of Hodgkin's disease in children. Cancer Treat. Rep. 66:977, 1982.)

ment of a second malignant tumor, but rather the specific chemotherapeutic agents. Most series have reported MOPP chemotherapy experience. Preliminary data suggest ABVD is less carcinogenic than the MOPP combination.

PSYCHOSOCIAL IMPACT

Psychosocial problems observed among the Hodgkin's disease survivors have to date received little attention. Such difficulties may be especially disabling for young people who have been treated and who have an expected long-term disease-free survival. A study of 473 patients treated for Hodgkin's disease at Stanford is currently underway to identify the specific psychosocial problems that develop as a result of the diagnosis or treatment to quantitate their severity and to design appropriate intervention.[106] Among the total sample, a disruption in family life as measured by disruption in marital status was seen in 49%, slightly higher than the United States rate of divorce for first marriages (30%), but the same as the percentage of failure of U.S. marriages in a lifetime, 49% (US Centers for Disease Control, 1983). Examination of a patient's perception of his general health, energy level, and activity level revealed that 86% of patients felt that their health was good or excellent following treatment. Younger patients, from teenage years to 34 years of age, indicated a 12-month time for energy level to return to normal as compared to adults over age 34 who required 14 months for energy levels to return to normal.[106] As well, younger (under 30 years of age) patients had less decline in sexual activity than older patients (over 30 years of age). When a general decline in the interests and frequency in sexual activity during treatment did occur, the younger patients had return of sexual libido sooner. A correlate with loss of energy was a perception of feeling one's body image was impaired, or that one's physical attractiveness had decreased as a result of Hodgkin's disease. Younger patients had fewer activity- and energy-related problems, but had more work-related problems.[107] Further investigation into school and work performance among youngsters and adolescents treated for Hodgkin's disease will be necessary to understand the impact of the disease in these areas. The scant amount of data available in the area of psychosocial sequelae of Hodgkin's disease suggest that children are affected less severely than their adult counterparts. Yet, with increasingly effective therapeutic programs and continual refinement of treatment resulting in a reduction of chemotherapy and radiotherapy toxicities, the psychosocial aspects of long-term survivorship may become a more important and recognized complication among the long-term Hodgkin's disease survivors.

RISK VERSUS BENEFIT

Since the 1950s, deaths from childhood Hodgkin's disease have fallen by 80%; a dramatic reduction due almost entirely to improved forms of staging and treatment. This tribute has brought with it a cohort of long-term survivors who now are teaching us the price of our success—long-term complications. The consequence of survival is most remarkable among the pediatric population. Yet the major obstacle remains the disease itself. The challenge today requires devising approaches to improve and maintain a high quality of survival while minimizing complications of treatment. This task necessitates individualization of therapy to maximize efficacy while minimizing sequelae. With children, it becomes apparent that there is no standard recipe for management. Optimal approaches require judgement in staging and selectivity in treatment recommendations, for the risk-benefit ratio is a function of age of patient, stage and extent of disease, and tumor burden. In general, the potential complications from the disease, staging, and treatment have been minimized by modern approaches. Clinical staging procedures are considered routine and not difficult when performed in centers having large numbers of patients and demonstrated expertise. Surgical staging carries minimal morbidity; its value being to define which patients require aggressive treatment for advanced disease and in whom therapy can be lessened. Bacterial, viral, and fungal infections are a problem of immunocompromise and are related to aggressive treatment. Prophylactic antibiotics have been useful in diminishing postsplenectomy bacteremia and meningitis. Interference with growth and development is known to follow high-dose extended-field radiotherapy. This problem has been largely avoided by combined-modality programs in which radiotherapy doses and volumes can be reduced when successful chemotherapy programs are employed. Disturbance in organ function, most notably cardiopulmonary dysfunction, has been largely negated by use of modern-day radiotherapy equipment and techniques. When large tumors overlay normal tissues, combined-modality approaches allow lower radiation doses to be used successfully. The late effects of chemotherapy on organ function are still being determined. In general, reduced doses of both radiotherapy and chemotherapy are recommended when used in combination. Thyroid injury related to radiotherapy is minimized by using lower therapeutic doses and is easily remedied by replacement medication. Psychosocial disturbances have not been well characterized and may become more prominent with increasing attention given to this area. The two areas that represent serious and severe sequelae are sterility accompanying gonadal injury and the development of second malignant tumors. These problems require development of new modality programs using cytotoxic agents that cause less testicular injury and less risk of carcinogenesis. Many programs are under development to minimize this recognized injury.

While attention to the consequences of survival cannot be overemphasized, the major goal must be cure of the tumor. Nowhere in medicine is it more important to individualize management and approaches, recognizing the severity of the disease while remembering the cost of survivorship.

The consequences of survival among children with Hodgkin's disease could be well expressed by the following:

> As frightened Patients, when they want a Cure,
> Bid any Price, and any Pain endure:
> But when the doctor's Remedies appear,
> The Cure's too easy, and the Price too dear!
>
> Daniel Defoe, 1659–1731
> *The Time-Born Englishman,*
> *"Britannia"*

REFERENCES

1. Kaplan, H.S. Hodgkin's Disease. 2nd Ed. Cambridge, Harvard University Press, 1980.
2. Donaldson, S.S., Glatstein, E., Rosenberg, S.A. et al. Pediatric Hodgkin's disease. II. Results of therapy. Cancer 37:2436, 1976.
3. Cham, W.C. et al. Involved field radiation for early stage Hodgkin's disease in children. Preliminary results. Cancer 37:1625, 1976.
4. Botnick, L.E. et al. Stages I–III Hodgkin's disease in children. Results of staging and treatment. Cancer, 39:599, 1977.
5. Dearth, J.C. et al. Management of stages I to III Hodgkin's disease in children. J. Pediatr. 96:829, 1980.
6. Olweny, C.L.M. et al. Childhood Hodgkin's disease in Uganda. A ten year experience. Cancer 42:787, 1978.
7. Ekert, H. and Waters, K.D. Results of treatment of 18 children with Hodgkin's disease with MOPP chemotherapy as the only treatment modality. Med. Pediatr. Oncol. 11:322, 1983.
8. Jacobs, P. et al. Hodgkin's disease in children. A ten year experience in South Africa. Cancer 53:210, 1984.
9. Wilimas, J., Thompson, E., and Smith, K.L. Long-term results of treatment of children and adolescents with Hodgkin's disease. Cancer 46:2123, 1980.
10. Mauch, P.M. et al. An evaluation of long-term survival and treatment complications in children with Hodgkin's disease. Cancer 51:925, 1983.
11. Lange, B. and Littman, P. Management of Hodgkin's disease in children and adolescents. Cancer 51:1371, 1983.
12. Bayle-Weisgerber, C. et al. Hodgkin's disease in children. Results of therapy in a mixed group of 178 clinical and pathologically staged patients over 13 years. Cancer 54:215, 1984.
13. Jereb, B. et al. Involved field (IF) irradiation with or without chemotherapy in the management of children with Hodgkin's disease. Med. Pediatr. Oncol. 12:325, 1984.
14. Donaldson, S.S. Pediatric Hodgkin's disease: Focus on the future. In Status of the Curability of Childhood Cancers. Edited by J. vanEys and M.P. Sullivan. New York, Raven Press, 1980.
15. Donaldson, S.S. and Kaplan, H.S. A survey of pediatric Hodgkin's disease at Stanford University: Results of therapy and quality of survival. In Malignant Lymphomas. Etiology, Immunology, Pa-

thology, Treatment. Edited by S.A. Rosenberg and H.S. Kaplan. New York, Academic Press, 1982.
16. Jenkin, D. et al. Hodgkin's disease in children: Treatment with low dose radiation and MOPP without staging laparotomy. A preliminary report. Cancer 44:80, 1979.
17. Jenkin, R.D.T. and Berry, M.P. Hodgkin's disease in children. Semin. Oncol. 7:202, 1980.
18. Jenkin, D. et al. Hodgkin's disease in children: Treatment results with MOPP and low-dose, extended-field irradiation. Cancer Treat. Rep. 66:949, 1982.
19. MacMahon, B. Epidemiology of Hodgkin's disease. Cancer Res. 26:1159, 1966.
20. Fraumeni, J.F., Jr. and Li, F.P. Hodgkin's disease in childhood: an epidemiologic study. J.N.C.I. 42:681, 1969.
21. Aghai, E., Brenner, H., and Ramot, B. Childhood Hodgkin's disease in Israel. A study of 17 cases. Cancer 36:2138, 1975.
22. Smith, I.E. et al. Hodgkin's disease in children. Br. J. Cancer 36:120, 1977.
23. Vianna, N.J., Davies, J.N.P., Polan, A.K. et al. Familial Hodgkin's disease: an environmental and genetic disorder. Lancet 2:854, 1974.
24. Gutensohn, N., Cole, P., and Li, F.P. Sibship size and Hodgkin's disease. N. Engl. J. Med. 292:1025, 1975.
25. Gutensohn, N. and Cole, P. Childhood social environment and Hodgkin's disease. N. Engl. J. Med. 304:135, 1981.
26. Vianna, N.J., Greenwald, P., and Davies, J.N.P. Extended epidemic of Hodgkin's disease in high-school students. Lancet 1:1209, 1971.
27. Vianna, N.J. et al. Hodgkin's disease: cases with features of a community outbreak. Ann. Intern. Med. 77:169, 1972.
28. Tan, C. et al. Chediak-Higashi syndrome in a child with Hodgkin's disease. Am. J. Dis. Child. 121:135, 1971.
29. Harris, V.J. and Seeler, R.A. Ataxia-telangiectasia and Hodgkin's disease. Cancer 32:1415, 1973.
30. Pritchard, J. et al. The effects of radiation therapy for Hodgkin's disease in a child with ataxia telangiectasia. A clinical, biological and pathologic study. Cancer 50:877, 1982.
31. McCormick, D.P., Meyer, W.J., and Nesbit, M.E. Coexistence of Hodgkin's disease and Down's syndrome. Am. J. Dis. Child. 122:71, 1971.
32. Strum, S.B. and Rappaport, H. Hodgkin's disease in the first decade of life. Pediatrics 46:748, 1970.
33. Poppema, S. and Lennert, K. Hodgkin's disease in childhood. Histopathologic classification in relation to age and sex. Cancer 45:1443, 1980.
34. Parker, B.R., Castellino, R.A., and Kaplan, H.S. Pediatric Hodgkin's disease. I. Radiographic evaluation. Cancer 37:2430, 1976.
35. Tessmer, C.F., Hrgovcic, M., and Wilbur, J. Serum copper in Hodgkin's disease in children. Cancer 31:303, 1973.
36. Wilimas, J., Thompson, E., and Smith, K.L. Value of serum copper levels and erythrocyte sedimentation rates as indicators of disease activity in children with Hodgkin's disease. Cancer 42:1929, 1978.
37. Dunnick, N.R., Parker, B.R., and Castellino, R.A. Pediatric lymphography: Performance, interpretation, and accuracy in 193 consecutive children. Am. J. Roentgenol. 129:639, 1977.
38. Castellino, R.A., Bergiron, C., and Markovits, P. Repeat lymphography in children with Hodgkin's disease. Cancer 38:90, 1976.
39. Daneman, A., Martin, D.J., Fitz, C.R. et al. Computed tomography and lymphogram correlation in children with Hodgkin's disease. J. Comput. Tomogr. 7:115, 1983.
40. Castellino, R.A. et al. Computed tomography, lymphography, and staging laparotomy: Correlations in initial staging of Hodgkin's disease. Am. J. Roentgenol. 143:37, 1984.
41. Silverman, S., DeNardo, G.L., Glatstein, E. et al. Evaluation of the liver and spleen in Hodgkin's disease, II. The value of splenic scintigraphy. Am. J. Med. 52:362, 1972.
42. Horn, N.L., Ray, G.R., and Kriss, J.P. Gallium-67, citrate scanning in Hodgkin's disease and non-Hodgkin's lymphoma. Cancer 37:250, 1976.
43. Russell, K.R., Donaldson, S.S., Cox, R.S. et al. Childhood Hodgkin's disease: Patterns of relapse. J. Clin. Oncol. 2:80, 1984.
44. Donaldson, S.S. and Kaplan, H.S. Complications of treatment of Hodgkin's disease in children. Cancer Treat. Rep. 66:977, 1982.
45. LeFloch, O., Donaldson, S.S., and Kaplan, H.S. Pregnancy following oophoropexy and total nodal irradiation in women with Hodgkin's disease. Cancer 38:2263, 1976.
46. Green, D.M. et al. Staging laparotomy with splenectomy in children and adolescents with Hodgkin's disease. A review. Cancer Treat. Rev. 10:23, 1983.
47. Robinette, C.D. and Fraumeni, J.P., Jr. Splenectomy and subsequent mortality in veterans of the 1933–45 war. Lancet 2:127, 1977.
48. Nomikos, I.N. Is sepsis the only possible harmful consequence of splenectomy? N. Engl. J. Med. 311:198, 1984.
49. Boles, E.T., Haase, G.M., and Hamoudi, A.B. Partial splenectomy in staging laparotomy for Hodgkin's disease: An alternative approach. J. Pediatr. Surg. 13:581, 1978.
50. Dearth, J.C. et al. Partial splenectomy for staging Hodgkin's disease: Risk of false-negative results. N. Engl. J. Med 299:345, 1978.
51. Grosfeld, J.L. and Ranochak, J.E. Are hemisplenectomy and/or primary splenic repair feasible? J. Pediatr. Surg. 11:419, 1976.
52. Dailey, M., Coleman, C.N., and Kaplan, H.S. Functional asplenia in patients undergoing splenic irradiation. A case report and a review of autopsy cases. N. Engl. J. Med. 302:215, 1980.
53. Coleman, C.N. et al. Functional hyposplenia after splenic irradiation for Hodgkin's disease. Ann. Intern. Med. 96:44, 1982.
54. Donaldson, S.S., Glatstein, E., and Vosti, K.L. Bac-

54. [continued] terial infections in pediatric Hodgkin's disease: Relationship to radiotherapy, chemotherapy, and splenectomy. Cancer 41:1949, 1978.
55. Chilcote, R.R. et al. Septicemia and meningitis in children splenectomized for Hodgkin's disease. N. Engl. J. Med. 295:798, 1976.
56. Desser, R.K. and Ultmann, J.E. Risk of severe infection in patients with Hodgkin's disease or lymphoma after diagnostic laparotomy and splenectomy. Ann. Intern. Med. 77:143, 1972.
57. Donaldson, S.S. et al. Response to pneumococcal vaccine among children with Hodgkin's disease. Rev. Infect. Dis. 3:S133, 1981.
58. Reboul F., Donaldson, S.S., and Kaplan, H.S. Herpes zoster and varicella infections in children with Hodgkin's disease: An analysis of contributing factors. Cancer 41:95, 1978.
59. Goodman, R., Jaffe, N., Filler, R. et al. Herpes zoster in children with stage I–III Hodgkin's disease. Radiology 118:429, 1976.
60. Probert, J.C. and Parker, B.R. The effects of radiation therapy on bone growth. Radiology 114:155, 1975.
61. Probert, J.C., Parker, B.R., and Kaplan, H.S. Growth retardation in children after megavoltage irradiation of the spine. Cancer 32:634, 1973.
62. Wilimas, J., Thompson, E., and Smith, K.L. Long-term results of treatment of children and adolescents with Hodgkin's disease. Cancer 46:2123, 1980.
63. Silverman, C.L. et al. Slipped capital epiphyses in irradiated children: Dose, volume and age relationships. Int. J. Radiat. Oncol. Biol. Phys. 7:1357, 1981.
64. Wolf, E. et al. Slipped femoral capital epiphysis as a sequela to childhood irradiation for malignant tumors. Radiology 125:781, 1977.
65. Prosnitz, L.R. et al. Avascular necrosis of bone in Hodgkin's disease patients treated with combined modality therapy. Cancer 47:2793, 1981.
66. Morris, L.L., Cassady, J.R., and Jaffe, N. Sternal changes following mediastinal irradiation for childhood Hodgkin's disease. Radiology 115:701, 1975.
67. Pui, C. et al. Hydrocele formation in patients with Hodgkin's disease. Cancer 51:2301, 1983.
68. Carmel, R.J. and Kaplan, H.S. Mantle irradiation in Hodgkin's disease. An analysis of technique, tumor eradication, and complications. Cancer, 37:2813, 1976.
69. Castellino, R.A. et al. Latent radiation injury of lung or heart activated by steroid withdrawal. Ann. Intern. Med. 80:593, 1974.
70. Stewart, J.R. and Fajardo, L.F. Radiation-induced heart disease: clinical and experimental aspects. Radiol. Clin. North Am. 9:511, 1971.
71. Stewart, J.R. et al. Radiation-induced heart disease, a study of twenty-five patients. Radiology 89:302, 1967.
72. McReynolds, R.A., Gold, G.L., and Robert, W.C. Coronary heart disease after mediastinal irradiation for Hodgkin's disease. Am. J. Med. 60:99, 1976.
73. Fajardo, L.F. Radiation-induced coronary artery disease. Chest 71:563, 1977.
74. Fuks, Z. et al. Long-term effects of external radiation on the pituitary and thyroid glands. Cancer 37:1152, 1976.
75. Slanina, J., Musshoff, K., Rahner, T. et al. Long-term side effects in irradiated patients with Hodgkin's disease. Int. J. Radiat. Oncol. Biol. Phys. 2:1, 1977.
76. Nelson, D.F., Reddy, K.V., O'Mara, R.E. et al. Thyroid abnormalities following neck irradiation for Hodgkin's disease. Cancer 42:2553, 1978.
77. Glaststein, E. et al. Alterations in serum thyrotropin (TSH) and thyroid function following radiotherapy in patients with malignant lymphoma. J. Clin. Endocrinol. Metab. 32:833, 1971.
78. Schimpff, S.C. et al. Radiation-related thyroid dysfunction: Implications for the treatment of Hodgkin's disease. Ann. Int. Med. 92:91, 1980.
79. Smith, R.E. et al. Thyroid function after mantle irradiation in Hodgkin's disease. JAMA 245:46, 1981.
80. Tamura, K., Shimaoka, K., and Friedman, M. Thyroid abnormalities associated with treatment of malignant lymphoma. Cancer 47:2704, 1981.
81. Ramsay, N. et al. Thyroid dysfunction in pediatric patients after mantle field radiation therapy for Hodgkin's disease. (Abstract) Proc. Am. Assoc. Clin. Oncol. 19:331, 1978.
82. Green, D.M. et al. Thyroid function in pediatric patients after neck irradiation for Hodgkin's disease. Med. Pediatr. Oncol. 8:127, 1980.
83. Shalet, S.M. et al.: Thyroid dysfunction following external irradiation to the neck for Hodgkin's disease in childhood. Clin. Radiol. 28:511, 1977.
84. Constine, L.S. et al. Thyroid dysfunction after radiotherapy in children with Hodgkin's disease. Cancer 53:878, 1984.
85. Constine, L.S. and McDougall, I.R. Radiation therapy for Hodgkin's disease followed by hypothyroidism and then Graves' hyperthyroidism. Clin. Nucl. Med. 7:69, 1982.
86. McDougall, I.R. et al. Thyroid carcinoma after high-dose external radiotherapy for Hodgkin's disease. Report of three cases. Cancer 45:2056, 1980.
87. Horning, S.J., Hoppe, R.T., Kaplan, H.S. et al. Female reproductive potential after treatment for Hodgkin's disease. N. Engl. J. Med. 304:1377, 1981.
88. Sherins, R., Winokur, S., DeVita, V.T. et al. Surprisingly high risk of functional castration in women receiving chemotherapy for lymphoma. (Abstract) Clin. Res. 23:343A, 1975.
89. Chapman, R.M., Sutcliffe, S.B., and Malpas, J.S. Cytotoxic-induced ovarian failure in women with Hodgkin's disease. I. Hormone function. JAMA 242:1877, 1979.
90. Pedrick, T.J. and Hoppe, R.T. Recovery of spermatogenesis following pelvic irradiation for Hodgkin's disease. Int. J. Radiat. Oncol. Biol. Phys. 12:117, 1986.
91. Thar, T.L. and Million, R.R. Complications of radiation treatment of Hodgkin's disease. Semin. Oncol. 7:174, 1980.
92. Chapman, R.M. et al. Cyclical combination chemotherapy and gonadal function. Retrospective study in males. Lancet 1:285, 1979.

93. Sherins, R.J. and DeVita, V.T. Effect of drug treatment for lymphoma on male reproductive capacity. Studies of men in remission after therapy. Ann. Intern. Med. 79:216, 1973.
94. Sherins, R.J., Olweny, S.L.M., and Ziegler, J.L. Gynecomastia and gonadal dysfunction in adolescent boys treated with combination chemotherapy for Hodgkin's disease. N. Engl. J. Med. 299:12, 1978.
95. da Cunha, M.F. et al. Recovery of spermatogenesis after treatment for Hodgkin's disease: Limiting dose of MOPP chemotherapy. J. Clin. Oncol. 2:571, 1984.
96. Santoro, A. et al. Comparative results and toxicity of MOPP vs. ABVD combined with radiotherapy (RT) in PS IIB, III(A,B) Hodgkin's disease (HD). (Abstract) Proc. Am. Soc. Clin. Oncol. 2:223, 1983.
97. Thachil, J.V., Jewett, M.A.S., and Rider, W.D. The effects of cancer and cancer therapy on male fertility. J. Urol. 126:141, 1981.
98. DeVita, V.T. The consequences of the chemotherapy of Hodgkin's disease: The 10th David A. Karnofsky Memorial Lecture. Cancer 47:1, 1981.
99. Coleman, C.N. et al. Leukemias, non-Hodgkin's lymphomas and solid tumors in patients treated for Hodgkin's disease. Cancer Surv. 1:733, 1982.
100. Valagussa, P. et al. Absence of treatment-induced second neoplasms after ABVD in Hodgkin's disease. Blood 59:488, 1982.
101. Coltman, C.A. and Dixon, D.O. Second malignancies complicating Hodgkin's disease. A southwest oncology group 10-year follow-up. Cancer Treat. Rep. 66:1023, 1982.
102. Glicksman, A.S. et al. Second malignant neoplasm in patients successfully treated for Hodgkin's disease: A cancer and leukemia group B study. Cancer Treat. Rep. 66:1035, 1982.
103. Tester, W.J. et al. Second malignant neoplasm complicating Hodgkin's disease: The National Cancer Institute experience. J. Clin. Oncol. 2:762, 1984.
104. Grunwald, H.W. and Rosner, F. Acute myeloid leukemia following treatment of Hodgkin's disease. Cancer 50:676, 1982.
105. Halperin, E.C., Greenberg, M.S., and Suit, H.D. Sarcoma of bone and soft tissue following treatment of Hodgkin's disease. Cancer 53:232, 1984.
106. Fobair, P. et al. Psychosocial problems among survivors of Hodgkin's patients. J. Clin. Oncol. 4:805, 1986.
107. Bloom, J. et al. Outlook and social functioning of long term survivors of Hodgkin's disease (HD). (Abstract) Proc. Am. Soc. Clin. Oncol. 3:76, 1984.

CHAPTER 19

Hodgkin's Disease Survivorship: Psychosocial Consequences

KAROLYNN SIEGEL
GRACE H. CHRIST

The ravages of Hodgkin's disease and the harrowing side-effects of its treatment are so much a part of the popular conception of cancer that little thought is usually given to the myriad kinds of psychosocial distress that may occur in the period following successful therapy. Indeed, the period of recovery following a life threatening illness is often idealized.[1] The general lack of awareness and understanding among the public of the types of residual psychosocial difficulties recovered cancer patients may experience is frequently a cause of frustration and further distress to this population. Survivors are frequently reminded how "lucky" they are to be alive, to have eluded the death sentence that most of the public reflexively associates with a diagnosis of cancer. In the face of these circumstances, Hodgkin's disease patients and other cancer survivors often feel unable to assert their needs or express their resentment and anger over the social, psychologic, and physical sequelae of their illness and its treatment.

Even with their physicians, they may worry that they will be regarded as ungrateful or neurotic if they communicate any of their dissatisfactions or concerns about their lives following successful treatment. The attitude that the physician has saved their life and all else is irrelevant, or at least insignificant by comparison, is often present. It is felt to be inappropriate to burden him with one's psychosocial problems of adjustment.

The fact that this illness commonly occurs at an early stage of life is another important aspect of the anguish it brings. Young adulthood is a period when the individual formulates goals and aspirations. Abundant opportunities seem to exist. Hodgkin's disease seems to suddenly impose an extraordinary burden that can significantly compromise future achievements.

Another source of stress for recovered cancer patients is that, as Smith has pointed out, our culture values individuals who emerge from a crisis "without missing a beat."[1] The notion that following diagnosis and successful treatment for cancer one can "pick up where he left off" is simply inconsistent with the experience of the overwhelming majority of survivors. Instead, the illness constitutes a major discontinuity in their life and brings about lasting changes in the way they view themselves and their future possibilities.[2]

The experience of having cancer constitutes what has been called a "psychosocial transition."[3] Psychosocial transitions, such as becoming a parent or bereavement, require a series of evolving adaptations and often result in lasting changes in one's self-concept, values, roles, and time perspective. The individual is in essence transformed by the experience and cannot return to his former sense of self. Such is the nature of the experience of having had cancer. The impact seems to be enduring, although it is sometimes subtle.

We describe some of the ways in which surviving Hodgkin's disease may alter the individual's sense of himself and his outlook on life, as well as some of the common psychosocial sequelae of survivorship. Interventions that can facilitate positive long-term adjustment are also discussed. Our observations rest on several sources of knowledge, including our own clinical work—both individually and in groups—with this patient population, reported research on long-term adjustment following treatment for cancer, and the findings of an in-depth study we recently completed of 47 Hodgkin's disease patients (mean age 32.2; 70% female) off treatment for at least one year (median time off treatment, 4 years).[4] Most of the patients from our own study were under the care of one Memorial Hospital physician. While this circumstance, together with the relatively small sample size, suggest limitations on the generalizability of the findings, their convergence with the observations of other investigators and clinicians would argue for their essential validity. While most of the studies reported in the literature do not deal specifically with Hodgkin's disease patients, a significant amount of agreement across studies and in our own observations suggests some "universal" concomitants of surviving cancer. Therefore, we shall refer to these studies later in the chapter.

LIFE-CYCLE CONSIDERATIONS

Many of the sources of psychosocial distress cancer patients must confront are similar, regardless of diagnosis (e.g., fears of recurrence, abandonment, and death). The stage of life in which the illness first occurs, however, influences the particular adult developmental problems that may result. Several contemporary theories of adult development have gained prominence and have achieved a considerable degree of empirical validation.[5,6,7] A brief review of these theories will help set our discussion of the consequences of the illness in the perspective of the life-cycle tasks most young Hodgkin's disease patients are struggling to accomplish at the time of their diagnosis and treatment.

Erikson[5] has proposed a developmental model of the eight stages of man. Each stage is organized around a crucial developmental issue conceptualized as a polarity.[6] Of particular interest to the present discussion are Erikson's stages five and six. In stage five, adolescence (ages 12 to 20), the individual is confronted with the tension between identity versus role confusion. The task of the adolescent is to separate from his parents, become self-reliant, and forge a new sense of identity. The tendency to experience regression and dependency in the face of a serious illness can significantly impede the achievement of the task of separation from parents. As we shall discuss below, recovered cancer patients often resist giving up the privileges—including that of dependency—of the sick role.

In stage six, young adulthood (ages 21 to 39), the conflict is between the issues of intimacy versus isolation or self-absorption. True intimacy in Erikson's terms refers to the capacity to experience another person's needs as being important as one's own.[6] As one enters young adulthood, he leaves the security of the family and peer group. The young adult must assume a more active role in creating opportunities for establishing social relationships. Low self-esteem can interfere with the individual's ability to initiate new relationships and isolation and self-absorption may result.[6] The damaged sense of self that many cancer patients experience following their illness can readily contribute to a sense of inferiority, which can seriously hamper the individual's capacity to engage in reciprocal relationships. Mages and Mendelsohn[2] found the resolution of the intimacy versus isolation conflict was greatly complicated by cancer patients' heightened needs for support and comfort.

Levinson[7] has proposed another model of adult development similar in its broad outlines to Erikson's, but emphasizing somewhat different issues. It should be pointed out that Levinson's model is based on intensive study of 40 adult males. In his conception, the basic adult developmental process is the creation of the individual life structure—the underlying design of a person's life at a given time.[8] Adult development alternates between sequential periods of stability and transition. The early adult transition occurs approximately between the ages of 17 and 22. Here, as in Erikson's stage five, the principal task is to establish one's independence from parents. Between the ages of 23 and 28 the individual enters the adult world. The relevant tasks are choosing an occupation and forming enduring intimate relationships, often including marriage and a family. At this stage, the individual establishes his first stable adult-life structures.

The next stage in Levinson's schema is the age 30 transition (ages 28 to 33). The central task is to question and modify initial life structures set down in the preceding stage. Those individuals whose life structure up to this time has not incorporated occupational and romantic commitments, tend to feel great pressure to do so at the age 30 transition. Between the ages of 33 and 40 the individual builds a second life structure and the culmination of early adulthood is marked. This is the period of settling down and focusing on achieving goals and aspirations.

It is easy to envision how having cancer can complicate the accomplishment of these normative adult developmental tasks. The interference with the establishment of self-reliance has already been commented on above. The creation of stable life structures, including the commitment to career and a family life, can be difficult to achieve in light of the persistent uncertainty about one's future well-being and a low sense of control over events. A long-term commitment to a career with the accompanying willingness to defer gratification is harder for the young adult to develop in the face of a seemingly precarious future. In a mutual support group for Hodgkin's disease patients at Memorial Hospital, the social worker has observed that group members tend to perceive their peers as successfully proceeding in accomplishing all the age-appropriate tasks, while they are often unable to recognize the growth and development going on within themselves as they move through the period of treatment and recovery.[9] Instead they feel their lives are in suspension or abeyance. These perceptions can create feelings of inadequacy and be a source of great distress to these young adults.

Having set the problem of survivorship in a larger context of developmental tasks and conflicts, let us now turn to an examination of some of the long-term consequences that have been found to be associated with successful treatment for Hodgkin's disease. We shall begin with a discussion of some of the general issues raised by survivors and then go on to explore the impact of survivorship in specific realms, such as work, interpersonal relationships, and psychosocial adjustment.

THE TRANSITION FROM PATIENT TO SURVIVOR

As Mullan has pointed out, "No one really knows when he or she passes the line from cancer patient to cancer survivor."[10] While patients often voice the importance they assign to having attained the five-year survival status, the change in self-definition is not so simply achieved. In a study of 22 cancer patients who had completed treatment 5 to 20 years earlier, it was found that only one half considered themselves cured.[11] Mages and Mendelsohn[2] have also pointed out that cancer rarely has a certain end, save in death. In our own study, we phrased the issue somewhat differently. We asked respondents if they thought of themselves as "having Hodgkin's disease now" or as "having had it in the past." The majority, almost 80%, said they had had it in the past. Nevertheless, a few of these added that while intellectually they wanted to say it was in the past, occasionally they experienced emotions related to the disease that made it feel like a present threat.

Following treatment for cancer, patients are often reluctant to relinquish the sick role and its prerogatives. The termination of treatment, with the implicit demand for a resumption of normal activities, is frequently experienced as an extremely stressful period for cancer patients. During the treatment stage, patients focus energy to deal with the immediate threat to life. Individuals find it easy to mobilize their coping capacities at that time. Once treatment is over, however, patients can feel directionless and let down. It is not uncommon for patients to report depression and anxiety in this post-treatment period. Confusion and embarrassment over these feelings may inhibit the individual from discussing them with others. Smith[1] has noted how the glorification of the recovery period can hamper the identification of important patient needs. In part, this distress is a manifestation of ambivalence about the cessation of treatment.[12] Being on active treatment provides patients with some sense of control over their disease. The end of treatment leaves them feeling completely passive and defenseless to the ravages of the disease.

Patients often cling to the sick role for a period of time following treatment because though their physician informs them they can resume their former activities, they continue to feel ill, lethargic, and apprehensive.[12] Equally important is the patient's fear of the loss of social support once he is perceived as having "recovered." The often sudden withdrawal of intense emotional support during the period of recovery and afterward contributes to a feeling of isolation in many patients.[12]

Maher[12] has identified some of the anomic aspects of cancer recovery. An anomic situation is one in which few or no established norms guide behavior and as a result the individual feels confused, insecure, and anxious. She points out that recovered patients suddenly lose an important goal that has given a focus, meaning, and purpose to their daily strivings—the goal of achieving remission. With the end of treatment, the patient may find his status unclear and confusing. O'Neill[13] has also pointed out the concept of the recovered cancer patient is still relatively new. Society continues to equate cancer with death. As a result, there are no clear expectations or norms regarding how the cancer survivor should act, feel, or be treated by others. Finally, the fear of recurrence—especially in the first months following the end of treatment—prevents many individuals from accepting that they have recovered from the illness.[13] This fear is so pervasive and enduring it deserves closer examination.

FEAR OF RECURRENCE

The fear of cancer recurrence is virtually a ubiquitous phenomenon among recovered patients. Mages and Mendelsohn[2] found that even 6 years following treatment, cancer patients manifested persistent underlying feelings of uneasiness and vulnerability. This is consistent with the findings of numerous other investigators[10,12-16] who have generally found fear of recurrence to be almost universally present among recovered cancer patients. While there is some evidence that this concern diminishes over time as the individual remains disease-free, the consensus is that it never dissipates completely. Furthermore, the latent anxiety can be quickly reactivated by such events as follow-up visits to the doctor or the appearance of new (unrelated) symptoms.[2,15,17] Koocher[16] has observed that anniversary reactions (e.g., significant emotional reactions at the time of the year when diagnosis occurred or successful treatment ended) and what he calls developmental marker events (e.g., social events or achievements that underscore growth or advancement, such as graduations or marriages) also have the capacity to rekindle feelings of uncertainty and renew anxiety about recurrence.

This anxiety is often generalized and creates heightened concern about all physical functions and a preoccupation with one's body.[13,17] One study[14] of 104 cancer survivors who had completed treatment at least one year earlier found that the only significant differences between the recovered patients and controls were a lower sense of self-control and more general health worries in the former group. As Maher has pointed out, the likelihood of recurrence seems to exist by definition for the patient "in remission."[12] Cancer survivors experience an enduring sense of enhanced vulnerability and of living a precarious existence.

In our own study of Hodgkin's disease survivors, we found that almost all our respondents were worried about the possibility of recurrence, although most of those 2 or more years off treatment had reached the point where they only thought of it occasionally. Consistent with what has been found in other survivor groups, anxiety and concern were usually triggered by visits to the doctor or the appearance of some new physical symptom. Other events likely to arouse worry included learning about someone experiencing a relapse or hearing or reading about cancer in the mass media. There were a small number of individuals in our study who confessed thinking about recurrence almost constantly and checking their lymph glands continually. A few also expressed worry about the development of a new cancer as a long-term consequence of their treatment for Hodgkin's disease. In a study of 60 male Hodgkin's disease patients (mean age = 31.6) at least 6 months off treatment (50% were 2½ years or more post-treatment), Cella found that two thirds reported that physical symptoms were distressing to them because they evoked fears of recurrence.[17]

Our clinical observations with this patient population also confirm the pervasiveness of fears of recurrence among cancer survivors. Although the passage of time seems to enable many patients to grow more confident about recovery and cure, lurking anxiety persists, although less intrusively. Because reminders of the threat of cancer are abundant in our daily lives, the potential for the reactivation of their anxiety is always close at hand. Nevertheless, patients try to draw some reassurance from reaching certain benchmarks, such as the 5-year survival mark.

We have found that the residual anxiety experienced after a period of a year or more off treatment is usually not so great as to interfere with the resumption of normal daily activities. It is, however, often sufficient to make survivors feel that while they may seem as vigorous and healthy as their peers, their sense of well-being is more precarious. The facts that the etiology of cancer is not well understood and that the disease has no clear onset only serve to heighten their sense of vulnerability. Even for those who say they believe that after 5 years their chances of a recurrence are no greater than another individual's chances of developing cancer for the first time, the defense of denial ("it can't happen to me") that can be effectively employed by most individuals who have never had cancer is no longer available to survivors. Uncertainty about their life expectancy and the future often leads these individuals to reassess their priorities. Some of the kinds of shifts in goals and outlook that have been observed are discussed below.

REDEFINITION OF PRIORITIES AND GOALS

Most cancer survivors report permanent changes in their view of themselves and their future.[7] For many, the confrontation with their own mortality caused them to reassess their values and reorder priorities. In general, there is a shift away from materialistic goals and a heightened emphasis on humanistic values.[1] Concomitantly, there is also a greater focus on establishing meaningful personal aspirations rather than merely adopting the dominant societal goals. Survivors also report an augmented appreciation of life since their illness.[10,14,15,17,18] In his study of male Hodgkin's disease patients, Cella[17] found among survivors a significantly greater increase in their appreciation of life following their illness than age-matched controls reported following a stressful experience (of their own definition) in their own lives. A greater acceptance of death and their own mortality has also been noted among survivors.[14]

Another study of long-term (3- and 6-year) survivors found that respondents felt that their ambition, drive, and the striving for achievement and recognition had diminished since their illness.[2] At the same time, they experienced themselves as more tolerant and more concerned about others. There seemed to be evidence of a more constricted involvement in the external world and a greater focus on home life, family, and friends. These findings are consistent with our own observations. About two thirds of the survivors we interviewed reported changes in their goals and priorities as a result of the illness. Among the changes most frequently mentioned were a decreased emphasis on accumulating money and a greater valuing of time, family, friends, health, and enjoyment of the present. Several women indicated that they had become more assertive and willing to put their own needs first since their illness. In our own study, as in others,[10,14] survivors felt better about themselves as a result of these value shifts.

VOCATIONAL ADJUSTMENT

We have observed that the impact of the illness on the individual's career aspirations varies considerably among Hodgkin's disease survivors we have studied. A few indicated that having successfully coped with the vicissitudes of the diagnosis of cancer and treatment, they felt more confident to deal with the stresses of a demanding career or profession. As a result, they raised their aspirations. A smaller number decided that faced with an uncertain future they preferred to adopt more modest goals, assuring more time with their families and more time to enjoy life. The majority felt they had not changed their career goals and aspirations in light of their illness. We found, however, that a significant proportion expressed a heightened desire following their illness to do something important and meaningful with their lives and to "make something of themselves."

In a study of 403 Hodgkin's survivors (mean age of 36, median time of treatment, approximately 9 years), Fobair et al.[18] found that 81% of those employed said that their work ambition was either greater than before their illness or unchanged. The remaining 19% reported less ambition.

In Cella's study of Hodgkin's disease survivors, 27% of the respondents felt their careers had been compromised as a result of their illness.[17] They conceded regret that they had avoided taking chances and pursuing opportunities because of an unwillingness to risk job security and a loss of insurance benefits.

Cella also found that, on average, respondents were working 5.7 hours less a week than before their diagnosis.[17] While no explanation for this finding was offered, it might in part be accounted for by the lower energy levels some patients report months and even years after treatment. Of the recovered patients studied, 57% said that they felt they had not regained premorbid levels of stamina. Length of time off treatment was not related to this feeling of reduced energy. An alternative explanation would be that the work activities were less valued after the illness, with more emphasis being placed on the enjoyment of leisure time.

In a study of 25 Hodgkin's disease patients in remission (88% in remission one year or longer) Goldman[19] found more men than women declined in their occupational functioning following their illness. Those patients over 40 years of age were more likely to report a decline in functioning than younger subjects.

Fobair et al.[18] found that 42% of their survivor sample reported work-related problems that they attributed to their illness. Among the most frequently cited difficulties were: denial of insurance (11%); not being offered a job (12%); and conflicts with supervisors or co-workers (12%).

In a study of 41 Hodgkin's survivors (median age, 26, median time from diagnosis, 12 years) Wasserman et al.[20] found that 21% of their sample reported job discrimination associated with their illness. Difficulties obtaining health insurance were experienced by 39% of the survivors, and problems acquiring life insurance were twice as common (80%).

Approximately 11% of our sample of survivors indicated they had been denied company offered health insurance because of their illness, and 6% said their employment was terminated because of their illness. None felt they had ever been denied a promotion because of their illness, although about 8% believed they had missed an opportunity for such things as a job transfer or a chance to work on a particular project because of their illness.

While only 8% said they had ever experienced discrimination by their coworkers, we found in our interviews that the large majority (about two thirds) did not tell their coworkers about their medical history. Most simply felt it was "none of their business" or "irrelevant." Whether these were the real reasons or whether they were insecure about how their coworkers would react is not clear. It did seem, however, that most were willing to reveal information about their illness if it came up naturally or seemed relevant. Almost all those who did tell coworkers felt that they perceived no difference in the treatment they received from them. Cases in which they felt the co-workers were more considerate and protective toward them were the few exceptions to this. In only a couple of instances was there a feeling that co-workers seemed uncomfortable with the respondent after learning about their illness. Male survivors in Cella's study also felt, with only a few exceptions, that they were not treated differently by employers or co-workers as a result of their illness.[17]

When we asked our survivors to rate how satisfied they were with their jobs, almost half (48%) were "delighted" or "pleased" and another 33% indicated they were "mostly satisfied." This represents high levels of job satisfaction, comparable to rates of satisfaction in the general population.[21]

Therefore, the evidence is that while the majority of Hodgkin's disease survivors seem to have attained satisfying employment situations, a significant proportion have encountered various kinds of job-related difficulties that they attribute to the illness. However, some of the problems survivors report, such as coworker discrimination or being passed over for certain job opportunities, may in some instances be more imagined than real; or it may represent patients' tendency not to compete for certain positions or assignments because of anticipated discrimination or feared loss of security and benefits. For example, in the Hodgkin's patient self-help group at Memorial Hospital, the social worker encountered a member whose lifelong ambition was to become a policeman.[9] After his illness, however, he assumed he would not be accepted as a candidate at the police academy despite his strong physical condition and current good health. He believed he would not be able to compete successfully for such a physically demanding occupation with "healthy" applicants. After much encouragement and support from the group, he applied and was accepted for training as a police officer. Currently, he is a N.Y.C. transit officer and performs capably in that position.

PSYCHOSOCIAL ADJUSTMENT

Available data on the psychosocial consequences of survivorship are characterized by some inconsistency. In a study of 3- and 6-year survivors, Mages and Mendelsohn found that most reported little change in their level of dysphoric affect or nervousness, although chronic underlying feelings of uneasiness and vulnerability did emerge.[2] Cella's study of male Hodgkin's disease survivors revealed that the mean score of his patient group on a global index of psychiatric symptomatology was one standard deviation above the score of the measure's principal normative nonpatient sample, but also nearly one standard deviation below the mean score of a sample of 425 male psychiatric outpatients.[17] Scores on the symptom index did tend to be higher in the patient subgroups that had more recently completed treatment, although group differences were not significant. Fobair et al. found that 18% of their patients had scores indicative of clinical levels of depression, a proportion comparable to that observed in general community samples.[18]

It should be mentioned that a number of studies[17,18,21,22] have observed diminished energy levels in cancer patients for months and years following treatment. There has been some feeling expressed in the literature that persistent lethargy might be a depressive equivalent rather than merely a result of treatment.

Among our own study participants, 22% reported a decrease in sexual interest since their illness, but another 12% indicated greater interest. Concerning levels of sexual activity, we found 21% reported a decline, but a comparable proportion reported an increase. There was evidence of general satisfaction with their sex life expressed by our survivors, with 57% giving a high satisfaction rating. In fact, about a third of the survivors suspected that their sex life was better than most of their peers'.

In the study by Fobair et al., 26% of the subjects felt that their physical attractiveness had diminished as a result of their diagnosis and treatment.[18] An equal proportion indicated that their interest in sex had changed since their illness. Of these, 71% (74 cases) reported less interest. Sexual interest was more likely to return to normal as the length of time since completed treatment increased. A little more than a third of the sample (36%) reported a decrease in sexual activity. About half (56%) of these respondents attributed the decline to their diagnosis or treatment.

Cella found no significant differences between his survivors and controls on their ratings of sexual and marital satisfaction.[17] In addition, 44% of his respondents reported improved sexual functioning after their treatment, and only 18% reported poorer performance. He did, however, find lowered intimacy motivation scores and some evidence of more constricted sexual fantasies in his patient group than among the controls on the Thematic Apperception Test (TAT). This is significant, because on the self-report measures his subjects may have been able to discern the behaviors and feelings being investigated. On the projective TAT, however, intimacy motivation was measured more indirectly and it was not clear to subjects what was being examined. Therefore, it is possible that his male survivors gave what they felt were responses that represented good adjustment on the self-report measures, while the projective TAT test reflected underlying feelings of interpersonal withdrawal of which they might be unaware.

Chapman et al. examined 47 male Hodgkin's disease patients.[23] Most were interviewed before therapy and then again after treatment had been completed. Twenty-one of the respondents answered questions regarding libido and sexual activity. Of these, one half indicated that their libido had never returned to its preillness level. A similar study by the same investigators[24] looked at 41 female Hodgkin's patients. Information concerning libido and sexual functioning before (this time using retrospective items) and after treatment was provided by 37 of the respondents. Following treatment, 73% of the women stated they had mild or no libido as compared to 8% before treatment. In a larger study,[25] the libido and sexual performance of 74 male Hodgkin's patients (median time off treatment was approximately 27 months) were studied. Of the 54 men who completed the questionnaire, 25 (46%) reported a persistent decline in libido. Few, however, expressed distress over this outcome.

Related to the issue of sexual interest and satisfaction is the issue of body image. Cancer patients often express the feeling that as a result of their illness they are left "damaged." Even in the absence of visible mutilation they experience themselves as not whole or in some way impaired. The psychosocial consequences of solid tumors, such as those leading to a mastectomy or amputation, have been studied and examined much more than systemic tumors like Hodgkin's disease. The former are palpable and as a result we have found they permit the patient to psychologically focus on a diseased part of their body, and yet at the same time retain a sense of a healthy part as well. In the case of systemic tumors, on the other hand, the disease often seems all pervasive and consuming.

In our study of Hodgkin's disease survivors, we found that 24% said they felt less attractive physically since their diagnosis, while 9% said they felt more attractive. A sense of loss of an intactness of self[13] and anger at their bodies for having failed or betrayed them[15] are common emotions among cancer patients. Even the treatment is generally experienced as an assault on one's body.[2] Shanfeld found among his survivor group a continuing sense of damage that would be passed on to future generations.[15] The subjective sense of impairment recovered cancer patients may experience often causes them to avoid intimate relationships and the fear of rejection. Based on their study of survivors 3 and 6 years after treatment, Mages and Mendelsohn concluded that following cancer intimate sexual relationships suffer, even in emotionally well adjusted individuals.[2] They suggest that sexual activity seems to make the cancer survivor especially vulnerable to poignant feelings of damage, defect, and loss.

Among our group of Hodgkin's disease survivors, an optimistic outlook on life was prevalent. A full 96% agreed with the statement that they feel hopeful about the future. Ninety percent affirmed that they expected to live to a "ripe old age." And only about 15% agreed with the statement that, "When you have Hodgkin's disease the future seems pretty bleak."

It should be noted that evidence is accumulating that suggests women cope better with the illness and its treatment than men. In Kennedy's study of survivors, males were observed to have higher mean stress reactivity scores than females.[10] Mages and Mendelsohn found that regardless of age, cancer seemed to have a more negative impact on men than women.[2] They were more likely to blame others for their difficulties, withdraw from social activities, and engage in self-destructive activities. Another study that interviewed recently recovered patients (6 and 12 months after diagnosis) and long-term survivors (3 and 6 years after diagnosis) found that in both groups men showed more negative changes in the realms of work and social relationships.[26]

Various explanations have been proposed for these sex-related differences. A greater readiness among women to seek out and use social support is one possible reason for their apparently more effective coping.[24] Another is that women are more accustomed to, and therefore more accepting of, bodily change.[2] Finally, it has been suggested that because self-reliance is a societal expectation for men, they experience greater distress over the dependency engendered by the illness.[2]

In summary, while psychosocial distress persists among recovered cancer patients, it generally does not reach sufficient levels to significantly impair daily functioning; rather, it seems to create a kind of undercurrent that to a greater or lesser extent compromises a sustained sense of well being and personal adequacy. The large majority, nevertheless, maintain an optimistic outlook on life. Undoubtedly, some of this optimism is at the price of a denial of true feelings of worry about future health.

INTERPERSONAL RELATIONSHIPS

We have already shown how the psychosocial sequelae of the illness can interfere with recovered cancer patients' capacity to form intimate relationships. This and other changes brought about in the realm of interpersonal relationships are among the most significant and far-reaching consequences of the illness. Cancer evokes intense and complex emotional responses, not just in the affected individual, but in those close to him as well. Ambivalence, anger, resentment, and discomfort cause them to behave in ways that often add to the emotional distress of the patient.[26]

For example, cancer may elicit feelings of aversion because of the physical mutilation and deterioration associated with the disease. To those the patient interacts with, cancer may connote "decaying," being "dirty," or being "contagious." It also evokes a sense of vulnerability in others because of its uncertain etiology, the widespread fear of developing the disease, and irrational fears of contagion.[27,28] These feelings often cause individuals to physically avoid the cancer patient or withdraw from social interaction with him. The patient experiences such reactions as painful rejections or desertions. An accompanying sense of loss of sexual attractiveness and self-esteem usually ensues.[29,30]

Other problems in interpersonal relations brought about by the response to the illness of significant others concerns communication. Family members, friends, and even medical personnel frequently avoid discussions of the patient's feelings because of their preconceptions that remaining optimistic and distracting him from thoughts of the illness are most beneficial. Their continual discouragement of open communication and attempts at reassurance leave the patient feeling hurt, misunderstood, and isolated.[27] He may even eventually come to feel that the way to maintain what limited support is available to him from his family and friends is to mask his anxiety and depression and present himself as coping effectively.[31] Furthermore, even though family members intellectually comprehend that the patient has recovered, they often tend to be overprotective, suppressing their anger and negative feelings.[13] Patients' own perception that talking about their negative feelings or distress will be interpreted as a sign of poor coping creates another barrier to communication.

Again, the findings from our study were mixed on the issue of the impact of the illness on interpersonal relationships. Most said they felt there had been no change in their relationships with close friends as a result of the illness. However, a group of survivors (17%) acknowledged losing some friends who were uncomfortable with their illness and who tended to avoid or neglect the patient during and after treatment. Many said that they had not revealed their past illness to any new close friends that they had made since ending treatment. In contrast to respondents' impressions that in the large majority of cases their relationships with close friends were not altered as a result of their illness, most did feel that their relationships with more casual acquaintances and "people in general" had been affected by the illness. They reported that others frequently viewed them as "freaks," "contagious," or among the "walking dead" when they heard of their cancer. On the other hand, a few reported that others regarded them as "strong" and treated them with more respect for having struggled with their illness. In fact, all but one of our respondents agreed with the statement that other people admired them for the way they coped with cancer.

Admiration for patients' courage and perseverance in the face of a horrifying life-threatening illness, however, does not preclude feelings on the part of others of uneasiness and discomfort in the presence of a cancer patient. Indeed, 47% of the same respondents indicated that they believed most people do not feel comfortable around someone with such an illness. And almost half agreed with this statement: "The fewer people who know I have Hodgkin's disease the better." Consistent with this impression is the finding that the large majority of the survivors we interviewed said they did not tell new friends or social acquaintances about their illness. Some of these individuals indicated that they do eventually disclose their illness at a later point when a certain degree of closeness has been achieved. Yet coexisting with feelings of hesitancy about how others will react to them when they learn of the illness, is the belief among 85% of the survivors that it doesn't seem to matter to most people that they had Hodgkin's disease.

Cella's[17] Hodgkin's disease survivor group experienced more positive changes in their interpersonal relationships than negative changes as a result of their illness. In the post-treatment period, 23% felt their family relationships had improved, while only 13% said they had worsened. When asked about changed relationships with a mate or significant other, 35% felt the relationship had gotten better and only 22% felt it had deteriorated. The quality of relationships with friends was deemed to have improved after treatment in 25% of the cases and declined in only 13%.

Some patients do report changes in the way they are treated by family, friends, and employers following their recovery.[12] As mentioned previously, O'Neill[13] pointed out that even family members who comprehend intellectually that the patient is recovered may continue to be over-protective. Angry or negative feelings may be suppressed in a belief these are harmful to the patient. Unfortunately, one consequence of this behavior on the part of family members is to make the patient feel that he also cannot express his negative emotions.

Our in-depth interviews with survivors revealed that among those who were married at the time of the illness, about half felt strongly that the marriage had been strengthened as a result of having gone through the crisis together. Some expressed that having handled this experience together they and their spouse felt confident to deal with any future problems. Others perceived no change in their marital relationship. Fobair et al.,[18] however, found that among their sample of Hodgkin's disease survivors, 49% (34 of 69) of those who were married at the time of diagnosis and later separated or divorced, attributed the marital disruption to their disease.

Those who were seeing someone at the time of the diagnosis generally felt it did not significantly strain or change the relationship. A few did end the relationship as a result of the illness. It seems possible in a couple of instances that the patient feared eventual rejection and felt more able to deal with the loss if the patient terminated the relationship.

Self-esteem is another important dimension of psychosocial adjustment. Most patients experience a lasting change in their self-image. While some recovered patients may experience enhanced self-esteem for having coped effectively with the illness and treatment, many, perhaps most, felt diminished by the experience. We have already touched on the issue of self-image in relation to the sense of "damage" or impairment many cancer patients report. This problem is especially salient in young adults (who account for the large proportion of Hodgkin's disease patients) because they are at a stage in life where dating and mating are central social activities. Therefore, they are especially sensitive to any feeling of loss of attractiveness or desirability.

In our interviews and group work with Hodgkin's disease patients, we have found that temporary or permanent sterility and interference with other gonadal functions, which may result from antineoplastic drugs, can also have a significant adverse impact on self-esteem. Among those who were unmarried at the time of their illness, the feeling was occasionally expressed (and we suspect often harbored) that they were an unacceptable mate because of their possible incapacity to bear children. About 20% agreed with this statement: "People willing to marry someone with Hodgkin's disease are few and far between." The wording of this item, however, did not cause our respondents to focus on the issue of infertility and marriageability. Even among those who had regained fertility, many feared that offspring might suffer birth defects as a result of their prior treatments. This fear that they might produce damaged children also contributed greatly to a sense of not being a desirable partner.

While most denied feeling overtly stigmatized or shunned as a result of having had cancer, a significant minority of the patients felt reduced in the eyes of others as a result of the illness. In a study of recovered Hodgkin's disease patients run at Memorial Hospital, many felt inadequate when competing with peers.

PSYCHOSOCIAL INTERVENTIONS

In the previous section, psychologic and social stresses that affect the sense of well-being and quality of life of survivors of Hodgkin's disease were identified. While these stressors do not interfere with the ability of the majority of survivors to function adequately, either in work or in social relationships, they are impediments to the functioning of a minority of patients and present serious adaptive challenges to all patients.

Several kinds of psychosocial interventions have been suggested as means of forestalling adverse patient reactions to their illness and mitigating their distress. These include:

1. Earlier discussion with the patient about potential psychosocial effects of the disease and its treatment.[16,32,27]
2. Facilitation of open communication between patient and family and patient/family and the health care staff.[32,27]
3. Early intervention with psychologically or socially vulnerable patients who may be more profoundly affected by illness-related stresses.[27]
4. Encouragement of patients meeting with other Hodgkin's disease patients, either individually or in groups.[32,27]

In addition, several important questions must be addressed in order to develop an intervention model. What are the goals of psychosocial interventions? When, during the course of the patient's treatment and rehabilitation, should interventions be provided? Who should receive the interventions? all patients or only those with identified problems? What interventions will be most cost-effective as well as supportive of Hodgkin's disease patients' long term adjustment (e.g., patient advocacy, education, group counseling, individual counseling, behavioral treatments, etc.)?

These issues will be addressed through a description of interventions that: (1) Improve staff/patient interaction and communication; (2) Identify patients at high risk for adjustment problems; (3) Provide psychosocial support at crisis points in the illness; and (4) Provide psychosocial support during the survivor period.

IMPROVING STAFF-PATIENT INTERACTION AND COMMUNICATION

The development of open and constructive communication with the patient is one of the most controversial areas in the treatment of Hodgkin's patients. Physicians and other health-care professionals have tended in the past to be reluctant to give patients information about the thoughts, feelings, and emotions that are likely to accompany the disease and its treatment. In fact, little was known about patients' long-term reactions before recent studies identified psychosocial consequences in Hodgkin's disease and other cancer survivors. As one observer stated: "It is often believed that such discussions will increase the likelihood that the patient will experience the emotion or side effects in question . . ."[26] Studies show this is unlikely, and further, that patients appreciate anticipatory information and praise physicians for providing it to them.[33,34] Patients often express great anger about not being told of physical side effects when they later occur. A 29-year-old woman was distraught over not knowing of her possible sterility resulting from treatment. She felt deprived of the right to make the decision to risk sterility in order to save her life. Her anger about not being given that control seriously impeded her psychologic adjustment to this treatment consequence.

Several authors strongly support the notion that helping Hodgkin's disease patients anticipate possible psychosocial effects of cancer will in itself give them an increased sense of control over their lives and reduce their anxieties.[34] Such preparation may prevent patients from perceiving themselves as weak or poorly adjusted as, for example, when they find they are upset on the anniversary of their diagnosis. It will also prevent them from feeling shocked when they find they cannot be admitted to the army or that insurance companies are reluctant to cover them. Rather, they can view these as likely problems that can and need to be managed.

With the improved prognosis of Hodgkin's disease, health-care professionals have tended to focus on the optimistic prognosis, at times inadvertently denying the realities of the patient's experience subsequent to diagnosis and treatment. While it is appropriate for most patients with Hodgkin's disease to expect long-term survival, they cannot ignore the potentially fatal nature of this disease or its meaning to the patient, his family and friends, and society in general. The patient should be hopeful about the ultimate outcome; he will not die. He must, however, also deal with the transition from being a healthy young adult to one who has the potential to be chronically or fatally ill. Cancer is not like a broken leg from which one can expect to recover fully with no possibility of later medical problems, side-effects, or psychologic or social consequences.

Minimizing the significance of having a life-threatening illness like cancer is a two-edged sword. It can have some positive effects on patients' coping (i.e., it encourages patients to be hopeful and to feel less concerned). For example, an adolescent patient at Memorial was overheard saying the following: "Having cancer here is like having the common cold anywhere else." However, in the extreme, trivializing the illness fails to provide the patient with an appropriate conceptual framework within which he can address the real problems confronting him; he may feel discouraged from seeking help for problems that he believes are a result of his own personal deficiency and inability to cope successfully with what has inadvertently been presented as a relatively minor adaptive challenge.

As the prognosis for cancer improves, staff should express increasingly hopeful attitudes, but guard against a natural tendency to trivialize an experience that still constitutes a major adaptive challenge for the patient. Staff attitudes and perceptions, as demonstrated in ongoing interactions with the patient, are critical psychosocial interventions throughout the illness and treatment. These attitudes should reflect optimism and hopefulness about survival and support of the patients' coping efforts, but also communicate a realistic appraisal of the nature of patients' reactions and the adaptational tasks they confront. At the same time, it should be emphasized that problems caused by the illness are manageable. Communication that encourages openness about both facts and feelings is one of the most effective ways of facilitating patients' coping and assuring access to needed services. In short, health-care staff may need to change the emphasis of their communication with Hodgkin's disease patients from an exclusive focus on survival to one that more adequately addresses the quality of survival.

IDENTIFICATION OF PATIENTS AT HIGH RISK FOR ADJUSTMENT PROBLEMS

Assessment of the patient's social and psychologic vulnerability is critical during the diagnostic phase. The health professional needs to screen patients to identify factors that have been found to be correlated with poor adjustment outcomes in the professional literature and clinical practice. These include: the presence of previous psychopathology in the patient; the excessive use of drugs or alcohol to cope with stress; the absence of reliable social supports; limited insurance or finances; a family history of Hodgkin's or other kinds of cancer.[35–38] These more vulnerable patients can be urged to participate in ongoing group or individual counseling programs at the treatment center or to seek the assistance of a mental-health professional in the community. More intensive interventions for highly vulnerable patients should be viewed as supplemental to the routine interventions provided to all patients at the illness crisis points described below. The post-treatment period may be an especially critical time for intervention with the more vulnerable patient because psychologically troubled individuals are reported to function well during acute crises, but have difficulty coping with chronic stress.

INTERVENTIONS AT CRISIS POINTS IN THE ILLNESS

Preparation for survivorship needs to occur from the point of diagnosis through treatment and treatment termination. At diagnosis, interventions should focus on initiating the patient's acceptance of the reality of the disease, including its vocational, personal, and social consequences, and facilitating the development of a hopeful but realistic perception of it. At this time, the patient must be helped to accept his body's changed condition and to begin to learn to live with the increased uncertainty this means in his life.

During the treatment phase, psychosocial interventions should focus on continuing to clarify the nature of the illness, and on helping the patient ultimately to attain an equilibrium between a constructive awareness of body functioning and preoccupation with body symptoms. The optimistic prognosis associated with Hodgkin's disease makes these patients no less concerned about the effects of treatment on their bodies. They require continuous clarification of the difference between the symptoms of Hodgkin's disease and the side-effects of the treatment. Young adults are especially worried about being able to conceive and bear children following treatment. Therefore, consideration of possible sterility and use of a sperm bank are further preparations for survivorship during treatment.

Treatment termination is one of the most critical times for intervention with the survivor. Patients almost universally report heightened anxiety at this time because of the cessation of intense medical surveillance (the loss of an activity to control the disease), and worry about returning to normal activities with an altered body and a changed perception of themselves. At treatment termination, the patient can be helped to prepare for societal reactions and barriers that will occur as he strives to normalize his life. These occurrences may reactivate the patient's self-doubts and misperceptions of himself as more damaged than he in fact is. Survivorship involves repeatedly mastering these insecurities and misperceptions. At treatment termination, information of a hopeful nature can also be reiterated, and includes such facts as the improved life expectancy of Hodgkin's patients and the increasing number of healthy children born to patients off treatment with no recurrence of the disease in the patient/mother. Information about available resources can also be given to patients at treatment termination so that they know where to turn when questions arise. They need to be encouraged to continue open communication with the health-care staff after they terminate treatment. Group meetings also provide information and support patients as they move back into society and begin the process of relinquishing the patient role.

A lack of synchrony between the coping of the patient and the family has been observed at treatment termination. The family is often eager for the patient to return to usual activities so they can be relieved of the painful anxiety about his health and possible death. The patient, on the other hand, needs time to integrate the changes the illness and treatment have made in his body, his view of himself and his life, and his relationships with family, friends, colleagues, and society in general. During treatment, the patient's energies are focused on managing the stresses of the treatment process. Therefore, the immediate post-treatment period is often one in which the patient requires time to reorganize his life. Excessive pressure from the family to be "normal" again can increase the patient's anxiety rather than support his reentry process. On the other hand, families that continue to relate to the patient as a sick person can also make it difficult for him to relinquish the patient role. This unevenness has been called dis–synchrony in coping between patient and family.[39] As patient and family become aware of their different coping tasks and needs, they are often able to adapt without feeling they are failing themselves or each other. Families may also benefit from educational and supportive help at this crisis point in the patient's illness.

INTERVENTIONS WITH SURVIVORS

For all patients, the goal of the survivorship period is to regain premorbid levels of functioning and to mitigate the impact of the physical, psychologic, and social stresses caused by the illness that can reduce the quality of their lives. As evidenced in our group at Memorial Sloan-Kettering Cancer Center, patients struggle with passivity, which seems to be related to a lowered self-esteem and a lack of self-confidence. The two major themes of the group discussions are helping patients become more assertive in their work and career pursuits and developing and maintaining adequate social participation. Interventions during this period include patient advocacy and use of the media, patient-to-patient contact, and ongoing communication between patients and the health care staff.

PATIENT ADVOCACY AND USE OF THE MEDIA

Coping with the reactions of family, friends, and society is a major challenge for the survivor. Many people still view the diagnosis of cancer as a certain death sentence, although the prognosis for cancers such as Hodgkin's disease has dramatically improved. Some employers still worry about absenteeism, and are reluctant to invest in training individuals they incorrectly perceive as dying. Because of these misperceptions, the patient must often keep this information concealed from an employer, especially a potential employer, and from coworkers. Patients may be unable to leave jobs they have outgrown because they fear they will lose benefits and be unable to obtain new health and life insurance. They may have to work part time in order to protect the employer from having to furnish benefits, or they may seek employment only in large organizations that can afford to provide some medical insurance to patients diagnosed with cancer. The constraints imposed by the need to maintain insurance benefits presents a special problem for the younger adult who is in the beginning stages of his career when mobility is often a requisite to career advancement.

Support of legislation to eliminate discrimination against patients is a critical intervention. Even with existing laws, however, patients can be helped to appeal discriminatory acts in ways that allow them to continue working with an employer and maintain good will.

The media can be a powerful force for changing societal attitudes. The media can be used to change societal misperceptions about Hodgkin's disease. Programs should highlight the extended life span of the survivor as well as the minimal work disruption that can result from ongoing treatment, similar to work disruption caused by other chronic illnesses. The increased productivity gained from an individual who views work as a privilege, as he views life, needs to be emphasized. Patients are often effective in media programs, although professionals must help them anticipate all possible outcomes of such public revelations.

PATIENT-TO-PATIENT CONTACT

When a veteran patient shares his experiential knowledge of the disease and its treatment, it inspires hope in the patient and also provides a realistic view of treatment and rehabilitation.[40] While research has not demonstrated that an encounter with the veteran patient reduces anxiety or depression, it is almost universally reported as a helpful experience by patients.[41,42,43] In larger treatment centers, patient contact with a veteran can take place within regularly scheduled groups and so facilitate the process. During the post-treatment period, these groups help individuals who are immobilized by depression and anxiety begin problem solving and provide a forum for patient advocacy for those encountering immovable societal barriers. Some patients attend groups on an ongoing basis while others use them only at points of crisis, high stress periods, or for particular discussion topics. In areas where there are few Hodgkin's disease patients, individual patient contacts can be arranged through the center or through national groups for Hodgkin's disease patients. Information about such groups can be obtained through the National Cancer Institute or the American Cancer Society.

ONGOING COMMUNICATION WITH HEALTH-CARE STAFF

Ongoing communication with other patients and with the health-care staff is experienced as helpful by many survivors and may be provided through the groups described above, periodic workshop meetings, individual follow-up contacts, or newsletter communications. In addition to providing help with coping, communication can serve to update information about the disease, its treatment, and late effects. One center has developed a quarterly newsletter that contains current medical information as well as articles by patients about how they are coping with survivorship and managing the problems it presents to them.[44] Optimally, the survivor's psychosocial functioning will also be assessed at the time of regular medical check-ups. While this may not always be feasible because of time constraints, the physician can use the appointment as an opportunity to reinforce the availability of supportive resources and to identify obvious functional problems.

In summary, preparation for survivorship needs to begin at the time of diagnosis through treatment and treatment termination. The patient must be assisted to accept his body's changed condition, to cope with the special problems this creates for him, and to learn to live with the increased uncertainty the illness introduces into his life. At treatment termination, he is helped to prepare for societal reactions and barriers that will occur in his efforts to normalize his life again. Survivorship involves repeatedly mastering self-doubts and misperceptions reactivated by these experiences. More vulnerable patients may require intensive psychosocial interventions during the post-treatment period in order to cope with these chronic stresses. The most critical interventions throughout the illness and treatment are the attitudes and interactions of the health-care staff. These attitudes need to reflect optimism and hopefulness, but also a realistic perception of the nature of patients' reactions and the coping tasks confronting them in society. Patients need to know these tasks are challenging, but can be successfully mastered. Health-care staff should avoid a tendency to focus exclusively on the good prognosis, which may inadvertently trivialize the patient's struggle. Rather, communication should also center around the quality of the patient's life during both the treatment and the post-treatment periods.

Society has been slow to integrate the improved prognosis of Hodgkin's disease patients into its perception of them and into its employment and insurance policies. Barriers to their full participation in society still exist. Patient advocacy with use of the media and the support of post-treatment groups and "veteran" patients is essential to the final goal: the ability to participate in life, in work, and in the pursuit of happiness.

REFERENCES

1. Smith, D.W. Survival of Illness. New York, Springer, 1981.
2. Mages, N.L. and Mendelsohn, G.A. Effects of cancer on patients' lives: A personological approach. In Health Psychology—A Handbook. Edited by G.C. Stone, F. Cohen, and N.E. Adler. San Francisco, Jossey-Bass, 1979.
3. Parkes, C.M. Psycho-social transitions: A field for study. Soc. Sci. Med. 33:101, 1970.
4. Siegel, K. and Christ, G. Sexual and interpersonal adjustment among Hodgkin's disease survivors. Grant from the Lymphoma Foundation, New York, 1982.
5. Erikson, E. Childhood and Society. New York, W.W. Norton, 1963.
6. Colarusso, C.A. and Nemiroff, R.A. Adult Development: A New Dimension in Psychodynamic Theory and Practice. New York, Plenum Press, 1981.
7. Levinson, D.J. et al. The Seasons of a Man's Life. New York, Alfred A. Knopf, 1978.
8. Newton, P.M. and Levinson, D.J. Crises in adult development. In Outpatient Psychiatry: Diagnosis and Treatment. Edited by A. Lazara. Baltimore, Williams and Wilkins, 1979.
9. Wall, M. Psychosocial issues in a long-term group for individuals with Hodgkin's Disease. Presentation at Leukemia Society. Tampa, Florida, 1984.
10. Mullan, F. Re-entry: The educational needs of the cancer survivor. Health Educ. Q. 10:88, 1984.
11. Kennedy, B.J., Tellegen, A., Kennedy, S. et al. Psychological response of patients cured of advanced cancer. Cancer 38:2184, 1976.
12. Maher, E.L. Anomic aspects of recovery from cancer. Soc. Sci. Med. 16:907, 1982.
13. O'Neill, M.P. Psychological aspects of cancer recovery. Cancer 36:271, 1975.
14. Schmale, A.H. et al. Well-being of cancer survivors. Psychosom. Med. 45:163, 1983.
15. Shanfeld, S.B. On surviving cancer: Psychological considerations. Comp. Psychiatry 21:128, 1980.
16. Koocher, G.P. The Crisis of Survival. In Childhood Cancer: Impact on the Family. Edited by A.E. Christ and K. Flomenhaft. New York, Plenum Press, 1984.
17. Cella, D.F. and Tross, S. Psychological adjustment to survival from Hodgkin's disease. J. Consult. Clin. Psychol. In press.
18. Fobair, P.A., Hoppe, R.T., Bloom, J.R. et al. Psychosocial problems among survivors of Hodgkin's disease. J. Clin. Oncol. 4:805, 1986.
19. Goldman, B.S. The resocialization of Hodgkin's disease patients in remission. University of Maryland School of Social Work and Community Planning, Thesis, 1978.
20. Wasserman, A., Wilimas, J., Fairclough, D. Psychosocial late effects of long-term survivors of childhood/adolescent Hodgkin's disease. Paper presented at American Society for Clinical Oncology. Los Angeles, California, 1986.
21. Andrews, F.M. and Witney, S.B. Social Indications of Well-Being: Americans' Perceptions of Quality of Life. New York, Plenum, 1976.
22. Greenleigh Associates, Inc. Report on the social, economic and psychological needs of cancer patients in California: Major findings and implications. San Francisco, American Cancer Society, California Division, 1979.
23. Chapman, R.M., Sutcliff, S.B., and Malpas, J.S. Male gonadal dysfunction in Hodgkin's Disease. JAMA 245:1323, 1981.
24. Chapman, R.M., Sutcliff, S.B., and Malpas, J.S. Cytotoxic-induced ovarian failure in Hodgkin's Disease: Effects on sexual function. JAMA 242:1882, 1979.
25. Chapman, R.M. et al. Cyclical combination chemotherapy and gonadal function. Lancet 1:287, 1979.
26. Freidenbergs, I. et al. Psychosocial aspects of living with cancer: A review of the literature. Int. J. Psychiatry Med. 11:303, 1981–82.
27. Wortman, C.B. and Dunkel-Schetter, C. Interpersonal relationships and cancer: A theoretic analysis. J. Soc. Issues 35:120, 1979.
28. Knopf, A. Changes in women's opinions about cancer. Soc. Sci. Med. 10:191, 1976.
29. Dyk, R.B. and Sutherland, A.M. Adaptation of the spouse and other family members of the colostomy patient. Cancer 9:123, 1956.
30. Bahnson, C.B. Psychological and emotional issues in cancer: Psychotherapeutic cure of the cancer patient. Semin. Oncol. 2:293, 1975.
31. Rollin, B. First You Cry. Philadelphia, Lippincott, 1976.
32. Fobair, P. and Mages, N.L. Psychosocial Morbidity Among Cancer Patient Survivors. In Living and Dying with Cancer. Edited by P. Ahmed. New York, Elsevier, 1981.
33. McIntosh, J. Processes of communication, information seeking and control associated with cancer: A selective review of the literature. Soc. Sci. Med. 8:167–187, 1974.
34. Cassileth, B., Zufkis, R., Sutton-Smith, K. et al. Information and participation preferences among cancer patients. Ann. Intern. Med. 92:832–836, 1980.
35. Weisman, A.G. Early diagnosis of vulnerability in cancer patients. Am. J. Med. Sci. 271:187–196, 1976.

36. Schonfield, J.J. Psychological factors related to delayed return to an earlier life-style in successfully treated cancer patients. J. Psychosomat. Res. 16:41–46, 1972.
37. Bloom, J.R. Social support, accommodation to stress and adjustment to breast cancer. Soc. Sci. Med. 16:1329–1338, 1982.
38. Morris, T., Greer, S., and White, P. Psychological and social adjustment to mastectomy. Cancer, 40:2381–2387, 1977.
39. Christ, G.H. A psychosocial assessment framework for cancer patients and their families. Health Soc. Work 8:57–64 (1), 1983.
40. Mantell, Joanne E. Cancer patient visitor programs: A case for accountability. J. Psychosoc. Oncol. 1:45–58.
41. Mantell, J., Kleiman, M.A., and Alexander, E.S. Social Work and Self-help Groups. Social Work 1:86–100, 1976.
42. Chesler, M. Patterns of participation in a self-help group for parents of children with cancer. Journal of Psychosocial Oncology (in press).
43. Rogers, T.F., Bauman, L.J., and Metzger, L.M. An assessment of the Reach to Recovery program. Cancer. 35:116–124, 1985.
44. Soiffer, B. History of Hodgkin. Surviving 9:3, November, 1984.

CHAPTER 20

Late Iatrogenesis: Legal Aspects

H. RICHARD BERESFORD

Oncologists presumably tell their patients that aggressive treatment of cancer poses both short and long-term hazards. But the extent of disclosure and patients' perceptions of risks may vary considerably. When treatment is administered under experimental protocols, disclosure of risks tends to be encyclopedic. Patients may not comprehend how likely a particular harm is or how much they will suffer if it eventuates, no matter how exhaustive the disclosure. Yet they can hardly be unaware that treatment itself may be a source of future trouble. Where accepted or nonexperimental treatments are offered, disclosure of risks may be less formalistic and detailed and seemingly trivial or rare risks may go unmentioned. Also, treatments may be more optimistically presented than in the context of an experimental protocol, and both physicians and patients may prefer to overlook their dangerous potential. Nevertheless, it is probable that most mentally competent patients who receive conventional radiation, chemotherapy, or other treatments for what they know to be malignant disease understand that treatment is a two-edged sword.

This chapter explores legal aspects of the process by which patients or subjects of experimental trials are made aware of the harms that cancer treatment may cause. Existing legal formulations of the doctrine of informed consent are briefly summarized, followed by a more focussed view of how the doctrine may operate in the context of late iatrogenesis. Most attention is given to the problem of communicating about risks that are improbable, uncertain, or speculative and that may not materialize until months to years after treatment is finished. The matter of how to avoid suits for malpractice in connection with treating cancer is not directly addressed, but the chapter closes with consideration of a hypothetical lawsuit arising out of late iatrogenesis. This may suggest some practical steps for reducing exposure to liability.

LAW OF INFORMED CONSENT

GENERAL CONSIDERATIONS

The doctrine of informed consent evokes varied responses among those who concern themselves with its applications. The busy practitioner, already sensitized to concerns about liability, may believe that its principal effect is to add still another string to the bow of the malpractice lawyer. The clinical researcher may see it as a device for making consent forms so prolix that they fail to communicate what an experiment is all about. Other physicians, be they practitioners or researchers, may view the doctrine as establishing a laudable standard but may nevertheless believe that it complicates relations with patients and has little influence on choices they make.[1] Yet to many physicians, ethicists, and social commentators, it is central to the quality of the relationship between physician and patient and failure to honor it violates a fundamental right of self-determination. Allowing for such differences in attitudes, most physicians apparently agree that they ought to explain to patients why treatments are being given and what harm these treatments may cause.[2] This apparent consensus has not, however, stilled criticism that physicians often pay no more than lip service to the notion of informed consent and fail to share with patients knowledge of the uncertainty inherent in many treatments.[3,4]

The law of informed consent has developed out of litigation of malpractice claims against physicians and hospitals. Until recent years, there has been little legislation on the subject.[5] Federal administrative regulations relating to government-supported biomedical research specify elements of informed consent with respect to subjects of research.[6] These regulatory standards are derived from judicial decisions, but seem to provide broader protections than do most judicial rules. They are not used for imposing personal liability on individual physicians, and the most severe sanction for noncompliance is loss of federal funding for research. Nevertheless, these administrative standards provide useful guidelines to any physician concerned with the sufficiency of a patient's consent to treatment, be it investigational or conventional.

In a provocative analysis, Katz has traced the somewhat halting evolution of the doctrine of informed consent in the American legal system.[3] He observes that early judicial decisions[7,8] emphasized only the physician's duty to tell patients what was planned and paid little heed to the process by which consent to treatment was actually obtained. Later cases[9,10] recognized that the doctrine also calls for the free exercise of patients' right to self-determination, but indicated that the adequacy of disclosure should be determined by reference to practice among physicians, the so-called professional standard. The most expansive cases held that lawfulness of disclosure must be judged from a patient's perspective, not from the standpoint of what doctors customarily tell their patients.[11,12] From these cases emerged the principle that only disclosure of information that a patient deems material to a decision is legally sufficient.

Katz interprets recent cases[13–15] as regressive because of their stress on the primacy of medical professional standards in judging the adequacy of disclosure. Moreover, recent legislation has tended to limit the scope of the doctrine, either by adopting professional standards of disclosure or by requiring disclosures of only the most extreme risks of treatment.[5] Despite fluctuations in legal doctrines, concerns about liability may, if anything, cause many physicians to be expansive in their descriptions of the dangers of medical treatment. Thus, whatever legal rules apply, underdisclosure of risks may not be the problem it once was. In any event, available data indicate that failure to obtain informed consent is seldom a basis for judgements against physicians in malpractice suits.[3,17]

LIABILITY FOR FAILURE TO OBTAIN INFORMED CONSENT

Malpractice. In most states, claims relating to informed consent are considered under the law of medical malpractice. This means that a claimant must prove that a physician negligently failed to obtain informed consent and that this wrongful conduct caused harm. The test of whether a physician's conduct is negligent is based on his conformity to reasonable or accepted standards of medical practice. In most states, therefore, courts evaluate physicians' conduct in obtaining informed consent by reference to what other comparable physicians would have done in a similar situation. But as previously indicated, some courts rely on medical professional standards only to establish the risks of a particular treatment, and judge adequacy of disclosure by determining if risks material to a patient's decision were in fact disclosed.[11,12]

These differing formulations of when disclosure is legally adequate can be criticized for providing insufficient guidance to conscientious physicians and for making meaningless distinctions.[16] While they may not produce different outcomes in practice, the latter patient-oriented standard offers a court greater leeway in weighing the adequacy of disclosure. To illustrate, suppose that doctor A tells patient B that drug D may cause anemia but fails to mention that it rarely may cause severe diarrhea. If B develops severe diarrhea after taking D, B may wish to sue A. In state Y, which has a professional standard of disclosure, B would probably not prevail if A could show that other physicians in Y do not customarily disclose the risk of diarrhea. But in state Z, which has a lay standard of disclosure, B might prevail by convincing a court that he would have rejected treatment with D had he known about a small risk of diarrhea, regardless of the fact that physicians in Z do not customarily disclose this particular risk.

Proof of nondisclosure of a legally significant risk is only the first step in establishing liability for malpractice. The claimant must also show that the nondisclosure itself resulted in harm. This requires proof that nonconsensual treatment was injurious and that the claimant would have refused treatment had disclosure been adequate. Thus, in the preceding example, B must establish both that D, not some other factor, caused his diarrhea and that had A told him of the risk of diarrhea, he would have refused to take it. A mere allegation that he would not have taken D does not suffice. Courts ordinarily impose an "objective" standard under which a claimant must show that a "reasonable" person in the claimant's position would have declined treatment if adequately informed.[11,12,17]

In summary, to win a malpractice suit based on lack of informed consent, a claimant must prove that a physician wrongfully failed to disclose a known risk, that the undisclosed risk materialized and was injurious, and that had the risk been disclosed he would have refused treatment (Table 20–1). This account of a claimant's formal burden of proof should suggest why it is difficult to win a malpractice suit based solely on a lack of informed consent. It should also suggest why it might be especially difficult for a claimant to prevail if an undisclosed risk is one that is speculative, rare, or only dimly perceived by knowledgeable physicians.

Battery. In a few states, failure to obtain informed consent gives rise to a claim for battery (wrongful touching).[18] Thus, if a claimant establishes that a physician did not secure his consent to a particular procedure, the physician is deemed to have committed a battery. The harm lies in the nonconsensual contact and the claimant need not prove that the physician violated accepted standards of disclosure.[19] As a practical matter, suit for battery is improbable unless a significant injury has occurred, because the amount of recoverable damages would be small when the only harm is a nonconsensual but otherwise harmless contact.

Invasion of Privacy. If a physician wrongfully discloses confidential information obtained in the course of treatment or research, as by identifying a patient in a publication without permission, the patient may be entitled to recover probable damages from the physician.[20] The theory of liability is that the physician has breached a fiduciary duty to protect the patient's privacy. Claims based on this theory are uncommon, but they highlight the way in which the law protects important interests, other than those related to physical well-being, of vulnerable persons. Such claims do not, strictly speaking, rest on lack of informed consent. At the same time, they do illustrate the law's attempt to remedy harms arising out of certain failures to respect personal autonomy.

Table 20–1. Elements of Liability for Failure to Obtain Informed Consent to Treatment

1. Proof that defendant physician failed to disclose risk
   a. That comparable physicians would have disclosed
   b. That was material to patient's decision
2. Proof that undisclosed risk materialized and caused harm measurable in monetary terms
3. Proof that had risk been lawfully disclosed, patient would have refused treatment

DAMAGES FOR FAILURE TO OBTAIN INFORMED CONSENT

Once a claimant proves lack of informed consent, the remedy is compensation in damages for provable harm. Unless the harm is substantial, however, a suit for damages is unlikely. Costs of pursuing the claim may exceed recoverable damages and, under the prevailing contingent fee system for compensating claimants' attorneys, little incentive would exist for a lawyer to press a claim that would yield only nominal damages.

Assuming that a claim is pursued, the measure of damage is the harm directly attributable to the physician's failure to obtain informed consent. Suppose, for example, that a physician performs a laparotomy for clinical staging in a patient with Hodgkin's disease without disclosing a small risk of postoperative infection. Suppose further that infection indeed occurs, resulting in several days of abdominal pain, treatment with antibiotics, and added hospitalization. If the operation was clinically appropriate and the surgeon was not negligent in performing it, the only remaining basis for a professional liability claim is lack of informed consent. Potentially recoverable damages would include costs of additional medical care occasioned by the infection and an allocation for general damages, such as "pain and suffering." If the claimant can convince a court that he would not have consented to a laparotomy had he been advised that one uncommon but known risk was infection, he might recover several thousand dollars were a lawyer willing to pursue the claim. Recoverable damages—and a lawyer's incentive to press the claim—would rise if the infection resulted in prolonged severe disability or death.

Accepting, for the sake of argument, that physicians often fail to obtain informed consent, legally provable harm attributable to this failure is probably uncommon. Saying this does not overlook the ethical myopia involved in ignoring a patient's right of self-determination. It simply indicates that quantifiable injury to patients is more likely to result from unskillful conduct than from insensitivity to patients' rights. Insensitivity of this sort may nevertheless fuel a malpractice claim, one element of which is an allegation that a physician failed to obtain informed consent to potentially harmful treatment. Supporting this suggestion is the frequent inclusion in formal complaints that initiate malpractice litigation of counts alleging lack of informed consent. Even though these claims are largely unsuccessful in the sense of yielding big recoveries of damages, neither claimants nor their lawyers necessarily regard them as trivial or nuisance items.

INFORMED CONSENT AND LATE IATROGENESIS

SCOPE OF THE PROBLEM

The concern here is with those side effects of cancer therapy that are serious (even catastrophic), but which appear months to years later. Examples include development of additional cancers, compromised immunologic function, cognitive impairment, peripheral neuropathies, and endocrine disorders. The incidence and pathogenesis of these late effects may be poorly understood, and it is foreseeable that currently unappreciated disorders will complicate potent therapies now in use or being developed. These treatments may be offered as potentially curative, but more likely will be deemed palliative, experimental, or a "last resort" for those with no other therapeutic options. Thus, the therapeutic context has distinctive elements: fearful illness, toxic treatments, and unknowable consequences. Tidy application of legal principles in this context is difficult. Yet it may be useful to consider how legal doctrines relating to informed consent might operate. To this end, the following sections consider legal overtones of the relationship between cancer patient and oncologist, what disclosures of therapeutic risks law seems to require, legal implications of the distinction between treatment and research, and potential civil liabilities of physicians whose patients develop major late complications from anticancer therapy.

RELATIONSHIP OF CANCER PATIENT AND ONCOLOGIST

Knowledge that one has cancer impacts on attitudes towards the attending physician.

But whether a patient views a physician as a caring parental figure, a potential savior, a distant technocrat, or a relentless bearer of bad tidings, law regards the physician as a relatively powerful person who must exercise professional competence and respect certain rights of patients. In conventional legalese, the physician must meet reasonable or accepted standards of medical practice, including obtaining of informed consent for risky treatments. Whether these standards are met in a particular case is determined by reference to what other comparable physicians would have done. Thus, an oncologist's conduct toward a patient is usually measured by how other oncologists would have responded in a similar situation, not by some abstract formulation or by the opinions of physicians untrained in oncology. A modification of this principle is the previously noted ruling of some courts that adequacy of disclosure is measured by the patient's need to know.[11,12]

These legal formulations imply a deference to medical professional standards in evaluating alleged misconduct by a physician. But where informed consent is at issue, a court may ask not only whether risks were adequately disclosed, but also ask whether it was reasonable for a physician to conclude that a frightened, ill, and poorly educated patient understood the disclosed risks and willingly ageed to incur them.[21] In other words, both personal attributes of a patient and the nature of the interaction with the physician may be analyzed in deciding the adequacy of consent. Any hint of coercion or misrepresentation will raise an inference that the physician failed to meet the duty of disclosure or to respect the patient's right to decide. By the same token, law does not require that physicians be error free in obtaining consent, only that they conduct themselves reasonably and in good faith.

The oncologist who diagnoses cancer, conveys a worrisome prognosis, and proposes potentially dangerous treatments surely evokes a complex emotional response in a patient. How this response is handled may have much to do with whether the patient obtains a realistic grasp of outlook and options and makes appropriate choices. Mere recitals of prognostic data or various risks of treatment, while informative in a narrow sense, may fail to convey a balanced view of how an oncologist actually assesses the situation. Yet it is this assessment that a patient needs to exercise an informed choice. A "laundry list" of complications of treatment may, for example, distort the threat of side effects and evoke rejection of palliative or even curative therapy. The oncologist thus must tread the fine line between defensive "crepe-hanging" and underdisclosure of potentially severe risks. This seemingly requires comprehensive knowledge, much time, and considerable sensitivity. Yet if one agrees that obtaining informed consent is both a moral and legal imperative, nothing less will suffice.

RISK DISCLOSURE

No simple formula describes what risks of treatment must be disclosed. In general, if a treatment is known to cause death or severe disability these facts must be disclosed. A court might uphold nondisclosure of a grave risk if its incidence is less than 1%. But if such a remote risk in fact materializes, judge and jury might be sympathetic to a claimant's contention that treatment would have been refused had the risk been disclosed. The law of most states would, however, require evidence that other comparable physicians customarily disclose such remote risks before finding nondisclosure culpable. In any event, once a patient is informed that treatment may be lethal or disabling, logic suggests that exhaustive disclosure of lesser potential risks is not required except for those risks that commonly materialize and cause distress. On the other hand, a strict autonomy model would require that a patient receive the fullest possible disclosure and that the physician not try to substitute professional judgement for that of the patient as to what risks are important for the patient to know about. Similarly, it is not legally justifiable to limit disclosure of significant risks because a physician wishes to protect a patient from the emotional distress that knowledge of such risks might engender. The exceptions are when the physician can demonstrate that disclosure would probably worsen the patient's condition or evoke refusal of urgently needed treatment.[11,12,17]

The duty of disclosure does not extend to

speculative or unforeseeable risks. Thus, if drug D is known to cause bone-marrow depression, but is not known to cause disabling peripheral neuropathy that sometimes occurs in patients who are receiving D along with unequivocally neurotoxic agents, the prescriber of D need not disclose neuropathy as one of its side effects. Similarly, if unexplained peripheral neuropathies occur in patients receiving D to the same extent as in age-matched persons not receiving D, the physician does not have an obvious legal duty to disclose this fact (even though the physician may elect to disclose the association). Suppose, however, that no published study has implicated D in neuropathies, but the association of D with neuropathies has been reported at clinical oncology meetings. While charging a physician with unpublished or unconfirmed knowledge may seem unfair, specialists in oncology are expected to know more about cancer chemotherapy than other physicians. Thus, the oncologist who fails to disclose toxicity, for which there is some credible evidence, may be vulnerable to claims based on a lack of informed consent, especially in a state where case law emphasizes a patient's right to know information that is material to a therapeutic choice.

The growing use of combination chemotherapies poses a distinctive problem relating to disclosure. While toxicities of individual drugs may be well defined, synergistic effects of combinations may be both profound and difficult to foretell. Beyond a sort of disclaimer that multidrug regimens may have additional and severe side effects beyond those that may occur with each individual drug, a physician can say little more. Practically speaking, it is probable that the major toxicities of individual agents used in the combination will have been disclosed, and a patient will be well-aware that treatment is a dangerous undertaking. Therefore, disclosure that merely alludes to presently unforeseeable, but possibly major future hazards (such as development of a second cancer), does not appear legally wanting. Indeed once the uncertainty about late effects is disclosed, it would seem inappropriate, even antitherapeutic, to discuss particular speculative risks.

CONSENT IN RESEARCH

If a patient becomes a subject of clinical research, the relationship between patient and physician takes on a different cast. No longer is the physician entirely motivated by the welfare of the individual patient (notwithstanding that benefit to patients in general is the goal of most clinical research). The investigator is testing a hypothesis (i.e., that a particular drug is effective against a particular cancer), and the patient is a vehicle for confirming or rejecting the hypothesis. Once the doctor/patient relationship is viewed in this way, the doctrine of informed consent assumes greater significance. For example, federal regulations applicable to government-funded clinical research require extensive written disclosure of risks, limit the extent to which research can be conducted in children or others whose competence to consent is doubtful, and mandate participation by institutional review boards (IRB) in oversight of the consent process.[6] The riskier the research, the greater the mandated safeguards. Moreover, even if federal standards are not specifically applicable, it can be anticipated that state officials or judges will refer to federal standards in evaluating adequacy of consents to participate in research.

It is not always self-evident when a particular treatment constitutes research and hence may be judged by more exacting legal standards. For example, drugs that are FDA-approved and in general use for specified conditions may be prescribed for certain other conditions if there is some evidence they may be helpful (e.g., some tricyclic antidepressants are apparently effective analgesics). In this situation, risks are likely to be similar regardless of the condition for which a drug is prescribed. But if prescription is designed as a test of a drug's effectiveness, a conservative approach is to advise the patient that treatment is experimental, tailor disclosure accordingly, and secure approval from an appropriate IRB. The indications for such an approach increase in proportion to the toxicity of the particular agent.

The fact that physicians classify some forms of frank experimentation as treatment may occasionally influence law's response. In a recent well publicized malpractice suit against a cardiac surgeon, a federal appellate court ruled that implant of a mechanical ventricular assist device in a patient was not an experiment, even though the device had never been used in humans nor extensively tested in animals.[22] The surgeon asserted that the implant was used solely for the purpose of treating the patient's end-stage heart disease, more specifically to sustain cardiac function pending heart transplantation. The court agreed that the therapeutic rationale for the novel procedure removed it from the realm of experimentation. This ruling was crucial to the defendant surgeon because it left the case to be resolved under conventional principles of malpractice law. The patient's surviving wife thus was left with the burden of proving that the surgeon's conduct was unreasonable. Because she could find no expert to testify on the adequacy of disclosure of risks of the implant, the suit failed. While the court's ruling suggests that research that has a substantial therapeutic goal will be scrutinized less closely than explicitly nontherapeutic research, this interpretation may be unwise if risks of "treatment" are great. Even if federal regulations do not apply (as with respect to nonfederally supported activities in private institutions), it should not be assumed that courts will uncritically accept a characterization of research as treatment.

In litigation arising out of an alleged failure to obtain informed consent, the issue of whether research or treatment is involved may be a factor in the outcome. More pivotal, however, is whether disclosure is adequate in the context of a risk-benefit appraisal. If a particular therapy is frankly experimental, a patient is entitled to know that certain risks are being taken for uncertain gain. Thus, both the known hazards and the unpredictable nature of benefits, if any, should be conveyed. If they are, then disclosure is legally adequate no matter how experimental the treatment. On the other hand, underdisclosure of known risks, overemphasis of potential benefits, or a combination of the two, may foster liability even if treatment is clearly nonexperimental.

LITIGATING LATE IATROGENESIS

To illustrate the operation of informed consent doctrines in a lawsuit based on failure to disclose a risk of cancer treatment that later materializes, assume the following marginally plausible facts:

X, diagnosed as having disseminated Hodgkin's disease at age 18, agrees to receive radiation and chemotherapy under a clinical research protocol. He is informed by Doctor Y that treatment might cause severe disability or death and he signs a detailed consent form that lists in detail the side effects of the component treatments. No mention is made of any possibility he might develop another cancer as a result of treatment. The treatment is effective and 5 years after treatment he is free of Hodgkin's disease. Eight years after treatment he develops an acute leukemia. After aggressive treatment, great suffering, and large medical expenses, remission of the acute leukemia occurs. X then reads in the newspapers that leukemia and other cancers have occurred in some persons "cured" of earlier leukemia and lymphomas. He consults Lawyer Z, a noted malpractice attorney, who obtains a copy of the earlier consent form and contacts an oncologist who expresses a willingness to testify that the treatment for Hodgkin's disease probably caused X's acute leukemia. Z must then decide whether there is a basis for filing a malpractice suit against Y, based on Y's failure to obtain informed consent from X before beginning treatment for Hodgkin's disease.

As will become evident, it is improbable that X's suit would succeed. Z would thus be well advised to decline to file the suit, or at least should refrain from investing substantial resources in pursuing the claim. But consideration of X's claim illustrates how a lawyer might approach a claim based on late iatrogenesis and how the law of informed consent functions in malpractice litigation.

Z's decision to take X's case may be influenced by several factors. One is the provability of harm attributable to Y's alleged failure to obtain informed consent. If Z follows the customary practice of representing X on a contingent fee basis, Z would want to be convinced that the chance of recovering damages is good enough to justify pursuing the claim. Willingness of an oncologist to testify as to the causal relationship between treatment of Hodgkin's disease and the later leukemia is essential because Z would need a rationale for holding Y responsible for the expenses and suffering X incurred from leukemia. Z would also want to satisfy himself that the consent form for the experimental treatment of Hodgkin's disease could not be interpreted as disclosing any risk of a possible second cancer. In addition, Z would want reassurance that X will be a credible witness in court. Success in a lawsuit will depend on persuading a court (or Y's malpractice insurer) that had X only known that the particular experimental treatment of his Hodgkin's disease might cause another cancer, he would have rejected the treatment. Z would also want to determine if there were any data available to Y at the time he treated X for Hodgkin's disease that leukemia was a possible risk of treatment. If no such data were extant, Z would have no basis for contending that Y had a duty to disclose a risk of a second cancer.

Assuming Z concludes that X and his medical experts will be persuasive witnesses, he may be inclined to bring suit against Y even if major legal hurdles exist. One such hurdle is the statute of limitations.[23] In some states, so-called "repose statutes" bar claims not filed within a specified time (usually 1 to 3 years) after an alleged injury. In the hypothetical case, the injury in question occurred when X's Hodgkin's disease was treated, 8 years before the leukemia appeared. Thus, the claim might be barred in those states with "repose statutes." In other states, however, the statute of limitations does not begin to run until an injury is or should have been discovered. This means that, as to X, the statute would not start to run until X discovered that his leukemia may have been caused by his previous treatment. Another hurdle might be a legal climate unfavorable to claims based on lack of informed consent. While informed consent claims are generally recognized, judicial decisions or legislation may restrict the scope of such claims.[5,22]

If Z files suit against Y on behalf of X, Y will be forced to seek legal assistance. Ordinarily, Y's malpractice insurer will provide legal counsel, but Y may prefer to retain a lawyer of his choice. In any event, Y's lawyer will evaluate the legal basis of X's claim, secure an opinion from an oncologist about the medical aspects of the claim, and then recommend a course of action to Y. If it is concluded that the claim lacks merit, Y's lawyer will probably recommend resisting the claim vigorously and eschewing negotiations to settle the claim out of court. Otherwise, Y's lawyer may suggest that efforts be made to settle the claim for the lowest possible sum. If the claim is somehow perceived as meritorious, the settlement figure will be proportionally higher. In fact, most malpractice claims are settled out of court, with the extent and difficulty of negotiations usually depending on the amount of money at issue.

If a suit proceeds to trial, the full panoply of legal procedures and rules will apply. As previously indicated, X must prove certain elements to win a suit against Y based on lack of informed consent. Each element must be established by a preponderance of evidence; in effect, X must convince a court that it is more probable than not that his version is correct as to each element. Thus, X must show that (1) Y knew or should have known that a future cancer was a risk of the treatment he prescribed for X; (2) Y wrongfully failed to disclose this risk to X; (3) he, X, would have refused the treatment had he been informed of this risk; (4) because he agreed to treatment he incurred leukemia; and (5) the leukemia caused injury calculable in monetary terms.

This summary of X's burden of proof suggests why X is unlikely to prevail. Proving that Y knew or should have known of the risk of leukemia would require convincing testimony from oncologists that this was a known risk at the time treatment was prescribed. To establish that Y did not adequately disclose risks of treatment, X must convince a court that Y's disclosure that death might result from treatment did not give X sufficient warning of the dangers of treatment. X must also show that his knowledge that a future cancer might result from treatment would have caused him to reject treatment, even though he was undissuaded by the disclosed risk of death. Even if X could prove all this, he must still show that the treatment itself caused the leukemia, not some other factor. Finally, X must establish that he should be compensated in money for the side effects of a treatment without which he probably would have died.

Other scenarios relating to late iatrogenesis can be envisioned (e.g., dementia after radiotherapy of brain cancer and permanent immunodeficiency after multidrug chemotherapy). But should they become a focus of legal inquiry, the issues will likely resemble those explored in the hypothetical case. From a medical standpoint, the key questions are the state of scientific knowledge about risks when treatment was administered and the relationship of a late-appearing disorder to the original anticancer therapy. From a legal standpoint, the central considerations are the extent to which known risks were actually disclosed, the impact of an inadequate disclosure on a patient's decision to accept treatment, and the appropriate measure of damages for harm resulting from life-saving treatments.

Law requires physicians to tell patients if treatment may be dangerous so that patients may exercise their right to accept or reject it. How much physicians must disclose and by what standards the adequacy of disclosure is judged may be uncertain, and it may be difficult to determine if patients fully comprehend even the most careful disclosures. Yet a perception that a "true" informed consent seldom occurs is not a lawful justification for nondisclosure, nor is a belief that a patient should be spared the anxiety of knowing that a potentially helpful treatment may cause serious harm. It is justifiable, however, to omit disclosure of risks that are speculative, improbable, or so ill-designed that there is no medical consensus that they exist.

Where late iatrogenesis is a concern, it may be justifiable to disclose no more than that long-range effects of complex, potent treatments are unpredictable but may be serious. Specificity of disclosure beyond that would depend on what data are reasonably available to prescribing physicians at the time disclosure is made. For example, if there is substantial evidence that a particular chemotherapeutic regimen carries with it a small but definite risk of a second cancer, disclosure of this risk seems advisable. It is probable that most patients who accept treatments that may cause major late effects already understand that the treatments are dangerous, even life-threatening, and may affect many organ systems. Nevertheless, full respect for their rights of self-determination requires disclosing any information that may influence their choice, including a known risk of another malignancy at some future time.

Even if a particular disclosure is inadequate, a physician is not necessarily subjected to liability. To sustain a claim for damages, a claimant must prove quantifiable injury and that, had disclosure been adequate, the harmful treatment would have been rejected. Many claimants have found it difficult to satisfy the burden of proving these elements, and judgements against physicians based solely on lack of informed consent are uncommon. This hardly suggests, however, that all legally defensible nondisclosures are ethically tolerable or of no practical consequence. Such omissions may lead to the filing of malpractice suits, may engender anger and cynicism among patients and other concerned persons, and may provoke judges or legislators to change legal doctrines so that nondisclosures are more readily punishable. Thus, giving careful attention to the process by which risks are disclosed may both enhance physician/patient relationships and prevent malpractice claims.[4]

REFERENCES

1. Ingelfinger, F. Informed (but uneducated) consent. N. Engl. J. Med. 287:465, 1972.
2. President's Commission for the Study of Ethical Problems in Medicine and Biomedical and Behavioral Research: Making Health Care Decisions. Washington, D.C., U.S. Government Printing Office, 1982, pp. 72–111.
3. Katz, J. The Silent World of Doctor and Patient, New York, The Free Press, 1984.
4. Gutheil, T.G., Bursztjan, H., and Brodsky, A. Malpractice prevention through the sharing of uncertainty. N. Engl. J. Med. 311:49, 1984.
5. Meisel, A. and Kabnick, L. Informed consent to medical treatment: an analysis of recent legislation. University of Pittsburgh Law Review 41:407, 1980.
6. Department of Health and Human Services: Protection of Human Subjects. 45 Code of Federal Regulations 46.101–46.117, 1981.
7. *Pratt v. Davis,* 118 Ill. App. 161 (1905).
8. *Schloendorff v. New York Hospital,* 211, New York 125 (1914).
9. *Hunt v. Bradshaw,* 88 S.E. 2d 762 (North Carolina 1955).
10. *Nathanson v. Kline,* 350 P. 2d 1093 (Kansas 1960).
11. *Canterbury v. Spence,* 464 F. 2d. 772 (District of Columbia Cir. 1972).
12. *Cobbs v. Grant,* 502 P. 2d 1 (California 1972).

13. *MacMullen v. Vaughan*, 227 S.E. 2d 40 (Georgia 1976).
14. *Woolley v. Henderson*, 418 A. 2d 1123 (Maine 1980).
15. *Malloy v. Shanahan*, 421 A. 2d 803 (Pennsylvania Super. 1980).
16. Plant, M. The decline of "informed consent." Washington and Lee Law Review 35:91, 1978.
17. President's Commission for the Study of Ethical Problems in Medicine and Biomedical and Behavioral Research: Making Health Care Decisions. Washington, D.C., U.S. Government Printing Office, 1982, pp. 23–27.
18. Waltz, J.R. and Inbau, F.E. Medical Jurisprudence. New York, Macmillan, 1971, pp. 152–156.
19. *Woods v. Brumlop*, 277 P. 2d 520 (New Mexico 1962).
20. Waltz, J.R. and Inbau, F.E. Medical Jurisprudence. New York, Macmillan, 1971, pp. 270–281.
21. Note: Informed consent: From disclosure to patient participation in medical decision-making. Northwestern Law Review 76:172, 1981.
22. *Karp v. Cooley*, 493 F. 2d 408 (5th Cir, 1974).
23. Note: The fairness and constitutionality of statutes of limitations for toxic tort suits. Harvard Law Review 96:1683, 1983.

Summary and Analysis

MORTIMER J. LACHER
JOHN R. REDMAN

PROGRESS TOWARD LONG SURVIVAL

In 1977, Dr. Franz J. Ingelfinger, Editor of *The New England Journal of Medicine,* wrote that physicians were failures at truly providing a longer life for our patients. Therefore, it was implied, practicing physicians should just concentrate on palliation, because trying to actually extend life was hopeless.[1]

"Perhaps the role of the doctor as reliever, rather than as healer should be accentuated to mitigate any disappointment that he [the practitioner] cannot appreciably reorient mortality or morbidity trends. In brief, tremendously important as they are, health statistics appear somewhat irrelevant to the ordinary purposes of patient care, which deal with the hope of an individual human being that his troubles will be ameliorated."[1]

Ingelfinger began his commentary with a cutting aphorism attributed to a world-famous biochemist, Lawrence Henderson: "Somewhere between 1910 and 1912 in this country, . . . a random patient, with a random disease, consulting a doctor chosen at random had, for the first time in the history of mankind, a better than fifty-fifty chance of profiting from the encounter." "Henderson's words," Ingelfinger said, "imply progress after 1912, but whether or not consultations between patients and doctors appreciably affected the statistics of health (i.e., morbidity and mortality curves) is still questioned. . . . That health statistics do not particularly reflect what doctors do in the hospital or office should not cause much consternation or even surprise."[1]

Unfortunately, Ingelfinger didn't live long enough to witness our realization of the prolonged useful survival of the Hodgkin's patient. He did not count on the changes in mortality trends wrought by our treatment of patients for Hodgkin's disease. Today, we would be terribly disturbed if our personal statistics did not reflect the tremendous advance we had fashioned with regard to the improvement in survival for the Hodgkin's patient.

IATROGENIC DISEASE CANCELS OUT PROGRESS

"Let us assume," Ingelfinger says, "that 80 per cent of patients have either self-limited disorders or conditions not improvable, even by modern medicine. The physician's actions, unless harmful, will therefore not affect the basic course of such conditions. In slightly over 10 percent of cases, however, medical intervention is dramatically successful, whether surgeon repairs bones or removes stones, the internist uses antibiotics or palliative measures (e.g., insulin, vitamin B_{12}) appropriately, or the pediatrician eliminates a food that an enzyme-deficient infant cannot absorb or metabolize. But, alas, in the final 9 percent, give or take a point or two, the doctor may diagnose or treat inadequately, or he may just have bad luck. Whatever the reason, the patient ends up with iatrogenic problems. So the balance of accounts ends up marginally on the positive side of zero. Henderson was right, but barely so."[1]

Ingelfinger presumes that progress in medical treatment that prolongs life is mitigated by, and even canceled out by, the iatrogenic effects of the treatment itself. Ingelfinger strikes the medical practitioner where it hurts the most: first he impugns the practitioner's overall ability to save patients' lives that definitely would have been lost if left to chance. He then says that not only are the advances in therapy marginal, but in the process of their application the "patient ends up with iatrogenic problems" and is thereby lost anyway.[1]

Fortunately, those of us who decided to care for cancer patients did not begin wrapped in Ingelfinger's cloak of philosophical pessimism about what we can or cannot do to prolong life in a useful manner. By not accepting the terrible odds stacked against us, we have successfully moved forward in our quest to treat and cure patients with Hodgkin's disease. In the process, we have on the one hand, disproved Ingelfinger's cynical negativism by significantly prolonging survival for the majority of Hodgkin's patients. On the other hand, we have fulfilled his prophecy by causing iatrogenic problems.

The good news is that we have appropriate treatments even for some of the iatrogenically induced problems. It is wonderful to know that, although at least as many as 60% of patients develop compensated hypothyroidism after radiation therapy to the neck area, the disorder can be considered "trivial" because we now recognize it, diagnose it early, and easily correct the problem.

MORTALITY STATISTICS HAVE BEEN REORIENTED FOR HODGKIN'S PATIENTS

Of course it is the physician's role always to deliver hope, but it is our higher calling to go beyond that role and deliver long life as well. We have significantly improved morbidity and mortality statistics for Hodgkin's patients in the past 20 years. At the same time every patient that we "cure" (or who lives beyond what might have been expected if left only to chance) is simultaneously disadvantaged in some way. None of our current treatments are completely innocuous.

On the other hand, not everything that occurs to the Hodgkin's patient after treatment is iatrogenic. Once the patient has recovered from the acute side effects of therapy, the late complications do not rest exclusively on what the physician had to do to achieve the good results. Surely the patient's ultimate course of life does not lie exclusively in the physician's hands. There is an internal driving force of nature that we have no control over. For instance, it is probable that we partly inherit Hodgkin's disease or at least the tendency to "catch" it. The same inheritance factor probably holds true for the development of second malignant neoplasms in the Hodgkin's population. All second malignant neoplasms do not originate from the side effects of therapy. A portion appear to arise from chance alone or from the tendency of the Hodgkin's patient to get other malignancies.

That we have changed the previous course of nature is not in doubt. We are now, for example, able to observe an increased birth rate among Hodgkin's patients after their disease is successfully treated with extensive radiation and chemotherapy, whereas prior to our current treatment methods this phenomenon was uncommon. What consequences this will ultimately have on the offspring is still unknown. No serious consequences have been observed so far, but the period of observation and the numbers of patients available for analysis are still limited.

During the 1940s and into the early 1960s, Hodgkin's disease was considered an almost uniformly fatal malignancy. Only 30 years ago, long survival was still limited to a lucky few.[2] The more intensive therapies introduced in the early 1970s changed that outlook. The immediate improvement in achieving long survival was a function of more effective initial radiation treatment, but probably more important was the application of both primary and salvage multidrug chemotherapy. The survival data at the University of Rochester Cancer Center epitomizes the general experience. In Stages IA and IIA supradiaphragmatic Hodgkin's disease, "Patients treated during the 1970s . . . had a substantially better prognosis than similar patients treated during the 1960s. At 12 years, disease-free survival improved from 38% to 65% and survival improved from 37% to 82%."[3]

The initial success of primary radiation therapy hinged on the use of "prophylactic" contiguous field irradiation.[4,5] Most of the Hodgkin's patients presented with an obvious tumor that appeared to be limited to areas above the diaphragm. When it became clear that at least 30% or more of patients actually had tumor below the diaphragm as well, "prophylactic" subdiaphragmatic irradiation was introduced as part of the primary radiation therapy protocols, even when tumor could not be identified below the diaphragm; this change in protocol was spearheaded by the initial study of laparotomy/splenectomy conducted by Glatstein et al. in 1969.[6]

Although the primary "academic" purpose of the more extensive radiation treatment was to provide "prophylactic" therapy, in reality Hodgkin's disease was being treated actively at multiple primary sites. The fact is we are unable to diagnose absolutely the presence of Hodgkin's tumors in all of the areas we are treating. In the past, in order to dramatically improve the Hodgkin's patient survival rate, we learned to treat patients as if there was more tumor than met the eye. Now that we have improved overall survival dramatically, we are starting to refine our methods to limit the therapy (and its potential side effects) as much as possible.

NEW CHEMOTHERAPY USHERED IN THE AGE OF CONTINUING SURVIVAL

Radiation therapy alone was insufficient to truly advance the long-term survival of Hodgkin's patients because it could not address effectively almost all relapsing patients or those patients whose tumors were not sufficiently anatomically restricted to fit into rigid radiation fields. Relapse after primary radiation therapy had always been a more formidable problem than anyone cared to acknowledge, even when the radiation included the large extensive fields presumed to be "curative" and was given in "ideal" doses through which no Hodgkin's tumor could survive or relapse. Analysis of the Stanford data concerning late relapses shows a 32% relapse rate among patients treated with primary radiation.[7]

Fortunately, effective single-agent chemotherapies were being discovered. These included nitrogen mustard, chlorambucil, thiotepa, vinblastine, vincristine, procarbazine, and cyclophosphamide. Combinations of these drugs then appeared on the scene: from the initially successful two-drug combination of vinblastine and chlorambucil[8] to the variations of four-drug therapies known as MOPP, which included mechlorethamine (nitrogen mustard), vincristine, procarbazine, and prednisone;[9] or the so-called C-MOPP, which used cyclophosphamide instead of nitrogen mustard (COPP); TOPP, which used thiotepa instead of nitrogen mustard; MVPP, which used vinblastine instead of vincristine (Oncovin): and TVPP (which used thiotepa, vinblastine, vincristine, prednisone and procarbazine). The success of these multidrug regimens truly changed the survival rate in previously hopeless situations. Later doxorubicin and bleomycin were discovered, and these drugs became incorporated in extremely effective additional multidrug combinations of four and eight (ABVD,[10] ABVD/MOPP, ABVP/TOPP).

Every "new" therapy must be treated with caution because of potentially dangerous late and serious side effects. So far, the most important single effect of intense radiation and multidrug chemotherapy has been to achieve long survival for the majority of patients and the side effects generally have not been immediately life threatening and are amenable to adjustments.

CURRENT TREATMENT PLANS ARE FAR FROM PERFECT

The Hodgkin's tumor is still a formidable enemy, and premature death still strikes a significant number of patients. Because of this, the risks of treatment with potentially late serious side effects must still be part of the therapeutic plan, provided the therapy can primarily extend life that is compatible with a high quality. It is estimated conservatively that approximately 70% of all Hodgkin's patients and only 50% of those presenting with more aggressive disease can achieve long survival (10 years or more) using radiation therapy alone, radiation plus combination chemotherapy, or in those with advanced disease, combination chemotherapy alone.

EARLY DEATH STILL THREATENS A HIGH PERCENTAGE OF HODGKIN'S PATIENTS

The fact must be conceded that some patients absolutely do not respond to currently available treatment, and these failures must not be taken as a sign of incompetence on the part of practicing physicians. Even the best hands experience a persistent failure rate, and only new therapy, yet to be discovered, will change this.

Today, the major reason for the treatment failure of some Hodgkin's patients usually has little to do with insufficient dosages of administered medication. Some patients do not respond to "ideal" primary treatment, and some relapse and die of Hodgkin's disease after complete remission intervals of months to many years. More likely the reason for failure is the phenomenon hinted at by Ferrant et al.: "The poor response to combined modality treatment of patients with B symptoms and a large mediastinal mass would suggest that the biologic behavior of their disease might be different. . ."[11] To help these patients we will have to wait for the development of new drugs and new drug combinations. Whether they are newly developed adaptive immunotherapies or "ordinary" chemotherapeutic agents to be used singly or in combinations remains to be discovered.

TIME-DOSE FACTORS IN CHEMOTHERAPY

Too many have implied that "more is better" when administering cancer chemotherapy. The implication that physicians who reduce dosages listed in a protocol may be "gambling" with the patient's duration of survival, or that the most serious side-effect of chemotherapy aimed at cure may be death from inadequate doses, is loaded with unfair innuendo and requires proper analysis. Alan J. Dembo supplied that analysis in his editorial in the *Journal of Clinical Oncology*.[12] He reviewed the report by Levin and Hryniuk[13] that showed a correlation between the planned dose intensities, especially of cisplatin-based regimens, and the observed median survival times and advanced ovarian cancer response rates. Dembo stated, "The methodology used in their analysis with its numerous assumptions permits the inferences drawn from their results to be viewed only as hypothesis-generating and not as proof."[12]

Dembo continued, ". . . failure to make the distinction between hypothesis and proof has two principal dangers for the reader: the first is that the dose-intensity concept will be used to justify an indiscriminate more-is-better approach to chemotherapy; the second is that the concept will be dismissed for lack of hard evidence and its potential value overlooked."[12]

In summary, the more-is-better philosophy is still generally unproven and must still be tested from tumor to tumor, from drug to drug, and from combination to combination. In Dembo's words: ". . . acceptance that the dose-intensity hypothesis needs to be tested and the concept expanded upon provides new avenues for clinical research at the same time as it highlights gaps in our knowledge. As far as tumor control is concerned, we need to know: (1) The ideal *total* dose of drug. Is there a ceiling total dose above which no benefit accrues? (2) The ideal overall *duration* of the treatment course. Is there a minimum time below which the benefits of intensification are lost? Is there a maximum overall time past which tumor cell proliferation and spontaneous and acquired drug resistance negate the benefits of a higher cumulative total dose? (3) The importance of *scheduling*."

The same questions must be asked concerning the dose-limiting toxicities of chemotherapy. That is, what must be learned about dose-intensity, scheduling, and duration of treatment course with regard to therapeutic effect must also be measured against the early and late toxicity of the chemotherapy itself. After all, it may be the iatrogenic toxic death, caused by too much of a good thing, that sets the ultimate limits on how much of a drug we can finally administer.

IN THE ACTUARIAL SENSE OF "CURABILITY," HODGKIN'S DISEASE IS CURABLE

The fact that we may consider Hodgkin's disease to be potentially "curable" does not mean that every patient with Hodgkin's disease can be cured or will be cured. As already conceded, some patients defy all treatment and die from Hodgkin's disease or its complications. These patients are usually those who repeatedly fail to respond to all the methods of treatment now at our disposal. They may never respond sufficiently to any treatment at any time, or they may initially respond, only to relapse at a later date and then die of Hodgkin's disease. Therefore, when we use the word "curable," what we mean is what Eason meant by curable.[14] That is, that even if patients are still dying of Hodgkin's disease, on an overall basis, we have moved all patients into the normal life expectancy curve of their peers. Some will die early, some later. Some will die of disorders totally unrelated to Hodgkin's disease or its treatment; others will die of disorders stemming from the effects of treatment. Some will even die at a much later date (i.e., 25 years later) of "relapsing" or "recurring" Hodgkin's disease. It is now hoped the majority, however, will die of what may be euphemistically called "natural causes" and that their median survival will be similar to that of their peers.

In the space of 25 years, the prognosis for almost all age groups of Hodgkin's patients has improved dramatically. In particular, the pediatric age group (under 14 years of age) has now fared so well with regard to survival, as Donaldson pointed out in Chapter 18, that there is no longer any reason to think of their overall prognosis as unfavorable. In fact, every effort is now being made to adjust the therapy[15] to prevent growth defects induced by maximal radiation treatment.

To mitigate the effects of radiation therapy, pediatricians are now treating their young Hodgkin's patients routinely with a primary combination of radiation and chemotherapy, limiting the dose of the radiation therapy, and adding multidrug chemotherapy combinations. Despite past fears concerning the use of primary combined radiation therapy and chemotherapy for patients with Hodgkin's disease, Donaldson and Link recently concluded, as did others years before, that "the experience from Stanford validates the effectiveness of the low-dose radiotherapy and chemotherapy approach by providing long-term follow-up data. . . " This use of combined radiation therapy and combination chemotherapy as primary therapy is now considered appropriate for the majority of children with Hodgkin's disease.[15]

To achieve a high percentage of survival at 5 years in a child's life is important but not spectacular. It remains to be seen what 10, 15, and 25 years or more of survival will bring in the way of late complications to the pediatric Hodgkin's population.

HODGKIN'S IN THE ELDERLY

Hodgkin's disease is not as successfully treated in the elderly as in children. Eghbali et al.[16] analyzed a group of 30 patients over the age of 70. They reported: "In five cases the treatment could be held responsible for death. Eleven patients died of Hodgkin's disease within a 36 month period. Five patients are alive and the nine other patients died from other causes." The median survival in this age group was 15 months. Over a 20-year period, from January 1962 to December 1981, this group of elderly patients represented 6.9% of all the patients treated (30 of 430).[16]

The study by Austin-Seymour et al., concerning the treatment of Hodgkin's disease in patients over 60 years old,[17] clearly showed that "elderly patients with Hodgkin's disease pose unique problems. . ."and that "they often present with advanced disease and other medical problems that cause difficulties in the proper staging and treatment of their disease. When treated aggressively, half of the elderly patients have acute complications during treatment, including significant leukopenia, thrombocytopenia and weight loss. [Older] patients with advanced disease were rarely cured even with optimal therapy. All these factors confirm that older age is a poor prognostic indicator."[17] What is "optimal" for the younger Hodgkin's patient is clearly not "optimal" for the older patient.

The older patient with Hodgkin's disease has a poor prognosis merely because of his age at onset. In addition, the intense therapy currently needed to achieve success is not well tolerated in the elderly. For these patients, the most important complications of survival may be related to the immediate acute effects of treatment. In the absence of long-term survivors among the elderly Hodgkin's patients, concern over the late side effects of therapy is a moot issue. In the elderly, it is possible that modest therapy could achieve more reasonable and even excellent palliation. Every effort should be made to avoid the phenomenon of debilitating treatment-related side effects and early death caused by an aggressive treatment approach in elderly patients who clearly do not tolerate or ultimately benefit from such aggressive treatment.

If historical analysis is going to be of benefit, we must learn to avoid a 20% treatment-related death rate in the elderly. What is necessary to extend the low median survival past 15 months in this group of patients remains to be learned. In the absence of long-term survivors in the elderly population with Hodgkin's disease, there is little reason to be overly concerned with the late complications of therapy. Our concern must be associated with the acute toxicities, and our goals must center around gentler methods of successfully treating the older patient. Their poor prognosis is partly due to their poor tolerance for the current aggressive therapies. In addition, as Austin-Seymour et al. have suggested, there must be ". . . a different natural history of the disease in older people."

RELAPSING HODGKIN'S DISEASE IS STILL A SERIOUS AND UNSOLVED CONSEQUENCE OF SURVIVAL

In 1985, Herman et al.[7] reviewed the late relapse among patients treated for Hodgkin's disease at Stanford University. They noted that, of 1360 consecutive patients, 1312 (96%) had complete remission, but 424 patients had a relapse. Fifty-five patients had relapses 36 months or more after completion of therapy. The actuarial risk of relapse in patients disease-free 3 years after therapy was 12.9%; what might seem odd is that the patients who had a significant increase in late relapses started with limited Stage I disease. Furthermore, patients who had late relapses had nodular sclerosis Hodgkin's disease significantly more often and tended to have mixed cellularity Hodgkin's disease less often than did patients who had earlier relapses. "Thus, patients with early stage disease and nodular sclerosis subtype, both of which have been correlated previously with a good prognosis, appear to be at risk of relapse for a longer period than patients with more aggressive or widespread disease."[7]

Especially with our currently improved and more realistic understanding of what can happen to the Hodgkin's survivor, the need for prolonged surveillance of patients for late relapse as well as other potential complications of survival after treatment cannot be overemphasized.

Drs. Hung, Jhung, and Anagnostou reported a case of recurrence of Hodgkin's disease 29 years after remission. It was their opinion that this represented the longest period between remission and "relapse" ever recorded to date.[18] More than 10 years ago we recorded late-relapsing Hodgkin's disease in a patient 16 years after remission. Only a handful of cases with elapsed time from remission to relapse greater than 16 years have been recorded. As the life expectancy of more and more Hodgkin's patients improves, it would appear reasonable to predict that this type of relapse will become more common.

LEUKEMIA AND SECONDARY SOLID TUMORS AFTER THERAPY FOR HODGKIN'S DISEASE

In 1982, Longo, Young, and DeVita[19] noted that the Stanford studies indicated a 15% improvement in survival using the combined modality (chemotherapy and radiation therapy) approach for "early-stage" Hodgkin's disease. They worried, however, that this improvement in survival would be offset by an increase in treatment-induced leukemia "that might be expected using that approach."[19] Of course, they were not alone in their concern. In fact, it was fashionable to condemn initial combined radiation and multidrug chemotherapy, particularly because leukemia was supposed to occur after this therapy. The presumption that treatment-induced leukemia would severely impact on survival turned out to be more imagined than real.

The physicians at the National Cancer Institute set up a prospective follow-up study of their patients treated with MOPP to record the morphologic changes in the bone marrow that they anticipated would precede the development of the leukemias they had initially predicted.[20] Instead of discovering that their initial ominous predictions had come true, they discovered that the rate of leukemia development faltered. After 11 years of observation, they now predict that in the surviving patient the incidence of secondary acute nonlymphocytic leukemia (ANLL) and myelodysplastic syndromes approaches the background incidence rate anticipated in a normal cohort of individuals.

Although the post-treatment development of leukemia has been particularly stressed, presumably primarily related to the addition of multidrug chemotherapy (and especially MOPP given for relapsing Hodgkin's disease after an initial remission induced by primary radiation therapy), it now seems much less important than originally feared. Furthermore, the development of acute leukemia in Hodgkin's patients never did seriously impact the overall survival data because the majority of patients with ANLL were relapsing Hodgkin's patients who could not be controlled in any way.

Succinctly put, Blayney et al. conclude the following: "The projection that an increasing fraction of long-term survivors would die from leukemia was premature. With longer follow-up it appears that the incidence of leukemia falls, following a second-order rather than a linear regression model. The decrease in treatment-related risk after 11 years should reinforce the aggressive approach to this once uniformly fatal disease."[20] All of which seems to prove that long survival does not carry with it a unique seed of latent destruction by leukemia, even if the survival was achieved by using multidrug chemotherapy.

If, as the new National Cancer Institute data by Blayney et al. suggest, the Hodgkin's survivor lives longer and the incidence of secondary leukemia actually diminishes to the point where it is no different than that in the general population, can the same be said for the development of secondary solid tumors? Probably not.

THE RISING INCIDENCE OF THE LATE OCCURRENCE OF "SOLID" MALIGNANT NEOPLASMS

All data indicate that the incidence of secondary solid tumors will occur at a much higher rate than expected. The cause for this is probably a late effect of radiation therapy plus the possibility that the Hodgkin's patient may have a genetic tendency to produce other malignancies.

Schottenfeld (Chapter 1) says that "No clear pattern of risk of sarcomas and carcinomas after treatment in Hodgkin's disease patients has appeared in published cohort studies. An important limitation in this regard, however, has been the concentration of person-years during the initial 10-year period of follow-up. Follow-up over longer intervals will be necessary before reliable estimates of risk for various solid tumors can be derived."

In the study by Boivin et al.,[21] the relative risk of all cancers, other than leukemia, did not significantly increase during the first decade after treatment (based on 10,195 person-years of observation). For the post-treatment interval of 10 to 38 years, however, a statistically significant risk of 20.0 relative to general population incidence rates was obtained for those patients who had intensive radiotherapy alone (no intensive chemotherapy).

Jorgen H. Olsen[22] evaluated the risk of developing a second cancer after developing a primary cancer in childhood by examining the population of Denmark from 1943 to 1980. Among a total of 5319 cases of primary cancer in childhood, followed until patient death or the end of 1980, 23 secondary tumors were observed (O) against an expected (E) figure of 6.5, corresponding to an O/E ratio of 4.4. That is, "a cancer diagnosed early in life, i.e., before the end of the 14th year, significantly increased the risk of later tumor occurrence with a factor of 3 to 4. The excess risk varies greatly according to the time elapsed since date of first tumor diagnosis, as the risk is found to be increased more than 10 times initially and thereafter gradually reduces to a level of 2.5 times the expected outcome in the period of 10 years or more since first malignancy."[22] Olsen concluded that the results of his analysis were in concert with other earlier observations that the development of a primary tumor in childhood increased the risk of developing a second tumor later in life. The magnitude of the risk depended on the time since first tumor diagnosis, with a negative time trend ranging from a 12-fold increase in close relation to first diagnosis to a 2.5-fold increase after 10 or more years from first diagnosis.

Bucking the more popular simplistic conclusion that the second malignant tumor was induced by the treatment, Olsen further concluded that "although treatment directed at the primary tumor may constitute a potential carcinogenic risk, this could not explain the observed excess risk of second cancer following cancer in childhood." Olsen indicated that the observations made in his study were compatible with a hypothesis ". . . proposed by Knudson on the possible role of prezygotic mutations with a subsequent risk of developing cancer in early life and multiple primaries in the same persons." The presumption that it is the treatment itself that is the main culprit in causing the second malignancy in the Hodgkin's patient must be tempered by observations such as Olsen's, which imply that the genetic make up of the cancer patient also plays a role in the development of second primary tumors in this population.

CANCER BOOMERANG

Tucker et al.[23] reported the results of an analysis of 1507 patients with Hodgkin's disease treated at Stanford University Medical Center since 1968. Eighty-three second cancers were recorded more than one year after diagnosis, as compared with the 15.9 expected on rates in the general population. The Stanford data showed that, among their population of patients, no patient developed leukemia after 9 years of follow-up and therefore the cumulative risk of leukemia reached a plateau level of 3.3%. However, a serious long-term problem was associated with the development of solid tumors and the risk of the development of solid tumors continued to increase after the risk of leukemia had reached a plateau. "The high risk of solid tumors long after there is any evidence of Hodgkin's disease underscores the importance of continued monitoring of the patients, with careful evaluation of medical symptoms." Tucker et al. warned: "Since alkylating agents increase the risk of leukemia, and radiation contributes mainly to other cancers, future treatment protocols should attempt to reduce the most serious consequences of therapy without compromising the excellent survival."[23]

The dangers from radiation therapy with regard to the development of second primary solid tumors may be greater than currently estimated, judging by the recent re-evaluation of the effects of the radiation exposure on the atomic bomb survivors.[24] "Risk estimates are also being revised in light of the new cancer mortality data among the atomic bomb survivors, which according to Upton, 'are causing total risk to appear much larger than it did a few years ago.' In the past 11 years the number of excess deaths among survivors has risen from about 100 to 300. The increase is occurring because the population is reaching the age when cancers typically occur. As the incidence of 'normal' cancers increases with age, so too does the incidence of excess cancers. Japanese women heavily exposed to radiation as children who are now in their 40s . . . are showing a marked increase in breast cancer . . . [These] data are also showing that the relative risk is greater for those who were exposed in utero or as children than it is for those exposed as adults."[24]

"When the mortality data and new dosimetry are combined, says Sinclair, radiation risks appear to be a factor of 2 or 3 higher than earlier estimates. For the young, risk could be up by a factor of 5 or 6, he suspects. And if the dose-response curve turns out to be linear, the risk estimate would rise by a factor of 2 again."[24]

CARDIAC EFFECTS OF HODGKIN'S DISEASE THERAPY

LATE EFFECTS OF MEDIASTINAL RADIATION

Loeffler, Mauch, and Hellman noted in Chapter 2 that, "while the acute effects of radiation therapy in the treatment of Hodgkin's disease are usually reversible and transient, late effects due to impaired function of radiation induced injury of normal tissues are not." They concluded: "Fortunately, the vast majority of late effects are not severe and only a very small proportion of patients develop major complications leading to permanent disability or death." Unfortunately, as our long-term survivors continue to increase and the time of follow-up grows longer and longer, it may turn out that a significant proportion of patients will develop major late cardiac complications of radiation therapy.

Clearly, mediastinal irradiation given as treatment for malignant diseases causes cardiac damage. Up until the 1980s, a wide range of complications, such as different forms of pericarditis, valvular abnormalities, restrictive cardiomyopathy, and coronary artery stenosis, have been reported as case reports or autopsy-based studies, and only a few studies have included a clinical series of patients. Therefore, the rate and significance of late cardiac complications are not known. Now that larger clinical evaluation studies are becoming more frequent, however, we will soon have a better understanding of how dangerous the radiation therapy is to the mediastinum.

Gomez et al.[25] evaluated heart size and function after radiation therapy to the mediastinum in patients with Hodgkin's disease using an equally weighted anterior-posterior technique. They studied first-pass left ventricular ejection fraction (LVEF) performed with ^{99m}Tc pertechnetate in 55 patients 30 to 120 months after radiation therapy of the mediastinum and compared this with the LVEF of 20 normal controls. They concluded that "the control group had a significantly higher LVEF than the group of patients who had received RT to the mediastinum. No correlation was observed between changes in their parameters and the use of adjuvant, salvage, or no chemotherapy after mediastinal RT."[25]

Although none of these patients presented with congestive heart failure or constrictive pericarditis, the analysis by Gomez et al. indicates a subclinical cardiomyopathy in more than one-half of the patients who received radiation therapy to the mediastinum. This clearly suggests that the incidence of heart damage after mediastinal radiation therapy will be higher than expected.[25]

Pohjola-Sintonen et al.[26] studied 28 patients younger than age 40 who were treated for Hodgkin's disease with mediastinal irradiation; the patients were examined no less than 5 years after the irradiation in order to evaluate the frequency of cardiac abnormalities. They found that 12 patients (43%) had had some pericardial event after radiation: a diagnosed pericarditis, remarkably increased heart volume, or a conspicuous change of cardiac silhouette, suggesting pericardial fluid. Fifty percent of the patients complained of symptoms, and 46% had to stop the exercise test on a low level because of chest pain, dyspnea, or general fatigue. "In two patients a severe coronary artery disease was found. One died suddenly after an acute myocardial infarction and the other had a large anterior AMI."[26] Nineteen of 28 patients had some abnormal cardiac findings, but only three were considered serious.

Perrault et al.[27] studied echocardiographic abnormalities 5 years or more after cardiac radiation. A total of 41 patients with Hodgkin's disease and seminoma in remission were subjected to echocardiography. "The abnormalities detected included pericardial thickening in 70%, thickening of the aortic and/or mitral valves in 28%, right ventricular dilatation or hypokinesis in 39%, and left ventricular dysfunction in 39%. In the 23 patients treated by an upper mantle technique with shielding, the incidence of right ventricular abnormalities and valvular thickening was significantly lower than in patients treated with modified techniques."[27] Although there was a lower prevalence of left-sided valvular thickening and right ventricular anormalities in patients treated by modern techniques of upper mantle irradiation, the current "standard" radiation technique of weighted anterior and posterior fields was not devoid of long-term complications, since valvular thickening was seen in 2 (9%) of 22 and right ventricular abnormalities in 5 (24%) of 21 patients. Although none of these patients had symptoms of valvular dysfunction or right ventricular failure, longer follow-up of a greater number of patients is required to assess the long-term hemodynamic implications of these observations.

Clearly, the effects of treatment for Hodgkin's disease are different in different age groups, and it may turn out that radiation to the heart in children and adolescents may be less damaging than its effects in adults.

Green et al. conducted cardiac evaluations on 28 children and adolescents treated for Hodgkin's disease with mediastinal irradiation using an equally weighted anterior-posterior megavoltage technique. The patients were aged 11 to 27 at the time of cardiac evaluation. So far, with a median follow-up of 90 months, none were found to have any significant cardiac dysfunction. Pericardial thickening, however, was demonstrated on echocardiograms from 12 of the 28 patients (42.9%). Thickening was more frequent among those patients observed for 72 months or more than among those with shorter follow-up.[28] Green et al. concluded that "cardiac dysfunction is an infrequent sequela of mediastinal irradiation following treatment using an equally weighted, anterior-posterior technique. [However] Longitudinal study of these patients will be necessary to determine the clinical significance and evolution of the occult pericardial thickening that was identified."[28]

LATE CHEMOTHERAPEUTIC DAMAGE TO THE HEART

Although opinions or interpretations of the existing data may differ about the seriousness of later effects of therapeutic mediastinal irradiation, there is little disagreement concerning the potentially life-threatening effects of the anthracycline drugs such as doxorubicin (Adriamycin). In Chapter 12, Gerling et al. comment: "The chronic toxic effects of anthracyclines result in the most important adverse clinical syndrome associated with these agents. Patients may present with rapidly progressive biventricular congestive heart failure following the insidious onset of symptoms weeks to months after administration of the last dose of doxorubicin. The occurrence of symptomatic congestive heart failure secondary to anthracycline cardiomyopathy is associated with a 50 to 60% early mortality. The incidence of clinically apparent congestive heart failure in patients treated with anthracyclines clearly depends on the total cumulative dose administered. In 1973, Lefrak suggested limitation of the total dose of doxorubicin to less than 550 mg/M^2 based on the incidence of ventricular failure of 0.27% in patients receiving less than 550 mg/M^2 and 30% in patients receiving greater than 550 mg/M^2. Recent evidence using invasive and noninvasive assessments of cardiac function and structure suggest that chronic cardiac toxicity occurs more frequently and at lower doses than had been appreciated earlier. Whereas only 1 to 2% of patients have overt evidence of congestive heart failure at a dose of 550 mg/M^2, more than 50% of asymptomatic patients have physiologic or pathologic evidence of cardiac damage."

It is possible that the cardiotoxic side effects of doxorubicin can be ameliorated by a change in the dose schedule. Since the schedule of doxorubicin administration has an impact on the development of congestive failure, Gerling et al in Chapter 12 comment that data from Weiss, Chlebowski, Von Hoff, Torti, and Lehga and their colleagues suggest that patients treated with smaller doses on a weekly schedule or by continuous infusion have a lower incidence of congestive heart failure than patients receiving larger doses every three weeks. "The decrease in cardiotoxic complications with the more frequent dosing schedule is attributed to lower peak doxorubicin concentrations." If this is true and the lower weekly doses do not compromise the therapeutic effect, obviously it makes sense to set up weekly lower dose schedules of doxorubicin for the treatment of Hodgkin's disease.

CARDIOPULMONARY SIDE EFFECTS

Like it or not, it must be concluded that, at least in adults, mantle field radiation therapy carries a significant risk of cardiopulmonary damage, even when using "modern" radiation techniques. If a third of patients treated with mantle field radiation with or without chemotherapy already can be identified to have cardiopulmonary dysfunction, there will never be fewer, and the risk is that as time goes by a higher percentage of patients will manifest the effects of late radiation damage.

RENAL DAMAGE AFTER THERAPY

Part of the debate over the value of initial splenectomy in the treatment of Hodgkin's patients involved the concern that treating the spleen with radiation therapy might seriously compromise the left kidney and renal function in general. This has not happened. Le Bourgeois et al.[29] studied the effects of irradiation on the spleen in lymphoma patients and thus far failed to find any serious permanent consequences of radiation treatment.

Neither compensatory hypertrophy nor changes in the overall kidney function were noted, although the upper pole of the left kidney became nonfunctional. The impact, if any, on long survival remains to be seen. These authors concluded that radiotherapy has proved its efficiency in splenic involvement in Hodgkin's disease, and that serious renal side effects secondary to this radiation treatment were lacking. However, "on the other hand morbidity was shown to occur in 5% of cases after splenectomy," and therefore, "from these data, [they] proposed to prefer radiotherapy rather than surgery for splenic treatment."

INFECTION

The majority of serious infections encountered in adults treated for Hodgkin's disease, with or without their spleens intact, have been associated with periods of retreatment for relapsing or progressive tumor and associated with chemotherapeutic leukopenia and suppression of immune function.[30-32] In Chapter 18, Donaldson notes: "Yet in the Stanford series, 52% of the episodes of serious bacterial infection in [splenectomized] children occurred months or years following completion of treatment among a population presumed to be cured of their Hodgkin's disease. Infection in this setting has been observed as an initial event at 13 years following therapy, with 4 of 12 of the treatment episodes being fatal." It is this group of 12 patients originally reported by Donaldson and Kaplan[33] that were "perhaps more alarming" because these patients developed their serious infections months and even years following completion of treatment, in a population presumed to be cured of Hodgkin's disease. In the Stanford experience, four of the off-treatment episodes were fatal resulting in a mortality rate for the whole group of 4%. It is the splenectomized patient with Hodgkin's disease who is at special risk for developing a late fatal sepsis.

POSTSPLENECTOMY SEPSIS

Askergren and Bjorkholm analyzed postsplenectomy septicemia in Hodgkin's disease.[34] They observed that "the immediate complications of diagnostic laparotomy with splenectomy appear to be few. However, the equally important assessment of long-term risks is more difficult." By studying the frequency of splenectomy and nonsplenectomy septicemia during a 10-year period in the Stockholm area and comparing the results with splenectomized and nonsplenectomized Hodgkin's patients, they concluded (in part) that "since no non-splenectomized control HD patients developed septicemia the contribution of splenectomy per se to the lowered resistance to infection should be substantial." That is, the chemotherapy and the radiation therapy were not implicated in inducing immunodeficiency leading to septicemia, but the septicemia was a complication of the splenectomy itself.

Furthermore, any estimates of dangerous infections following splenectomy were always presumed to be underestimated because the risk of developing septicemia appears to persist for decades. In the study of Askergren and Bjorkholm, pneumococci were the only causative agent of septicemia in HD patients and pneumococcal infection also dominated among patients splenectomized for other reasons. They considered the risk of septicemia to be "entirely confined to pneumococcal infection . . ." and that "the overall risk in splenectomized persons of developing septicemia was 34 times higher than in the normal population." It was their impression that their study merely extended observations already made by others.

Although one report attributes the development of splenic atrophy and dysfunction to splenic irradiation as a significant contributing factor in the cause of overwhelming infection 12 years after successful treatment for Hodgkin's disease,[35] so far it is the splenectomized patient and not the merely irradiated patient who seems to be in the greatest danger of developing late fatal sepsis, most commonly inflicted by the encapsulated bacteria (especially pneumococci). A cautious attitude, however, would also consider all patients who have had splenic irradiation to be at risk of developing overwhelming pneumococcal sepsis, although actual observations of patients so afflicted are, practically speaking, extremely rare.

Because the predominant organisms identified as causing the serious bacterial infections are penicillin-sensitive, the routine use of prophylactic antibiotics in children with previous splenectomy should be considered. Recommendations for postsplenectomy prophylactic antibiotic therapy have varied and are evolving; exactly what physicians should recommend is still not absolutely certain.

In 1983, Rosner and Zarrabi[36] reviewed 145 postsplenectomy infections in 115 patients with Hodgkin's disease and noted that most of the infections presented clinically as pneumonia, septicemia, meningitis, or a combination of these with the most common offending organisms being pneumococci. Of the 115 patients, 50 were said to have died as a result of the infection, and at least 78 episodes of infection occurred in 48 patients who were in complete remission at the time of the infection. At that time it was their recommendation that prophylactic penicillin should be administered at least for 3 years and possibly indefinitely, since postsplenectomy infections can occur many years later; they also recommended that pneumococcal vaccine should also be given before any chemotherapy or radiotherapy is initiated.

In 1984, Zarrabi and Rosner[37] reviewed the case reports of 47 adults with serious infections following splenectomy for trauma. They concluded that fulminant sepsis after splenectomy for trauma in the absence of Hodgkin's disease in adults is also a potential risk and that all such patients should receive penicillin prophylaxis and pneumococcal vaccine.

In 1986, the same authors[38] observed that, although all splenectomized individuals are at risk of developing pneumococcal sepsis, most reports fail to mention how many patients are given prophylactic penicillin therapy. Thus it is really impossible to evaluate the usefulness of penicillin prophylaxis. They reviewed 14 reported cases of postsplenectomy bacterial sepsis in patients receiving prophylactic penicillin therapy. In only 5 cases did the patients have a penicillin-sensitive pneumococcal infection. On the presumption that penicillin prophylaxis might prevent at least some cases of infection, it was now recommended that treatment be carried on for a lifetime.

The absence of data concerning prophylactic antibiotic therapy in splenectomized Hodgkin's patients is summarized by Chou et al.[39] in their report from the Memorial Sloan-Kettering Cancer Center on severe pneumococcal infections in patients with neoplastic disease: "Since splenectomized children at Memorial Hospital receiving prophylactic penicillin have experienced no episodes of pneumococcal bacteremia, we should consider administering prophylactic penicillin to all splenectomized patients with underlying neoplastic disease in addition to giving pneumococcal vaccine. However, there are no controlled studies to support this recommendation or the exact length of time to continue penicillin prophylaxis after splenectomy."

It is clear that neither the optimal dose, nor the optimal duration of antibiotic administration is known. It is not even certain, in the absence of any controlled studies, that penicillin prophylaxis is definitely helpful. Furthermore, the probability that patients will not and cannot fully comply with the taking of a daily dose of medication complicates and hinders any analysis of the data. In addition, even in splenectomized patients presumed to be taking penicillin prophylactically, penicillin-sensitive infections still occur. The chance of developing an allergic reaction to the penicillin must also be taken into account. All things considered, and for whatever the interpretation, the fact is that serious infections in children in the Stanford series (Chapter 18) dropped from 13 to 1% after penicillin prophylaxis was recommended.

THE VALUE OF PNEUMOCOCCAL VACCINE

As it has evolved, the pneumococcal vaccine does not appear adequate to provide long-term protection for the splenectomized Hodgkin's patient. Any confusion concerning the use of pneumococcal vaccine is magnified by statements such as that by Armstrong and Minamoto (Chapter 6): "The efficacy of the vaccine is therefore questionable, but administration prior to treatment with radiotherapy and chemotherapy is recommended."

Although Shapiro and Clemens[40] found that "pneumococcal vaccine confers substantial protection against systemic pneumococcal infections of the elderly and patients with illnesses associated with a moderate increased risk of pneumococcal infections," they also found that "the vaccine's efficacy was 77% for patients at moderately increased risk of pneumococcal infections, [and] 0% for patients who were severely immunocompromised." Their conclusions were at variance to other large randomized trials done in institutionalized and elderly American populations, since these other studies, Shapiro and Clemens noted, "yielded inconclusive evidence about the value of the vaccine." Shapiro and Clemens also reviewed the confusion presented by the Center for Disease Control reports, one of which suggested "that the vaccine may have little efficacy for patients with many of the high-risk conditions for which the vaccine is recommended."

The rarity of pneumococcal infections in general makes any study of the efficacy of the pneumococcal vaccine difficult to interpret. Even though nearly 15,000 subjects were enrolled in the two trials that ". . . found no statistically significant reduction among vaccinees in the frequencies of systemic pneumococcal infection, pneumonia, pneumonia associated with the isolation of pneumococci from sputum, or deaths from putative pneumococcal infection," according to Shapiro and Clemens there was a question of the statistical accuracy of the studies.

Although Shapiro and Clemens were inclined to recommend the use of the pneumococcal vaccine as efficacious, they hedged their reommendation based on their own data as "a single case-controlled study cannot prove that a vaccine is effective, and more studies are needed to validate our findings."

With regard to the clinical usefulness of the pneumococcal vaccine, it seems to be the case that vaccination might not to be absolutely scientifically useful, but if it does no harm, what's to lose by giving it? The point must then be made that if you do not administer the vaccine, there is evidence that you have done no harm and have not missed helping the patient, and if you do give the pneumococcal vaccine, you may have helped but there is no definite proof that it was beneficial or that you have actually assisted the patient in fighting off a pneumococcal infection.

Five years after the first administration of the previously employed dodecavalent pneumococcal vaccine, its effectiveness, especially in immunocompromised patients, splenectomized patients, or patients subsequently treated for Hodgkin's disease, is not clear. The newest pneumococcal vaccine now contains purified capsular polysaccharide from the 23 types of Streptococcus pneumoniae that are responsible for about 90% of recent bacteremic pneumococcal infection in this country. Despite this and "even with current antibiotic therapy, the mortality rate in high-risk patients hospitalized with pneumococcal bacteremia has remained higher than 25%" according to the review in the Medical Letter on Drugs and Therapeutics.[41] Their commentator indicates that the titers of pneumococcal antibody have been reported to persist for up to five years following immunization, and that the vaccine has been about 60 to 75%

effective in people with normal immune systems, including the elderly, but severely immunocompromised patients apparently are not protected.

They warned that mild erythema and pain at the injection site occur in up to half of recipients after a single dose; fever, arthralgia, and rash have been uncommon. However, because more severe local reactions have occurred after a second dose, more than one dose is not recommended, even for patients who received an older vaccine that contained fewer pneumococcal types.

In the Position Paper on Pneumococcal Vaccine by the Health and Public Policy Committee of the American College of Physicians,[42] it is noted that "the vaccine is safe," but that "local transient side effects, which may include discomfort, erythema, an induration, occur in up to 40% of recipients. Systemic side effects are infrequent and rarely severe. Fever, myalgias, and severe local reactions have been reported at a rate of five doses per million." However, "the incidence of severe local and systemic reactions is increased with revaccination."

"Recipients" of the pneumococcal vaccine, they advise, "should be informed that although the vaccine will reduce the risk of pneumococcal pneumonia substantially, it will not eliminate the risk completely. The 23 capsular-type polysaccharide antigens included in the vaccine are responsible for approximately 85% of bacteremic pneumococcal pneumonia, and several are related immunologically to types not included in the vaccine that account for additional cases of the disease. However, as with any vaccine, protection against disease caused by these types is not absolute."

Patients with Hodgkin's disease, among other disorders, are "at an increased risk of developing and succumbing to pneumococcal infection, but may not respond to the vaccine." It was the view of the Public Policy Committee that these patients may be offered the vaccine but should be informed of their potential inability to respond to it and thus be protected by it.

It seems clear that, at this writing, the recommendation is that "revaccination is not advised at this time because of the increased incidence of severe local and systemic reactions that may occur." Yet, as confusing as it may seem, the Committee of the American College of Physicians still left some room for revaccination with the newer pneumococcal vaccine in splenectomized Hodgkin's patients with the following statement: "Given the marginal additional protection offered by the new vaccine over the previous formulation, revaccination with the 23-valent vaccine generally is not recommended for people who have received the 14 valent vaccine. However, the vaccine's use may be warranted in specific persons in whom the benefits of revaccination with the new vaccine are thought to exceed the risks, such as patients who have had splenectomies."

A few years previously in recommendations made by the Immunization Practices Advisory Committee of the Centers for Disease Control, Atlanta, Georgia,[43] it was clearly stated that "Pneumococcal vaccine should be given *only once* [emphasis theirs] to adults. Arthus reactions and systemic reactions have been common among adults given second doses and are thought to result from localized antigen-antibody reactions. Therefore, second or booster doses are *not* [emphasis theirs] recommended. Data on revaccination of children are not yet sufficient to provide a basis for comment."

"Persons who have received the 14-valent pneumococcal vaccine should *not* [emphasis theirs] be revaccinated with the 23-valent vaccine, because the modest increase in coverage does not warrant the possible increased risk of adverse reactions."[43]

Donaldson and Link recently stated[15] that "we do not rely on pneumococcal vaccine as the sole protection [to prevent serious bacterial infection] because of the variability of immune responses and the poor duration of response to the vaccine."

THE VALUE OF ACYCLOVIR AND VARICELLA-ZOSTER IMMUNE GLOBULIN

Acute herpes zoster is a common cause of morbidity in Hodgkin's patients. It can result in the development of chronic pain (post–herpes neuralgia syndrome) and visceral dissemination. The search for an effective antiviral treatment continues, and acyclovir may be the first readily useful available drug. Administering intravenous acyclovir early in the course of herpes zoster infection (usually within 3 days of the onset of rash) over a period of 7 days, Balfour and his collaborators[44] concluded that "effective treatment of acute herpes zoster appears to be at hand" and that now work had to be directed toward refining the dose and administration intervals. The data supporting their conclusion, however, is a bit shaky.

In their study, acyclovir was not especially effective in controlling acute pain or the postherpetic neuralgia syndrome. The reality is that the results only "favored acyclovir," but the differences between acyclovir and placebo were not statistically significant. Therefore, any sweeping conclusions must still be considered subjective, because the impeccably recorded graphs[44] indicated that the relationship between the placebo and the acyclovir recipients with regard to the "development of new lesions," "lesions not scabbed," "pain," and "virus cultured from lesions" failed to show any clear differences between the two groups. The curves for the two groups are almost superimposable, and the authors concluded that "none of the differences are significant by the Breslow test." There was also some evidence that the acyclovir as administered intravenously in this study, was toxic in its ability to cause decreased renal function, hypotension, and other less important reactions. Because acyclovir probably does have some beneficial effect, it allows some hope for the control of herpes zoster virus, but it represents just a beginning.

Also confusing are the recommendations for the use of varicella-zoster immune globulin (VZIG) in adults exposed to chickenpox. In the first statement of the Immunization Practices Advisory Committee of the Centers for Disease Control in Atlanta, Georgia, originally published in Morbidity and Mortality Weekly Report and then in the Annals of Internal Medicine,[45] the committee concluded that "varicella-zoster immune globulin is not known to be useful in treating clinical varicella or zoster or in preventing disseminated zoster, and it is not recommended for such use." Its most important primary use is for passive immunization of susceptible, immunocompromised children with primary immunodeficiency disorders and neoplastic diseases and children currently receiving immunosuppressive treatment. VZIG definitely seems to work in children; its value in adults is much less clear.

The recommendations for the use of VZIG in adults includes its possible use in immunocompromised adults, normal adults, and pregnant women, although the data and the experience to recommend its use are mostly theoretical. For instance, the committee states that, in pregnant women, ". . . there is no evidence that administration of VZIG to a susceptible, pregnant woman will prevent viremia, fetal infection, or congenital varicella syndrome. Because most immunosuppressed persons who receive VZIG after a significant exposure develop modified clinical disease or subclinical infection, it is theoretically possible that VZIG may prevent or suppress clinical disease in the normal mother without preventing fetal infection and disease."

"In the absence of evidence that VZIG can prevent congenital varicella syndrome or neonatal varicella, the primary indication for VZIG in pregnant women is to prevent complications of varicella in a susceptible adult patient rather than to prevent intrauterine infection. Neonates born to mothers who develop varicella within the 5 days preceding or 48 hours after delivery should receive VZIG regardless of whether the mother received VZIG."

Furthermore, since "varicella-zoster immune globulin has not been evaluated as a prophylactic measure for prevention or attenuation of varicella in normal or immunocompromised adults," data does not exist with which to calculate the appropriate dose in adults. It is stated therefore that "it seems likely that 625 units should be sufficient to prevent or modify infection in normal adults. Higher doses may be needed in immunocompromised adults."[45]

Adverse events after the use of VZIG have been recorded, but severe reactions such as angioneurotic edema and anaphylactic shock, are "rare" (less than 0.1%).

Should VZIG be used in adults? The conclusion is similar to that for the pneumovaccine issue: If it can do no harm, why not use it? Jus because it cannot clearly be shown to do any good is no reason not to use it—it might be useful. Until some evidence for the usefulness and appropriate dose of VZIG in adults is established, however, the practitioner should not be condemned for failing to use it. On the other hand, if it is used and for some reason causes a severe side effect, the practitioner should not be condemned as VZIG has been recommended for use by some even in the absence of any data that indicate its effectiveness in adults.

Since the recent development of intravenous immune globulin, it has been found to modify the severity of at least one virus (cytomegalovirus) that attacks immune suppressed patients,[46] and therefore intravenous immune globulin might be considered for an experimental trial against herpes zoster infections. Herpes zoster occurs in about 20 to 30% of Hodgkin's patients, and a proportion of these patients develop the post-herpes neuralgia syndrome, which appears to last for a lifetime. There is still no clear treatment available. The hope remains that herpes zoster infection might respond to some extent to acyclovir and that eventually it will be treatable with more effective antiviral agents before it gains a strong foothold in the host.

IMMUNOCOMPETENCE IN HODGKIN'S DISEASE

Bjorkholm, Holm, and Mellstedt (Chapter 5) provide us with some insights into the immunologic puzzle of Hodgkin's disease. Long-term survivors after treatment for Hodgkin's disease are characterized by having T-cell lymphocytopenia and impairment of T-cell functions. Although it seemed that these immunodeficiencies could be attributed primarily to the effects of therapy, they may actually be genetically determined.

The high familial incidence of Hodgkin's disease led to the concept that Hodgkin's disease is partially genetically determined. One way to approach this issue is through the analysis of immunologic aberrations that characterize Hodgkin's disease. Bjorkholm, Holm and Mellstedt pose the following issues: "1. Is the immunodefect in 'cured' Hodgkin's disease patients acquired? If so, is it secondary to the tumor- or disease-associated factors that may promote and perpetuate a state of immunologic imbalance in predisposed individuals? 2. Is the immunodeficiency an inherited (genetic?) characteristic of Hodgkin's disease patients? If so, it might be detected in relatives. Moreover, it may predispose one to developing the disease and may modulate its course. An inherited immunodeficiency may also be latent and precipitated by the disease or other factors. Early immunologic aging may contribute."

After studying healthy relatives to Hodgkin's patients, it was concluded that ". . . otherwise healthy persons with a first-degree relative with Hodgkin's disease display a significantly increased frequency of T-cell impairment. These findings have led us to hypothesize that a state of T-cell impairment existed in certain patients prior to the evolution of Hodgkin's disease."

Attempting to look into the future of the long-surviving Hodgkin's patient, they address themselves to the following: "Another, and in many aspects more important, issue is whether treatment and its detrimental immunologic effects may enhance a conceivable constitutional risk to develop Hodgkin's disease. In other words, are Hodgkin's patients more prone to develop de novo Hodgkin's disease than the normal population? This might be anticipated if there is a constitutional/genetic basis for the evolution of Hodgkin's disease. To fully resolve this issue, not only Hodgkin's disease-specific markers in general, but also clonal markers will be needed. In the future, molecular genetic analyses will be demanded to differentiate between relapsing and de novo Hodgkin's disease. What we call late relapses are relatively rare 5 years or more following successful treatment. However, limited numbers of patients have survived 15 years or more following the introduction of modern radiotherapy and chemotherapy. Consequently, it remains to be seen whether this patient category will retain its low probability of 'relapse.' "

The immunologic effects of pretreatment splenectomy were also reviewed by Bjorkholm, Holm, and Mellstedt in Chapter 5.

They wrote "no immediate reduction of serum IgM was observed after splenectomy. A progressive fall in serum IgM after radiotherapy and cytotoxic drug therapy observed in long-term survivors was slightly potentiated by prior splenectomy." They concluded, ". . . splenectomy seems to protect patients from therapy-induced lymphocytopenia and it contributes to the delayed reduction of serum IgM. No major changes in delayed skin hypersensitivity of T-cell functions in vitro can be ascribed to splenectomy. The asplenic state, reduced IgM levels, and possibly impaired B-cell responses contribute to the persistent life-long threat of overwhelming postsplenectomy infections in splenectomized patients with Hodgkin's disease."

STAGING AND SPLENECTOMY

The spleen remains an organ that is impossible to assess accurately until it is removed for meticulous pathologic examination. The determination of splenic involvement cannot be made by inspection at laparoscopy (peritoneoscopy will never substitute for laparotomy/splenectomy, for as DeVita and his colleagues[47] once noted, "Splenectomy cannot be performed through a peritoneoscope . . ."), or palpation of the spleen, or by currently available imaging techniques. The entire spleen must be studied with serial sectioning at millimeter intervals. Even after such meticulous analysis, Hodgkin's disease might still be present and not be diagnosed.

A major problem associated with staging laparotomy and splenectomy is the incomplete information obtained, whether by the casual surgeon who only rarely performs this procedure or even by the meticulous, experienced surgeon. The technique of exploration in this special situation cannot be equated with a simple splenectomy. Much more information is being sought. The more extensive surgery required to explore the retroperitoneal space properly must be anticipated in advance. The surgeon should thoroughly acquaint himself with the preoperative lymphangiogram (all patients with Hodgkin's disease should have a lymphangiogram prior to laparotomy unless there is some absolute contraindication to the procedure). The surgeon is responsible for the systematic removal of the spleen, liver biopsy samples, node samples, and in some instances transposition of the ovaries. Appendectomy is usually performed as part of the procedure, because if a postoperative abdominal crisis occurs, it is extremely helpful to know that the appendix has been removed.[48]

The surgeon must systematically mark each area of dissection to assist the postoperative evaluation of the work accomplished at surgery (were the suspicious nodes visualized on the preoperative lymphangiogram actually removed?) and to assist the radiation therapist in future treatment planning. Despite the most meticulous surgery, the failure to obtain complete node samples must be anticipated. Partly because there is still a high probability that Hodgkin's tumor was missed and left behind even after the most meticulous staging laparotomy/splenectomy has been declared "negative" that almost all treatment programs for Hodgkin's disease include extended radiation fields with or without the use of combined chemotherapy as primary treatment.[49,50]

Assessing the risk versus the benefit of primary diagnostic surgical staging laparotomy/splenectomy and accounting for the post-surgical complications will probably become moot issues as the movement toward ending staging laparotomy/splenectomy takes hold.[51-55] Especially among the pediatric Hodgkin's population, staging laparotomy/splenectomy has already been abandoned, because these patients are being treated with combined modality therapy (limited radiation therapy and multidrug chemotherapy) as primary therapy.[54] Staging surgery is becoming very selective, rather than "routine."

Some investigators continue to rely upon operative staging of most children to establish a staging category, but then treat their young patients with combined radiation therapy and chemotherapy as primary treatment anyway.[55] The current preference to use combined radiation therapy and multidrug chemotherapy as primary therapy of Hodgkin's disease in children is based on the discovery that primary intensive radiation therapy alone resulted not only in growth abnormalities, primarily affecting the vertebral growth centers in susceptible children, but that combined initial radiation/chemotherapy approach appears to have improved overall survival while reducing the complications. For many pediatric oncologists, this protocol also ended the need to perform a staging laparotomy/splenectomy.

Bergsagel et al. of the Ontario Cancer Clinic and the Princess Margaret Hospital[52] reviewed their survival data on treating adult Hodgkin's patients without a policy of laparotomy staging, and they compared their results with the Stanford data using staging laparotomy.[57] These authors came to the "general conclusion that two widely different policies of investigating and treating patients with Hodgkin's disease have resulted in similar survival results. . . "

In prospective randomized studies, Gomez et al.[53] and Askergren et al.[57] analyzed the prognostic effect of diagnostic splenectomy in Hodgkin's disease and found that it did not improve prognosis. "Rather," Askergren et al. concluded, "it may lead to surgical complications, increased risk of severe infections and may be associated with earlier relapse of disease."[57]

As mentioned in Chapter 15 by Zimbalist and Shike, if laparotomy is avoided, then bowel obstruction related to adhesions, which were reported to range between 3 and 4% in various series following the surgical procedure, can be eliminated completely. The surgical mortality associated with laparotomy alone should not be totally ignored.

Another important factor in assessing the value of staging laparotomy prior to therapy is the fact that less than 10% of cases may be "down-staged" while 20% are "up-staged" after laparotomy. To allay fears that patients might be overtreated because of incorrect clinical staging, under the best circumstances, less than 10% of pediatric patients would be affected (7.5% or 10/133 were "down-staged" in the Stanford pediatric series).[53] This presumes, of course, that analysis of the laparotomy material is so meticulous that tumors are never missed and the surgical techniques are so perfect that no abnormal node is ever overlooked.

Evaluation of the results of treatment might also be unfairly influenced if clinically staged patients treated before the advent of "modern" radiation and chemotherapy regimens are compared to patients treated more currently. The review of pediatric Hodgkin's patients from Stanford University is an example of this type of comparison.[58] They compared the results of treatment of a cohort of patients (46 out of 133) who were diagnosed before July 1968, and who did not have laparotomy but who also might not have benefitted from advances in chemotherapy.

Conclusions based on this type of selective retrospective comparison might have been foregone even before any analysis was made. Relapsing patients treated prior to 1968 could not benefit from the advances made in salvage chemotherapy. Even the primary radiation therapy may not have been up to modern standards in the pre-1968, clinically assessed patients. Therefore, the presentation of a "fact" that pediatric "patients who were clinically staged and managed with primary radiation have only a 69% survival (p = 0.05)" when compared to laparotomy-staged pediatric patients, of whom "86% are alive at 10 years after primary radiation with chemotherapy reserved for relapse compared with 90% managed by planned combined modality therapy (p = 0.62)"[58] must be judged on the basis of the bias of the primary data itself.

CAN SPLENECTOMY AND ITS LATE COMPLICATIONS BE AVOIDED?

It has been implied that "careful staging" and laparotomy/splenectomy were necessary for improved survival results. Neither in the pediatric nor the adult populations with Hodgkin's disease is the staging laparotomy/splenectomy per se a clear factor that results in long survival.[52–54,57] More likely, it was the discovery, after staging laparotomy was first performed, that more tumor existed below the diaphragm than anyone had ever expected that led to the use of more extensive primary radiation and chemotherapy. The more intense and more extended primary radiation therapy plus additional primary chemotherapy is the reason for the improved survival, not the laparotomy/splenectomy per se. Removal of the spleen itself has not had a salutary therapeutic influence; in fact, the concern is the opposite. Does removal of the spleen, for instance, make surviving Hodgkin's patients more vulnerable to unusual infections for the rest of their lives?

STAGING LAPAROTOMY PER SE DOES NOT INFLUENCE SURVIVAL IN A POSITIVE WAY

According to Donaldson (Chapter 5), among children subjected to staging laparotomy, the subset aged 10 years and less have a 5-year relapse-free survival of 83%, and adolescents aged 11 years or more, like their adult counterparts, have only a 61% relapse-free 5-year survival rate. On the other hand, in a large series of children from France, Bayle-Weisgerber et al.[59] matched the generally achieved actuarial survival rate for all patients of 90% at 5 years and 81% at 10 years despite the fact that only 30 of 178 patients in this series were subjected to laparotomy. It is now expected that a 90% overall 5-year survival rate can be achieved in children by utilizing reduced radiotherapy volumes and doses plus multidrug chemotherapy without surgical staging.

Sutcliffe et al.,[49] from the Princess Margaret Hospital in Toronto, Canada, summarized the reasons why the staging laparotomy taught us to treat apparently localized Hodgkin's disease more extensively, indicating that the laparotomy/splenectomy was not in itself the reason for the current experience of improved survival. They commented: "The following circumstances must, however, be acknowledged: (1) that the risk of upper abdominal disease in clinical stages I and II Hodgkin's disease is now generally accepted, (2) that institutions reporting the most favorable control rates with radiation treat upper abdominal nodes despite negative laparotomy results, (3) that upper abdominal relapse occurs in patients with pathologic stages I and II supradiaphragmatic disease at an unacceptable level when 'mantle' radiation alone is used, and (4) that adverse features within the designation of supradiaphragmatic stages I and II disease are also recognized to be important determinants of treatment strategy."

Thus, not only does effective radiation treatment strategy necessitate incorporation of anatomic sites in excess of those defined by laparotomy, but optimal treatment strategy increasingly incorporates clinical information in addition to "stage" of disease. These views are similar to the analysis of data from the University of Rochester Cancer Center by Zagars and Rubin[31] that the "striking therapeuic gains in Stage IA and IIA supradiaphragmatic HD [resulted] from the use of prophylactic periaortic XRT [radiotherapy] and MAC [multiagent chemotherapy] salvage for relapsing patients."

In time, we will dispense with the staging laparotomy/splenectomy as a diagnostic tool for all patients with Hodgkin's disease. "Extensive surgery to define the extent of disease below the diaphragm should no longer be necessary if chemotherapy proves capable of reaching all possible foci of disease" and the laparotomy/splenectomy procedure "will eventually be recalled only as a milestone in the history of Hodgkin's disease management, important at one time but abandoned because it was no longer needed."[60]

PREGNANCY AFTER TREATMENT

Thirty-five years ago, in what might be considered the early dawn of the effective treatment of Hodgkin's disease, Barry, Diamond and Craver analyzed the data concerning the influence of pregnancy on the course of Hodgkin's disease on all patients "reporting clinical onset of symptoms between the childbearing years of 18 and 40" who had been admitted to the Memorial Hospital and James Ewing Hospital between 1910 and 1959.[61] The major purpose of this analysis was to help answer the dilemma concerning "the influence of pregnancy on the course of Hodgkin's disease," which had been "a source of controversy for many decades." It is a credit to their careful analysis that their conclusions are still true today. That is, pregnancy has no adverse effect on either the course or longevity of patients with Hodgkin's disease, nor is there evidence that being born to a mother who had Hodgkin's disease or who was successfully treated for Hodgkin's disease adversely affects the health of the infant. The subtle, long-term late effects of these pregnancies and their issue are still unknown.

Barry et al. asked the question: "But what should one say to the young woman with Hodgkin's disease who wants to become pregnant?"[61] It is in the answer to this question that the effects of time and the marked improvement in life expectancy of all patients become apparent and we part company with the past: Only in 1962 did Barry et al. comment: "Advising the young woman suffering from an incurable disease but deeply desirous of having children is difficult at best. Even though pregnancy itself may do no demonstrable harm, the morbidity of the disease itself must be taken into consideration." Today we take such an optimistic view of the potential for long survival of the Hodgkin's patient that the word "incurable" never passes our lips. Once the patient has completed the primary course of therapy, we generally advise that she should go about her business in a "normal" fashion. That, of course, includes her getting pregnant as suits her social instincts.

On the other hand, the advice of Barry, Diamond, and Craver to the patient with active disease is still sound and worth following. Chronically relapsing patients with Hodgkin's disease would be ill-advised to become pregnant. The authors' view that "certainly a woman with active disease during the first and second year of illness should be advised against entering pregnancy" is based on the observation that poorly controlled, chronically relapsing patients are continually faced with the prospect of repetitive bouts of sickness even if they survive for long periods. Practically speaking, women who find themselves caught up in the monumental task of trying to survive recurring bouts of relapsing Hodgkin's disease do not usually seek to become pregnant. But since so many of our patients now enter complete remission after radiation, or radiation and chemotherapy, little in the way of medical contraindications exist for those who want to get pregnant.

The opinion that "castration commonly appears to be the price of cure in patients treated with chemotherapy for Hodgkin's disease," which has been emphasized by Chapman,[62] Sutcliffe,[63] and Waxman,[64] applies primarily to women who require extensive multidrug chemotherapy to stay alive. Sterility is an unfortunate side effect of Hodgkin's treatment that is difficult to avoid in certain individuals. Most vulnerable are male patients. The average female Hodgkin's patient, however, retains fertility despite most therapy.

FERTILITY IN FEMALE HODGKIN'S PATIENTS

Female patients treated primarily with radiation therapy that avoids direct irradiation of the ovaries, even with the addition of chemotherapy, retain a high level of fertility. Different chemotherapy regimens have different effects on the ovaries, and the least amount of chemotherapy is usually better. Amazingly, female fertility persisted after primary treatment using combined radiation and chemotherapy (combining thiotepa, vinblastine, vincristine, prednisone, and procarbazine) over a period of 6 months,[65] or after radiation therapy and MOPP (nitrogen mustard, Oncovin, prednisone, and procarbazine) primarily for a period of 3 months,[66] or after a wide variety of chemotherapies and varying radiation fields.[67] However, in women over the age of 25 in one series[68] and over the age of 30 in other series,[65-67] the frequency of amenorrhea definitely increased when the patients received a variety of different multidrug chemotherapies.

FERTILITY IN MALE HODGKIN'S PATIENTS

In men, the story is different. Evidence shows that prior to any therapy but after the diagnosis of Hodgkin's disease, as many as 70% of men may have abnormal semen with a decreased chance for fertility.[69] When their sperm was tested for density and motility in anticipation of cryopreservation prior to treatment, a decreased number of motile sperm as well as a poor grade of motility was discovered.[70]

As few as 20% of men have any sperm present after completion of various chemotherapeutic regimens. The type of chemotherapy and the amount of drug does make a difference to the outcome. By limiting the MOPP chemotherapy to three cycles or less, da Cunha et al.[71] showed that recovery of spermatogenesis following treatment-induced azoospermia was significantly higher. After giving more than three cycles of MOPP, "recovery of spermatogenesis is rare or absent." Other therapies, such as TVPP[72] and ABVD, have been reported to result in less gonadal toxicity than MOPP.[73]

Because of a high probability of inducing sterility after chemotherapy, every effort should be made to cryopreserve sperm before treatment in anticipation of future attempts at artificial insemination. In two different analyses,[70,74] successful artificial insemination was accomplished in Hodgkin's patients. Three out of 15 patients attempting artificial insemination in Redman's group of Hodgkin's patients were successful.

Not every male patient who undergoes radiation therapy or combination chemotherapy and radiation therapy wants to have any or more children. Lacher and Toner[72] analyzed 30 men with a median age of 27.5 years who received primary treatment of Hodgkin's disease with sequential radiation therapy and multidrug chemotherapy. All patients received radiation therapy and six months of sequential chemotherapy (thiotepa, vinblastine, vincristine, procarbazine, prednisone, prednisolone) as their primary treatment. Twenty-six patients (87%) are presently surviving. The median survival from the time of diagnosis is 64.7 months (range: 13 months to 111.4 months). Twenty-five patients are in their first complete remission; one patient relapsed 31 months postdiagnosis and is presently being treated with multidrug chemotherapy.

Before being diagnosed with Hodgkin's disease, 16 patients were married and interested in having children. The wives of 14 of these patients had 24 pregnancies (23 births and 1 miscarriage) prior to the diagnosis of Hodgkin's disease. Five patients married after the completion of therapy, bringing the number of married patients who had completed therapy to 21. Only 10 of the 21 married patients were interested in having children. Seven patients already had established families and 4 were too sick to even consider the problem of fertility. Five of the ten patients or 50% of those actually desiring to have children successfully impregnated their wives, producing six normal births.

The ability of men to father children after treatment for Hodgkin's disease may be greater than previously thought provided the type of chemotherapy administered gives them the chance. Limiting the cycles of MOPP therapy[73] or using an alternative chemotherapy to MOPP is one way to accomplish this. We recognize that the results of Hodgkin's treatment are imperfect and that not every patient can have both a treatment that saves life and a treatment that also guarantees the preservation of fertility.

SPERM BANKING DOES NOT APPEAR TO INCREASE CONGENITAL ABNORMALITIES

In a review concerning the general usefulness of sperm banking, Rothman noted that "in a recent series of 520 children resulting from insemination with frozen sperm, one percent had congenital abnormalities and eight percent resulted in spontaneous abortions. These percentages are lower than those that occur in the general population. Human sperm stored for up to 10 years have been effective in conception."[75]

IS HODGKIN'S DISEASE INHERITED?

In Chapter 11 it was noted that "A large number of families have been reported to have multiple occurrences of Hodgkin's disease. The risk of a patient's first-order relatives developing Hodgkin's disease has been estimated as threefold to ninefold. A relative risk of 7.1 was found for siblings in another study," and "a recent analysis in Scotland found a four-fold increase in deaths due to Hodgkin's disease among first- and second-degree relatives of patients."

Redman et al. also concluded in Chapter 11 that "there is a genetic basis for Hodgkin's disease but the magnitude is not great." Inheritance is a factor in the development of Hodgkin's disease, but to what degree is poorly understood.

TREATMENT PLANNING FOR HODGKIN'S DISEASE WILL ALWAYS BE EVOLVING UNTIL THE ABSOLUTELY BEST TECHNIQUES ARE DETERMINED

We understand and recognize the seriousness of the potential late side effects of the therapy for Hodgkin's disease and will always subject our results to constant long-term analysis. This will result in adjustments in the treatment techniques as more knowledge and even newer techniques are learned. Sacroscanct views and pronouncements about exactly what is right and what is wrong must be viewed with some philosophical leeway until the final word is in.

The changes in attitude toward the use of combined radiation therapy and chemotherapy provide a good example of this evolution. Initially it was touted that leukemia would overwhelm Hodgkin's patients treated primarily with combined radiation and chemotherapy. Now, in fact, the use of combined radiation therapy and chemotherapy has become a common recommended primary therapy.

Cunningham et al.,[76] for instance, in their review of the long-term complications of MOPP chemotherapy in patients with Hodgkin's disease made the observation that ". . . it appears that stage IIIA patients treated with initial combined radiation therapy and chemotherapy may have a better survival than patients treated with radiation therapy alone, with chemotherapy reserved for relapse. This indicates that, for stage IIIA patients, MOPP may not be as effective for relapse as for initial use."

In 1984, Dorreen et al.[77] reported concerning the management of Stage II supradiaphragmatic Hodgkin's disease at St. Bartholomew's Hospital, London, England. They concluded that, despite the striking heterogeneity within a single substage of Hodgkin's disease (Stage II), there was an adverse influence on mediastinal/hilar disease on freedom from relapse following mantle radiation therapy that extended beyond a consideration of the tumor volume alone. Their results suggested that the presence of any intrathoracic disease is a poor prognostic factor of major importance. They pointed out that "it is likely that all such patients require intensification of primary treatment aimed at permanent sterilization of disease. Although modifications of RT might achieve this goal, the use of MVPP and adjuvant mantle RT has resulted in significant 'cure' rates for patients with otherwise unfavorable presentations of nodal disease."

In 1987, Willet et al.[78] reported that "extensive disease, as estimated by the number of sites of involvement at presentation, degree of splenic involvement, extent of intra-abdominal disease or mediastinal involvement, did not reveal statistically significant prognostic subgroups for relapse. It is currently recommended that patients with Stage 3A Hodgkin's disease receive six cycles of multiagent chemotherapy and mantle and para-aortic irradiation."

Jenkin et al.[54] led the movement to end staging splenectomy in children and to treat almost all of them immediately with combined limited radiation and multidrug chemotherapy. Donaldson and Link of Stanford[15] have now joined in that movement in at least a partial way, by more selectively using staging laparotomy/splenectomy and by treating their pediatric patients with primary combined limited radiation therapy plus multidrug chemotherapy.

Therefore, despite initial fears concerning the potential development of secondary leukemia in patients with Hodgkin's disease, it appears that primary combined radiation therapy and chemotherapy constitute the best approach for at least 70% of the patients. The development of leukemia per se has turned out not to be as much of a problem for the Hodgkin's disease patient as the late development of solid tumors. The development of solid tumors is probably primarily associated with the radiation therapy rather than the chemotherapy. Therefore, limiting radiation therapy, and possibly even eliminating it in time may be the goal for the future.

THE CURRENT TREATMENTS DO CREATE UNIQUE LATE SERIOUS SIDE EFFECTS, BUT THE OVERALL IMPACT FOR THE MAJORITY OF HODGKIN'S PATIENTS HAS BEEN THE ACHIEVEMENT OF LONG SURVIVAL

By using formidable, potentially toxic therapeutic techniques of high-dose large-field radiation therapy and multidrug chemotherapy we have significantly prolonged the lives of the majority of the patients with Hodgkin's disease. In the beginning our goals were clear. Our old techniques of low-energy, limited-field radiation therapy and limited or non-existent chemotherapy had not allowed the majority of Hodgkin's patients to achieve long survival. Late complications or side-effects were not a problem, as not enough patients survived long enough for us to develop a great concern about this problem. We tried, therefore, at first without counting the possible late price to be paid, to get people with all stages of Hodgkin's disease to survive as long as possible. We have partially achieved that goal, and for the first time in history we will have a substantial number of patients entering "real time" survival periods of ten plus years.

Now we are just beginning to determine the cost of that initial flush of success. Clinical evaluation studies are just beginning to appear that investigate the delayed effects of the treatment itself (surgery-laparotomy/splenectomy, radiation therapy, chemotherapy) on the survivors. Since a large cohort of Hodgkin's survivors have not yet lived for 15 years since the end of their treatment, most studies currently being reported refer to a limited number of patients followed for very short periods of their lives. Obviously, this limited follow-up time can only underestimate the potential seriousness of the side effects.

We recognize that the therapy that we have employed to achieve long survival for the majority of patients is damaging to multiple organ systems. Because we have been able to indulge in the good results with a large number of long survivors, we must now take a closer look at what iatrogenic disease we may have introduced and determine how we can change our therapy to improve survival and reduce both the early and late side effects. For example, adjustments in the primary treatment of children, in particular, have already been adopted to reduce or eliminate some of the unwanted late side effects of radiation therapy. Meanwhile, we must accept the fact that in the process of "curing" we are also damaging, and it remains to be seen just how much damage has been done.

The final exact treatment for every Hodgkin's patient is still in flux. Eventually the least toxic therapies will be identified (or discovered in the future), and these will be chosen as the treatment of choice.

REFERENCES

1. Ingelfinger, F.J. Health: A matter of statistics or feeling? N. Engl. J. Med. 296:448–449, 1977.
2. Lacher, M.J. Long survival in Hodgkin's disease. Ann. Int. Med. 70:7–17, 1969.
3. Zagars, G., and Rubin, P. Hodgkin's disease stages IA and IIA. A long term follow-up study on the gains achieved by modern therapy. Cancer 56:1905–1912, 1985.
4. Peters, V.M. Prophylactic treatment of adjacent areas in Hodgkin's disease. Cancer Res. 26:1232–1240, 1966.
5. Kaplan, H.S. The radical radiotherapy of regionally localized Hodgkin's disease. Radiology 78:553–561, 1962.
6. Glatstein, E., Guernsey, J.M., Rosenberg, S.A., Kaplan, H.S. The value of laparotomy and splenectomy in the staging of Hodgkin's disease. Cancer 24:709–718, 1969.
7. Herman, T.S., Hoppe, R.T., Donaldson, M.D., et al. Late relapse among patients treated for Hodgkin's. Ann. Intern. Med. 102:292–297, 1985.
8. Lacher, M.J., and Durant, J.T. Combined vinblastine and chlorambucil therapy of Hodgkin's disease. Ann. Intern. Med. 62:468–476, 1965.
9. DeVita, V.T., Jr., Simon, R.M., Hubbard, S.M., et al. Curability of advanced Hodgkin's disease with chemotherapy: Long-term follow-up of MOPP treated patients at the National Cancer Institute. Ann. Intern. Med. 92:587–595, 1980.
10. Bonnadonna, G., Zucali, R., Monfardini, S., et al. Combination chemotherapy of Hodgkin's disease wih adriamycin, bleomycin, vinblastine, and imidazole carboxamide versus MOPP. Cancer 36:252–259, 1975.
11. Ferrant, A., Vincent, H., Binon, J., et al. Combined modality therapy for mediastinal Hodgkin's disease—prognostic significance of constitutional symptoms and size of disease. Cancer 55:317–322, 1985.
12. Dembo, A.J.: Editorial. Time dose factors in chemotherapy: Expanding the concept of dose-intensity. Clin. Oncol. 5:694–696, 1987.
13. Levin, L., and Hryniuk, W.M. Dose intensity analysis of chemotherapy regimens in ovarian carcinoma. J. Clin. Oncol. 5:456–469, 1987.
14. Easson, E.C. Long-term results of radical radiotherapy in Hodgkin's disease. Cancer Res. 27:1244–1249, 1966.
15. Donaldson, S.S., and Link, M.P. Combined modality treatment with low-dose radiation and MOPP chemotherapy for children with Hodgkin's disease. J. Clin. Oncol. 5:742–749, 1987.

16. Eghbali, H., Hoerni-Simon, G., de Mascarel, I., et al. Hodgkin's disease in the elderly. Cancer 53:2191–2193, 1984.
17. Austin-Seymour, M.M., Hoppe, R.T., Cox, R.S., et al. Hodgkin's disease in patients over sixty years old. Ann. Intern. Med. 100:13–18, 1984.
18. Hung, S.J., Jhung, J.W., and Anagnostou, A.A. Recurrence of Hodgkin's disease 29 years later. Cancer 61:186–188, 1988.
19. Longo, D.L., Young, R.C., and DeVita, V.T., Jr. Chemotherapy for Hodgkin's disease: The remaining challenges. Cancer Treat. Rep. 66:928–936, 1982.
20. Blayney, D.W., Longo, D.L., Young, R.C., et al. Decreasing risk of leukemia with prolonged follow-up after chemotherapy and radiotherapy for Hodgkin's disease. N. Engl. J. Med. 316:710–714, 1987.
21. Boivin, J.F., Hutchison, G.B., Lyden, M., et al. Second primary cancers following treatment for Hodgkin's disease. JNCI 72(2):233–241 1984.
22. Olsen, J.H. Risk of second cancer after cancer in childhood. Cancer 57:2250–2254, 1986.
23. Tucker, M.A., Coleman, M.D., Cox, R.S,. et al. Risk of second cancers after treatment for Hodgkin's disease. N. Engl. J. Med. 318:76–81, 1988.
24. Research News: Atomic bomb doses reassessed. Science 238:1649–1651, 1987.
25. Gomez, G.A., Park, J.J., Panahon, A.M., et al. Heart size and function after radiation therapy to the mediastinum in patients with Hodgkin's disease. Cancer Treat. Rep. 67:1099–1103, 1983.
26. Pohjola-Sinonen, S., Totterman, K.-J., Salmo, M., and Siltanen, P. Late cardiac effects of mediastinal radiotherapy in patients with Hodgkin's disease. Cancer 60:31–37, 1987.
27. Perrault, D.J., Levy, M., Herman, J.D., et al. Echocardiographic abnormalities following cardiac radiation. J. Clin. Oncol. 3:546–551, 1985.
28. Green, D.M., Gingell, R.L., Pearce J., et al. The effect of mediastinal irradiation on cardiac function of patients treated during childhood and adolescence for Hodgkin's disease. J. Clin. Oncol. 5:239–245, 1987.
29. Le Bourgeois, J.P., Meignan, M., Parmentier C., Tubiana, M. Renal consequences of irradiation of the spleen in lymphoma patients. Br. J. Radiol. 52:56–60, 1979.
30. Casazza A.R., Duvall, C.P., and Carbone, P.P. Summary of infectious complications occurring in patients with Hodgkin's disease. Cancer Res. 26:1290–1296, 1966.
31. Schimpff, S.C., O'Connell, M.J., Greene, W.H., and Wiernik, P.H. Infections in 92 splenectomized patients with Hodgkin's disease: A clinical review. Amer. J. Med. 59:695–701, 1975.
32. Ahmed, M.D., Lacher, M.J., Lyden, M., et al. Infections in Hodgkin's disease: An analysis of risk factors. Unpublished data, 1987.
33. Donaldson, S.S., and Kaplan, H.S. Complications of treatment of Hodgkin's disease in children. Cancer Treat. Rep. 66:977–989, 1982.
34. Askergren, J., and Bjorkholm, M. Post-splenectomy septicemia in Hodgkin's disease and other disorders. Acta Chir. Scand. 146:569–575, 1980.
35. Coleman, C.N., McDougall, I.R., Daily, M.O., et al. Functional hyposplenia after splenic irradiation for Hodgkin's disease. Ann. Intern. Med. 96:44–47, 1982.
36. Rosner, F., and Zarrabi, M.H. Late infections following splenectomy in Hodgkin's disease. Cancer Invest. 1:57–65, 1983.
37. Zarrabi, M.H., and Rosner, F. Serious infections in adults following splenectomy for trauma. Arch. Intern. Med. 144:1421–1424, 1984.
38. Zarrabi, M.H., and Rosner, F. Rarity of failure of penicillin prophylaxis to prevent postsplenectomy sepsis. Arch. Intern. Med. 146:1207–1208, 1986.
39. Chou, M., Brown, A.E., Blevins, A., Armstrong, D. Severe pneumococcal infection in patients with neoplastic disease. Cancer 51:1546–1550, 1983.
40. Shapio, E.D., and Clemens, J.D. A controlled evaluation of the protective efficacy of pneumococcal vaccine for patients at high risk of serious pneumococcal infections. Ann. Intern. Med. 101:325–330, 1984.
41. The Medical Letter on Drugs and Therapeutics: Routine Immunization for Adults. Pneumococcal vaccine. 27:99, 1985.
42. Position Paper on Pneumococcal Vaccine by the Health and Public Policy Committee of the American College of Physicians, Philadelphia, Pennsylvania. Ann. Intern. Med. 104:118–120, 1986.
43. Update: Pneumococcal polysaccharide vaccine usage—United States. Recommendation of the Immunization Practices Advisory Committee. Ann. Intern. Med. 101:348–350, 1984.
44. Balfour, H.H., Jr., Bean, B., Laskin, O.L., et al. Acyclovir halts progression of Herpes zoster in immunocompromised patients. N. Engl. J. Med. 308:1448–1453, 1983.
45. Centers for Disease Control, Department of Health and Human Services, Immunization Practices Advisory Committee. Varicella-zoster immune globulin for the prevention of chickenpox. Ann. Intern. Med. 100:859–865, 1984.
46. Winston, D.J., Ho, W.G., Lin, C.L., et al. Intravenous immune globulin for prevention of cytomegalovirus infection and interstitial pneumonia after bone marrow transplantation. Ann. Intern. Med. 106:12–18, 1987.
47. Devita, V.T. Jr., Bagley, C.M., Goodell, B., et al. Peritoneoscopy in the staging of Hodgkin's disease. Cancer Res. 31:1746–1750, 1970.
48. Paglia, M., Hertz, R.E.L. Surgical technique for laparotomy and splenectomy in Hodgkin's disease. In Hodgkin's Disease, edited by M.J. Lacher, New York, John Wiley & Sons, 1976.
49. Sutcliffe, S.B., Gospodorowicz, M.K., Bergsagel, D.E., et al. Prognostic groups for management of localized Hodgkin's disease. J. Clin. Oncol. 3:393–401, 1985.
50. Lacher, M.J. Staging laparotomy in patients with Hodgkin's disease. In Hodgkin's Disease, edited by M.J. Lacher, New York, John Wiley & Sons, 1976.
51. Lacher, M.J. Routine staging laparotomy for patients with Hodgkin's disease is no longer necessary. Cancer Invest. 1:93–99, 1983.
52. Bergsagel, D.E., Alison, R.E., Bean, H.A., et al. Re-

sults of treating Hodgkin's disease without a policy of laparotomy staging. Cancer Treat. Rep. 66:717–731, 1982.
53. Gomez, G.A., Reese P.A., Nava, H., et al. Staging laparotomy and splenectomy in early Hodgkin's disease. No therapeutic benefit. Am. J. Med. 77:205–210, 1984.
54. Jenkin, D., Chan, H., Freedman, M., et al. Hodgkin's disease in children: Treatment results with MOPP and low-dose, extended-field irradiation. Cancer Treat. Rep. 66:949–959, 1982.
55. Kaplan, H.S. Hodgkin's Disease. 2nd ed., Cambridge, MA, Harvard University Press, 1980, p. 689.
56. Donaldson, S.S., and Link, M.P. Combined modality treatment with low-dose radiation and MOPP chemotherapy for children with Hodgkin's disease. J. Clin. Oncol. 5:742–749, 1987.
57. Askergren, J., Bjorkholm, M., Holm, G., et al. Prognostic effect of early diagnostic splenectomy in Hodgkin's disease. A randomized trial. Br. J. Cancer 42:284–290, 1980.
58. Russell, K.J., Donaldson, S.S., Cox, R.S., and Kaplan, H.S. Childhood Hodgkin's disease: Patterns of relapse. J. Clin. Oncol. 2:80–87, 1984.
59. Bayle-Weisgerber C., et al. Hodgkin's disease in children. Results of therapy in a mixed group of 178 clinical and pathologically staged patients over 13 years. Cancer 54:215–222, 1984.
60. Lacher, M.J. Laparotomy and splenectomy in Hodgkin's disease. Hosp. Pract. 6(8):87–100, 1971.
61. Barry, R.M., Diamond, H.D., and Craver, L.F. Influence of pregnancy on the course of Hodgkin's disease. Am. J. Obstet. Gynecol. 84:445–454, 1962.
62. Chapman, R.M., Sutcliffe, S.B., and Malpas, J.S. Cytotoxic-induced ovarian failure in women with Hodgkin's disease: Hormone function. JAMA 242:1877–1881, 1979.
63. Sutcliffe, S.B. Cytotoxic chemotherapy and gonadal function in patients with Hodgkin's disease. JAMA 242:1898–1899, 1979.
64. Waxman, J.H.X., Terry, Y.A., Wrigley, P.F.M., et al. Gonadal function in Hodgkin's disease: Long-term follow-up of chemotherapy. Br. Med. J. 285:1612–1613, 1982.
65. Lacher, M.J., and Toner, K. Pregnancies and menstrual function before and after combined radiation (RT) and chemotherapy (TVPP) for Hodgkin's disease. Cancer Invest. 4:93–100, 1986.
66. Andrieu, J.M., Ochoa-Molina, M.E. Menstrual cycle, pregnancies and offspring before and after MOPP therapy for Hodgkin's disease. Cancer 52:435–438, 1983.
67. Horning, S.J., Hoppe, R.T., Kaplan, H.S., et al. Female reproductive potential after treatment for Hodgkin's disease. N. Engl. J. Med. 304:1377–1382, 1981.
68. Schilsky, R.L., Sherins, R.J., Hubbard, S.M., et al. Long-term follow-up of ovarian function in women treated with MOPP chemotherapy for Hodgkin's disease. Am. J. Med. 71:552–556, 1981.
69. Reed, E., Sanger, W.G., Armitage, J.O. Results of semen cryopreservation in young men with testicular carcinoma and lymphoma. J. Clin. Oncol. 4:537–539, 1986.
70. Redman, J.R., Bajorunas, D.R., Goldstein, M.C., et al. Semen cryopreservation and artificial insemination for Hodgkin's disease. J. Clin. Oncol. 5:233–238, 1987.
71. da Cunha, M.F., Meistrich, M.L., Fuller, L.M., et al. Recovery of spermatogenesis after treatment for Hodgkin's disease: Limiting dose of MOPP chemotherapy. J. Clin. Oncol. 2:571–577, 1984.
72. Lacher, M.J., and Toner, K. Evaluation of the impact of combined radiation therapy and chemotherapy using thiotepa, vinblastine, vincristine, prednisone, procarbazine (RT/TVPP) on reproductive system of male Hodgkin's patients. Proc. Am. Soc. Clin. Oncol., 1985 (Abstr.).
73. Santoro, A., Viviana, S., Zucali, R., et al. Comparative results and toxicity of MOPP vs ABVD combined with radiotherapy (RT) in PS IIB, III(A, B) Hodgkin's disease (HD). Proc. Am. Soc. Clin. Oncol. 2:223, 1983 (Abstr).
74. Henry, W.F., Stredonska, J., Jones, C.R., et al. Semen analysis in testicular cancer and Hodgkin's disease: Pre- and post-treatment finding and implications for cryopreservation. Br. J. Urol. 55:769–773, 1983.
75. Rothman, C.M. The usefulness of sperm banking. CA 30:186–188, 1980.
76. Cunningham, Mauch, Rosenthal, and Canellos. Long-term complications of MOPP/chemotherapy in patients with Hodgkin's disease. Cancer Treat. Rep. 66:1015–1022, 1982.
77. Dorreen, M.S., Wrigley, P.F.M., Laidlow, J.M., et al. The management of stage II supradiaphragmatic Hodgkin's disease at St. Bartholomew's Hospital. A retrospective review of 114 previously untreated patients over 14 years. Cancer 54:2882–2888, 1984.
78. Willet, C.G., Linggood, R.M., Meyer, J., et al. Results of treatment of stage 3A Hodgkin's disease. Cancer 59:27–30, 1987.

INDEX

Page numbers in *italics* indicate figures; numbers followed by "t" indicate tables.

Abdomen
   infections of, 159-161
Abortion
   therapeutic
      recommendations for, 254, 255
ABVD regimen
   gonadal toxicity of, 53
   leukemia and, 91
   mutagenicity of, 55
Acne
   steroid, 338
Acquired immunodeficiency syndrome (AIDS)
   Hodgkin's disease and, 73, 163
Actinomycin D
   radiation nephropathy and, 311
Acyclovir
   for herpes simplex, 175
   for herpes zoster, 175
   for varicella, 175
   prophylactic use of, 164, 176, 176t
   value of
      summary and analysis, 423-424
Adipocyte(s)
   in hematopoiesis, 65, 66t
Adriamycin. *See* Doxorubicin
Age. *See also* Child(ren); Elderly
   damage to ovarian function and, 6, 42
   immune function changes associated with, 117-119
   prognosis and, 363-364, *364*
   radiation-induced hypothyroidism and, 226-227
   second primary cancers and, 14, 15t
   treatment-induced leukemia and, 48, 91
Alkaline phosphatase
   clinical significance of
      in children, 367
Alkylating agent(s). *See also* particular drugs
   effects of
      on embryo and fetus, 251
      on hematopoiesis, 67
   leukemia and, 71
   mechanism of action of, 19, 126
   neurotoxicity of, 208, 209t
Alopecia. *See* Hair loss
Aminopterin
   effects on embryo and fetus, 251
Amphotericin B
   for cryptococcal meningitis, 155-156
   intrathecal administration of, 155
   intraventricular administration of, 155-156
Amyloidosis
   in Hodgkin's disease, 307-308

Anemia
   acquired sideroblastic
      in Hodgkin's disease, 66
   immunohemolytic. *See* Immunohemolytic anemia
   in treatment-related hypothyroidism, 69
   in untreated Hodgkin's disease, 66
   refractory, with excess blasts (RAEB), *83*, 83-85
Antibiotic(s). *See also* particular drugs
   effects on embryo and fetus, 251
   neurotoxicity of, 209t, 211
   prophylactic, 164
      after splenectomy, 421-422
      for children, 371
Antibody response. *See* Immunity, antibody-mediated
Antidiuretic hormone
   syndrome of inappropriate secretion of (SIADH)
      with vincristine therapy, 312
Anti-inflammatory drug(s). *See also* Corticosteroid(s); particular drugs
   in radiation enteritis management, 320
Antimetabolite(s). *See also* particular drugs
   effects of
      on embryo and fetus, 251
      on hematopoiesis, 67
   leukemia and, 72
Arteriosclerosis. *See also* Coronary artery disease
   radiation-induced
      in carotid artery, 207
      in peripheral vascular system, 282-283
Asparaginase
   thyroid function and, 227-228
Aspergillus species
   antimicrobial agents of choice for, 160t
   central nervous system infection by, 213
Ataxia-telangiectasia
   Hodgkin's disease and, 365
Autoimmune disease
   cutaneous
      with Hodgkin's disease, 332-333
   hematologic
      in Hodgkin's disease, 73-80
   thyroid
      radiation-induced hypothyroidism and, 228-229
Autoimmune hemolytic anemia. *See* Immunohemolytic anemia
Autoimmune neutropenia, 80
Avascular necrosis, 4-5, 187-192, *191*, 373
   clinical features of, 190
   conditions associated with, 190t
   etiology of, 189-190, 190t
   pathophysiology of, 190

Avascular necrosis *(Continued)*
  prevention of, 192
  radiographic findings in, 190-192, *192-193*
  treatment of, 5, 192

B lymphocyte(s)
  chemotherapy's effects on, 127
  function of
    in untreated Hodgkin's disease, 115
    radiation therapy's effects on, 120, 121, 122
    in nonlymphoid cancers, 124
    splenectomy's effects on, 131
Bacteria. *See also* particular organisms
  causing interstitial pneumonia, 159t
  infection by
    cutaneous, 340
    in children, 371-372, 372t
    with predilection for Hodgkin's disease patients, 152t
Battery
  failure to obtain informed consent and, 402
BCG immunization
  effects of, 132
BCNU (carmustine)
  nephrotoxicity of, 312
  neurotoxicity of, 209t, 212
  pulmonary toxicity of, 57
Beau's lines
  with chemotherapy, 337
Benzene
  leukemia and, 71
Bladder
  cyclophosphamide damage to, 312-313
  radiation injury to, 311-312
Bleomycin
  autoimmune phenomena associated with, 338
  effects on collagen formation, 338
  hair loss with, 336
  hyperpigmentation due to, 336-337
  hypersensitivity reaction to, 338
  liver damage due to, 324
  nail changes due to, 336-337
  neurotoxicity of, 209t, 211
  pulmonary toxicity of, 56-57, 301, *302-303*
    in children, 374
    pathophysiology of, 57
  radiation therapy with
    cutaneous complications and, 339
    pulmonary complications and, 38
    renal complications and, 311
  stomatitis due to, 336
Body image, 390-391
Bone atrophy
  radiation-induced, 185, *186*
Bone growth
  chemotherapy's effects on, 373
  herpes zoster's effects on, 351
  radiation's effects on, 4-5, 347-351, 372-373, 373t
Bone marrow. *See* Marrow
Brachial plexus
  radiation damage to, 40-41, 205-206
Brain
  infection of. *See* Encephalitis
  radiation damage to, 204
Brain abscess
  Nocardia, 156, 213
Breastfeeding
  during chemotherapy, 257
Brown-Séquard syndrome
  radiation-induced, 205
Busulfan

effects of
  on embryo and fetus, 251
  on hematopoiesis, 67
  pulmonary toxicity of, 57

Cancer(s). *See also* Carcinoma; Lymphoma(s); Sarcoma
  bladder
    cyclophosphamide and, 313
  childhood
    radiation exposure in utero and, 247
  incidence of
    in pregnancy, 244-245
  nonlymphoid
    chemotherapy's effects on lymphocytes in, 128
    radiation therapy's effects on lymphocytes in, 123-124
  risk of
    in offspring of survivors, 256
  second primary. *See* Second malignancy(-ies)
  thyroid. *See* Thyroid carcinoma
Candida albicans
  antimicrobial agents of choice for, 160t
  pulmonary infection with, *158*
  skin infections with, 161
  stomatopharyngitis due to, 157
Candida neoformans
  skin infections with, 161
Candida species. *See also Candida albicans*
  antimicrobial agents of choice for, 160t
  cutaneous infections with, 161
  gastrointestinal infection with, 325
  urinary-tract infection with, 161
Candida tropicalis
  antimicrobial agents of choice for, 160t
Carcinoma
  basal cell
    of skin, 341, *342*
  post-treatment
    epidemiology of, 24-25
  squamous cell
    of skin, 341
  thyroid. *See* Thyroid carcinoma
Cardiac disease. *See also* Cardiomyopathy
  compensated hypothyroidism and, 230
  conduction system
    radiation-induced, 281-282
  valvular
    radiation-induced, 282
Cardiac pacemaker(s)
  radiation's effects on, 282
Cardiomyopathy
  doxorubicin (Adriamycin), 56, 284-291
    acute, 286
    clinical manifestations of, 286
    detection of, 286-289, *288-289*
    mechanisms of, 284-285
    mediastinal radiation and, 35
    pathologic changes in, 57, 285-286
    renal function and, 308
    risk factors for, 289-290, *290*
    summary and analysis, 419
    treatment of, 290-291
  radiation-induced, 275-278
    clinical manifestations of, 277-278
    constrictive pericarditis vs., 278
    diagnosis of, 278, *279-280*
    pathogenesis of, 275-277, *276*
Cardiovascular complication(s), 267-295. *See also* Cardiomyopathy; Pericardial disease

in children, 374-375
   of chemotherapy, 56, 284-292
   of radiation therapy, 33-35, 268-284
      dose and, 283
      mechanisms of, 269-270
      prevention of, 283-284
      summary and analysis, 418-420
Caries. *See* Radiation caries
Carmustine. *See* BCNU
Carotid artery disease
   radiation-induced, 207
Case-control design
   epidemiologic studies using, 16, 16t
CCNU (lomustine)
   neurotoxicity of, 209t, 212
Cellulitis
   chemical, 337, *337*
Central nervous system
   infections of, 152-157, *153-154*, *156*, 213-215
   radiation damage to, 40, 204-205
Cerebral atrophy
   radiation-induced, 204
Chédiak-Higashi syndrome
   Hodgkin's disease and, 365
Chemical compound(s)
   leukemia and, 71
Chemotherapy, 47-62. *See also* particular drugs
   agents used in, 208t
      neurotoxicity of, 209t
   bone growth alterations due to, 373
   breastfeeding during, 257
   cardiovascular complications of, 56, 284-292
      in children, 375
      summary and analysis, 419
   combined
      risk disclosure in, 405
   cutaneous complications of, 335-338, 336t
   effects of
      on embryo and fetus, 250-254, 252t-253t
      on hematopoiesis, 67
   genitourinary complications of, 312-313
   gonadal toxicity of, 52t, 52-54
      in children, 375-376
   immunologic effects of, 55-56, 126-128
   intestinal damage from, 324-326
   leukemia after, 48-52, 50t, 71, 91
   liver and pancreatic damage from, 323-324
   mutagenic effects of, 54-55
   nephrotoxicity of, 312
   neurologic complications of, 207-213
   osteoporosis due to, 185
   pathophysiology of late effects of, 57
   preconception
      effects on progeny, 254, 256-257, 258t-260t
   protective effect of
      against radiation-induced autoimmune thyroiditis, 227, 228
   psychosocial and psychosexual sequelae of, 56
   pulmonary damage due to, 301
      in children, 374
   radiation therapy with. *See* Combined modality therapy
   renal complications of, 312-313
   second malignancies due to, 47-52
   thyroid function and, 227-228
   time-dose factors in, 413-414
Chickenpox. *See* Varicella
Child(ren)
   bone and soft-tissue growth alterations in, 372-374, 373t

cardiac and pulmonary sequelae in, 374-375
clinical staging in, 366-370, *367-368*
curability of, 414
endocrine complications in, 375-376
Hodgkin's disease in, 363-382
   epidemiologic, genetic and familial factors in, 365
   histopathology of, 365-366, 366t
   sites of involvement in, 366, *368*
psychosocial complications in, 378
second malignancies in, 376-378, 377t
surgical staging in, 370
summary and analysis, 426-427
Chlorambucil (Leukeran)
   effects of
      on embryo and fetus, 251
      on hematopoiesis, 67
   leukemia and, 71
   neurotoxicity of, 209t, 210
Chloramphenicol
   leukemia and, 71
Chlorhexidine
   in caries prevention, 356
Clostridial sepsis, 159
Cobalt irradiation
   penumbra with, 31
Coccidioides immitis
   antimicrobial agents of choice for, 160t
   cutaneous infection with, 340
Colitis
   radiation-induced, 319
Colony stimulating factor(s) (CSF), 65
Colony-forming cell(s), 65
Combined modality therapy
   cutaneous complications of, 338-339
   effects on hematopoiesis, 67
   leukemia and, 48, 51t, 91
   lower radiation dose with, 30
   pericardial disease in, 271
   pulmonary complications of, 37-38
   radiation nephropathy in, 310-311
   thyroid function and, 227, 228
Communication
   staff-patient, 394-395
   after completion of treatment, 397
Complement
   therapy's effects on, 129
Computed tomography (CT)
   in children, 369
Constrictive pericarditis
   radiation-induced. *See under* Radiation pericarditis
Copper
   serum levels of
      in children, 367
Coronary artery disease
   radiation-induced, 34, 278-281
      in children, 374
Corticocerebellar degeneration, 216
Corticosteroid(s). *See also* particular drugs
   avascular necrosis and, 189-190
   cutaneous reactions to, 338
   effects of
      on embryo and fetus, 251
      on hematopoiesis, 67
   iatrogenic osteoporosis and, 185
   immunosuppressive effects of, 126-127
   in radiation enteritis management, 320-321
   in radiation pneumonitis management, 37, 297-298
   intestinal damage from, 325
   pancreatitis due to, 324
   withdrawal of

Corticosteroid(s) *(Continued)*
  radiation pneumonitis and, 37, 299-301, *300*
  radiation recall and, 269
Counseling
  for survivors, 395-396
  on pregnancy, 257-261
  patient-to-patient, 397
Cranial nerve(s)
  radiation damage to, 207
"Crescent sign"
  in avascular necrosis, 190, *192*
Cryptococcus neoformans
  antimicrobial agents of choice for, 160t
  cutaneous infection with, 340
  meningitis due to, 152, *153*, 154-156, 213
Cyclophosphamide (Cytoxan)
  activation of, 19
  bladder toxicity of, 312-313
  cardiotoxicity of, 291
  doxorubicin cardiomyopathy and, 56
  effects of
    on embryo and fetus, 251
    on hematopoiesis, 67
  for male patients
    effects on offspring, 254
  gonadal toxicity of, 53
  hair loss with, 336
  immunosuppressive effects of, 126
  in breast milk, 257
  leukemia and, 71
  nephrotoxicity of, 312
  neurotoxicity of, 209t, 210
  radiation therapy with
    pulmonary complications and, 38
    renal complications and, 311
  stomatitis due to, 336
Cystitis
  hemorrhagic
    with cyclophosphamide therapy, 312-313
    with MOPP, 313
  radiation
    acute, 311
    chronic, 311-312
Cytomegalovirus infection
  central nervous system, 214
  cutaneous, 340
  prophylaxis of, 176t
  rash due to, 162
Cytosine arabinoside
  effects on embryo and fetus, 251
  for refractory anemia with excess blasts, 85
  for treatment-induced leukemia, 93
Cytoxan. *See* Cyclophosphamide

Dacarbazine. *See* DTIC
Daunomycin
  effects on embryo and fetus, 251
Delayed hypersensitivity
  in Hodgkin's disease, 112-113
    disease activity and, 133
    therapy's effects on, 128
  reactions to chemotherapeutic agents, 337-338
Dental complication(s), 346-362
Dermatitis
  radiation-induced, 334-335, *335*
Dermatomyositis, 332
Diabetes mellitus
  juvenile
    preceding Hodgkin's disease, 375
Dimethyltriazeneimidazole carboxamide. *See* DTIC

Down's syndrome
  Hodgkin's disease and, 365
Doxorubicin (Adriamycin)
  cardiotoxicity of. *See under* Cardiomyopathy
  chemical cellulitis due to, 337
  chemical phlebitis due to, 337
  delayed hypersensitivity reaction to, 337-338
  effects on embryo and fetus, 251
  enhancement of radiation effects by, 339
  gonadal toxicity of, 53
  hair loss with, 335-336
  hyperpigmentation due to, 337
  in breast milk, 257
  liver damage due to, 324
  neurotoxicity of, 209t, 211
  radiation recall with, 269
  radiation therapy with
    cardiomyopathy and, 35
    pulmonary complications and, 38
    renal complications and, 311
  stomatitis due to, 336
DTIC (dacarbazine)
  chemical phlebitis due to, 337
  liver damage due to, 324
  neurotoxicity of, 209t, 212-213
  photosensitivity reaction to, 338
Dysmyelopoiesis. *See* Myelodysplasia

Elderly
  Hodgkin's disease in, 414-415
Embryo. *See also* Fetus
  cytotoxic drugs' effects on, 250-254
  radiation's effects on, 246-250
Encephalitis
  herpes-simplex, 157, 214
  measles, 157, 214
  Toxoplasma, 156, 214
Encephalomyelitis, 215-216
Endocrine complication(s), 222-266
  in children, 375-376
Endothelial cell(s)
  in hematopoiesis, 65, 66t
Enteritis
  radiation-induced. *See* Radiation enteritis
Enterococcus(-i)
  urinary-tract infection due to, 161
Epidemiology
  of second primary cancers, 11-26
    case-control design in, 16, 16t
    illustrative problem, 13-16, 14t-16t
    methodology of study of, 11-13
    power and sample size in, 14-16, 16t
    summary of study results, 16-25, *18*, 20t-23t
Epstein-Barr virus (EBV)
  Hodgkin's disease and, 173
  in nonHodgkin's lymphoma, 98-99
Erikson, E.
  developmental model of, 384-385
Erythroleukemia, 84
Erythropoietin, 66
Esophagus
  radiation damage to, 28, 319
Estrogen replacement therapy
  hematopoiesis and, 69
Ethiodol
  lymphangiography using
    radiation-induced hypothyroidism and, 39, 225
Euthyroid sick syndrome, 223

Femoral head
  avascular necrosis of. *See* Avascular necrosis
Fertility, 6
  female
    chemotherapy and, 54
    radiation and, 42
    radiation-induced hypothyroidism and, 229
    summary and analysis, 429
    treatment in childhood and, 375-376
  male
    chemotherapy and, 52t, 53-54
    Hodgkin's disease and, 6
    radiation and, 42
    summary and analysis, 429-430
    treatment in childhood and, 376
Fetus
  cytotoxic drugs' effects on, 250-254, 252t-253t
  Hodgkin disease's effect on, 245-246
  metastasis to, 245-246
  radiation exposure of
    with diagnostic procedures, 247t
    with mantle field irradiation, 250t
    with therapeutic irradiation, 250
  radiation's effects on, 246-250, 248t-249t
Fever
  Hodgkin's disease vs. infection as cause of, 151-152
Fibroblast(s)
  in hematopoiesis, 65-66, 66t
Flucytosine
  for cryptococcal meningitis, 155
Fluoride
  topical
    for radiation caries prevention, 354-356
5-Fluorouracil
  effects on embryo and fetus, 251
  thyroid function and, 227
Folic acid
  in hematopoiesis, 66
Fracture(s)
  radiation therapy and, 185
Fungus(-i). *See also* particular organisms
  causing interstitial pneumonia, 159t
  cutaneous infections due to, 340
  with predilection for Hodgkin's disease patients, 152t

Gastrointestinal tract
  complications involving, 316-330
  second malignancies involving, 326
Glomerulonephritis
  with Hodgkin's disease, 307
Gonadal toxicity, 6
  from chemotherapy, 52t, 52-54
  from radiation, 41-42
  in children, 375-376
  summary and analysis, 429-430
Graft versus host disease, 72
Graves' disease
  radiation-induced, 38-39, 231-232
Guillain-Barré syndrome, 217

Haemophilus influenzae
  cutaneous infection due to, 340
  meningitis due to, 156
Hair loss
  with chemotherapy, 335-336
  with radiation, 334
Hashimoto's thyroiditis
  radiation-induced, 39

thyroidal Hodgkin's disease and, 223
Health-care professional(s)
  communication with patients, 394-395
    after completion of treatment, 397
Heart
  treatment-induced damage to. *See* Cardiovascular complication(s)
Heart block
  radiation-induced, 281-282
Heart disease. *See* Cardiac disease
Hematologic complication(s), 63-111
Hematopoiesis
  chemotherapy's effects on, 67
  leukemic
    biology of, 69-72
  normal, 63-66
    abnormalities of, induced by Hodgkin's disease and its therapy, 66-69
    nutritional and endocrine factors in, 66
Hematopoietic stem cell(s) (HSC), 63-65
  cryopreservation of, 65
Hematopoietic tissue
  acute effects of Hodgkin's disease therapy on, 63t
  chronic effects of Hodgkin's disease therapy on, 64t
  expansion of, during stress, 64-65
  normal
    production of, 63-64, *64*
Hemithyroidectomy
  radiation-induced hypothyroidism and, 227
Hemolytic anemia
  autoimmune. *See* Immunohemolytic anemia
Hemorrhagic cystitis
  with cyclophosphamide therapy, 312-313
  with MOPP, 313
Henderson, Lawrence, 410
Hepatitis
  radiation-induced, 321-323
Herpes simplex
  central nervous system infection due to, 157, 214
  cutaneous infection due to, 161, 162, 340
  gastrointestinal tract infection due to
    during chemotherapy, 325-326
  incidence and predisposing effects on incidence of, 173
  prophylaxis of, 176, 176t
  stomatitis due to, 157
  treatment of, 174t, 175
  visceral infection due to
    characteristics of, 173
Herpes zoster, 161-162, 339
  central nervous system involvement in, 157, 214
  characteristics of, 173
  disseminated, 214, 339, *340*
  effects on tooth and bone growth, 351, *352*
  in children, 372
  incidence of, 168-173, 170t-172t
  prophylaxis of, 176
  treatment of, 174t, 175
Histoplasma capsulatum
  antimicrobial agents of choice for, 160t
  cutaneous infection with, 340
Hodgkin's disease
  acquired immunodeficiency syndrome and, 73, 163
  curability of, 414
  cutaneous involvement in, 333, *333*
  de novo, in treated patient
    immunologic effects of treatment and, 134
  epidemiologic factors in, 365
  familial and genetic factors in, 137-138, 255-256, 365, 430

Hodgkin's disease *(Continued)*
  histopathology of
    in children, 365-366, 366t
  immunocompetence in, 112-117, 114t-116t, *117*, 118t
    summary and analysis, 425-426
  in children, 363-382
  in elderly, 414-415
  pathogenesis of
    immunologic impairment and, *130*, 138-139
  relapsing, 415
  renal involvement in, 306-307
  sites of involvement in
    in children, 366, *368*
  successfully treated
    immune function in, 132-133
  thyroid involvement in, 223
Humeral head
  avascular necrosis of. *See* Avascular necrosis
Humoral immunity. *See* Immunity, antibody-mediated
Hydrocele
  after radiation therapy, 373-374
Hydroxyurea
  in breast milk, 257
Hyperparathyroidism
  radiation and, 236-237
Hyperpigmentation
  with chemotherapy, 336-337
  with radiation therapy, 334
Hypersensitivity
  delayed. *See* Delayed hypersensitivity
Hyperthyroidism
  after radiation therapy, 231-232, 232t
  iodine administration and, 225
Hypoparathyroidism
  radiation and, 236
Hypothyroidism
  radiation-induced, 4, 38, 222-231
    clinical presentation of, 229
    compensated, 4, 38, 230
    hematologic abnormalities in, 69
    history of, 222-223
    in children, 375
    incidence of, 223, 224t
    potential factors leading to, 223-229
    potential relationship of, to other clinical settings, 229-230
    prevention of, 231
    recovery of euthyroid function in, 230
    renal function and, 308
    treatment of, 230-231

Ichthyosis
  acquired, 332
Immune function, 112-150
  activation of
    in Hodgkin's disease, 73-80
  after successful treatment, 132-133
  chemotherapy's effects on, 55-56
  confounding factors in studies of long-term survivors, 117-119
  impaired
    lymphocyte maldistribution as mechanism of, 136-137
    pathogenesis of Hodgkin's disease and, *130*, 138-139
  in untreated Hodgkin's disease, 55, 72, 112-117, 114t-116t, *117*, 118t
  leukemia and, 71-72
  normal age-related changes in, 117-119
  of family members of patients, 137-138

  post-treatment infection and, 134-135
  pre- and post-treatment
    prognosis and, 133
  radiation's effects on, 119-126
  second malignancies and, 133-134, 341-343
    interaction with radiation's effects, 43
  summary and analysis, 425-426
Immune thrombocytopenia, 74, 77-80, *78*, 79t-80t
  clinical features of, 77-78
  treatment of, 78-80
Immunity. *See also* Immune function
  antibody-mediated
    in untreated Hodgkin's disease, 115-117, 118t
    radiosensitivity of, 120
    therapy's effects on, 128-129
Immunocompetence. *See* Immune function
Immunoglobulin(s)
  serum levels of
    in untreated Hodgkin's disease, 117, 118t
    splenectomy's effects on, 131
Immunohemolytic anemia, 73-77, *74*, 75t-76t
  clinical picture of, 74-76
  treatment of, 77
Immunopotentiating therapy
  effects of, 131-132
Immunosuppressive therapy
  nonHodgkin's lymphoma and, 98
  second malignancies and, 341
  radiation-induced, 43
Infection(s), 151-167. *See also* particular diseases and pathogens
  antimicrobial agents of choice for, 160t
  central nervous system, 152-157, *153-154*, *156*, 213-215
  cutaneous, 161-162, 339-340
  in children, 370-372, 372t
  intra-abdominal, 159-161
  of mouth and pharynx, 157
  postsplenectomy, 162-163
  post-treatment immunodeficiency and, 134-135
  prevention and treatment of, 163-165
  pulmonary, 157-159
  regional, 152-162
  summary and analysis, 420-428
  urinary tract, 161
  viral. *See* Viral infection(s)
Infertility. *See* Fertility
Inflammatory reaction(s)
  in Hodgkin's disease
    therapy's effects on, 129
Informed consent
  failure to obtain
    damages for, 403
    liability for, 401-402, 402t
  in research, 405-406
  late iatrogenesis and, 403-408
  law of, 400-401
    evolution of, 401
  physician-patient relationship and, 403-404
  risk disclosure in, 404-405
Ingelfinger, Franz J.
  on progress in health care, 410-411
Interferon
  for varicella, 175
  prophylactic use of, 176
Interleukin-3, 65
  in leukemic hematopoiesis, 69
Interpersonal relationship(s), 391-393
Invasion of privacy
  lawsuits based on, 402

Iron
  in hematopoiesis, 66
Irradiation. *See* Radiation; Radiation therapy

Jawbone
  osteoradionecrosis of. *See under* Osteoradionecrosis

Kaposi's sarcoma, 342, *342*
Kidney(s)
  complications involving. *See* Renal complication(s)
  impaired function of
    radiation-induced cardiac and thyroid disease and, 308
Kyphoscoliosis
  due to radiation damage to spine, 183-184, *184*

Laparoscopy
  for staging, 317
Laparotomy
  complications of, 316-317
  in children, 370
  summary and analysis, 426-428
Legal issues, 400-409
Leukemia
  biology of, 69-72
  chemical compounds inducing, 71
  chemotherapy and, 48-52, 50t, 71, 91
  chronic myelomonocytic, 84
  cytogenetic alterations in, 18-19, 70, 92t
  genetic and constitutional influences in, 71
  oncogenes in, 70
  radiation and, 48, 49t, 70-71
  treatment-induced, *83-84*, 85-98, 86t-87t
    clinical characteristics of, 18-19, 48-52
    diagnosis of, 92
    epidemiologic studies of, 17-24, 20t-23t
    immunodeficiency and, 133-134
    in children, 376-377
    overall survival and, 2-3, 415-416
    risk of, 48, 49t-51t, 85-91, 88t-90t
    treatment of, 52, 92-98, 94t-95t
    types of, 91, 92t
Leukemic cell(s)
  chromosomal abnormalities in, 70, 92t
Leukemic hematopoiesis
  biology of, 69-72
Leukeran. *See* Chlorambucil
Leukocytosis
  in Hodgkin's disease, 66-67
Levamisole
  effects of, 132
Levinson, D. J.
  developmental model of, 385
Lhermitte's syndrome, 40, 205
Life-table survival method(s)
  epidemiologic studies using, 12-13
Listeria monocytogenes
  antimicrobial agents of choice for, 160t
  meningitis due to, 152-154, *154*, 213
Liver
  damage to
    from chemotherapy, 323-324
    from radiation, 321-323
Lomustine (CCNU)
  neurotoxicity of, 209t, 212
Lumbosacral plexus
  radiation damage to, 206-207

Lung(s)
  complications involving. *See* Pulmonary complication(s)
  radiation therapy to
    protective blocks in, 33, 298-299, 299t
Lymphadenopathy
  assessment of
    in children, 366, *367-368*
  massive
    radiation dose for, 30
Lymphangiography
  in pregnancy, 254
  radiation-induced hypothyroidism and, 39, 225-226, 226t
Lymphocyte(s)
  function of
    age dependency of, 115, *117*
    chemotherapy's effects on, 127-128
    clinical correlations of, 115
    in untreated Hodgkin's disease, 113
    splenectomy's effects on, 131
  in vivo activation of
    after curative treatment, 129
    clinical correlations of, 115
    in untreated Hodgkin's disease, 113-115, 116t
  maldistribution of
    as mechanism of immunodeficiency in Hodgkin's disease, 136-137
  radiation therapy's effects on
    in nonHodgkin's lymphoma, 124-126
    in nonlymphoid cancers, 123-124
  subpopulations of
    chemotherapy's effects on, 127
    in untreated Hodgkin's disease, 113, 115t
    radiation therapy's effects on, 120-122, 121t, *122*
    radiosensitivity of, 120
    splenectomy's effects on, 130-131
Lymphocytopenia
  clinical correlations of, 115
  in untreated Hodgkin's disease, 113, 114t-115t
  radiation-induced, 119
Lymphography
  in children, 368-369
Lymphokine(s), 65
Lymphoma(s). *See also* NonHodgkin's lymphoma
  cutaneous
    in Hodgkin's disease, 342-343
  cutaneous involvement in, 333
Lymphopoiesis
  abnormalities of
    in Hodgkin's disease, 72-73

Malignancy(-ies). *See* Cancer(s)
  second primary. *See* Second malignancy(-ies)
Malpractice
  failure to obtain informed consent and, 401-402
Mandible
  osteoradionecrosis of. *See under* Osteoradionecrosis
Mantle field irradiation, 31-33, *32*
  modification of
    to prevent radiation pneumonitis, 37, 298-299
    thin lung block technique for, 298-299, 299t
Marrow
  cryopreservation of, 65, 98
  regeneration of
    after radiation therapy, 68
  stromal elements of
    in hematopoiesis, 65-66, 66t
  transplantation of

Marrow *(Continued)*
    for treatment-induced leukemia, 93-98
"Marrow-failure cocktail," 82
Measles
    central nervous system infection due to, 157, 214
    rash due to, 162
Mechlorethamine. *See* Nitrogen mustard
Media
    educational programs using, 397
Megavoltage therapy, 30-31
Melanoma
    of skin, 341-342, *342*
Melphalan
    effects on hematopoiesis, 67
    leukemia and, 71
Meningitis, 152-157, *153-154, 156,* 213
Menopause
    premature
        osteoporosis and, 185
6-Mercaptopurine (6-MP)
    effects on embryo and fetus, 251
    liver damage due to, 324
Methotrexate (MTX)
    effects on embryo and fetus, 251
    in breast milk, 257
    intestinal damage due to, 324
    liver damage due to, 324
    neurotoxicity of, 209t, 213
Methylcholanthrene
    leukemia and, 71
Microcephaly
    after radiation exposure in utero, 246
Microorganism(s). *See also* particular organisms
    causing interstitial pneumonia, 159t
    with predilection for Hodgkin's disease patients, 152t
Mitomycin C
    cardiotoxicity of doxorubicin and, 56
Moniliasis. *See Candida* species
Monocyte(s)
    therapy's effects on, 129
MOPP regimen
    gonadal toxicity of, 52t, 53
        in children, 376
    hemorrhagic cystitis with, 313
    intestinal damage from, 324-325
    second malignancies and
        in children, 377-378
6-MP. *See* 6-Mercaptopurine
MTX. *See* Methotrexate
Mucormycosis
    rhinocerebral, 157
Muehrke's lines
    with chemotherapy, 337
Mycobacterium tuberculosis. See also Tuberculosis
    antimicrobial agents of choice for, 160t
Mycosis fungoides
    in Hodgkin's disease, 99
Myelitis
    radiation-induced, 40
Myelodysplasia, 80-85. *See also* Refractory anemia with excess blasts (RAEB)
    clinical features of, 81
    cytogenetic abnormalities in, 82-83, 92t
    laboratory evaluation of, 81, *82*
    treatment of, 82-83
Myokymia
    in radiation plexopathy, 206

Nail changes
    with chemotherapy, 337

Nephritis
    radiation-induced. *See* Radiation nephropathy
Nephropathy
    radiation-induced. *See* Radiation nephropathy
Nephrotic syndrome
    in Hodgkin's disease, 307
    renal vein thrombosis and, 308
Neurologic complication(s), 203-221
    infectious, 152-157, 213-215
    of chemotherapy, 207-213
        pathophysiology of, 57
    of radiation therapy, 40-41, 204-207
        symptom-free interval before onset of, 3-4
    paraneoplastic, 215-217
Neutropenia
    autoimmune, 80
Neutrophil(s)
    therapy's effects on, 129
Nitrogen mustard (mechlorethamine)
    amyloidosis and, 308
    chemical cellulitis due to, 337
    chemical phlebitis due to, 337
    effects on embryo and fetus, 251
    gonadal toxicity of, 53
    hair loss with, 336
    hypersensitivity reaction to, 338
    mutagenicity of, 55
    neurotoxicity of, 208-210, 209t
    pulmonary damage due to, 301
Nitrosourea(s)
    leukemia and, 71
    neurotoxicity of, 212
Nocardia asteroides
    antimicrobial agents of choice for, 160t
    central nervous system infection due to, 156, 213
    pulmonary infection due to, 158, *158*
NonHodgkin's lymphoma
    hypothyroidism after radiation treatment for, 224t
    lymphocyte function in, 124-125
    of thyroid gland, 223
    radiation therapy's effects on lymphocytes in, 124-126
    thyroid carcinoma after treatment of, 234t-235t
    treatment-induced, 2, 52, 96t-97t, 98-99
        epidemiology of, 24

Oncogene(s), 70
Oncologist(s)
    patient's relationship to
        informed consent and, 403-404
Oophoropexy
    before pelvic irradiation, 42, 375
Ophthalmopathy
    after radiation therapy, 38-39, 231-232, 232t
Optic neuropathy
    radiation-induced, 207
Oral contraceptive(s)
    protective effect of, on ovarian function, 54
Orthovoltage therapy
    drawbacks of, 30
Osteitis
    radiation-induced, 185
Osteochondroma
    radiation-induced, 193, *194,* 194t
Osteomyelitis
    reactive tuberculous
        after radiation therapy, 185-187, *187*
Osteonecrosis
    of femoral or humeral head. *See* Avascular necrosis

radiation-induced
of jawbone. *See under* Osteoradionecrosis
Osteoporosis
iatrogenic
causes of, 185
localized
radiation therapy and, 185
Osteoradionecrosis
of jawbone, 357-360, *361*, 361
incidence of, 357-358, 358t
pathogenesis of, 358-360
Ovary(-ies)
chemotherapy's effects on, 54
radiation therapy's effects on, 42
treatment's effects on
in children, 375-376

Pacemaker(s)
radiation's effects on, 282
Pancreas
damage to
from chemotherapy, 324
dysfunction of
preceding Hodgkin's disease, 375
Para-aortic field, 31-32
modification of
to prevent radiation nephritis, 41
Paraneoplastic syndrome(s)
cutaneous, 332-333
neurologic, 215-217
Parasite(s)
causing interstitial pneumonia, 159t
with predilection for Hodgkin's disease patients, 152t
Parathyroid disease
radiation-induced, 236-237
Patient advocacy, 395-396
Patient education
on pregnancy, 257-261
Patient-to-patient contact
value of, 397
Pelvic nodal field, 31
testicular damage from, 41-42
Penicillin prophylaxis, 164
after splenectomy, 421-422
for children, 371
Pentamidine isethionate
for *Pneumocystis carinii* pneumonia, 159
Pericardial disease
radiation-induced, 34, 270-275. *See also* Radiation pericarditis
chronic, 273, 274-275
factors influencing, 270-271
histopathologic description of, 271
radiation-induced hypothyroidism and, 229
Pericardiectomy, 275
Pericarditis
radiation-induced. *See* Radiation pericarditis
Peripheral nerve(s)
paraneoplastic syndrome involving, 216-217
radiation damage to, 40-41, 205-207
radiation-induced tumors of, 41, 207
Peripheral vascular disease
of carotid artery, 207
radiation-induced, 282-283
Person-years at risk
epidemiologic studies using, 11-12
Pharyngitis, 157
Phenylbutazone
leukemia and, 71

Phlebitis
chemical, 337
Photosensitivity reaction(s)
with chemotherapy, 338
Placenta
metastasis to, 245-246
Plant alkaloid(s). *See* Vinblastine; Vinca alkaloid(s); Vincristine
Platelet associated immunoglobulin, 77
Platinum
thyroid function and, 228
Pneumococcal vaccine
response to
in Hodgkin's disease, 164
value of
in children, 371-372
summary and analysis, 422-423
Pneumococcus
meningitis due to, 156, *156*
Pneumocystis carinii
antimicrobial agents of choice for, 160t
pulmonary infection with, 158-159
in children, 372
Pneumonia, 157-159
interstitial
organisms causing, 159t
Pneumonitis
radiation-induced. *See* Radiation pneumonitis
Pneumothorax, 304
Polymorphonuclear leukocyte(s)
therapy's effects on, 129
Port film(s), 31, 32
Prednisone
avascular necrosis and, 189-190
cutaneous reactions to, 338
for radiation pneumonitis, 301
immunosuppressive effects of, 126
mutagenicity of, 55
neurotoxicity of, 209t
Pregnancy, 244-266. *See also* Fetus
after completion of treatment, 255-257, 258t-260t
for pediatric patients, 376
summary and analysis, 428-430
timing of, 257
cancer incidence in, 244-245
chemotherapy during, 250-254, 252t-253t
effect on Hodgkin's disease, 245
Hodgkin's disease incidence in, 245
management of Hodgkin's disease during, 254-255
maternal outcome and, 255
patient education and counseling on, 257-261
radiation therapy during, 248t-250t, 250
radiation-induced hypothyroidism and, 229-230
Preleukemia
frequency of
in Hodgkin's disease, 80-81
Privacy
invasion of
lawsuits based on, 402
Procarbazine
activation of, 19
effects on embryo and fetus, 251
gonadal toxicity of, 53
hypersensitivity reaction to, 338
leukemia and, 71
liver damage due to, 324
mutagenicity of, 52, 54-55
neurotoxicity of, 209t, 212
pulmonary toxicity of, 57, 301
stomatitis due to, 336

Prognosis
  for children, 363-364, *364*
  pre- and post-treatment immune status and, 133
  pruritus and, 331-332
Progressive multifocal leukoencephalopathy, 157, 214-215
Progressive radiation myelopathy, 205
Prostacyclin
  radiation's effects on, 270
Pruritus
  in Hodgkin's disease, 331-332
Pseudomonas aeruginosa
  pharyngitis due to, 157
Psychosocial consequence(s), 383-399
  gender differences in, 391
  identification of patients at risk for adjustment problems, 395
  in children, 378
  interventions for, 393-398
  of chemotherapy, 56
Psychosocial transition(s), 384
Pulmonary complication(s), 296-305
  in children, 374
  of chemotherapy, 56-57, 301
  of radiation therapy, 35-38, *36*, 296-301, 301-304
Pulmonary fibrosis, 37, 301-304, 303t
  spontaneous pneumothorax and, 304

Radiation. *See also* Radiation therapy
  biologic effects of, 19
  dose of
    cardiovascular complications and, 283
    hypothyroidism and, 223-225
    intestinal injury and, 318
    liver damage and, 322
    radiation pneumonitis and, 298-299, 299t
  effects on immune system, 119-126
  fetal exposure to
    effects of, 246-250, 248t-249t
    with diagnostic procedures, 247t
    with mantle field irradiation, 250t
    with therapeutic irradiation, 250
  leukemia and, 70-71
  tissues most sensitive to, 19
Radiation caries, 351-356, 361, *361*
  prevention of, 354-356
Radiation cystitis
  acute, 311
  chronic, 311-312
Radiation enteritis
  chronic, 319
    clinical manifestations of, 319, 321
    prevention of, 320
    staging laparotomy and, 317
Radiation hepatitis, 321-323
Radiation myelitis, 40
Radiation nephropathy, 41, 308-311
  acute, 310
  chronic, 311
  clinical manifestations and treatment of, 310-311
  pathology of, 309-310
Radiation osteitis, 185
Radiation pericarditis, 34-35
  acute, 271-273
    differential diagnosis of, 272
    management of, 275
    natural history of, 272-273
    renal function and, 308
  constrictive, 34, 273-274
    management of, 275
    restrictive cardiomyopathy vs., 278
  mechanism of, 270
  nonconstrictive, 34
Radiation pneumonitis, *36*, 36-38, 296-301
  clinical picture of, 298-299
  drug effects in, 299-301, *300*
  histopathology of, 298
  risk of, 36, 37
  signs and symptoms of, 296-297, 297t, *297*
  treatment modification for prevention of, 37, 298-299
  treatment of, 37, 297-298
Radiation recall, 269, 339
Radiation sarcoma. *See under* Sarcoma
Radiation therapy, 27-46
  acute effects of, 28
  bone tumors due to, 192-199, 196t-197t
  "boosting" dose in, 30
  cardiovascular complications of, 33-35, 268-284
    clinical results of, 270-284
    history of, 268-269
    in children, 374-375
    mechanisms of, 269-270
    prevention of, 283-284
    summary and analysis, 418-419
  carotid artery disease due to, 207
  chemotherapy with. *See* Combined modality therapy
  cobalt
    penumbra with, 31
  cutaneous malignancy after, 340-343
  cyclophosphamide bladder toxicity and, 312-313
  damage to spine from, 183-184
  distant effect of
    on marrow, 68
  doses for, 29-30
    fractionation of, 30
    in combined modality therapy, 30
    recurrence rate and, *29*, 29-30
  doxorubicin cardiomyopathy and, 35
  during pregnancy, 248t-250t, 250
  effects on hematopoiesis, 68-69
  fields for, 31-33, *32*
    opposing, 33
  genitourinary complications of, 311-312
  intestinal complications of, 317-319
    acute, 318-319
    chronic, 319
    management of, 319-321
  late effects of
    mechanism of, 28-29
  leukemia and, 19-24, 48, 49t, 90-91
  liver damage due to, 321-323
  localization and planning procedures for, 31-33, *32*
  megavoltage, 30-31
  neurologic complications of, 40-41, 204-207
  orthovoltage
    drawbacks of, 30
  ovarian function and, 42
    in children, 375-376
  parathyroid disease due to, 236-237
  physical and technical considerations in, 29-33
  preconception
    effects on progeny, 256-257, 258t-260t
  protective blocks in, *32*, 32-33
  pulmonary complications of, 35-38, *36*
    in children, 374
  renal complications of, 41, 308-312
  rest periods in, 33
  risk-benefit considerations in, 28, *28*
  second malignancies and, 42-43, 417-418

"shrinking-field technique" in, 33
skeletal damage due to, 183-200, 348-350
  in children, 372-373, 373t
  pathophysiology of, 182-183
skin damage due to, 333-335, *335*
testicular function and, 41-42
  in children, 376
thin lung block technique in, 298-299, 299t
thyroid abnormalities due to, 38-40, 222-236. *See also* Hypothyroidism, radiation-induced
  in children, 375
to thymus
  effects on immune function, 120
tooth development changes due to, 347-351, *350*
Radiodermatitis
  chronic, 334-335, *335*
Rash
  due to viral infection, 162
"Recall" phenomenon, 269, 337, 339
Recurrence
  fear of, 386-387
Refractory anemia with excess blasts (RAEB), *83*, 83-85
  treatment of, 84-85
Refractory anemia with excess blasts in transformation (RAEBIT), 84
Remote effect syndrome(s). *See* Paraneoplastic syndrome(s)
Renal artery stenosis
  after radiation, 311
Renal complication(s), 306-315
  of chemotherapy, 312-313
  of Hodgkin's disease, 306-308
  of radiation therapy, 41, 308-312
  summary and analysis, 420
Renal function
  impaired
    radiation-induced cardiac and thyroid disease and, 308
Renal vein thrombosis
  in Hodgkin's disease, 308
Repose statutes
  late iatrogenesis lawsuits and, 407
Reproductive system. *See also* Pregnancy
  chemotherapy's effects on, 52t, 53-54
  radiation therapy's effects on, 41-42
  treatment's effects on
    in children, 375-376
    summary and analysis, 429-430
Research
  informed consent in, 405-406
Rheumatoid arthritis
  cyclophosphamide's effects on lymphocytes in, 128
  radiation therapy's effects on lymphocytes in, 124
Risk disclosure
  requirements for informed consent, 404-405

Salicylazosulfapyridine(s)
  in radiation enteritis management, 320
Salivary gland(s)
  radiation's effects on, 351-354
    caries development and, 353-354
Salmonella infection
  abdominal, 159
  antimicrobial agents of choice for, 160t
  central nervous system, 157
Sarcoma
  post-treatment
    epidemiology of, 24
  radiation, 194-199, 196t-197t, *199-200*

criteria for, 198
Schwannoma
  malignant
    radiation-induced, 41, 207
Scoliosis
  due to radiation damage to spine, 183-184, *184*
Second malignancy(-ies). *See also* Leukemia
  chemotherapy-induced, 47-52
  cutaneous, 340-343, 341t
  epidemiology of, 11-26
    case-control design in, 16, 16t
    illustrative problem, 13-16, 14t-16t
    methodology for study of, 11-13
    power and sample size in, 14-16, 16t
    summary of study results, 16-25, *18*, 20t-23t
  gastrointestinal tract, 326
  in children, 376-378, 377t
  legal issues, 400-409
  nonhematopoietic solid
    epidemiology of, 24-25
  radiation therapy and, 42-43
  relationship to treatment, 411, 417
  risk of
    immunodeficiency and, 133-134
  treatment-induced
    summary and analysis, 415-418
Self-esteem, 393
Sepsis, 162
  postsplenectomy
    summary and analysis, 420-422
Sexual interest, 389-391
Sézary syndrome, 343
Shingles. *See* Herpes zoster
"Shrinking-field technique," 33
Simulator
  in radiation therapy planning, 31-33, *32*
Skeletal complication(s), 182-202
  of radiation therapy, 183-200, 348-350
    in children, 372-373, 373t
    pathophysiology of, 182-183
Skin
  chemotherapy's effects on, 335-338, 336t
  complications involving, 331-345
  infections of, 161-162, 339-340
  involvement of
    in Hodgkin's disease, 333, *333*
  radiation damage to, 333-335, *335*
  second malignancies involving, 340-343, 341t
Slipped capital femoral epiphysis, 373
  radiation-induced, *188*, 188-189, 189t
Smallpox vaccine, 162
Solid tumor(s)
  second primary. *See* Second malignancy(-ies)
Sperm banking, 376
  congenital anomalies and, 430
Spinal cord
  radiation damage to, 40, 204-205
Spine
  radiation-induced damage to, 183-184, *184*
Spleen
  assessment of involvement of
    in children, 369, 370-371
    summary and analysis, 426-428
  irradiation of
    infection and, 421
    renal effects of, 420
  lymphocyte elimination by
    as mechanism of immunodeficiency in Hodgkin's disease, 136-137

Splenectomy
  effects of, 129-131
  for children, 370-371
  infection after, 55-56, 135, 162-163
    cutaneous, 340
  summary and analysis, 426-428
Staging
  clinical
    in children, 366-370, *367-368*
  summary and analysis, 426-428
  surgical, 316-317
    in children, 370
Staphylococcus aureus
  urinary-tract infection due to, 161
Statute of limitations
  late iatrogenesis lawsuits and, 407
Sterility. *See* Fertility
Steroid(s). *See* Corticosteroid(s)
Stomach
  radiation damage to, 319
  radiation tolerance of, 318
Stomatitis, 157
  with chemotherapy, 336
Streptococcus pneumoniae
  meningitis due to, 156, *156*
Streptococcus pyogenes
  stomatopharyngitis due to, 157
Strongyloides stercoralis
  abdominal infection due to, 159-161
  antimicrobial agents of choice for, 160t
  central nervous system infection due to, 157
Sulfadiazine
  for *Nocardia* brain abscess, 156
Support group(s)
  value of, 397
Survival analysis
  in epidemiologic studies, 13
Symptomatic pulmonary radiation reaction (SPRR), 298
Syndrome of inappropriate antidiuretic hormone (SIADH)
  with vincristine therapy, 312

T lymphocyte(s)
  chemotherapy's effects on, 127
  function of
    radiation therapy's effects on, 122-123, *123*
  persistent defect of
    after curative chemotherapy, 128
    mechanisms of, 135-137
  radiation therapy's effects on, 120-122, 121t
    in nonHodgkin's lymphoma, 125
    in nonlymphoid cancers, 124
  splenectomy's effects on, 131
  subpopulations of
    in untreated Hodgkin's disease, 113, 115t
  radiosensitivity of, 121, 121t
Taste
  radiation's effects on, 360
Testis(-es)
  chemotherapy's effects on, 53-54
  radiation therapy's effects on, 41-42
  treatment's effects on
    in children, 376
Testosterone
  in hematopoiesis, 66
Thalidomide
  for male patients
    effects on offspring, 254
Thiabendazole
  prophylactic use of, 164
Thin lung block technique, 298-299, 299t
6-Thioguanine
  effects on embryo and fetus, 251
Thiotepa
  effects on embryo and fetus, 251
Thrombocytopenia
  immune. *See* Immune thrombocytopenia
Thrombocytosis
  in Hodgkin's disease, 67
Thymus
  assessment of
    in children, 367-368
  fetal
    transplantation of, 132
  irradiation of
    effects on immune function, 120
Thyroid
  chemotherapy's effects on, 227-228
  function of
    in untreated Hodgkin's disease, 223
  Hodgkin's disease infiltrating, at time of diagnosis, 223
  radiation's effects on, 38-40, 222-236. *See also* Hypothyroidism
    in children, 375
Thyroid carcinoma
  compensated hypothyroidism and, 230
  radiation-induced, 39-40, 232-236, 234t-235t
  experimental studies of, 233
Thyroid hormone(s)
  in hematopoiesis, 66
Thyroid nodule(s)
  radiation-induced, 232
Thyroiditis
  Hashimoto's. *See* Hashimoto's thyroiditis
Thyroxine
  early administration of
    to prevent radiation-induced hypothyroidism, 38, 231
  in hematopoiesis, 66
Tinea cruris, 340
Tinea pedis, 340
Tooth(-eeth)
  development of
    herpes zoster's effects on, 351
    radiation's effects on, 347-351, *350*
  extraction of
    osteoradionecrosis and, 359-360
Toxoplasma gondii
  antimicrobial agents of choice for, 160t
  central nervous system infection due to, 156, 213-214
Treatment
  completion of
    psychosocial intervention at, 395-396
    psychosocial issues, 386
Triethylenemelamine
  effects on embryo and fetus, 251
Trimethoprim-sulfamethoxazole
  for *Pneumocystis carinii* pneumonia, 159
  prophylactic use of, 164
Trismus
  radiation-induced, 360-361
Tuberculosis, 157-158
  antimicrobial agents of choice for, 160t
  of spine
    after radiation therapy, 185-187, *187*
Tumor(s)
  second primary. *See* Second malignancy(-ies)

Ureter(s)
  radiosensitivity of, 311
Urinary tract
  chemotherapy's effects on, 312-313
  infections of, 161
  radiation's effects on, 311-312

Vaccination(s). See also Pneumococcal vaccine
  safety of
    in Hodgkin's disease, 164
    smallpox, 162
    varicella, 176
Vaccinia
  infection due to, 162
Varicella, 161-162
  in children, 372
  prophylaxis of, 176
  treatment of, 174t, 175
Varicella vaccine, 176
Varicella-zoster immune globulin (VZIG), 351
  recommendations for, 164, 176
  value of
    summary and analysis, 424-425
Varicella-zoster virus. See also Herpes zoster; Varicella
  infection with, 161-162
    in children, 372
Verruca vulgaris, 340
  in children, 372
Vidarabine
  for herpes simplex, 175
  for herpes zoster, 175
  for varicella, 175
Vinblastine
  chemical cellulitis due to, 337
  chemical phlebitis due to, 337
  effects on embryo and fetus, 251
  hair loss with, 336

neurotoxicity of, 209t, 211
photosensitivity reaction to, 338
radiation nephropathy and, 311
Vinca alkaloid(s). See also Vinblastine; Vincristine
  neurotoxicity of, 209t, 210
Vincristine
  chemical cellulitis due to, 337
  effects on embryo and fetus, 251
  hair loss with, 336
  intestinal damage from, 325
  mutagenicity of, 55
  nephrotoxicity of, 312
  neurotoxicity of, 209t, 210-211
  radiation nephropathy and, 311
  stomatitis due to, 336
Vindesine, 210
Viral infection(s), 168-181. See also particular diseases
  characteristics of, 173
  cutaneous, 339-340
  in children, 372
  prophylaxis of, 176, 176t
  treatment of, 173-175, 174t
Virus(es)
  causing interstitial pneumonia, 159t
  in chemical-induced leukemia, 71
  in radiation-induced leukemia, 70
  with predilection for Hodgkin's disease patients, 152t
Vitamin B_{12}
  in hematopoiesis, 66
Vocational adjustment, 388-389

Wart(s). See Verruca vulgaris

Xerostomia
  radiation-induced, 352-353

Zoster. See Herpes zoster